MAJOR MORPHOLOGIC GROUPS (CON[illegible]

ECZEMATOUS DISEASE

Prominent Excoriations or Lichenification
- *Atopic dermatitis: atopic dermatitis, neurodermatitis, lichen simplex chronicus*
- *Allergic contact dermatitis*

Inapparent Excoriations or Lichenification
- *Seborrheic dermatitis*
- *[illegible] dermatitis*

Other Eczematous Patterns
- *Hand, foot eczema*
- *Stasis dermatitis*
- *Nummular eczema*

TOPICAL CORTICOSTEROIDS BY POTENCY

GENERIC NAME	*BRAND NAMES*
I: Ultrapotent	
Clobetasol propionate 0.05%	*Temovate*
Betamethasone dipropionate 0.05% (ointment, gel, lotion)	*Diprolene*
Difluorasone diacetate 0.05% (ointment)	*Psorcon*
Halobetasol propionate 0.05%	*Ultravate*
II: High Potency	
Amcinonide 0.1% (ointment)	*Cyclocort*
Betamethasone dipropionate 0.05% (cream)	*Diprolene AF*
Betamethasone dipropionate 0.05% (ointment)	*Diprosone*
Desoximetasone 0.05% (gel) 0.025% (cream, ointment)	*Topicort*
Difluorasone diacetate 0.05% (cream)	*Psorcon*
Diflorasone diacetate 0.05% (ointment)	*Florone, Maxiflor*
Fluocinonide 0.05%	*Lidex*
Halcinonide 0.1% (cream)	*Halog*
Mometasone furoate 0.1% (ointment)	*Elocon*
III: High-Medium Potency	
Amcinonide 0.1% (cream, lotion)	*Cyclocort*
Betamethasone dipropionate 0.05% (cream)	*Diprosone*
Betamethasone valerate 0.1% (ointment)	*Valisone*
Diflorasone diacetate 0.05% (cream)	*Florone, Maxiflor*
Fluticasone propionate 0.005% (ointment)	*Cutivate*
Halcinonide 0.1% (ointment)	*Halog*
Triamcinolone 0.1% (ointment)	*Aristocort, Kenalog*
IV: Higher Midpotency	
Desoximetasone 0.05% cream	*Topicort LP*
Fluocinolone acetonide 0.025% (ointment)	*Synalar*
Hydrocortisone valerate 0.2% (ointment)	*Westcort*
Mometasone furoate 0.1% (cream)	*Elocon*
Triamcinolone 0.1% (cream)	*Aristocort, Kenalog*
V: Midpotency	
Betamethasone dipropionate 0.05% (lotion)	*Diprosone*
Betamethasone valerate 0.1% (cream, lotion)	*Valisone*
Fluticasone propionate 0.05% (cream)	*Cutivate*
Fluocinolone acetonide 0.025% (cream)	*Synalar*
Hydrocortisone butyrate 0.1% (cream)	*Locoid*
Hydrocortisone valerate 0.2% (cream)	*Westcort*
Triamcinolone 0.1% (lotion)	*Aristocort, Kenalog*
VI: Lower Midpotency	
Alclometasone dipropionate 0.05% (cream, ointment)	*Aclovate*
Desonide 0.05% (cream)	*Tridesilon, DesOwen*
Fluocinolone acetonide 0.01% (cream, lotion)	*Synalar*
VII: Low Potency	
Hydrocortisone 0.5%, 1%, 2.5%	*Hytone*

Dermatology
IN EMERGENCY CARE

Dermatology
IN EMERGENCY CARE

Libby Edwards, M.D.

Chief of Dermatology
Carolinas Medical Center
Charlotte, North Carolina
Associate Clinical Professor
Department of Dermatology
Bowman Gray School of Medicine of Wake Forest University
Winston-Salem, North Carolina

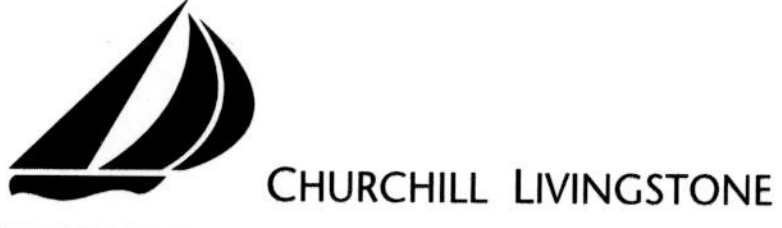
CHURCHILL LIVINGSTONE

New York, Edinburgh, London, Madrid, Melbourne, San Francisco, Tokyo

Library of Congress Cataloging-in-Publication Data

Edwards, Libby.
Dermatology in emergency care / Libby Edwards.
p. cm.
Includes bibliographical references and index.
ISBN 0-443-07952-8 (alk. paper)
1. Dermatology. 2. Medical emergencies. 3. Skin—Diseases.
I. Title.
[DNLM: 1. Skin Diseases. 2. Emergencies. WR 140 E26d 1997]
RL72.E39 1997
616.5´025—dc21
DNLM/DLC
for Library of Congress 97-13186
CIP

Distributed in the United Kingdom by Churchill Livingstone, Robert Stevenson House, 1–3 Baxter's Place, Leith Walk, Edinburgh EH1 3AF, and by associated companies, branches, and representatives throughout the world.

Medical knowledge is constantly changing. As new information becomes available, changes in treatment, procedures, equipment and the use of drugs become necessary. The editors/authors/contributors and the publishers have, as far as it is possible, taken care to ensure that the information given in this text is accurate and up to date. However, readers are strongly advised to confirm that the information, especially with regard to drug usage, complies with the latest legislation and standards of practice.

The Publishers have made every effort to trace the copyright holders for borrowed material. If they have inadvertently overlooked any, they will be pleased to make the necessary arrangements at the first opportunity.

Acquisitions Editor: *Sheila Khullar*
Assistant Editor: *Vicky Stapf*
Production Editor: *Rachel Klahr*
Production Supervisor: *Laura Mosberg Cohen*
Desktop Coordinator: *Alice Terry*
Cover Design: *Jeanette Jacobs*

Printed in Singapore

First published in 1997 7 6 5 4 3 2 1

To Clayton Samuel Owens
My best friend, personal copyeditor,
cheerleader, and husband

Preface

Even my mother, who remains under the delusion that I am perfect, thought that teaching dermatology to emergency health providers was bizarre. She and others asked questions such as "are there *any* dermatology emergencies?" In response, my reasons for this peculiar enterprise are as follows:

My definition (and yours) of an emergency differs from that of patients. The skin is visible, and frightening lesions—from a bleeding mole to new blisters—can be deemed an emergency by a patient, a spouse, or a parent. Also, intense pruritus or skin pain can become a psychological emergency, as anyone with severe urticaria will confirm.

I know from my practice that skin disease is regularly seen in emergency departments—at least it is at ours at Carolinas Medical Center. My Monday morning clinic consists primarily of patients referred from our emergency department over the previous week.

Finally, I was talked into giving dermatology courses at the annual Scientific Assembly of the American College of Emergency Physicians several years ago. I found emergency clinicians to be the most responsive and appreciative of any audience I have ever taught. I have since become a regular speaker at national ACEP meetings, smaller emergency medicine conferences, and individual training programs.

Dermatology in Emergency Care was written to address needs for emergency departments or office dermatology when patient contact is limited to one visit. For example, diseases are described by their morphologic appearance, so that the reader can turn to the chapter that discusses the causes and therapy of little blisters. Short tables describe, for most of the diseases and usually in one sentence, the clinical presentation. Accompanying lists give step-by-step instructions on how to treat the diseases in the emergency department and when follow-up is needed. Handouts designed to be photocopied and given to patients are provided for most diseases in an appendix at the end of the book. Hopefully, this will allow for a quick but adequate evaluation, precise therapy, and patient education.

I would like to know of any constructive comments for incorporation into future editions of this book. Detailed therapy of major catastrophes (yes, Mother, there are a few) are not a goal of this book. These are well covered in other sources, including emergency medicine textbooks. For example, necrotizing fasciitis also falls into the domain of surgery and infectious disease. The therapy of meningococcemia and Rocky Mountain spotted fever are well known. However, the skin manifestations and approaches to these diagnoses are less well known, and this is the thrust of the book in the realm of disasters with cutaneous findings.

This book is the product of several people. My husband, Clayton Owens, read and corrected typographic and medical errors, suggested clarifications, additions, and changes, and contributed a photograph of his apthous ulcer. My mother did quite a bit of weekend babysitting. My daughter has allowed photographs of her plantar wart, hand-foot-and-mouth disease, and flea bites to appear in this book. My secretary, Jeanette Parker, typed the first draft of this book outside of regular working hours. And my partner, Dr. Jennifer Helton, did my consults and critiqued parts of the manuscript.

Libby Edwards, M.D.

Contents

CHAPTER 1

Definitions and Principles of Diagnosis

Unlike most medical specialties, dermatology is a visual field of practice. In other areas of medicine, clinicians are dependent on a careful patient history as well as an integrated physical examination with corroborative testing to arrive at a diagnosis; however, the skin can easily be examined so that abnormalities can be directly observed, rather than inferred. This advantage frees the practitioner from dependence on the patient's own observations and from the results of expensive laboratory tests whose results may not be immediately available.

Although a thorough medical history is the mainstay for diagnosis in most areas of medicine, visibility of the skin relegates patient history to a secondary role. After the skin is examined, pertinent history can be obtained with selective questioning. Usually, this is limited to the duration of the condition, previous therapy and response, and the presence or absence of pain or pruritus.

Therefore, the success of diagnosis rests almost exclusively on the observational skills and interpretive ability of the examiner. The careful practitioner can correctly identify and treat many skin diseases. The purpose of this chapter is to familiarize the nondermatologist with a basic descriptive vocabulary and to allow that clinician to generate an appropriate differential diagnosis for the most commonly encountered or dangerous skin conditions.

DESCRIBING SKIN LESIONS

The ability to make a correct diagnosis requires knowledge of common dermatology vocabulary as well as its correct use. For example, the meaning of the term *maculopapular* is ambiguous. In fact, this term is often used because of its lack of precision; the practitioner cannot be held to a precise description when using an imprecise term. Does the clinician see papules or macules? Although both might be present, only one will be the primary lesion.

The noun descriptive of the type of lesion (e.g., papule, nodule, plaque, patch) is the cornerstone of description, to which modifiers are added (Table 1.1). Once the noun or nouns have been chosen, adjectives are added. Modifiers describing color and the presence of scale should always be included.

Types of Lesions

A *papule* is a small area, less than 1.5 cm, that is palpable. It may be raised, scaly, or crusted (Fig. 1.1). A *macule* is a small area (less than 1.5 cm) of color change only, such as a freckle. It is not palpable and has no—or only barely perceptible—surface change, such as scale. The active lesions of rash are generally composed of either macules or papules, but not both. A *plaque* (Fig. 1.2) is a lesion greater than 1.5 cm that is palpable (a large papule), and a *patch* (Fig. 1.3) is an area greater than 1.5 cm that is flat and not palpable (a large macule). A *nodule* is a papule with substantial 3-dimensional, or spherical, enlargement. A large nodule, greater than 1.5 cm is a *mass.*

A *blister* is a lesion that is filled with loculated fluid. If the lesion is punctured, fluid escapes, and the lesion collapses. A small blister of less than 1 cm is a *vesicle*, whereas a large blister is a *bulla.* A blister that is cloudy and filled with white fluid is called a *pustule.* A papule or plaque that is formed by edema is called a *wheal*, even though a wheal is filled with fluid, it does not collapse when punctured. Often, blisters are very fragile so the examiner will seldom see intact blisters; however, it is important to be aware of other skin lesions that

Table 1.1 Description

Nouns	
Papule, nodule, mass, plaque, macule, patch, blister, bulla, vesicle, collarette, pustule, wheal, erosion, excoriation, fissure, ulcer	
Adjectives	
Color	Red (or pink, violaceous, brown-red, purple), brown (or black, blue, tan), yellow (or orange), white, skin-colored
Surface character	Dome-shaped, flat-topped, scaling, hyperkeratotic, smooth, irregular, pebbly, cobblestoned, papillomatous, verrucous/warty, lichenified, crusted
Border character	Sharply demarcated, poorly demarcated, irregular, smooth
Location	Scalp, hands, antecubital, elbows/knees, perioral, etc.
Pattern	Dermatomal, photodistributed, acral, annular, arcuate

suggest previous blistering, such as round erosions and collarettes. Round or arcuate erosions, indicating confluence of circular lesions, represent blisters after the blister roof has been removed (Fig. 1.4). A *collarette* is a circular rim of scale that represents a remnant of the edges of the blister roof (Fig. 1.5).

An *erosion* is an area where the epidermis has been removed. A *fissure* is a linear crack or erosion that is too narrow to be easily identified as such and often is characterized simply by a red line. An *ulcer* is deeper than an erosion and extends at least into the dermis.

Scale refers to excess stratum corneum that is visible on the skin. *Psoriatic* scale is seen as flakiness and corresponds to the most common usage of the word scale. *Pityriasis* (from the Latin for "fine scale") scale is fine, powdery scale and easily overlooked by the unsophisticated observer (Fig. 1.2). Scraping the skin with a fingernail often raises this powdery scale and makes it more visible. *Lichenoid scale* is tightly adherent to the epidermis; the absence of air under the scale gives the surface a shiny rather than scaling appearance (Fig. 1.6). *Hyperkeratosis* results from an extreme

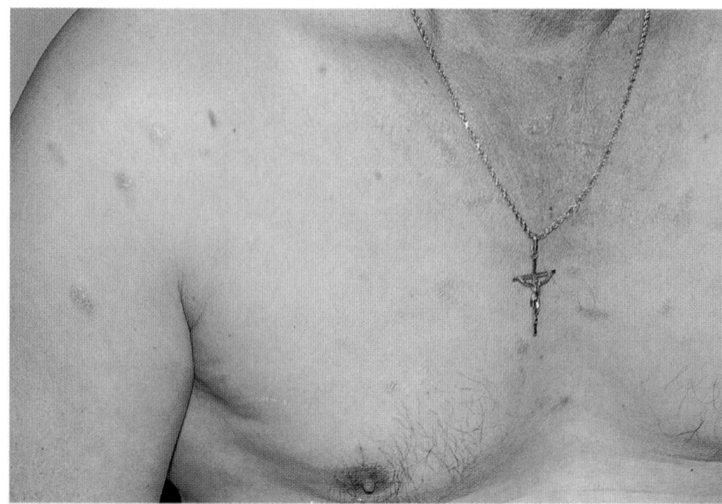

Figure 1.1 These nearly flat lesions of pityriasis rosea are papules rather than macules because of the presence of scale. If these lesions were large, they would be called plaques.

Figure 1.2 This lesion of pityriasis ("tinea") versicolor is a plaque, rather than a patch, because of the presence of fine pityriasis scale. The scale can be easier to appreciate if the surface of the skin is scratched with a fingernail. The sharp margination is characteristic of a papulosquamous disease, rather than eczema, where the eruption is produced by rubbing or scratching.

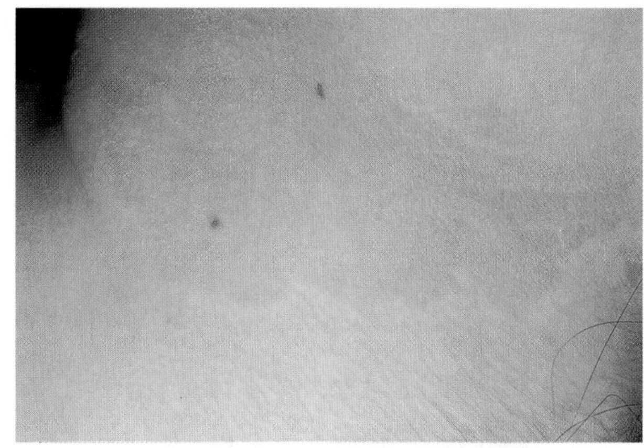

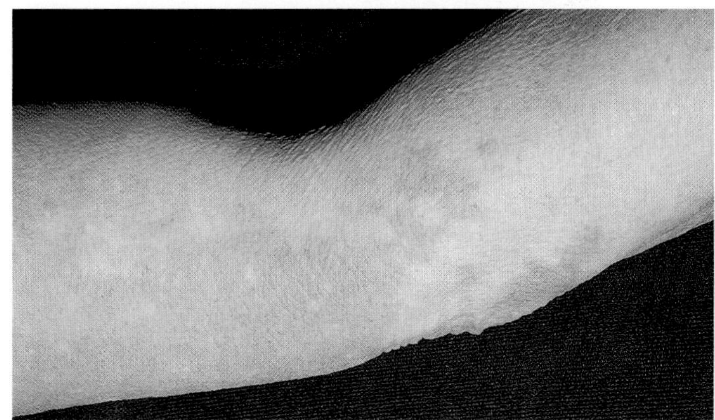

Figure 1.3 Depigmented area of color change only, without scale, texture change, elevation, or depression is called a patch because it is large; if it were smaller than about 1.5 cm, it would be called a macule. This patient has vitiligo.

Figure 1.4 Very round or arcuate erosions are also signs of previous blisters, as is true in this man with an early, vesicular form of bullous pemphigoid.

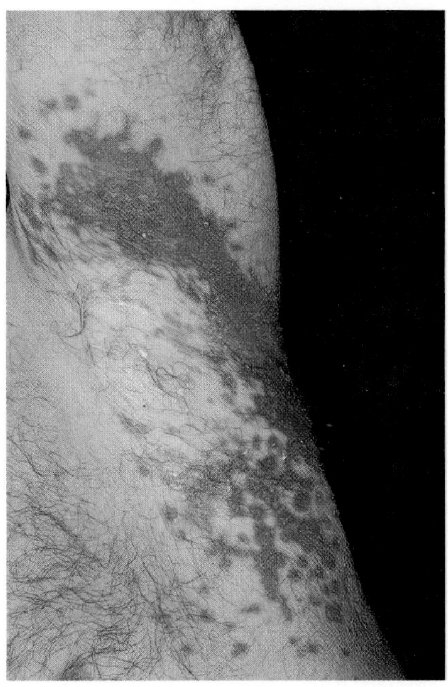

Figure 1.5 Collarettes (arrows) represent superficial pustles that have lost the blister roofs in this patient with pustular psoriasis.

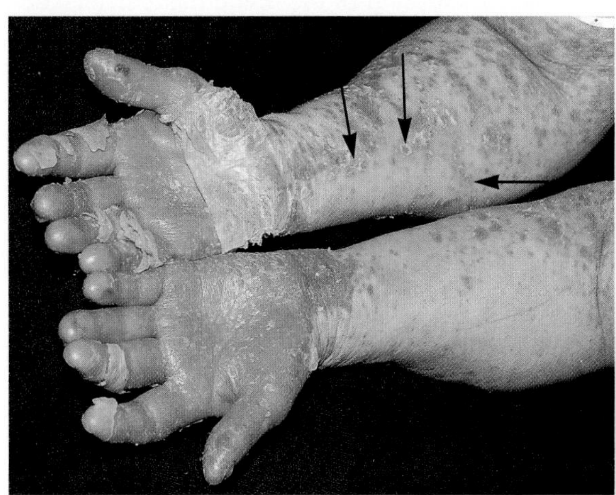

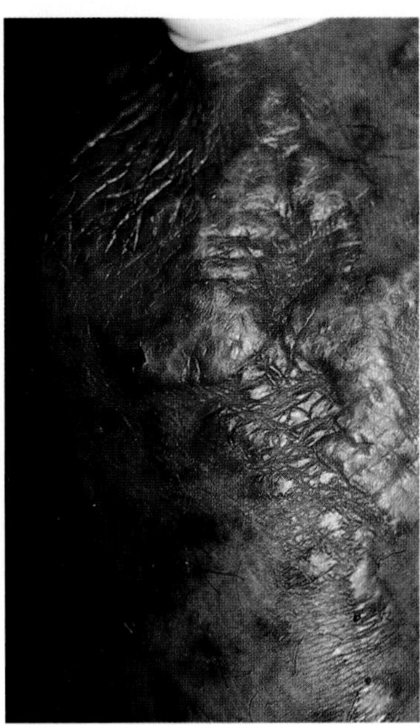

Figure 1.6 Lichenoid scale is closely adherent, so that it often appears shiny rather than scaly. Lichenoid scale is characteristic of lichen planus as seen here, and lichen simplex chronicus, or chronically rubbed skin.

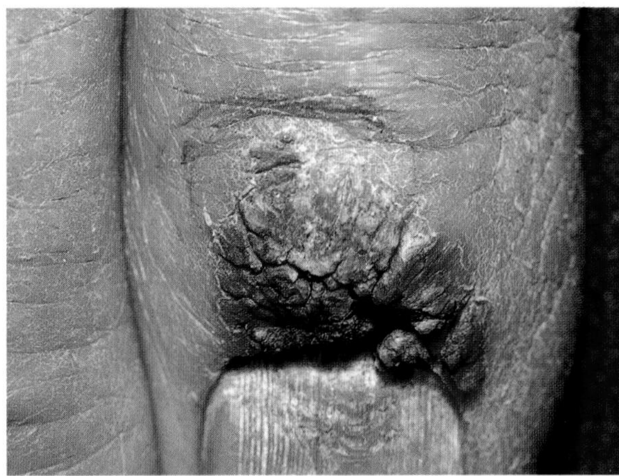

Figure 1.7 Verrucous, papillomatous, and warty are all terms used to describe the irregular, folded, hyperkeratotic surface of this squamous cell carcinoma initially misdiagnosed as a wart.

amount of retained scale and gives the skin a hard surface. When hyperkeratosis overlies a papillomatous lesion, the surface is called *verrucous* or *warty* (Fig. 1.7). Skin that has been thickened by rubbing so that the normal skin lines and surface texture are exaggerated is called *lichenified.*

Linear or angular erosions that have been produced by scratching or picking are called *excoriations.* Any disruption of the epidermal barrier, such as an erosion or fissure is likely to exhibit an overlying *crust,* a mixture of serum, scale, and sometimes blood (the lay term being "scab").

Color

Color is one of the most important elements of a description. Even the meager description, "pink macule," carries an enormous amount of information. This rash would consist of small, flat, inflamed lesions without scale, erosions, crust, or hyperkeratosis. Already, the differential diagnosis is fairly short. Although nuances in color can be very informative to the experienced dermatologist trying to differentiate among several inflammatory diseases, generalizing all colors into five categories serves most nondermatologists very well. Colors considered *red* include pink, purple, and brown-red. Blue, black, and tan are all categorized as *brown* lesions. Yellow and orange are considered *yellow,* and both milk-white (depigmented) lesions and those only somewhat lighter than surrounding skin color (hypopigmented) are termed *white* in this book. Skin lesions indistinguishable from surrounding skin color are referred to as *skin-colored.* It is important to remember that many skin-colored lesions are tumors that can easily become inflamed and thus secondarily red or pink, and this should be remembered when generating a differential diagnosis.

Other Elements of Descriptions

The surface character of a lesion is also very important unless it is implicit, as for a macule, patch, or blister. The surface can be described as flat-topped, dome-shaped, scaling, hyperkeratotic, smooth, irregular, cobblestoned, or papillomatous, for example.

For scaling red papules and plaques, and for pigmented lesions, the sharpness or fuzziness, and irregularity or smoothness of border characteristics

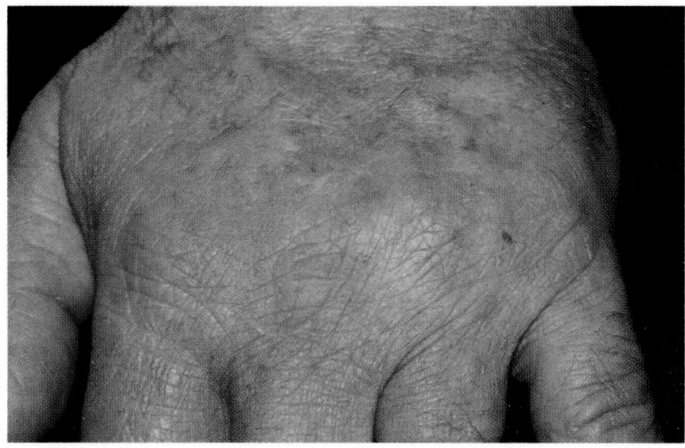

Figure 1.8 This red plaque of lichen simplex chronicus is covered with lichenoid scale and an erosion. It is poorly demarcated because it was produced by rubbing and scratching.

are important in differentiating among diseases within diagnostic categories (Figs. 1.2 and 1.8). The location is often important, not only in documenting the extent of disease, but in helping to make the diagnosis as well. For example, the elbows and knees are characteristic locations for psoriasis, while the antecubital and popliteal fossae are locations nearly pathognomonic for atopic dermatitis. When a distribution pattern is apparent, this should also be documented. Common patterns are dermatomal distribution, sun-exposed patterns, and acral locations.

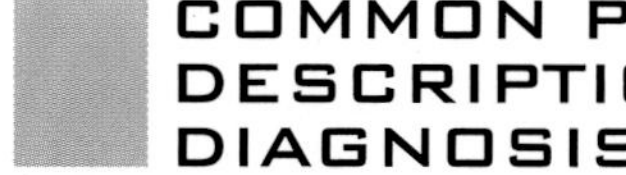

COMMON PITFALLS IN DESCRIPTION AND DIAGNOSIS

The presence or absence of scale is often crucial as a starting point for the generation of a differential diagnosis. Although the presence of copious psoriasiform scale rarely poses a problem, the detection of scale is sometimes difficult, and a high index of suspicion is required. Pityriasis and lichenoid scale (see above) do not appear as classic scale. Also, all scale can be difficult to detect if the patient bathes and washes scale off just before an examination, or if the patient applies lubricants, sticking scale to the surface of the skin so that it is less visible. In addition, partial treatment, such as with over-the-counter hydrocortisone, can minimize the appearance of scale. These are important areas to probe in the patient history if there is any question as to the presence of scale.

Some patients are naturally itchy individuals, generally those who are atopic (i.e., have a tendency toward allergies). These patients experience itching with almost any cutaneous inflammation or injury or sometimes even with benign tumors such as nevi or moles. Consequently, atopic patients often obscure the primary, underlying morphologic features with secondary changes from rubbing and scratching. Chronic rubbing and scratching produce eczema, also called dermatitis, characterized by redness, scaling, and either lichenification or excoriation. In addition, many patients will have tried over-the-counter therapies or medications and home remedies at the suggestion of family or friends, possibly producing changes associated with contact dermatitis, either irritant or allergic. Again, previous therapy, both prescribed and otherwise, are important questions in the history of some skin conditions. Occasionally, the underlying diagnosis cannot be made at an initial visit because of secondary changes. Usually, however, dangerous diagnoses can be eliminated, and the most likely diagnosis or diagnoses treated as such. Otherwise, a re-evaluation performed after eliminating those confusing variables is required.

Describing the skin of black patients presents unique difficulties. The most common difficulty in evaluating black skin is the identification of inflammation. Very often, even with intense inflammation, erythema is undetectable; it is usually manifested in black skin by apparent hyperpigmentation. A rule of thumb is that whenever scale or a rough texture to the skin is present, the skin lesion is inflamed. Occasionally, black skin manifests inflammation by lighter skin color, particularly with seborrheic dermatitis on the face. Once again, scale is generally present and is a reliable clue to the underlying inflammatory nature of the skin disease.

Black skin often thickens, or lichenifies, more easily than the skin of other races. Atopic dermatitis is common in these patients, but the thickened, lichenified, shiny, and hyperpigmented skin may be quite different in appearance from classic descriptions of atopic dermatitis.

Finally, many inflammatory skin diseases may occur in a follicular pattern in blacks that is uncommon in other races. For example, pityriasis rosea, secondary syphilis, and atopic dermatitis all may occur as 1 to 3 mm follicular papules over the trunk in blacks. Skin diseases that sometimes present atypically in black skin are each discussed in this book in their respective sections.

DEVELOPING A DIFFERENTIAL DIAGNOSIS BY MORPHOLOGIC GROUPING

Skin diseases are categorized by their morphologic appearance, rather than by their pathogenesis. Whereas most medical textbooks group diseases in sections under such headings as "infectious diseases," "metabolic diseases," "congenital abnormalities," or "autoimmune diseases," dermatology textbooks often present these diseases in sections with such headings as "blistering diseases," "pigmented diseases," and "papulosquamous disorders." Most skin diseases can be fitted into a specific morphologic group based on their description. The great majority of patients who walk into the general practitioner's office with a skin disease have a disease found in one of the 12 groups discussed in this book. Only common or dangerous diseases in each group are discussed in detail in this book, but short descriptions of other diseases are provided.

MAJOR MORPHOLOGIC GROUPS

- *Vesicular diseases*
- *Bullous diseases*
- *Hemorrhagic bullous/necrotic diseases*
- *Pustular lesions*
- *Skin-colored lesions*
- *White skin lesions*
- *Brown lesions*
- *Yellow lesions*
- *Red papules and nodules (dome-shaped, discrete lesions)*
- *Vascular reactions (flat-topped red lesions with tendency for confluence)*
- *Papulosquamous diseases (well-demarcated, scaling red diseases without significant crusting or erosions)*
- *Eczematous diseases (poorly demarcated, sscaling red diseases with crusting, erosions, or lichenification)*

Blistering Disease Groups

Although blistering diseases are among the easiest to categorize, the short-lived nature of these lesions means that the patient may not have clinically evident blisters when presenting to the practitioner. In addition, although the definition of a blister seems obvious to the clinician, even educated lay persons sometimes have a different mental image of a blister than the correct one. Therefore, the examiner must be sensitive to the presence of collarettes and round erosions (particularly on fragile mucous membranes, where blisters are especially transient) suggesting the presence of a primary blistering disorder, even despite a patient's denial of blistering.

Blistering diseases comprise 4 of 12 major morphologic groups. The first group is composed of *vesicular diseases*, including herpes simplex virus (HSV) infection, herpes zoster, varicella, insect bites, dyshidrosis, and allergic contact dermatitis. Thesecond group consists of *bullous diseases*, the most common disorders being bullous pemphigoid, severe allergic contact dermatitis, Stevens-Johnson syndrome/toxic epidermal necrolysis (TEN) and bullous impetigo. Blistering diseases characterized by hemorrhage, *hemorrhagic bullous/necrotic diseases*, include necrotizing fasciitis, leukocytoclastic vasculitis, brown recluse spider bites, and rattlesnake bites. The differentiation of

VESICULAR DISEASES

- *Herpes simplex virus infection*
- *Herpes zoster*
- *Varicella*
- *Hand, foot, and mouth disease*
- *Acute allergic contact dermatitis*
- *Dyshidrosis (pomphylox)*
- *Vesicular tinea*
- *Insect bites*
- *Rare causes of vesicles*
  - *Dermatitis herpetiformis*
  - *Chronic bullous disease of childhood*
  - *Scabies*

BULLOUS DISEASES
- *Bullous pemphigoid*
- *Cicatricial pemphigoid*
- *Pemphigus vulgaris*
- *Blistering erythema multiforme (erythema multiforme major, Stevens-Johnson syndrome, toxic epidermal necrolysis)*
- *Fixed drug eruption*
- *Staphylococcal scalded skin syndrome*
- *Acute allergic contact dermatitis*
- *Burns, thermal, chemical*
- *Edema blisters*
- *Diabetic bullae*
- *Coma/pressure blisters*

HEMORRHAGIC BULLOUS/ NECROTIC DISEASES
- *Necrotizing fasciitis and other necrotizing subcutaneous infections*
- *Vasculitis*
  - *Polyarteritis nodosa*
  - *Leukocytoclastic vasculitis*
  - *Other vasculitis*
- *Bullous pyoderma gangrenosum/ Sweet syndrome*
- *Brown recluse spider bite*
- *Pit viper snake bite*
- *Other causes*
  - *Herpes zoster infection*
  - *Trauma*

PUSTULAR DISEASES
- *Folliculitis*
  - *Staphylococcal folliculitis*
  - *Pseudomonas (hot tub) folliculitis*
  - *Sterile folliculitis*
  - *Fungal folliculitis*
- *Acne vulgaris*
- *Pustular psoriasis*
- *Reiter's disease*
- *Cutaneous candida*
- *Fire ant bites*
- *Intense dermal inflammation and infection*
- *Lesions that look, but are not, pustular*
  - *Old vesicles*
  - *Molluscum contagiosum*
  - *Milia*

the fourth group, *pustular diseases*, from vesicular diseases can sometimes be tricky, because any blister may become inflamed and attract white blood cells that produce a pustule, simply from the abnormal disruption of the skin. The practitioner should realize that the presence of pustules does not necessarily mean that the disease is primarily pustular, or that the disease is secondarily infected. If any clear vesicles or bullae are present, the diagnosis is almost certainly in the vesiculobullous category, rather than the pustular category. Pustular disorders are few, and include infection, acne, and pustular psoriasis.

Colored Lesions

Nonblistering nonred diseases are categorized by color. These include *skin-colored lesions* (mostly tumors), and *white lesions*, both depigmented (totally devoid of pigment) and hypopigmented (lighter than surrounding skin). The few lesions in the *yellow lesion* group result from the presence of lipids (xanthomas and necrobiosis lipoidica), the deposition of amyloid, or yellow surface crust

SKIN-COLORED DISEASES

Keratotic Papules
- *Warts*
- *Calluses and corns*
- *Actinic keratoses*
- *Squamous cell carcinomas*
- *Cutaneous horns*
- *Seborrheic keratoses*
- *Prurigo nodules*

Nonkeratotic Papules, Nodules, and Plaques
- *Intradermal nevi*
- *Neurofibromas*
- *Epidermal cysts*
- *Lipomas*
- *Genital warts*
- *Molluscum contagiosum*
- *Skin tags*
- *Basal cell carcinomas*
- *Sebaceous hyperplasia*
- *Squamous cell carcinomas*

WHITE LESIONS

White Macules and Patches
- *Vitiligo*
- *Piebaldism*
- *Albinism*
- *Postinflammatory hypopigmentation and depigmentation*
- *Achromic nevus (hypochromic nevus)*
- *Pityriasis "tinea" versicolor*
- *Lichen sclerosus et atrophicus*
- *Mucosal lichen planus*

White Papules and Nodules
- *Milia*
- *Molluscum contagiosum*
- *Calcinosis cutis*
- *Chronic cutaneous (discoid) lupus erythematosus*

YELLOW LESIONS

Smooth-Surfaced Lesions
- *Necrobiosis lipoidica (diabeticorum)*
- *Xanthomas*
  - *Xanthelasma*
  - *Eruptive xanthomas*
  - *Other*
- *Amyloidosis*
- *Sebaceous hyperplasia*
- *Colloid milium*

Crusted Lesions
- *Impetigo*
- *Actinic keratoses*

BROWN LESIONS

Brown Macules/Patches
- *Ephelides (freckles)*
- *Solar lentigo ("liver spots")*
- *Lentigo simplex*
- *Pityriasis "tinea" versicolor*
- *Café-au-lait spots*
- *Postinflammatory hyperpigmentation*
- *Fixed drug reaction*
- *Becker's nevus*
- *Melasma*
- *Futcher's lines*

(Continued)

Brown Papules/Plaques
- *Seborrheic keratoses*
- *Pigmented nevi (melanocytic nevi, "moles")*
  - *Acquired pigmented nevi*
  - *Congenital pigmented nevi*
  - *Atypical moles (dysplastic nevi)*
- *Malignant melanoma*
- *Dermatofibroma*
- *Prurigo nodules*
- *Bowenoid papulosis, pigmented Bowen's disease, pigmented intraepithelial neoplasia*

(impetigo). Diseases in the *brown lesions* group include melanocytic tumors and postinflammatory hyperpigmentation.

Red or Inflammatory Lesions

The remaining groups are either inflammatory or red as a result of abnormal blood vessels or bleeding. The *red papules and nodules* group is characterized by discrete, dome-shaped, nonscaling papules, including insect bites, cherry angiomas, skin lesions of sepsis, and secondarily inflamed skin-colored tumors. The only other red, nonscaling group is the *vascular reaction* group, comprising red, flat-topped, nonscaling, papules, macules, patches, and plaques with a tendency for lesions to coalesce. This group is one of the few groups almost all of whose diseases share the same pathogenesis. These are generally hypersensitivity reactions such as urticaria, erythema multiforme, and vasculitis.

The two groups characterized by both inflammation and scaling are the *papulosquamous* group and the *eczematous* group. Both morphologic types of rashes are inflamed and scaling. Although the differentiation is sometimes clear, factors such as those discussed under "common pitfalls" above can make diagnosis difficult, and diseases from both groups sometimes have to be considered in any individual patient. Papulosquamous diseases are characterized by red, scaling papules or plaques whose borders are sharply demarcated; evidence of rubbing or scratching (excoriation or lichenification) is absent. Atopic dermatitis and its variants are the main diseases that compose the

RED PAPULES AND NODULES

Noninfectious Inflammatory Papules and Nodules
- *Insect bites*
- *Granuloma annulare*
- *Sarcoidosis*
- *Rosacea*
- *Inflamed epidermal "sebaceous" cysts*
- *Hidradenitis suppurativa*
- *Cystic acne*
- *Dissecting cellulitis of the scalp*

Infectious Nodules
- *Granulomatous Infections*
  - *Deep fungal infections*
  - *Mycobacterial infections*
  - *Parasites*
- *Furuncules*
- *Hot tub folliculitis*
- *Sepsis*

Vascular Tumors
- *Cherry angiomas*
- *Capillary hemangiomas*
- *Kaposi sarcoma*
- *Pyogenic granulomas*

Lymphocytic Infiltrates
- *Leukemia and lymphoma*
- *Cutaneous lupus erythematosus*

Secondarily Inflamed Tumors
- *Intradermal nevi*
- *Basal cell carcinomas*
- *Squamous cell carcinomas*
- *Seborrheic keratoses*

eczematous group. These are very itchy diseases, and scratching or rubbing is generally responsible for their appearance. Eczema is sometimes referred to as "the itch that rashes," with redness, scale, excoriation, and lichenification the being visible evidence.

Other

Some dermatologic diseases cannot be categorized into one of these 12 morphologic groups. These special circumstances are discussed separately in this book. Prime examples are abnormalities of the hair and nails, as well as pain or itching with no visible findings. In addition, diseases sometimes present atypically, such as in a setting of immunosuppression, or when occurring on mucous membranes.

VASCULAR REACTIONS AND OTHER FLAT-TOPPED, NONSCALING LESIONS

Vascular Reactions
- *Urticaria*
- *Erythema multiforme*
- *Erythema nodosum*
- *Fixed drug eruption*
- *Gyrate erythema*
- *Leukocytoclastic vasculitis*

Other
- *Sunburn*
- *Cellulitis*
- *Erysipelas*
- *Nevus flammeus*
- *Actinic/steroid purpura*
- *Acute cutaneous lupus erythematosus*
- *Dermatomyositis*

PAPULOSQUAMOUS DISEASES

Large Plaques
- *Psoriasis*
- *Lupus erythematosus*
- *Fungal infection*

Small Plaques
- *Pityriasis rosea*
- *secondary syphilis (Lues)*
- *Lichen planus*
- *Psoriasis (guttate)*

Other Diseases
- *Pityriasis rubra pilaris*
- *Parapsoriasis*
- *Superficial basal cell carcinomas*
- *Bowen's disease (squamous cell carcinoma in situ)*
- *Paget's disease*

ECZEMATOUS DISEASE

Prominent Excoriations or Lichenification
- *Atopic dermatitis*
  - *Atopic dermatitis*
  - *Neurodermatitis*
  - *Lichen simplex chronicus*
- *Allergic contact dermatitis*

Inapparent Excoriations or Lichenification
- *Seborrheic dermatitis*
- *Irritant contact dermatitis*

Other Eczematous Patterns
- *Hand, foot eczema*
- *Stasis dermatitis*
- *Nummular eczema*

SUGGESTED READINGS

Lynch PJ: Dermatology. House Officer Series. 3rd Ed. Williams & Wilkins, Baltimore, 1994

This paperback book describes in more detail the diagnostic technique discussed in this chapter, and it also includes a discussion of those diseases most often encountered. There are no photographs.

Sams M, Lynch PJ (eds): Principles and Practice of Dermatology. 2nd Ed. Churchill Livingstone, New York, 1996

This one-volume textbook with all color, high-quality photographs is a multiauthored work that covers general dermatology and is directed to the primary care clinician.

Habif TP: Clinical Dermatology. A Color Guide to Diagnosis and Therapy. 2nd Ed. CV Mosby, St. Louis, 1990

This one-author textbook directed at the primary care clinician contains color photographs.

McDonald CJ, Scott DA: Dermatology in black patients. Dermatol Clin 6:343, 1988

An entire volume of Dermatologic Clinics, this book discusses the structural differences in black and white skin, characteristic reaction patterns and differences in morphology of diseases when occurring in black skin, and diseases characteristic of blacks.

Fitzpatrick TB, Eisen AZ, Wolff K, et al: Dermatology in General Medicine. 4th Ed. McGraw-Hill, New York, 1993

This weighty (in more ways than one) two-volume dermatology bible contains more basic science, pathogenesis, and detail than most nondermatologists would ever want to read, but information can be found here that is lacking in other texts.

CHAPTER 2

Diagnostic Procedures

Because skin diseases are usually visible, far fewer tests and procedures are required for the diagnosis than for most other specialties. However, experienced dermatologists are extremely adept at interpretation of the diagnostic procedures that are commonly performed. Although skin biopsies are generally not useful in the emergency department because of the time required for routine processing and interpretation, biopsy techniques are discussed in this chapter. However, the clinician should realize that, in emergency circumstances, a biopsy can be processed by frozen-section technique and some diseases ruled in or out, although optimal information is obtained from permanent, fixed specimens.

For the most part, excluding serology for syphilis and laboratory testing for systemic infections or autoimmune diseases, diagnostic procedures are limited to microscopic examination of skin scrapings or smears. Many generalists and medical students erroneously assume that the evaluation of a fungal preparation and an examination of a skin scraping for scabies are straightforward procedures that belong in the armamentarium of the general clinician. In actuality, these are difficult procedures to perform reliably, requiring months of experience with a seasoned teacher. In my experience from teaching medical students and primary care residents, nondermatologists should not trust their own interpretations of fungal, Tzanck, and scabies preparations; they should be wary also of trusting the results from other nondermatologists, or from a laboratory, in the absence of culture.

SKIN BIOPSY

Skin biopsies are extremely easy procedures to perform, requiring minimal education and experience. However, the usefulness of information gained depends on the biopsying practitioner and on his or her care in choosing the optimal site and the proper technique. Careful handling of the delicate skin and the listing of a differential diagnosis for the pathologist are also important.

Unless sutures are to be used, a skin biopsy need not be a sterile procedure, and nonsterile gloves and universal precautions are all that are required. When the skin is left open, the use of sterile gloves and sterilization of the skin is unimportant, as organisms have immediate access to the biopsy site after the procedure. However, for those punch biopsies performed on the face or other cosmetically critical areas, sutures are generally used to close the round hole into a less obvious linear scar. In these cases, the skin should be prepared and the procedure performed with the usual sterile technique.

Except over fingers and toes, the skin should be anesthetized definitively with lidocaine 1% with epinephrine. Although many surgeons also avoid the use of epinephrine over the nose, ears, and penis, very superficial instillation of anesthesia avoids problems with vasoconstriction over these areas. Even problems over the fingers and toes are rare, except in patients with significant peripheral vascular disease. For the patient who is extremely frightened of needles, or for children, eutectic mixture of local anesthesia (EMLA) cream can be applied initially to minimize the pain of injection. However, EMLA cream must be left on the skin, heaped up in a mound under occlusion, for 1 to 2 hours, to achieve significant anesthesia.

After the instillation of lidocaine with epinephrine, the clinician should wait at least 10 minutes before performing the biopsy, so that vasoconstriction from the epinephrine can occur and minimize bleeding, particularly for punch biopsies. However, if epinephrine is not added to the lidocaine, the biopsy should be performed immediately because the duration of this anesthesia is very short in the absence of vasoconstriction.

Biopsy Methods

A *shave skin biopsy* is performed either with a No. 15 scalpel or, by some experienced practitioners, with a hand-held razor blade. Holding the scalpel like a pen, with the other hand stabilizing the skin and elevating the lesion (Fig. 2.1), a portion of skin is removed that includes the epidermis and part of the dermis. A chemical cautery such as ferric chloride, ferrous subsulfate (Monsel solution), or silver nitrate can then be applied to stop the bleeding. The area is then covered with an adhesive plaster.

The skin *punch biopsy* is performed with a disposable Keye's punch instrument, most often a 3-mm diameter size. With one hand stabilizing the skin, the punch biopsy is applied to the skin with pressure and back-and-forth rotational movement to cut through the skin up to the hub of the punch instrument (Fig. 2.2). Sometimes the biopsy specimen lifts out with the punch instrument, but even more often the loosened specimen is still tethered at its base. When this occurs, the specimen should not be grasped with forceps that might crush the skin; rather, it should be speared with a needle and lifted gently so that curved iris scissors can detach the specimen at the base. A chemical cautery is then applied with a cotton-tipped applicator to the defect and the biopsy site covered with an adhesive plaster.

Figure 2.1 Tenting the skin up enables the surgeon to obtain a better sample of the skin to include adequate dermis. The shave biopsy does not extend to fat.

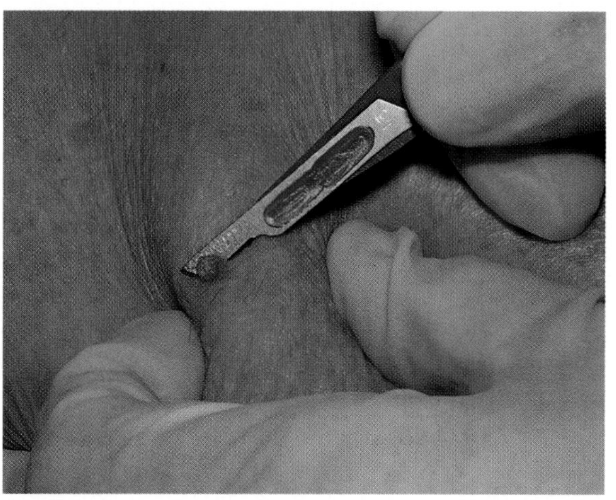

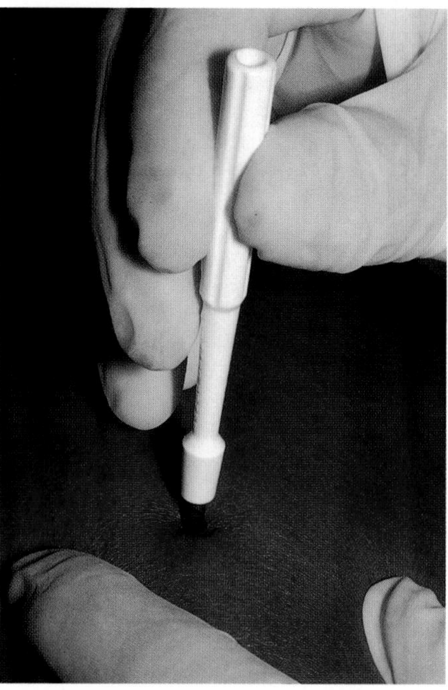

Figure 2.2 The punch biopsy instrument is held at a 90-degree angle to the skin and twisted into the skin up to the hub, so that a sample including epidermis, dermis, and superficial fat is obtained.

Pedunculated lesions can easily be removed by snipping at the base with curved iris scissors. This biopsy technique removes the lesion in its entirety with a very nice cosmetic result.

Deeper lesions extending into fat require an *incisional biopsy*. A narrow ellipse of skin extending into fat is removed and the defect repaired in two layers.

Choosing the Proper Biopsy Technique

Punch biopsies are the preferred method for inflammatory skin diseases. Histologic differentiation among some skin diseases depends on the extent, depth, and type of inflammatory cells. The punch biopsy is the only quick biopsy method that includes all layers of skin from the epidermis to the subcutaneous fat.

A punch-biopsy technique is also preferred for the diagnosis of recurrent skin cancer. However, this technique should be avoided if there is a high index of suspicion for primary (i.e., never treated) basal cell or squamous cell carcinoma because a full-thickness defect limits the quickest and least expensive options for later definitive therapy. In the case of primary skin cancer, a shave should be used, as discussed below.

The punch biopsy technique is also the preferred method for biopsying a possible malignant melanoma when removal of the entire lesion with excision and suture closure is not practical or if the diagnosis is tentative and removal of the entire lesion would cause significant cosmetic or financial repercussions. Incisional biopsies are not believed to be associated with an increased rate of metastases of melanoma, although this has been debated.[1]

Because the twisting motion required for penetration of the punch biopsy often shears a blister roof, a shave biopsy of an entire small vesicle or a shave biopsy that includes the edge of a bulla is preferred for blisters. A shave biopsy is also preferred for a primary basal cell or squamous cell carcinoma so that curettage and electrodesiccation is then possible for definitive removal. For shave biopsy of a squamous cell carcinoma or any hyperkeratotic lesion, the clinician should be very careful to include a significant portion of dermis. The clinician should avoid the temptation to remove the sometimes large hyperkeratotic, exophytic lump that yields no diagnosis unless the underlying cells that manufacture the keratin are included in the biopsy. A suspected malignant melanoma should not be biopsied by the shave method because transection of the tumor may not only be nondiagnostic, but may prevent later biopsies and procedures from yielding the correct diagnosis and prognostic thickness.

The scissors snip biopsy is generally reserved for pedunculated lesions such as skin tags and some genital warts.

Choosing the Biopsy Site

Lesions chosen for biopsy should be fresh when inflammatory (generally less than 2 days' duration), and without significant secondary change such as crusting or erosion. Involved skin near the edge of an inflammatory lesion is usually a good choice, as many plaques are actively extending peripherally.

The ideal biopsy method for blistering disease is the removal *in toto* of a small, fresh vesicle. Samples of old blisters may yield incorrect results because new epithelium regenerates over the dermis and under the blister roof, changing the histologic appearance after 1 or 2 days. If the blister is too large to remove totally with a shave, a portion of normal skin extending into the blister should be removed, so that the cleavage plane can be examined histologically. If there is a concern for immunobullous disease, an additional punch biopsy of adjacent normal-appearing skin should be taken and placed in Michele's solution or transport medium. A direct immunofluorescent test can be performed later on this tissue if indicated after interpretation of the routine biopsy. The skin can remain in reserve in these solutions for several days, and it can be discarded if the routine biopsy yields a definitive diagnosis not requiring this expensive immunofluorescent examination.

If an ulcer is to be biopsied, the very edge, where most of the biopsy sample contains intact epithelium, should be sampled. This is because many diagnoses require evaluation of the epidermis and upper dermal inflammatory characteristics. An erosion should be biopsied with the same clinical considerations in mind as for blisters and ulcers, to include the gradation of intact epithelium and the edge of the erosion.

FUNGAL PREPARATION

Because of the extensive experience required for correct interpretation of fungal preparations, this test has limited value as a tool for the nondermatologist. When the diagnosis is in question, and is important, a fungal culture also should be performed, since empirical therapy makes microscopic confirmation impossible for the dermatologist during follow-up. Alternatively, empirical therapy can be instituted but the patient instructed to discontinue therapy 1 week before re-evaluation by a dermatologist if response is incomplete.

To prepare the specimen, the skin is wiped with an alcohol swab or water, both to remove cream and to dampen scale, which then will adhere to the scalpel. A No. 15 scalpel blade is scraped across the surface at the periphery of the lesions—the area of greatest scale and concentration of the fungus. The debris on the blade is then scraped onto a microscope slide, and 1 or 2 drops of potassium hydroxide are added at a concentration of 10% to 20%. A coverslip is then affixed. To improve the ability of potassium hydroxide to dissolve nonfungal structures, accentuating the fungal hyphae and yeast, the specimen should be left for 10 to 15 minutes (occasionally much longer for thick scale or full-thickness skin). Alternatively, the specimen can be gently warmed over an alcohol flame (match flames deposit a brown substance on the bottom of the slide), or the potassium hydroxide can be premixed with dimethyl sulfoxide (DMSO). A drop or two of methylene blue is then added to the slide, facilitating visualization of the fungal elements.

The clinician should then press the coverslip firmly to the slide, to flatten and thin the specimen as much as possible, using a pencil eraser or the flat of a fingernail, rather than a finger pad, which leaves a fingerprint. The microscope condenser should be set at its lowest adjustment and the light set relatively low to enhance contrast. The undissolved fungal elements then stand out against the ghost outline of the skin cells. The low-power objective (× 40) should be used; lower power provides inadequate magnification and higher powers both reveal too many artifacts and require too long to examine the entire slide. A higher-power objective can be used to confirm the presence of hyphae and pseudohyphae in suspect formations. These structures are branching filaments of constant, rather than tapering, caliber, and they cross cell borders (Fig. 2.3). Yeast forms such as *Candida albicans* and *Malassezia furfur* or *Pityrosporum ovale*, the causative organism of pityriasis "tinea" versicolor, also show budding yeast forms.

Figure 2.3 Branching hyphae (arrow), compared here to hair and cotton fibers, are often much smaller than some examiners expect. When there is doubt, a fungal preparation can be sent to the laboratory or a culture obtained.

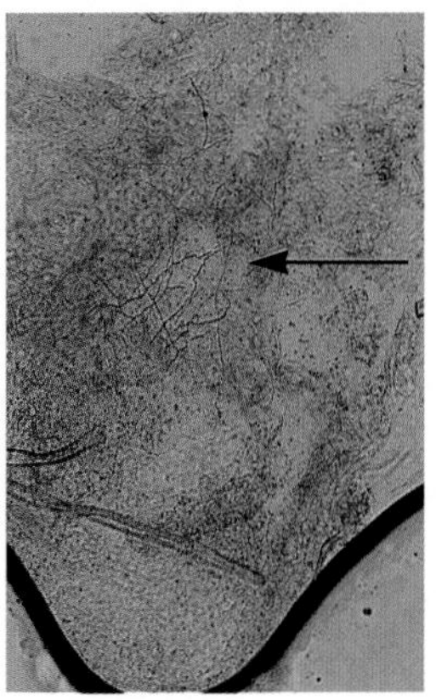

TZANCK PREPARATION

Somewhat easier to perform, but still requiring experience, is the Tzanck preparation. This is used primarily for confirmation of herpes simplex virus (HSV) infection or varicella zoster virus (VZV) infection. These viruses cause epidermal cells to form very large giant cells. The giant cells formed by the viral effect on epidermal cells are larger and more obvious structures than foreign body giant cells.

A fresh lesion is necessary. Either a recent erosion or an unroofed blister base should be scraped with a No. 15 scalpel blade. The exudate and material on the blade should then be spread thinly onto the microscope slide and allowed to dry. This slide can then be stained with Giemsa or any other rapid tissue stain.

The stained preparation should be scanned under the × 40 objective. Large epidermal cells with multiple nuclei indicate a positive finding for HSV infection (Fig. 2.4). This test does not distinguish between HSV infection and VZV infection.

Figure 2.4 The giant cells of a positive Tzanck preparation represent multinucleated epithelial cells that are much larger than surrounding inflammatory cells.

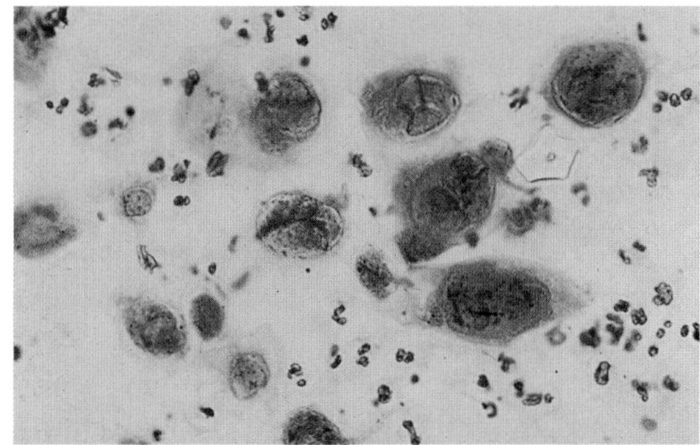

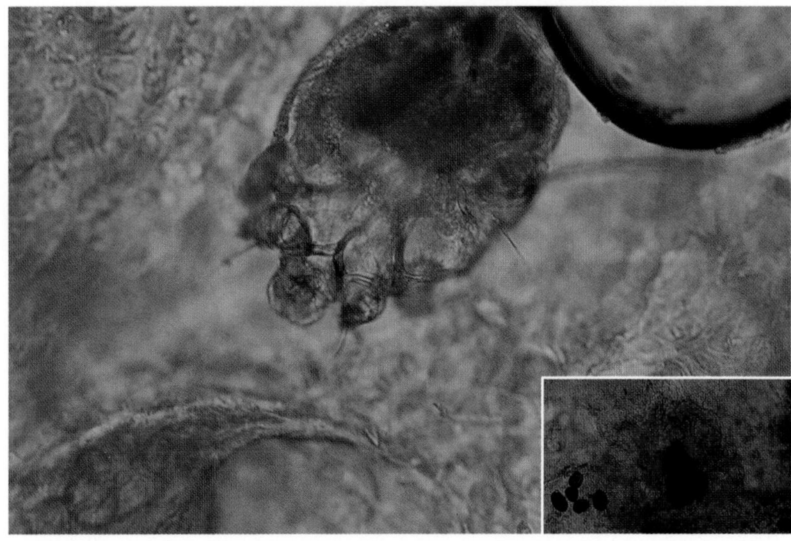

Figure 2.5 Although interpretation of a scabies preparation is easy when the mite is present, the choice of an appropriate site to sample, the vigorous scraping required, and the recognition of feces (inset) are more difficult.

SCABIES PREPARATION

Although the interpretation of a scabies preparation is relatively easy, it is difficult even for experienced practitioners to obtain the proper material. First, most patients have only a few mites over the entire skin surface, in spite of often extensive-appearing disease. Second, light scraping of the skin as done for a fungal preparation is inadequate for obtaining the mite or any other material diagnostic of scabies. Vigorous scraping is required. Even in very experienced hands, a scabies preparation produces a false-negative finding in about 40% of cases, so a negative scraping should not dissuade an examiner from the diagnosis.

The lesions with highest yield are those without excoriation or scale. Oval edematous or vesicular papules that are usually less than 3 mm in length (called "burrows") are the ideal lesions. These are found in highest concentration in digit web spaces, volar wrists, and skin folds. A firm scrape with a No. 15 blade or a curette sometimes drawing slight blood is usually required.

The specimen is then spread on the microscope slide and a coverslip affixed. The specimen is examined with a low-power (×10) objective because of the relatively large size of the mite and her ova. Identification of the mite, ova, or the dark brown globules of feces indicates a positive result (Fig. 2.5).

REFERENCE

1. Lever WF, Schaumburg-Lever G: Benign melanocytic tumors and malignant melanoma. p. 786. In: Histopathology of the Skin. 7th Ed. Lippincott-Raven, Philadelphia, 1990

CHAPTER 3

Medical Therapy

The management of skin diseases is gratifying because of the accessibility of skin that frequently allows for topical therapy, the visible nature of improvement, and the rewarding appreciation of the patient who is immediately aware of improvement. Often, a patient's skin disease has been ignored by clinicians who were more concerned about "real" medical problems, when the patient was bothered day-to-day by a pruritic eruption. Or, the patient's complaints were brushed off because the practitioner had no answers. Proper medical therapy extends beyond "if it is wet, dry it, and if it is dry, wet it," and can produce much more comfortable and happy patients.

PRINCIPLES OF TOPICAL THERAPY

A great advantage to therapy for skin disease is the accessibility of skin. Many medications can be delivered topically or with local injections rather than systemically, avoiding most adverse reactions that accompany systemic therapy. Not only is topical therapy an option, but often local therapies such as lubrication are essential and cannot be provided by systemic medication.

The diseases best suited for topical therapy are those that are superficial rather than deep (e.g., impetigo, rather than a furuncle) and limited in area. When diseases are extensive, deep, or exudative, systemic therapy is generally required.

Soaks

Soaks are often beneficial in the treatment of erosive exudative diseases. Soaks serve several purposes. First, the pain and itching associated with some inflammatory skin diseases are often partly due to exposed nerve endings. A wet environment helps soothe and bathe these nerve endings, minimizing pain and itching. Second, debridement of crust and exudate is achieved more easily following hydration and softening. Some clinicians are fond of wet-to-dry dressings that allow crust and necrotic debris to dry and adhere to dressings. When the dressing is removed, skin, crust, and debris are pulled off, and the wound is debrided. However, this method often causes excessive trauma. Gently soaking the area, rather than tearing off both necrotic and viable tissue, is less painful and decreases healing time. Third, soaks are occasionally used as a delivery system for medications. In spite of these beneficial effects, soaks are a short-term therapy. Repeated soaking is damaging to the skin, producing maceration and ultimately fissuring and inflammation, as natural oils that serve as intercellular "glue" are dissolved by the soaks.

Skin can be soaked by immersion, whereby the body part is placed in the fluid. This is easy for a limb; for a mobile patient even the entire area below the neck can be soaked in a bathtub or whirlpool. For an upper limb, or for a patient who is not mobile, soaks can be delivered by wet dressings. The affected area is wrapped loosely with a generous amount of soft gauze, which is then saturated. For hospitalized patients, intravenous tubing attached to a bag of fluid can be inserted into the gauze and left at a slow drip. For home soaking, a soft, absorbent towel or washcloth can be wrapped or placed over the affected area and repeatedly saturated.

BENEFITS OF SOAKS

- *Decrease pain, itching*
- *Debridement*
- *Delivery of medication*

The choice of an agent as a soak is not particularly important. Warm tap water is easily available and inexpensive and produces few adverse reactions. An aluminum acetate solution (Burow's solution, Domeboro) is popular and soothing as well. Soaks with povidone-iodine (Betadine) solution provide antibacterial activity. Colloidal oatmeal (Aveeno) added to water is very soothing and is known for its antipruritic properties.

Lubrication

Inflamed skin is often dry, cracked, and scaling. This fissuring with exposure of the normally protected dermis to the external environment perpetuates inflammation and irritation. Oils added to the skin cover fissures and erosions, soothing exposed nerve endings. As a result, the patient feels much more comfortable, and ongoing inflammation is minimized. Also, because keratinocytes actually migrate across the surface of an erosion, lubrication provides a moist environment that allows migration to occur more easily than would occur over a crusted or dried surface. Finally, when lubrication is applied over medication, the occlusive properties of the moisturizer promote absorption of the medication.

There are several basic principles for moisturization. A first principle in the use of moisturizers is that lubrication improves the appearance and often the symptoms in all scaling diseases.

The second principle is the thicker the better. Although patients generally prefer a lubricant that disappears after application to the skin, leaving the skin softer with an impression that the substance "soaked in," these thinner lotions actually evaporate because of the high concentrations of water and alcohol. The lubricating action of agents that leave a greasy residue is more marked and longer lasting. Thick emollients—those that do not pour and are generally packaged in jars rather than bottles—include Eucerin cream, petrolatum (Vaseline petroleum jelly), Aquaphor, Polysorb, and even vegetable shortening, such as Crisco. This latter preparation has the advantage of low cost, both the disadvantage and advantage of extreme greasiness, and a tendency to become rancid. Once the skin disease is better controlled, the patient can substitute a more cosmetically acceptable lotion. There are large numbers of these on the market, including Keri, Eucerin, Vaseline Intensive Care, and Lubriderm lotions, as well as many store brands.

Third, lubricants should be applied both over topical corticosteroids to promote absorption, and, in more severe disease, the more often the better. In particular, patients with eczema whose itching is worsened by dryness should apply a lubricant very frequently.

However, moisturization is avoided in naturally damp areas, such as the axillae and genital area, as it can promote maceration. Also, the face and scalp have a high concentration of sebaceous (oil) glands, and these areas usually do not require lubrication.

Many additives are popular with consumers, including aloe, vitamin E, jojoba, elastin, and collagen. There is no evidence that these substances have additional intrinsic properties. Some lubricants contain lactic acid, salicylic acid, or α-hydroxy acids, all of which dissolve scale and produce smoother skin. However, these acids can be irritating and can exacerbate some inflammatory diseases.

PRINCIPLES FOR LUBRICATION

- *Beneficial for scaling skin diseases*
- *Thick creams are more effective than lotions*
- *Apply over topical corticosteroid agents*
- *Apply as often as possible*
- *Avoid moisturizers on the face and skin folds*

Vehicles

Medications are formulated in a variety of vehicles designed to maximize delivery of the medication, lubricate, and provide cosmetic acceptability (Table 3.1). The choice of a vehicle depends on the disease to be treated, the degree of inflammation and erosions, and the area of the body. Nondermatologists sometimes disregard the importance of the proper vehicle and, although the medication may be quite appropriate, the wrong vehicle may delay or prevent healing. For example, an alcohol-containing lotion or gel over eroded or eczematized skin can exacerbate the underlying inflammation. If the prescribing physician does not indicate the vehicle, pharmacists usually dispense a cream, although sometimes more interesting vehicles are given to the patient.

Ointments Ointments are most often petrolatum (petroleum jelly) based. These greasy but soothing vehicles lack many of the alcohols, preservatives, and stabilizers required for other vehicles. This minimizes both irritant and allergic reactions. Ointments are more lubricating, but can produce maceration in damp areas or skin folds. Because of the oily nature of ointments, small amounts spread widely, making this vehicle economical. Ointments are also occlusive, so that active medications are better absorbed. For example, a corticosteroid ointment is more potent than the same corticosteroid cream in the same concentration.

Creams Creams are prepared from oils added to water, so that they are less greasy—and less moisturizing. Although creams are more cosmetically elegant than ointments, stabilizers and preservatives mixed with oils make this vehicle irritating to broken or badly inflamed skin, and there is an increased risk of allergic contact dermatitis. Creams are often preferred over the face or in skin folds, where skin is naturally damp or oily. Patients often prefer creams because they "rub in well," when actually the water and alcohols evaporate.

Gels, Lotions, and Solutions Gels, lotions, and solutions are very thin because these are almost entirely composed of alcohols and water. These are useful for very hairy areas, such as most scalps, where creams and ointments are difficult to apply, and between toe web spaces, where drying rather than lubricating agents are often required. Gels are also sometimes used on the oral mucosa. However, the high concentration of alcohol renders this vehicle irritating in general, and often actually painful on broken or sensitive skin, or over thin genital or axillary skin.

Although major corticosteroids are available in all vehicles, most other medications are only pro-

Table 3.1 Vehicles

VEHICLE	INGREDIENTS	ADVANTAGES	DISADVANTAGES	BEST USES
Ointments	Most often petrolatum	Moisturizing Few additives More potent delivery of medications Spreads farther	Greasy Macerating in damp areas	Very broken or inflamed skin Very dry skin
Creams	Oils in water, preservatives, stabilizers	Cosmetically elegant Less macerating	Irritates very inflamed or eroded skin Less moisturizing Increased risk of allergic contact dermatitis to additives	Face, skin folds Intact skin
Lotions, gels, solutions	Water and alcohol	Nongreasy Avoids maceration	Drying Irritating Increased risk of allergic contact dermatitis to additives	Hairy areas (scalp) Damp areas (toe web spaces) Oral mucosa

duced in one or two forms. For example, most antifungal medications are in cream or lotion bases but are not available in the more soothing ointment. I sometimes use nystatin ointment on skin infected with *Candida*, even though nystatin is less effective than the newer azoles, simply because the azoles are not available in an ointment base.

Vehicles are very carefully formulated by the pharmaceutical company. The biochemical characteristics of the vehicle and the medication must be complementary. The medication must remain suspended in the vehicle without precipitating, yet not be so well suspended that the medication is not released to the skin. Because of this, compounding medications into vehicles other than those designed by the company can yield a formulation with an unknown potency. For example, adding an antifungal medication to a topical steroid medication has the potential for improving or decreasing the absorption of either or both medications. Most dermatologists primarily prescribe formulations prepared by a pharmaceutical company.

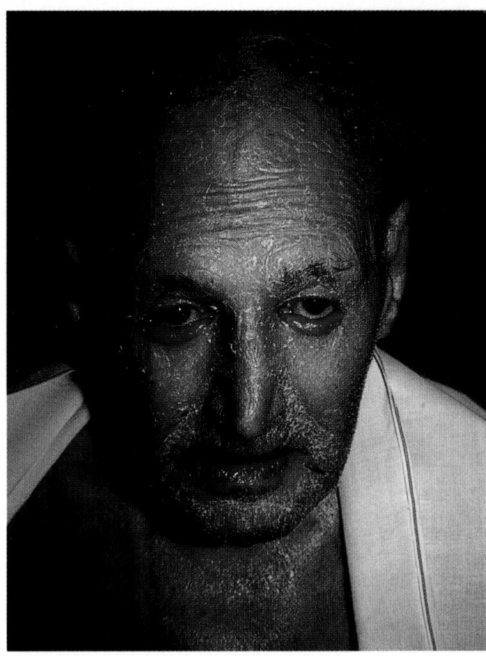

Figure 3.1 This elderly man has a long-standing history of untreated, severe atopic dermatitis, with generalized erythema and scale.

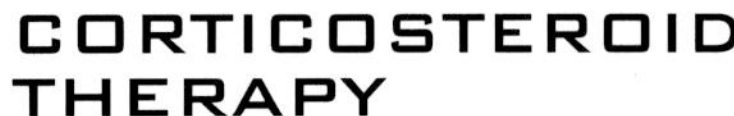

CORTICOSTEROID THERAPY

The therapy least understood by most nondermatologists is the use of corticosteroids for skin disease. Everyone knows the long-standing joke that all of dermatology is divided into steroid-responsive and steroid-unresponsive skin disease. Like many jokes, this one is funny because of the underlying truth—except that skin disease can actually be divided into one of three groups: very steroid responsive, moderately steroid responsive, and unresponsive to corticosteroids.

Appropriate Diseases for Corticosteroid Therapy

Atopic dermatitis (eczema, neurodermatitis, lichen simplex chronicus, dermatitis) and seborrheic dermatitis are the primary diseases that are very steroid responsive (Figs. 3.1 and 3.2). Corticosteroids are the treatment of choice and the only very effective therapy for these rashes. However, most other red, scaling diseases, such as those

Figure 3.2 The same patient as pictured in Figure 3.1, 2 days after hospitalization and treatment with topical corticosteroids under occlusion and sedation.

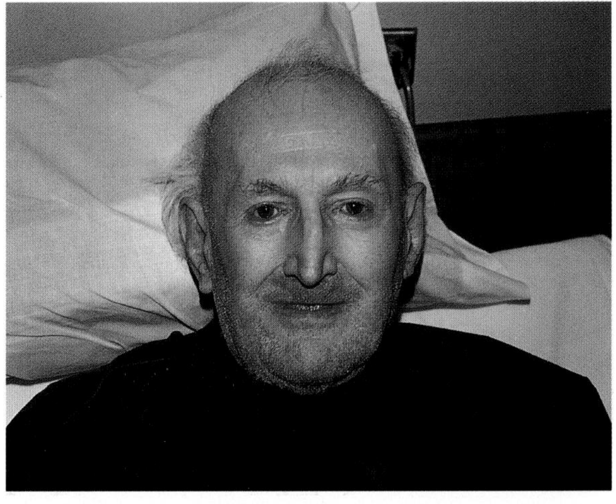

from the papulosquamous group, are improved with corticosteroids, although a higher potency is generally required. Psoriasis, lichen planus, and pityriasis rosea are all improved by topical corticosteroids, but corticosteroids rarely produce complete and lasting improvement. Although all red, scaling diseases improve to some degree with corticosteroids, this improvement does not indicate that corticosteroids are necessarily the best therapy. For example, patients with skin lesions of secondary syphilis, particularly those who are itchy, may experience significant improvement—although not clearing—with a topical corticosteroid. Certainly, corticosteroids are not the treatment of choice for secondary syphilis.

Corticosteroids are sometimes useful as well for relatively resistant inflammatory, nonscaling diseases such as sunburn and insect bites. However, improvement is often unimpressive, requiring higher-potency topical medications or systemic administration.

Topical Corticosteroid Therapy

Uncountable different corticosteroid preparations are available (Table 3.2). These represent seven different potencies and different brands of the same active medication, different vehicles, and different quantities. This confusing array of choices discourages many clinicians, but topical corticosteroid therapy can be simplified by a few general principles: choose one corticosteroid from each of three main potency classes; learn where on the body to use high-, mid-, and low-potency medications; and learn what circumstances are best treated with an ointment, cream, or lotion vehicle.

Potency In general, within the same general potency class, there are no particular medical advantages of one preparation over another. Topical corticosteroid therapy can be simplified by limiting one's repertoire to one widely and generically available corticosteroid of each major potency. This can be simplified even further by consolidating therapy into four rather than seven classes (Table 3.3). Very common choices include hydrocortisone 1% or 2.5% as a low-potency medication, triamcinolone 0.1% (Aristocort, Kenalog) as a mid-potency medication, and fluocinonide (Lidex) as a high-potency agent. Stating the 0.05% concentration when prescribing fluocinonide is unnecessary, as it is the only concentration available. All these medications are available in generic forms and therefore cost-effective, and all are carried essentially by all pharmacies. Generally, an ultrapotent (also called superpotent) corticosteroid should not be prescribed in the emergency department because of its remarkable potency. This newest class of steroids contains only one medication available in generic form, clobetasol propionate (Temovate), available only as a 0.05% preparation. Diprolene is an ultrapotent corticosteroid that some pharmacists mistakenly believe is available generically. The active medication, betamethasone dipropionate, is available generically but, unless compounded in an optimized vehicle found only with Diprolene, it is much less potent.

Vehicle Nearly all these corticosteroids are available in creams, ointments, and either solutions, gels, or lotions (see above section on vehicles). Generally, ointments are used for dry or extremely inflamed skin and for areas with broken skin. Creams are used in moist areas such as the body folds, and the face. Lotions, solutions, and gels are most useful on the scalp and oral mucosa. However, because there is no cosmetically elegant liquid form of triamcinolone, many dermatologists prescribe generic betamethasone valerate (Valisone) as a standard, reasonably priced, and cosmetically acceptable preparation for most steroid-responsive dermatoses of the scalp.

Corticosteroid combination products Several well-known medications contain both a corticosteroid and antifungal agents. Generally, these are shunned by dermatologists but are used extensively by nondermatologists. A middle ground is probably appropriate. Most popular is Lotrisone, a combination of a high-potency corticosteroid (betamethasone dipropionate) and an antifungal/anticandidal agent (clotrimazole). The advantages of this medication include the delivery of adequate therapy most of the time, even if the practitioner is unsure of whether the underlying problem is fungal, yeast, or any steroid-responsive dermatosis.

In addition, markedly inflammatory tinea and *Candida* improve more rapidly if treated during the first few days with an anti-inflammatory medication as well as an antifungal drug. The disadvantages of these medications include the confusion that occurs when the eruption does not completely clear. When the patient follows up with a dermatologist, that physician is unable to evaluate the

Table 3.2 Topical Corticosteroids by Potency[a]

GENERIC NAME	BRAND NAMES
I: Ultrapotent	
Clobetasol propionate 0.05%[b]	Temovate
Betamethasone dipropionate 0.05%[c] (ointment, gel, lotion)	Diprolene
Difluorasone diacetate 0.05%[c] (ointment)	Psorcon
Halobetasol propionate 0.05%	Ultravate
II: High Potency	
Amcinonide 0.1% (ointment)	Cyclocort
Betamethasone dipropionate[c] 0.05% (cream)	Diprolene AF
Betamethasone dipropionate[b] 0.05% (ointment)	Diprosone
Desoximetasone 0.05% (gel) 0.025% (cream, ointment)	Topicort
Difluorasone diacetate 0.05% (cream)	Psorcon
Diflorasone diacetate 0.05% (ointment)	Florone, Maxiflor
Fluocinonide[b] 0.05%	Lidex
Halcinonide 0.1% (cream)	Halog
Mometasone furoate 0.1% (ointment)	Elocon
III: High-Medium Potency	
Amcinonide 0.1% (cream, lotion)	Cyclocort
Betamethasone dipropionate[b] 0.05% (cream)	Diprosone
Betamethasone valerate[b] 0.1% (ointment)	Valisone
Diflorasone diacetate 0.05% (cream)	Florone, Maxiflor
Fluticasone propionate 0.005% (ointment)	Cutivate
Halcinonide 0.1% (ointment)	Halog
Triamcinolone 0.1%[b] (ointment)	Aristocort, Kenalog
IV: Higher Midpotency	
Desoximetasone 0.05% cream	Topicort LP
Fluocinolone acetonide 0.025% (ointment)	Synalar
Hydrocortisone valerate 0.2% (ointment)	Westcort
Mometasone furoate 0.1% (cream)	Elocon
Triamcinolone 0.1%[b] (cream)	Aristocort, Kenalog

(Continues)

Table 3.2 Topical Corticosteroids by Potency[a] (Continued)

GENERIC NAME	BRAND NAMES
V: Midpotency	
Betamethasone dipropionate[b] 0.05% (lotion)	Diprosone
Betamethasone valerate[b] 0.1% (cream, lotion)	Valisone
Fluticasone propionate 0.05% (cream)	Cutivate
Fluocinolone acetonide 0.025% (cream)	Synalar
Hydrocortisone butyrate 0.1% (cream)	Locoid
Hydrocortisone valerate 0.2% (cream)	Westcort
Triamcinolone 0.1%[b] (lotion)	Aristocort, Kenalog
VI: Lower Midpotency	
Alclometasone dipropionate 0.05% (cream, ointment)	Aclovate
Desonide 0.05% (cream)	Tridesilon, DesOwen
Fluocinolone acetonide 0.01% (cream, lotion)	Synalar
VII: Low Potency	
Hydrocortisone 0.5%, 1%, 2.5%[b,d]	Hytone

[a]There are differences among potencies of different vehicles of the same active medications, as well as differences among different brands of the same active medication. Different potencies are sometimes listed by different sources, none of which is referenced. These potencies are not documented in package inserts or the Physician's Desk Reference. For example, triamcinolone 0.1% cream is sometimes found in classes IV, V, or VI.

[b]Available in generic form.

[c]Available in other brands, but these are not of equivalent potency.

[d]Available over the counter.

skin because the clinical appearance has been modified and fungal smears and cultures rendered negative by partial treatment. In addition, the anti-inflammatory effects of corticosteroids are usually only required the first 2 or 3 days of treatment. However, with a combination medication, the corticosteroid is continued far longer than needed, interfering with the cure rate of the fungal infection (Fig. 3.3). Finally, betamethasone dipropionate is a high-potency corticosteroid that can cause significant atrophy with long-term use, particularly in the genital area. Mycolog II (triamcinolone and nystatin) has the additional disadvantage of containing nystatin as its antifungal agent, which only treats yeast infections, and not dermatophyte fungi such as tinea cruris or tinea pedis. Therefore, if this is used inappropriately on a fungal infection, the corticosteroid allows the dermatophyte to worsen and extend unopposed. Fortunately, the very common sensitizer, neomycin, has been removed from Mycolog II, so that allergic contact dermatitis is no longer a great concern. In general, patients with inflammatory fungal infections benefit more from a small tube of a corticosteroid used for the first few days, and a separate tube of an antifungal/anticandidal preparation to be used until the skin clears.

Pramosone cream, ointment, and lotion combine low-potency hydrocortisone with pramoxine hydrochloride, a local anesthetic that can immediately decrease itching. This is especially useful on thin skin, as for perianal pruritus.

Choosing an Appropriate Topical Corticosteroid A few simple principles allow the practitioner to choose an appropriate potency and vehicle (Table 3.3).

Table 3.3 Selected Topical Corticosteroids

POTENCY	COMMON PREPARATIONS	VEHICLES	USES
Low potency	Hydrocortisone 1%,[a] 2.5%	Ointment Cream Solution Lotion	Children Face Skin folds Mild disease
Mid potency	Triamcinolone 0.1% (Kenalog, Aristocort) (no "nice" liquid preparations) Betamethasone valerate 0.1%[b] (Valisone)	Ointment Cream Ointment Cream Lotion	Adult skin (nonfacial, nonintertriginous) More severe disease or disease unresponsive to hydrocortisone
High potency	Fluocinonide 0.05%[b] (Lidex)	Cream Ointment Gel Solution	Very lichenified skin Palms and soles
Ultrapotent	Clobetasol dipropionate 0.05%[b] (Temovate)	Cream Ointment Gel Scalp solution	Severe disease unresponsive to other topical corticosteroids to prevent need for systemic corticosteroids Avoid face, skin folds, children. Follow-up advised

[a]Available over the counter.
[b]Only available in one concentration, so no need to remember or record concentration on prescription.
[c]Must be prescribed by trade name, as generic is not equivalent because potency is a result of the vehicle.

In general, a low-potency corticosteroid preparation such as hydrocortisone is standard therapy for thin adult skin such as the face, and axillary and genital skin folds. Hydrocortisone is also first-line therapy for children or for very mild disease on any part of the body. Moderately steroid-responsive dermatoses (most diseases other than eczema or dermatitis) may require slightly higher potency in these settings.

A midpotency medication such as triamcinolone is the usual therapy for nonfacial and non-skin fold areas of the adult. Triamcinolone is also often used short-term on more severe disease or lichenified skin in those circumstances usually treated with hydrocortisone; for example lichenified skin in children, or severe disease over the face.

A high-potency corticosteroid such as fluocinonide is routinely used over the palms and soles, which are thicker and generally require a strong medication. A high-potency agent is also indicated for very lichenified or severe disease on other non-facial and non-skin fold adult skin.

An ultrapotent corticosteroid such as clobetasol propionate should be prescribed from the emergency department only for very short periods of time to avoid the necessity of systemic steroids. It

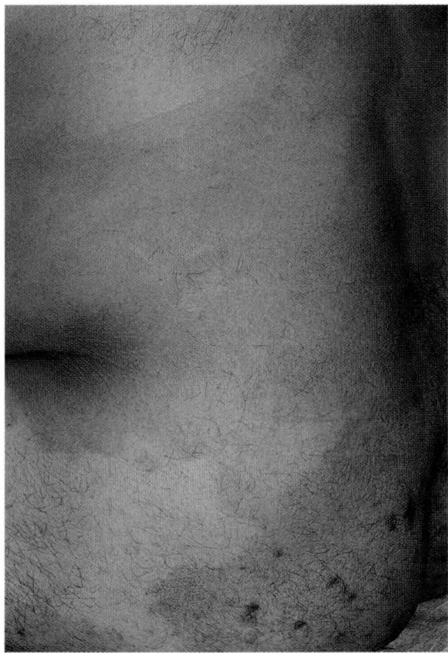

Figure 3.3 When dermatophyte infections are mistakenly treated with topical corticosteroids, the infection can extend, while the anti-inflammatory action of the steroid can change the clinical appearance.

is especially useful for eczematous changes over the hands or feet.

Hints to Simplify Prescribing Corticosteroids and Enhance Compliance All topical corticosteroids are applied twice daily and are usually covered with a moisturizer unless used in skin folds or on the face. Although each different medication and each different brand is supplied in different sizes, not all pharmacies carry every size of each medication. Therefore, it is often practical and quick to prescribe medications as "largest commercial size," which is usually about 60 g (about the size of a large tube of toothpaste), "smallest commercial size," which is usually about 15 g, or "medium commercial size."

Patients should also be given refills if a follow-up visit is not immediate or if the area to be covered is large. On the other hand, when the affected area is limited, potentially harmful medication, such as high-potency corticosteroids, should be prescribed as small size without refills. This both prevents adverse reactions and, since most of these patients should be seen by a dermatologist or their personal physician in follow-up, refills or changes can be made at that time.

Adverse Reactions to Topical Corticosteroids
Although topical steroids have many local and systemic side effects, short-term (3 weeks or shorter) use of topical corticosteroids is associated with remarkably few significant adverse reactions. Classic local side effects include atrophy or thinning of the skin that is manifested by a thin, smooth texture, visible telangiectasias, and, sometimes, striae (Fig. 3.4). Although atrophy improves with discontinuation of therapy, some residua can be permanent.

Some areas, particularly the face and vulva, are susceptible to the development of steroid dermatitis. This rosacea-like condition is characterized by

ADVERSE REACTIONS OF TOPICAL CORTICOSTEROIDS

Any area (naturally thin or occluded skin at higher risk)
- *Atrophy*
- *Striae*
- *Telangiectasias*
- *Hypopigmentation*
- *Worsening of dermatophyte infection*
- *Changed appearance of dermatophyte infection (tinea incognito)*
- *Allergic contact dermatitis*
- *Irritant contact dermatitis*

Trunk
- *Steroid acne*

Face, Vulva
- *Perioroficial dermatitis/steroid dermatitis*
- *Glaucoma (used near eyes)*
- *Cataracts (used chronically near eyes)*
- *Worsening of herpes keratitis*

Large Areas (especially when very inflamed or eroded)
- *Systemic absorption and all adverse reactions of systemic administration (see box on p. 28, Adverse Reactions to Systemic Corticosteroids)*

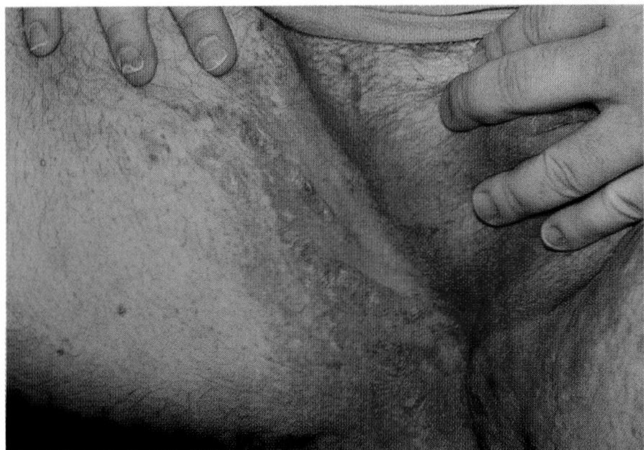

Figure 3.4 A well-known side effect of topical corticosteroids is atrophy and striae, which occur quickly in some patients and not at all in others.

erythema, burning, red papules, and sometimes pustules, often with scale.

Another occasional local complication of corticosteroid therapy is the exacerbation of fungal infections (Fig. 3.3). Topical steroids are occasionally and appropriately used for inflammatory fungal infection for the first few days, in conjunction with an antifungal agent to produce more rapid resolution of inflammation. At times, when the corticosteroid is not discontinued, or when a topical corticosteroid is used as treatment for a misdiagnosed fungal infection, fungal disease worsens. The area of disease may extend, and morphologic features can change as the fungus affects the deeper areas of hair follicles, producing papules and nodules.

When either very high-potency topical corticosteroids are used over large areas, or when even medium-potency corticosteroids are used over a significant area of very broken or inflamed skin, systemic absorption can occur and systemic adverse reactions are possible. If this occurs for several days, no particular harm will occur with the absorption of the equivalent of 20 or 30 mg of prednisone daily. However, patients who use topical corticosteroids in this setting for many months are at risk of adrenal suppression and all the other adverse reactions associated with chronic, systemic steroid use. Therefore, any patient who requires ongoing topical corticosteroid therapy for control of the disease should receive follow-up evaluation by either a generalist who is especially knowledgeable about skin disease or a dermatologist. The patient should be evaluated for the presence of adverse reactions and the possibility of decreasing the potency of corticosteroids.

Systemic Corticosteroids

Although most steroid-responsive skin diseases can be managed with topical corticosteroids, some situations require systemic therapy. Systemic corticosteroids can be administered orally, intramuscularly, or intravenously (Table 3.4).

Indications Very widespread or exudative skin disease often is better managed by systemic corti-

Table 3.4 Systemic Corticosteroids

MEDICATIONS	AVAILABLE PREPARATION	ROUTE	DOSING
Prednisone	1 mg, 2.5 mg, 5 mg, 10 mg, 20 mg, 50 mg	PO	40–60 mg every morning
	15 mg/5 ml		1–2 mg/kg/day children
Triamcinolone acetonide (Kenalog)	10 mg/ml, 40 mg/ml; both in 1-ml vials	IM	60–80 mg once
Methylprednisone (Solu-Medrol)	Multiple combinations	IV	250–500 mg q6h

costeroids during the first few days, if there are no significant contraindications. These patients are generally miserable, and systemic corticosteroids produce more rapid improvement than topical medication. At any rate, systemic absorption of topical corticosteroids is substantial when applied over very inflamed skin and over large areas. Blistering and eroded skin is usually best treated systemically until healing begins to occur. Absorption through a blister roof is minimal, and the application of topical creams and ointments to eroded areas can produce maceration. Papulosquamous diseases such as discoid lupus erythematosus, lichen planus, and pityriasis rosea, as well as other moderately responsive skin conditions such as sunburn respond far better to systemic corticosteroids than to topical corticosteroids. Although ongoing prednisone is fraught with possible serious adverse reactions, short bursts of prednisone sometimes can help initiate improvement that can be maintained with topical therapy.

Oral Corticosteroids Dermatologists generally prefer systemic corticosteroids administered orally, except for patients with life-threatening diseases that require hospital admission and intravenous therapy. Prednisone is extremely inexpensive, and the dose can be adjusted or discontinued on a day-to-day basis. Because prednisone is administered orally rather than intramuscularly, the occasional side effect of atrophy or abscess in an injection site is avoided. In addition, prednisone has the advantage of allowing a higher initial dosage than is generally delivered with intramuscular medication, while avoiding exposure of the adrenal glands to a full month of suppression as the intramuscular preparation is gradually absorbed. The most cost-effective and efficient method of treating with oral corticosteroids is not by a prepackaged tapering dose (Medrol Dosepak), but rather by the daily administration of 40 to 60 mg of prednisone to an adult and 1 to 2 mg/kg for a child, up to an adult dose. Most patients requiring systemic corticosteroids deserve followup, and a decision as to whether and how to taper the patient is best made at that time.

Intramuscular Corticosteroids Corticosteroids can also be administered as triamcinolone acetonide (Kenalog) intramuscularly at a usual adult dose of 60 to 80 mg. This medication is slowly absorbed. Maximum effect requires two or three days, and the effective highest daily dose is probably equivalent to 20 to 25 mg of prednisone, with gradual tapering over 1 month. Some clinicians prefer intramuscular administration for an acute allergic contact dermatitis. Strong reactions as occur with poison ivy or poison oak often flare when systemic corticosteroids are discontinued, and this automatic taper can be useful. However, other practitioners argue that prednisone delivers a faster and higher initial dose and that tapering can be achieved more safely and as effectively by substituting topical corticosteroids or alternate-day prednisone after an initial burst of oral prednisone.

Intravenous Corticosteroids Very ill patients and those with life-threatening or organ-threatening disease are usually best treated with intravenous therapy. Patients with very early toxic epidermal necrolysis who have been judged good candidates for corticosteroid therapy, patients with aggressive systemic leukocytoclastic vasculitis, and patients with severe pemphigus vulgaris are examples of instances where hospital admission with the intravenous administration of methylprednisolone (Solumedrol) is indicated. Patients generally receive up to one gram intravenously per day with the duration depending upon the disease and the patient's response.

Adverse Reactions Systemic corticosteroids are well tolerated short-term. Mood changes are the most common acute side effect, with most patients experiencing a sense of well being and increased energy. However, depression occurs in some, and frank psychosis is rare but occurs, especially in elderly patients. After several days, appetite often increases and an elevation of blood sugar and blood pressure can occur. These are generally not significant over the short term except in those with preexisting unstable diabetes mellitus or hypertension. Significant immunosuppression generally begins after about five days.

The chronic side effects of systemic corticosteroids are well known by most practitioners. These include immunosuppression, osteopenia, high blood pressure, diabetes mellitus, muscle

ADVERSE REACTIONS TO SYSTEMIC CORTICOSTEROIDS

Immediate (1–2 days)
- *Mood changes*
- *Psychosis*
- *Glaucoma*

Short Term (1–3 weeks)
- *Increased appetite*
- *Increased blood pressure*[a]
- *Increased blood sugar*[b]
- *Immunosuppression*
- *Edema*

Long Term (months)
- *Truncal obesity*
- *Loss of muscle*
- *Osteoporosis*
- *Cataracts*
- *Skin fragility (striae, purpura)*
- *Aseptic necrosis of femoral head*[c]
- *Hair loss*
- *Hirsutism*

[a]*Usually important over the short term only in patients with significant pre-existing hypertension.*
[b]*Usually important over the short term only in patients with significant pre-existing diabetes mellitus*
[c]*Rare reports of aseptic necrosis after short-term therapy.*

wasting, truncal obesity, hair loss, skin fragility resulting in purpura and striae, and adrenal suppression and atrophy. Aseptic necrosis of the hip can occur with shorter courses of corticosteroids but are more common in those treated with long-term medication.

ANTIPRURITIC THERAPY

The only effective antipruritic therapy is management that addresses the cause of pruritus. Although good oral and topical medications for pain relief are available, there are no specific therapies that alleviate itch. However, there are several topical agents that can minimize itching.

TOPICAL ANTIPRURITIC AGENTS

Antihistamines
- *Doxepin cream*
- *Diphenhydramine (no! no!)*

Anesthetics
- *Pramoxine HCl cream, ointment, solution*
- *Crotamiton cream*

Counter Irritants
- *Phenol, menthol, camphor*
- *Capsaicin cream*

Physical Agents–cooling
- *Water*
- *Calamine*
- *Alcohol (no! no!)*

Topical Antipruritic Therapy

Antihistamines Antihistamines are generally perceived as effective medications for itching. However, these medications are usually effective primarily when given orally for those diseases for which histamine plays a role, especially urticaria, or when given in sedating doses. Topical preparations have limited usefulness.

Two topical antihistamines are available. The first is diphenhydramine (Benadryl) cream. Unfortunately, although this medication is effective partly because of its topical anesthetic properties, it is also a potent sensitizer and should be avoided. In fact, it has now been removed from several common, over-the-counter preparations such as Caladryl. A newer addition is topical doxepin HCl (Zonalon). This 5% cream has been shown to decrease itching in patients with eczema (atopic dermatitis) when applied twice daily, but allergic contact dermatitis does occur.

Anesthetics Other topical anesthetics that are not antihistamines can be antipuritic at times. The most widely used is pramoxine hydrochloride (Prax). This medication is also available compounded with hydrocortisone 1% and 2.5% (Pramosone) cream, ointment, or lotion, so that steroid-responsive diseases have more immediate relief from these local anesthetics. Benzocaine

(Americaine) is another local anesthetic used primarily for pain. This is most effective on mucous membranes and, like diphenhydramine, is associated with a high risk of allergic contact dermatitis. Crotamiton (Eurax) lotion and cream have limited anesthetic, antipruritic properties.

Counterirritants Several topical preparations improve itching by their activity as counterirritants. Lotions can be mixed with menthol, camphor, and/or phenol. Sarna lotion is one such commercially available preparation. Capsaicin (Zostrix is available over the counter; Zostrix HP is available by prescription) although used primarily for neuropathic pain, is antipruritic for some diseases. It acts partly as a counterirritant and also by depleting substance P in peripheral sensory neurons. However, all counterirritants are irritating by definition and can exacerbate some conditions, such as eczema. They should be avoided in patients with very inflamed or eroded skin.

Cooling Just as heat generally increases itching, cooling the skin often improves itching. This can be achieved with cool soaks and alcohol, but both (especially the latter) tend to dry the skin and ultimately increase inflammation and itching. Therefore, soaks should only be used short term until more basic therapy to eliminate the problem has been established; alcohol generally should be avoided altogether. Calamine lotion is a time-honored preparation that is cooling but drying, so the clinician should take care that scaling conditions are not worsened by overdrying.

Oral Antipruritic Therapy

There are two main types of systemic medication for itching. For those patients with inflammation, oral prednisone is usually effective although potentially toxic (see section on systemic corticosteroids). Otherwise, except for some patients with urticaria that is responsive to antihistamines, itching can be controlled only with sedation, a reasonable nighttime therapy but with obvious daytime limitations. Corticosteroids are not curative, but only control symptoms until remission of the disease process occurs.

Sedation can be achieved with many different medications. Most clinicians prefer to use sedating antihistamines because of their safety. However, antihistamines have no inherent antipruritic properties. Therefore, most patients who are itching derive less benefit by the newer, nonsedating antihistamines. In addition, low doses of sedating antihistamines are often not particularly useful for itching. Hydroxyzine HCl (Atarax) and diphenhydramine (Benadryl) are older, inexpensive, and widely used sedating antihistamines. Although low doses every 4 to 6 hours around the clock sometimes control urticaria, doses of 25 to 100 mg of each are generally required to produce deep and comfortable sleep during the night.

Doxepin (Sinequan) and amitriptyline (Elavil) are tricyclic antidepressants with very strong antihistaminic and sedating effects. Doxepin has both a longer half-life and is a more potent antihistamine than either hydroxyzine HCl or diphenhydramine, making it a superior medication for nighttime itching. Tricyclic antidepressants also induce deeper sleep than most antihistamines, and sedation is longer lasting.[1] These medications have the added advantage of providing antidepressant effects in patients with pruritus who are also depressed or anxious. Patients should be warned about the anticholinergic effects of all these medications.

ANTIBIOTICS

Although the numbers of systemic antibiotics seem to increase daily, there are a very few that are used for skin diseases (Table 3.5). The more expensive, newer, broader spectrum, and much more expensive antibiotics have no particular advantage over these older, well-known agents for most patients.

Antibiotics are used by dermatologists in two clinical settings. First, as in other areas of medicine, antibiotics are used as antimicrobial agents, either to treat an established infection or to prevent infection in a wound. More confined to the realm of skin disease is the concept of some antibiotics as anti-inflammatory agents because of inhibitory effects on neutrophil chemotaxis. The most well-known diseases that benefit from these nonspecific

Table 3.5 Systemic Antibiotics for Skin Infections

MEDICATION	AVAILABLE PREPARATIONS	DOSE	DURATION
Cephalexin (Keflex)	250-, 500-mg tablets; 125, 250 mg/5 ml	500 mg bid or qid Children: 25–50 mg/kg/day, divided bid, qid	Until clear
Dicloxacillin	250, 500 mg; 125, 250 mg/5 ml	500 mg bid or qid Children: 12.5–50 mg/kg/day, divided bid, qid	Until clear
Erythromycin[a]	200-, 250-, 400-, 500-mg tablets; 125, 200, 250, 400 mg/5 ml	500 mg bid or qid Children: 30–50 mg/kg/day, divided bid, qid	Until clear
Ciprofloxacin	250, 500, 750 mg	500–750 mg/bid	Until clear

[a]High prevalence of *Staphylococcus aureus* resistance to erythromycin in some areas.

anti-inflammatory actions are acne, acne rosacea, and hidradenitis suppurativa.

Topical Antibiotics as Antimicrobial Agents

The only topical antibiotic that is unquestionably useful for frank infection is mupirocin (Bactroban) ointment. Although this is a potent antistaphylococcal agent that is very effective for impetigo and even slightly deeper infections, resistance can occur rapidly. An important role for mupirocin ointment is its ability to decrease nasopharyngeal carriage of *Staphylococcus aureus* when this medication is inserted into the nares four times a day for 5 days.[2]

A plethora of other topical antibiotics are useful for wound care and extremely minor infections. These include gentamicin ointment, Neosporin ointment (which contains neomycin, a potent sensitizer), Polysporin ointment, and Bacitracin ointment. More popular with surgeons than dermatologists are topical sulfas, including Sulfamylon and Silvadene. Sulfas in general are potent sensitizers, and, when applied over large areas, can exert effects due to systemic absorption, including leukopenia.

Topical Antibiotics as Anti-inflammatory Agents

Five commonly prescribed topical antibiotics are used for their anti-inflammatory properties. Benzoyl peroxide 5% and 10% creams and lotions; erythromycin 2% gels, pads, and solutions; clindamycin 2% solutions, gels, and lotions (Cleocin T); and sulfas (Sulfacet-R MVL lotion) significantly improve acne when used twice daily. Topical metronidazole (Metrogel) gel and cream are as effective as oral tetracycline for acne rosacea. The primary side effect of these medications is local irritation in some patients.

These topical antibiotics are generally not used for their effects on the treatment of infection of the skin, although metronidazole and clindamycin are available as vaginal preparations for their antibacterial effects. In addition to the relative ineffectiveness of these medications for the treatment and prevention of cutaneous infection, the vehicles in commercial preparations used for acne are alcohol-containing, so that use over very inflamed or broken, infected skin can be painful.

Oral Antibiotics

For widespread or anything other than mild disease, oral antibiotics are preferred to topical medication for both infections and inflammatory conditions such as acne, hidradenitis suppurativa, and acne rosacea.

Oral Antibiotics as Antimicrobial Agents The vast majority of bacterial skin infections are due to *Staphylococcus aureus*, with the few remaining infections primarily caused by α-hemolytic *streptococcus*. Therefore, when antibiotics are used specifically for skin infections, the usual antibiotics are cephalexin (Keflex), dicloxacillin, cloxacillin, and, in areas where *S. aureus* is generally not resistant, erythromycin (Table 3.5). The dose of each is 1 to 2 g a day, divided into two to four doses, with the duration depending on the disease and its severity.

Cephalexin is a cost-effective, very well-tolerated antibiotic that is often used as first-line therapy in skin infections. It is taken as 500 mg bid for minor infections with or without food and, although not frequent, allergic reactions or diarrhea are the most likely side effects.

Dicloxacillin and cloxacillin, also at doses of 250 mg qid or 500 mg bid are extraordinarily good antistaphylococcal medications, which also cover streptococcal skin infections. These medications are reasonably priced and well tolerated. The major drawback to dicloxacillin and cloxacillin are the allergenicity of penicillins.

Erythromycin at 500 mg bid is an antibiotic often used in dermatology as both an antistaphylococcal agent and an anti-inflammatory medication. It is particularly useful when the examiner is not sure whether the disease is primarily an infection or sterile inflammation, as can occur with chronic folliculitis. Although this is a relatively safe and inexpensive medication, there are several major disadvantages. First is the high frequency of abdominal cramping, diarrhea, and, less often, nausea. Second is the increasingly high prevalence of resistance of *S. aureus* to this medication. In addition, there are a number of medication interactions with erythromycin. Fortunately, allergy to erythromycin is uncommon.

Occasionally, particularly in skin areas that remain damp, *Pseudomonas aeruginosa* may play a role in skin disease. For these patients, therapy with ciprofloxacin (Cipro) 250 to 500 mg bid may be beneficial.

Oral Antibiotics as Anti-inflammatory Agents Acne vulgaris, acne rosacea, hidradenitis suppurativa, and bullous pemphigoid are all inflammatory diseases that are not primarily infectious, although bacteria may play a minor or complicating role. These diseases are often treated with antibiotics, which exhibit anti-inflammatory actions primarily by decreasing neutrophil chemotaxis (Table 3.6). Unlike the action of antibiotics in infection, the anti-inflammatory effects are much more delayed,

Table 3.6 Systemic Antibiotics for Inflammation (Acne, Hidradenitis Suppurativa)

MEDICATION	AVAILABLE PREPARATION	DOSE	DURATION
Tetracycline	250, 500 mg capsules	500 mg bid	Ongoing
Erythromycin	200, 250, 400, 500 mg	500 mg bid	Ongoing
Doxycycline	100 mg	100 mg bid	Ongoing
Minocycline	50, 100 mg	100 mg bid	Ongoing
Clindamycin	150 mg	150 mg bid	Ongoing

sometimes taking 1 to 2 months to show an effect. Patients should be warned that this delay is usual, since most expect more rapid improvement. Tetracycline and erythromycin 500 mg bid are safe, inexpensive, and usually effective. Tetracycline has the disadvantage of requiring an empty stomach for 2 hours before and 1 hour after dosing, and erythromycin causes gastrointestinal side effects in many patients. Doxycycline or minocycline at 100 mg bid is used for those who are not improved by, or who are intolerant to, tetracycline or erythromycin. Doxycycline and minocycline have fewer day-to-day disadvantages, although doxycycline causes photosensitivity in many patients, and minocycline is often associated with dizziness, much less often with (reversible) gray-blue discoloration of scars, and very rarely with a lupus-like syndrome.[3,4] Clindamycin 150 mg bid is also very beneficial, extremely well tolerated, and safe, as long as the patient is advised of the possibility of pseudomembranous colitis. Sulfas such as dapsone and trimethoprim-sulfamethoxazole are effective but they are potent sensitizers so that allergic reactions are common and can be severe.

ANTIFUNGAL AGENTS

Fungus infections of the skin are of three main varieties. First are the dermatophytes, superficial fungus infections characterized in microscopic examinations of skin scrapings by branching hyphae. Examples include tinea corporis, tinea cruris, and tinea pedis. These are local rather than systemic infections. The second type of fungal infection is the deep fungal infection. This includes cutaneous coccidioidomycosis, histoplasmosis, blastomycosis, and sporotrichosis. Some of these are blood-borne infections, and some are local but spread via lymphatics. These are much deeper and usually infect the dermis and subcutaneous fat. The third group includes yeast infections, manifested on microscopic preparation by hyphae, pseudohyphae, and budding yeast forms. The primary organisms responsible are *Candida albicans* and *Pityrosporum ovale (Malassazia furfur)*, the causative organism of pityriasis "tinea" versicolor. Only superficial dermatophyte and yeast infections are appropriately treated with topical agents.

Some antifungal medications are effective only for dermatophytes, and some are effective only for yeast forms. However, some of the newer medications are effective for both.

Topical Antifungal Therapy

Many topical antifungal medications are available, but differences among the newer preparations are minor (Table 3.7).

One of the oldest topical antifungal medications, *nystatin*, is effective only for yeast forms. This medication is applied four times a day and is effective for the vast majority of patients with *Candida* infection. Nystatin is available as a cream, ointment, and powder. Nystatin is not effective in the treatment of tinea infections, such as tinea cruris or tinea pedis. Amphotericin (Fungizone) cream and lotion is closely related to nystatin and exhibits good anticandidal effects, but it is not useful against dermatophytes.

Keratolytics are somewhat useful therapy for fungal infections. Selenium sulfide (Selsun) lotion applied nightly for 1 to 2 weeks is quite effective in the treatment of pityriasis "tinea" versicolor, although irritating and tiresome. Whitfield's ointment, which contains 3% salicylic acid is mildly fungistatic and sometimes used for tinea pedis.

Tolnaftate (Tinactin) solution, cream, and powder is an over-the-counter topical antifungal agent, well known to lay people, that is moderately useful for dermatophytes. It is primarily used for chronic control of tinea pedis and tinea cruris, but it is not effective against yeast infections.

Most of the newer medications are more effective than the classic standbys for superficial dermatophyte and yeast infections. Also, some are useful for both yeast and dermatophyte forms. Therefore, an unsure clinician can prescribe an active medication even when he is unsure of whether the infection is a dermatophyte or a yeast. The most widely used class of medication in this group is the *azoles*. These include the over-the-counter medications,

Table 3.7 Topical Antifungal Medications

MEDICATION	ACTIVE AGAINST *CANDIDA*	ACTIVE AGAINST DERMATOPHYTE	DOSING	OINTMENT	CREAM	SOLUTION/ LOTION	POWDER
Polyenes							
Nystatin[a]	Yes	No	qid	Yes	Yes	No	Yes
Amphotericin	Yes	No	qid	No	Yes	No	No
Azoles							
Miconazole[a,b]	Yes	Yes	bid	No	Yes	Yes	No
Clotrimazole[a,b]	Yes	Yes	bid	No	Yes	Yes	No
Ketoconazole	Yes	Yes	bid	No	Yes	Yes	No
Econazole[c]	Yes	Yes	bid	No	Yes	Yes	No
Oxiconazole[c]	Yes	Yes	bid	No	Yes	Yes	No
Sulconazole[c]	Yes	Yes	bid	No	Yes	Yes	No
Allylamines							
Naftifine[c]	Yes	Yes	bid	No	Yes	No	No
Terbinafine[c]	Yes	Yes	bid	No	Yes	No	No
Other							
Ciclopiroxolamine	Yes	Yes	bid	No	Yes	Yes	No
Tolnaftate[a,b]	No	Yes	qid	No	Yes	Yes	Yes
Undecylenate[a,b]	No	Yes	qid	Yes	No	No	Yes

[a]Available generically.
[b]Available over the counter.
[c]Once a day dosing, except for *Candida* and *Tinea pedis.*

clotrimazole (Lotrimin) and miconazole (Micatin), which require application four times a day. Newer related azoles are available only by prescription and require less frequent dosing. However, these azoles are available only in cream and liquid forms, which are irritating to extremely inflamed or broken skin, whereas nystatin is available as an ointment. An unrelated antifungal medication with similar effects is *ciclopirox olamine* (Loprox), which also exhibits mild antibacterial properties.

Naftifine (Naftin) cream and gel are useful for dermatophytes but less so for *Candida,* and *terbinafine* (Lamisil) cream is useful for both but more effective against dermatophytes. Topical terbinafine (Lamisil) has been shown to require shorter duration of therapy for dermatophyte infection as compared to azoles, with this medication requiring only 1 week to clear tinea pedis in many patients.[5] There is evidence that allylamines (terbinafine and naftifine) may be more effective than azoles, but these medications have not been compared extensively.[6]

Many of the above medications are available in solution form, which are particularly useful for control of chronic tinea pedis. This vehicle is beneficial for damp areas between the toes to prevent maceration, but solutions, lotions, and gels should not be used in other areas, particularly the genital area, because of the irritation caused by alcohol in a solution vehicle.

The two antifungal–corticosteroid combination medications are discussed in the section pertaining to topical corticosteroids.

Oral Antifungal Agents

Very extensive fungal disease, nail infections, and dermatophytes located in hairy areas or producing fungal folliculitis are not treated effectively with topical agents and require oral therapy (Table 3.8). Systemic and deep fungal infections also require systemic therapy, and the use of antifungal medications in these circumstances is beyond the scope of this book.

Griseofulvin

Griseofulvin is an old, well-known, oral medication that remains a first-line therapy for superficial dermatophyte infections. It has no activity against yeast. This medication is quite safe despite its much exaggerated reputation of causing bone marrow suppression and liver disease. Otherwise healthy people do not experience these adverse reactions, and most dermatologists do not follow patients with laboratory testing. However, griseofulvin very often causes nausea and other gastrointestinal symptoms, headache, and, less often, photosensitivity or hives. The usual dose of griseofulvin in adults is 500 mg twice a day with a fatty meal since this medication is fat soluble. The effective dose in children is higher than that

Table 3.8 Oral Antifungal Medications

GENERIC NAME	TRADE NAME	ACTIVE AGAINST	ADVERSE REACTIONS	ADULT DOSE	CHILD DOSE
Griseofulvin	Gris-PEG Grifulvin Grisactin	Dermatophytes (not yeast)	Headache GI upset Urticaria Photosensitivity	500 mg bid	10 mg/lb/day
Griseofulvin (ultramicrosize)	Grisactin Ultra Fulvicin P/G	Same as micro-size form	Same as micro-size form	330 mg bid	5 mg/lb/day
Ketoconazole	Nizoral	Dermatophytes Yeasts[a]	Liver toxicity[b] Medication interactions LFTs required[c]	100–200 mg/day	5–10 mg/kg/day
Fluconazole	Diflucan	Dermatophytes Yeasts[a]	Headache	100–200 mg/day	3–6 mg/kg/day
Itraconazole	Sporonox	Dermatophytes Yeasts[a]	Nausea Medication interactions[c]	200 mg/day for 4 mo (nail disease)	3–5 mg/kg/day
Terbinafine HCl	Lamisil	Dermatophytes	Rash	250 mg/day for 12 wk (nail disease)	

[a]Yeasts include both *Candida albicans* and *Pityrosporum ovale* ("tinea" pityriasis versicolor).

[b]Liver toxicity can be fatal, and now that safer medications are available, this medication is generally not used.

[c]Medication interactions occur with macrolide antibiotics and nonsedating antihistamines, sometimes producing fatal cardiac arrhythmias.

reported in the Physician's Desk Reference, and consists of 10 mg/lb (20 to 25 mg/kg) per day. Dosing of the ultramicrosize product is lower. Generally, laboratory testing to monitor the patient for hepatotoxicity or bone marrow suppression is not required.[7]

Ketoconazole

Ketoconazole (Nizoral) was the second oral antifungal medication available in the United States. Extraordinarily well tolerated on a day-to-day basis as compared to griseofulvin, this medication is effective against yeast, dermatophytes, and deep fungal infections. The usual dose for superficial skin infections and onychomycosis is 100 to 200 mg/day until the skin or nails appear normal. However, a major drawback to the medication is the occasional idiosyncratic hepatotoxicity that can be fatal. In addition, both ketoconazole and its close relative, itraconazole, produce serum elevations of some medications metabolized by the P-450 cytochrome system. The nonsedating antihistamines astemizole (Hismanal), and terfenadine (Seldane), as well as erythromycin and cisapride (Propulsid) are the major offenders, sometimes producing cardiac arrhythmias. Patients should be carefully warned about interactions with these medications and possible, as-yet-unidentified new drugs. Thus, with the more recent introduction of other oral azoles, ketoconazole is very rarely used except for extremely short courses in the treatment of pityriasis "tinea" versicolor or for patients who simply cannot afford the higher prices of the newer agents. Monthly liver function testing is required for patients taking ketoconazole.

Fluconazole

Fluconazole (Diflucan) is an oral antifungal medication approved by the Food and Drug Administration (FDA) for the treatment of deep fungal infections and mucocutaneous candidiasis. Although fluconazole does not have FDA indication approval for dermatophytes, it is quite effective and it is often used as second-line therapy for patients with cutaneous dermatophyte infections (except nails, which can be treated more efficiently with itraconazole) when griseofulvin is not tolerated. It lacks significant hepatotoxicity as compared to ketoconazole. Medication interactions, although certainly theoretically possible, are far less remarkable than with ketoconazole and itraconazole. Interactions with astemizole, terfenadine, erythromycin, and cisapride are not clinical problems at the usual therapeutic doses.[8] The usual dose of fluconazole for dermatophytes is 100 to 200 mg (3 to 6 mg/kg for children) per day until the skin appears clear. One dose of 150 mg is effective for vulvovaginal candidiasis. Side effects with fluconazole are very uncommon, but headaches, abdominal pain, and nausea occur in some, and hepatic necrosis (primarily in very ill patients) and severe allergic skin reactions have been reported.

Itraconazole

Itraconazole (Sporanox) is a related azole effective against dermatophytes, deep fungi, and yeast. This medication has approval by the FDA for the treatment of onychomycosis as well as deep fungal infections. Because itraconazole has a very strong affinity for keratin and is incorporated into the nail matrix, most nail infections can be cleared with a 4-month course of therapy at 200 mg/day, even though about 1 year is required for the nail to be completely replaced by new growth. Alternatively, itraconazole can be administered at 400 mg/day for the first week of each month for 4 months.[9] All other antifungal medications require that therapy be continued until the nail has grown out normally. Itraconazole is also effective for other dermatophyte infections such as tinea capitis or tinea corporis, but this requires daily or alternate-day dosing.[10,11] Dosing in children is 3 to 5 mg/kg/day.[12] Because the capsule is available in a 100 mg size only, modification of the dosing schedule may be required. For example, a child weighing 15 kg can be treated with itraconazole 100 mg every other day, with the capsule contents disguised in food. The most serious adverse reactions occur as the result of drug interaction (see above discussion of ketoconazole). Otherwise, the primary side effects of itraconazole include rash, abdominal discomfort, and nausea.

The newest addition to the systemic antifungal armamentarium in the United States is oral terbinafine (Lamisil). This medication is an allylamine that is very effective against dermatophytes and variably effective against yeast. This medication is well tolerated, with side effects occurring in about 11% of patients.[13] Gastrointestinal side effects account for the majority of side effects. Terbinafine is given at a dose of 250 mg/day.

Amphotericin

Amphotericin (Fungizone) is a medication that is extremely effective for systemic *Candida* infections, and it is also used in some deep fungal infections. Useful only as an intravenous or topical preparation, amphotericin is reserved for serious infections not controlled with the less toxic azoles. Sometimes dubbed "amphoterrible," this medication frequently causes fever and chills, with anaphylaxis and kidney failure less likely possibilities. This medication is never used in outpatient dermatology.

ANTIVIRAL AGENTS

Unfortunately, few specific antiviral agents are effective in skin diseases. Herpesviruses are the only viruses for which there is good therapy, and even in this case, medication does not prevent the latent phase. There are no topical therapies that produce clinically significant benefits.

Acyclovir

Acyclovir was the first oral agent available for the herpesviruses. This medication inhibits viral DNA synthesis without affecting host DNA formation. Side effects are limited to nausea in a small minority of patients. However, rapid intravenous infusion can produce crystallization of medication in the kidneys. The usual oral dose of acyclovir is 200 mg (or, in children, 5 mg/kg/dose) five times a day for active herpes simplex virus (HSV) infection, and 400 mg bid for ongoing suppression of recurrences.[14] Chronic suppressive acyclovir has also been shown to decrease asymptomatic viral shedding.[15] The early administration of acyclovir in patients with herpes zoster can ameliorate the disease somewhat.[16] The dose of acyclovir is 800 mg (or, in children, 20 mg/kg/dose) five times a day for varicella zoster virus (VZV) infections. This medication is useful primarily when given within the first 48 to 72 hours from onset of a HSV or herpes zoster infection, and some clinical trials examining the effect of acyclovir on chicken pox have enrolled patients within 24 hours of onset.

Famciclovir and Valacyclovir

More recently, famciclovir (Famvir) and valacyclovir (Valtrex) have become available. These are prodrugs, which are absorbed better than acyclovir. Once in the body, they converted almost immediately into acyclovir (valacyclovir) or penciclovir (famciclovir), the active metabolite. Their advantage over acyclovir is the less frequent dosing required. Acyclovir will be available in a generic form in the near future, and cost will become another advantage. Famciclovir is used at a dose of 500 mg tid for VZV infections, and 125 mg tid for HSV infections. The doses are valacyclovir 1,000 mg (two 500-mg caplets) tid for herpes zoster infections, and 500 mg bid for HSV. HSV infections resistant to acyclovir are also resistant to valacyclovir and famciclovir.

Foscarnet

Foscarnet, is often effective for those few immunosuppressed patients with acyclovir-resistant herpes simplex virus infection. Unfortunately, it is only used as an intravenous medication.

α-Interferon

α-Interferon is an injectable medication that exerts antiviral effects. Multiple local injections constitute useful therapy for condylomata acuminata.

Other viral therapies are primarily destructive, such as liquid nitrogen, salicylic acid, and podophyllum resin, all used for warts.

OTHER MEDICATIONS

The medications discussed briefly in this section have essentially no place in the management of dermatology patients in the emergency department. However, some patients on these medications find themselves in an emergency department.

Retinoids

Retinoids are vitamin A derivatives that are used primarily for skin disease. Two oral retinoids are available in the United States. The first is isotretinoin (Accutane), approved by the FDA for the treatment of recalcitrant cystic acne. However, it is also useful for a number of other diseases including cutaneous lupus erythematosus, some forms of psoriasis, and many skin diseases characterized by heavy scale or abnormalities of maturation of the epithelial cells. Etretinate (Tegison) is a similar medication used primarily for pustular and erythrodermic psoriasis. Like isotretinoin, it is also used for a variety of other scaling diseases unresponsive to more standard therapy.

Both medications are potent teratogens and, because etretinate is stored in body fat for years, this medication can produce birth defects long after it is discontinued. Cutaneous dryness and chapped lips are regular side effects of these retinoids. Less common side effects include precipitation of eczema, peeling of palms and soles, arthralgias and myalgias, and hair loss. A sensation of sticky skin, as well as cutaneous fragility, are additional adverse reactions associated with etretinate. Both medications increase serum levels of triglyceride. This elevation is generally minor in patients with baseline normal studies, but remarkable elevation can occur in those with pre-existing hypertriglyceridemia or in those who drink significant amounts of alcohol. Mild abnormalities of liver function tests occur in many patients, and long-term therapy is associated with exostoses and calcifications of ligaments in some cases. Obviously, patients receiving oral retinoids should be followed by a clinician familiar with the adverse reactions and necessary laboratory and radiologic studies needed for follow-up.

Tretinoin is a topical retinoid. This medication is available in two primary forms, with the first and oldest being Retin-A, which is used for comedonal acne. The second is compounded in a less irritating base (Renova), and has received FDA approval for the treatment of actinically induced wrinkles. These medications are applied at night to dry skin and rinsed off the next morning. A high sun protection factor (SPF) sunscreen should be used every morning since protective layers of stratum corneum are removed by this medication. Topical retinoids are generally avoided during pregnancy for theoretical reasons, although systemic absorption from topical therapy is extremely small.

Cytotoxic and Immunosuppressive Agents

Cytotoxic agents are used for a variety of skin diseases for their antiproliferative, immunosuppressive, and sometimes anti-inflammatory effects.

Methotrexate Methotrexate is one of the most commonly used oral agents. This medication is extraordinarily useful for the treatment of all forms of severe psoriasis. The dose ranges from 2.5 to 25 mg weekly because daily administration is far too toxic. Methotrexate has also been found to produce beneficial effects in some patients with bullous pemphigoid, sarcoidosis, and some other inflammatory diseases unresponsive to more standard therapies. The primary toxicities include bone marrow suppression and hepatotoxicity.

Azathioprine and Cyclophosphamide Azathioprine (Imuran) and cyclophosphamide (Cytoxan) are immunosuppressive medications that are often used as steroid-sparing agents in patients with bullous pemphigoid and pemphigus vulgaris and in combination with other medications for patients with some severe recalcitrant inflammatory diseases, such as atopic dermatitis, cutaneous lupus erythematosus, and lichen planus. These medications exhibit bone marrow toxicity, and chronic use confers an increased risk for leukemia and lymphoma. Additional concerns for patients treated with cyclophosphamide include a possibility of hemorrhagic cystitis and a late increased risk of bladder fibrosis and cancer, as well as a risk of infertility in male patients.

Hydroxychloroquine and Chloroquine The antimalarial agents, hydroxychloroquine (Plaquenil) and chloroquine also exert immune-modulating effects. These medications are treatments of choice for cutaneous lupus erythematosus and they have been reported beneficial for some patients with cutaneous sarcoidosis and lichen planus. Hydroxychloroquine usually controls the skin findings of porphyria cutanea tarda when administered in the extremely low dose of 200 mg twice per week, with higher doses sometimes producing hepatic necrosis in these patients. Otherwise, the primary adverse reaction associated with this medication is retinal toxicity, so that twice yearly examinations by an ophthalmologist are standard.

Cyclosporine Cyclosporine (Sandimmune) is an immune suppressant medication that is used primarily to prevent rejection of transplanted organs. However, cyclosporine also exerts powerful antipsoriatic effects. The profound nephrotoxicity of this medication serves to relegate it to use only in patients with severe psoriasis unresponsive to other therapies. Cyclosporine has also been reported beneficial for pyoderma gangrenosum, lichen planus, and aphthous ulcers. Cyclosporine is sometimes effective when applied to mucosal surfaces. Therefore, both oral and parenteral forms of cyclosporine sometimes improve oral lichen planus and aphthae.

Please see patient information handouts for this chapter, on pages 357 and 368.

REFERENCES

1. Savin JA, Paterson WD, Adam K et al: Effects of trimeprazine and trimipramine on nocturnal scratching in patients with atopic eczema. Arch Dermatol 115:313, 1979
2. Reagan DR et al: Elimination of coincident *Staphylococcal aureus* nasal and hand carriage with intranasal application of mupirocin calcium ointment. Ann Intern Med 114:101, 1991
3. Gough A, Chapman S, Wagstaff K et al: Minocycline-induced autoimmune hepatitis and systemic lupus erythematosus-like syndrome. BMJ 312:169, 1996
4. Goulden V, Glass D, Cunliffe WJ: Safety of long-term high-dose minocycline in the treatment of acne. Br J Dermatol 134:693, 1996
5. Bergstresser PR, Elewski B, Hanifin J et al: Topical terbinafine and clotrimazole in interdigital tinea pedis: a multicenter comparison of cure and relapse rates with 1- and 4-week treatment regimens. J Am Acad Dermatol 28: 648, 1993
6. Ablon G, Rosen T, Spedale J: Comparative efficacy of naftifine, oxiconazole, and terbinafine in short-term treatment of tinea pedis. Int J Dermatol 35:591, 1996
7. Sherertz EF: Are laboratory studies necessary for griseofulvin therapy? J Am Acad Dermatol 22: 1103, 1990
8. von Moltke LL, Greenblatt DJ, Duan SX et al: Inhibition of terfenadine metabolism in vitro by azole antifungal agents and by selective serotonin reuptake inhibitor antidepressants: relation to pharmacokinetic interactions in vivo. J Clin Psychopharmacol 16:104, 1996
9. De Doncker P, Decroix J, Pierard GE et al: Antifungal pulse therapy for onychomycosis: A pharmacokinetic and pharmacodynamic investigation of monthly cycles of 1 week pulse therapy with itraconazole. Arch Dermatol 132: 34, 1996
10. Haroon TS, Hussain I, Mahmood A et al: An open clinical pilot study of the efficacy and safety of oral terbinafine in dry non-inflammatory tinea capitis. Br J Dermatol 26:956, 1992
11. Degreef H: Itraconazole in the treatment of tinea capitis. Cutis 58:90, 1996
12. Elewski BE, Weil ML: Dermatophytes and superficial fungi. p. 155. In Sams WM Jr, Lynch PJ (eds): Principles and Practice of Dermatology, 2nd Ed. Churchill Livingstone, New York, 1996
13. Shear NH, Villars V, Marsolais C: Terbinafine: an oral and topical antifungal agent. Clin Dermatol 9:487, 1991

14. Goldberg LH, Kaufman R, Kurtz TO et al: Long-term suppression of recurrent genital herpes with acyclovir: a five year benchmark. Arch Dermatol 129:582, 1993

15. Wald A et al: Suppression of subclinical shedding of herpes simplex virus type 2 with acyclovir. Ann Intern Med 124:8, 1996

16. Huff JC, Bean B, Balfour HH Jr et al: Therapy of herpes zoster with oral acyclovir. Am J Med, suppl 2A. 85:84, 1988

SUGGESTED READINGS

General

Franz TJ, Lehman PA, Franz S, Guin JD: Comparative percutaneous absorption of lidane and permethrin. Arch Dermatol 132:901, 1996

Knowles SR, Shapira L, Shear NH: Serious adverse reactions induced by minocycline: report of 13 patients and review of the literature. Arch Dermatol 132:934, 1996

Maddin S, McLean DI (eds): Dermatologic Therapy. Dermatol Clin 11:1, 1993

Antipruritic Therapy

Herman LE, Bernhard JD: Antihistamine update. Dermatol Clin 9:603, 1991

Corticosteroid Therapy

Barnetson RSC, White AD: The use of corticosteroids in dermatological practice. Med J Aust 156: 428, 1992

Giannotti B, Pimpinelli N: Topical corticosteroids. Which drug and when. Drugs 44:65, 1992

Antifungal Therapy

Gupta AK, Sauder DN, Shear NH: Antifungal agents: an overview. Part I. J Am Acad Dermatol 30:677, 1994

Gupta AK, Sauder DN, Shear NH: Antifungal agents: an overview. Part II. J Am Acad Dermatol 30:911, 1994

Other Medications

Ho VC, Zloty DM: Immunosuppressive agents in dermatology. Dermatol Clin 11:73, 1993

Shalita AR, Fritsch PO: Retinoids: present and future. J Am Acad Dermatol, suppl. 27:S1, 1992

Wolverton SE: Monitoring for adverse effects from systemic drugs used in dermatology. J Am Acad Dermatol 26:661, 1992

CHAPTER 4

Vesicular Diseases

Vesicular diseases include those skin conditions characterized by the presence of small blisters, or vesicles. Because bullae, or large blisters, may begin as vesicles, occasionally bullous diseases should be considered in the differential diagnosis of vesicular diseases.

Diseases characterized by vesicles comprise a very heterogeneous group, including infectious diseases such as herpes simplex virus (HSV) infection, immune diseases such as acute allergic contact dermatitis, and physical injury such as thermal burns. These diseases can usually be distinguished on the basis of morphology, setting, body location, and, sometimes, culture. Occasionally, a biopsy is required, and the clinician should review the section in Chapter 2 pertaining to biopsy procedures, with special attention to suggestions that refer to the biopsy of blisters.

HERPES SIMPLEX VIRUS INFECTION

HSV infection is a well-known, extremely common viral skin infection. More than 85% of adults exhibit antibodies to the HSV, demonstrating the high prevalence of this infection in spite of a much lower rate of clinical infection.[1] Although HSV infection classically occurs over genitalia or on the lips, this infection can occur anywhere on the skin surface. Two types of HSV have been identified, with HSV type 1 (HSV-1) showing a predilection for the lip, and type 2 (HSV-2) for the genitalia. In general, clinicians have a very low index of suspicion for HSV infection when lesions occur elsewhere, even when the morphology is typical.

Clinical Manifestations

The symptoms and morphology of HSV infection vary according to the stage of the infection (i.e., primary versus recurrent) and the location. A primary HSV infection occurs within 3 to 14 days after exposure to the virus. The virus must be introduced into the deeper layers of the epidermis. For infection to occur, either the exposed skin must be broken, or a fragile, nonkeratinized surface such as genital epithelium must be inoculated in association with friction, as occurs during intercourse. Often, the primary infection is subclinical. When apparent, a primary infection consists of painful, multiple, scattered, discrete vesicles, with erosions occurring at the general site of inoculation. The clustering of vesicles or erosions so characteristic of a recurrent infection is absent. Because the vesicles are very superficial and fragile, crusts and erosions often outnumber the intact blisters (Figs. 4.1 and 4.2). When a primary HSV infection affects the genitalia, the vagina and cervix are often involved, producing a purulent vaginal discharge. Occasionally, pain can be so intense as to produce urinary retention. Primary HSV infection of the mouth, herpes stomatitis, is seen almost exclusively in children. Not only is the lip involved, but the oral mucosa and keratinized skin of the face surrounding the lips exhibit lesions as well (Fig. 4.3). Erosions, rather than intact vesicles, are seen on fragile moist mucous membranes such as the oral mucosa or vaginal introitus. Herpes stomatitis is characterized by 1- to 2-mm round erosions located over all mucous membrane areas, including the gingiva and hard palate.

Other physical findings and symptoms associated with a primary HSV infection include local

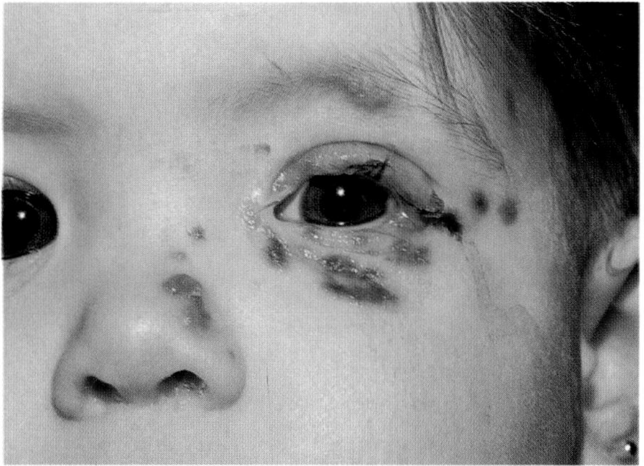

Figure 4.1 Although crusting is the most obvious finding in this child, who was initially diagnosed with impetigo, vesicles in the eyebrow are typical for HSV infection.

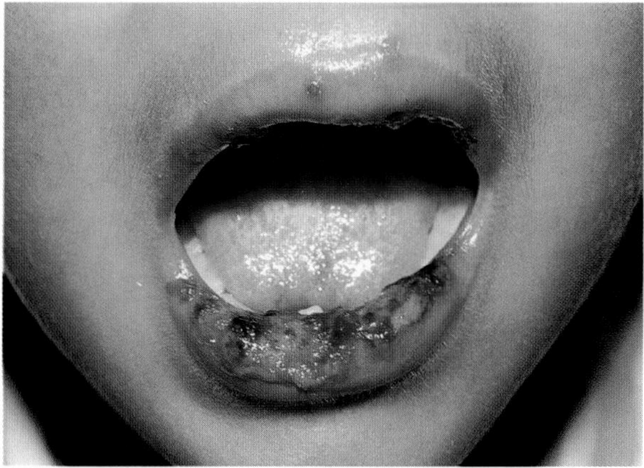

Figure 4.3 Herpes gingivostomatitis: a primary HSV infection of the mouth produces vesicles, erosions, and crusts over all areas of the oral mucosa, as well as on the outside of the lips and surrounding skin of the face.

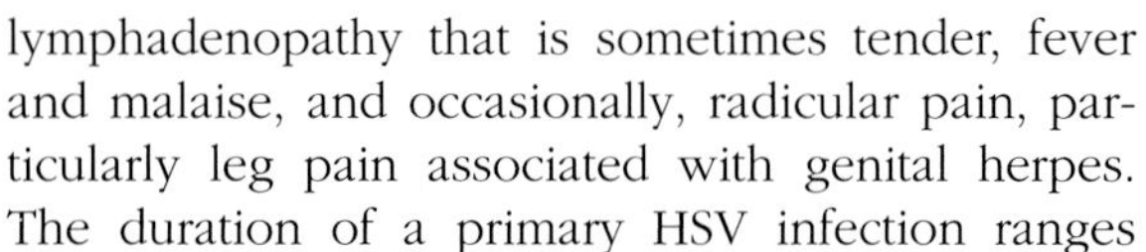

lymphadenopathy that is sometimes tender, fever and malaise, and occasionally, radicular pain, particularly leg pain associated with genital herpes. The duration of a primary HSV infection ranges from 1 to 3 weeks if untreated. Genital lesions require longer than orofacial lesions for healing.

Figure 4.2 Primary HSV infection: because the vulvar epithelium is very fragile, these vesicles rapidly disintegrated to form punched-out erosions that are scattered, rather than grouped.

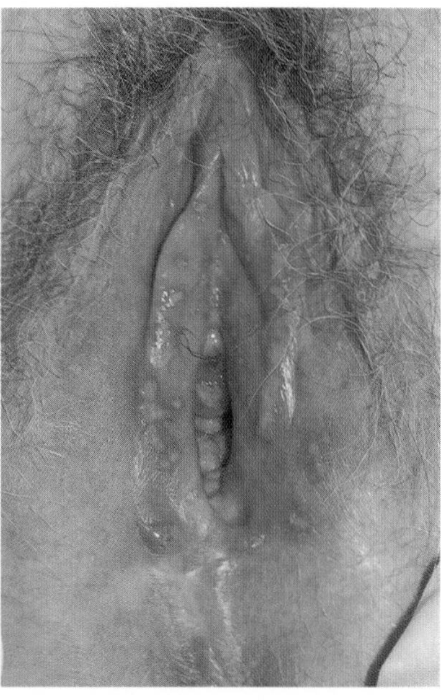

After a first episode of HSV infection, almost all patients experience recurrent episodes.[2] Often, patients—especially those with labial HSV infection—do not recognize their primary HSV infection, either because the outbreak was mild or because they experienced a truly subclinical infection. Thus, the first episode of recognized infection often presents with the clinical features of a recurrent episode. Recurrent HSV infection is characterized by grouped, coalescing vesicles on a pink base. Any blister can become cloudy after several days, so pustules are sometimes present without signifying secondary infection (Fig. 4.4). The affected area is usually, but not always, painful. On fragile skin, such as a lip, or the poorly keratinized skin of the vulva and uncircumcised glans penis, intact vesicles are generally not appreciated, while punched-out coalescing erosions are characteristic. Yellow crusting can occur, particularly on the face, raising concern for secondary impetiginization (Fig. 4.1). Occasionally, recurrent genital HSV infection presents as fissures, or linear erosions, requiring a high index of suspicion to make the correct diagnosis. In some areas, particularly the buttocks, recurrent HSV infection can be pruritic, and subsequent scratching can produce eczematous plaques that obscure the underlying vesicular

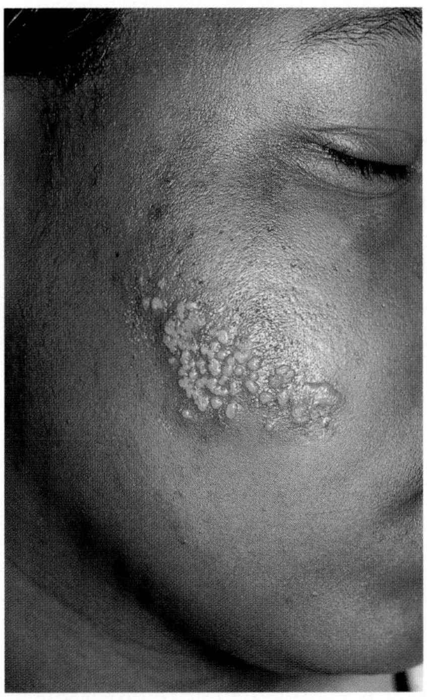

Figure 4.4 Recurrent HSV infection is characterized by grouped vesicles, pustules, or erosions on a red plaque.

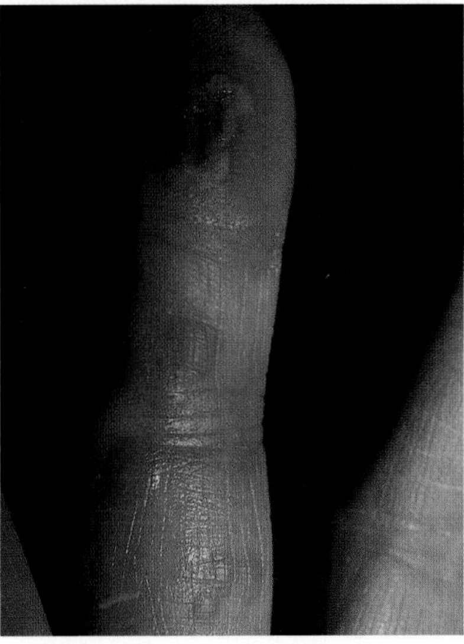

Figure 4.5 Herpetic whitlow. Recurrent HSV infection of the fingertip produces deep vesicles and pustules and often exhibits surrounding erythema and edema suggestive of a bacterial paronychia.

morphology of the disease. Scattered, poorly demarcated, hyperpigmented patches that represent postinflammatory hyperpigmentation from prior outbreaks are a subtle clue to this diagnosis.

Another area occasionally affected is the fingertip, where the infection is referred to as a herpetic whitlow (Fig. 4.5). The fingertip may be red and indurated, sometimes with deep vesicles or pustules. Not surprisingly, this condition is often misdiagnosed as a bacterial infection. Any area on the skin surface can be affected by HSV, and this infection should be considered whenever grouped vesicles, pustules, or punched-out erosions occur.

Constitutional symptoms, local lymphadenopathy, and pain are generally absent or much less marked with recurrent HSV infection than with primary infection. However, radicular pain may continue to accompany outbreaks, and local tingling, itching, or burning often precede recurrences.

The clinical appearance of HSV infection can be atypical in several situations. First, patients who are immunosuppressed do not contain their infection, so that it becomes ongoing, chronic, and ulcerative, rather than erosive. Ulcerative HSV infection is discussed further in Chapter 20, which addresses the immunosuppressed patient. Second, patients with pre-existing skin disease (classically, eczema) sometimes spread HSV infection evenly over the surface of the skin, a condition called *eczema herpeticum*, or Kaposi's varicelliform eruption. For example, a patient with HSV infection on the lip inoculates the virus into all the fissures and eroded areas of the skin, producing scattered monomorphous vesicles and punched-out erosions (Fig. 4.6). Third, the virus can be spread over the surface of the skin by trauma, as when HSV from a herpetic lip lesion is spread and inoculated into hair follicles by a razor as a result of shaving, producing *sycosis barbae* (Fig. 4.7). Again, circular erosions and follicular vesicles are scattered over the area, becoming reservoirs for the viral infection, which continues daily to be spread to other follicles.

Left untreated, recurrent HSV infection generally will resolve within 7 to 10 days, with longer resolution over the genitalia, where heat and dampness prolong the course as compared to the lip. The frequency of recurrences varies from fewer than once each year to twice a month.

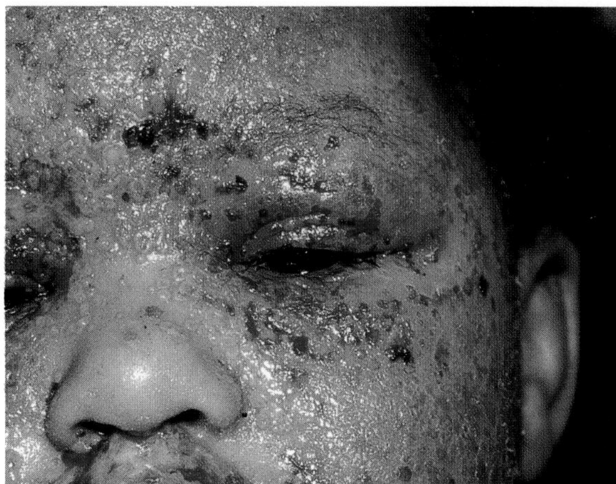

Figure 4.6 Eczema herpticum. Patients with eczema sometimes widely inoculate HSV within their inflamed, scaling skin to produce confluent blisters and coalescing, punched-out erosions.

Differential Diagnosis

The intraoral lesions of a primary oral HSV infection (herpes stomatitis) are sometimes confused with aphthous stomatitis. However, aphthous ulcers occur only within the mouth, sparing the external surface of the lips, the face, and also sparing mucous membranes over bone such as the gingivae and hard palate. HSV infection does not produce intraoral lesions, except during a first episode outbreak. Another cause of oral erosions that can sometimes be confused with HSV infection is hand, foot, and mouth disease, also a viral syndrome. Hand, foot, and mouth disease produces less pain and many fewer lesions and is confined to the mucous membrane of the mouth, rather than to the lips and face. In addition, associated vesicles usually appear on the hands and feet (see also Ch. 19).

Figure 4.7 Sycosis barbae. Herpes labialis can be spread to other areas of the face by shaving, where the razor spreads the virus to each hair follicle.

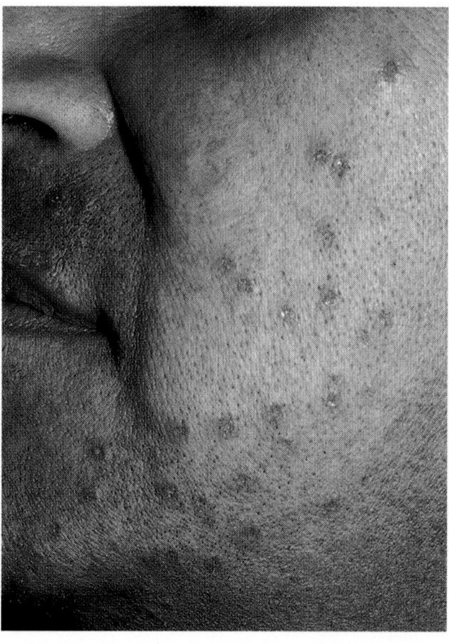

The erosions of typical genital HSV infection are usually too superficial and small to be confused with a syphilitic chancre or the lesions of chancroid or granuloma inguinale, although HSV in an immunosuppressed patient can be ulcerative (see Ch. 20). Occasionally, genital HSV infection can be confused with a *Candida* infection, another superficial blistering disease. These two diseases can generally be differentiated by their clinical presentations, although occasionally a culture or a microscopic smear (fungal preparation or Tzanck preparation) may be required.

Recurrent HSV infections over other areas of the body are most often confused with herpes zoster infections. However, herpes zoster infection is usually in a dermatomal distribution, most often in an older patient, and the individual vesicles tend to be larger and more coalescent, often containing hemorrhagic fluid. In addition, patients with HSV infection often have a prior history of similar lesions, whereas herpes zoster occurs only once. Neither a Tzanck smear nor a biopsy differentiates between herpes simplex and herpes zoster infection.

Yellow crusting that can sometimes occur after the rupture of vesicles can be confused with impetigo. Occasionally, bacterial superinfection does occur during or after an HSV infection, particularly around the mouth and nose (Fig. 4.1).

A firm diagnosis of HSV infection can usually be made on clinical grounds. However, when HSV occurs in the genital area, the psychological impact can be so great that laboratory confirmation is often beneficial. In the face of positive laboratory findings, the patient can have no lingering doubt, and future clinicians cannot question the diagnosis. Unfortunately, HSV cultures frequently exhibit false-negative findings, even when the base of a fresh blister is sampled. In addition, varying laboratory techniques and the all-too-common delay in handling of specimens produces false-negative results in many cases. Therefore, a negative culture should not dissuade the examiner from a diagnosis of HSV infection if he or she feels very strongly that this diagnosis is correct. Still, in most cases, a culture for HSV infection is adequate and accurate, as long as the specimen is transported immediately to the laboratory, and a positive culture confirms the clinical diagnosis

A biopsy of a vesicle is very sensitive and specific for herpesvirus, but it does not distinguish between changes from the HSV and the varicella-zoster virus (VZV). A Tzanck preparation is useful in experienced hands but is less definitive than a culture or biopsy; also, it does not differentiate between an HSV and a VZV infection.

Serologic testing for HSV antibodies generally is not helpful. Most adults exhibit antibodies to HSV, whether or not they have experienced clinical outbreaks.[1] Although negative serology can at times be useful, a HSV culture, a positive Tzanck smear, a biopsy, or the increasingly available and exquisitely sensitive polymerase chain reaction (PCR) technique for identifying HSV infections are much more reliable and direct.

Management

The only specific antiviral therapy with clinically significant benefits is oral therapy. Topical acyclovir (Zovirax) produces clinically insignificant shortening of the course of the primary HSV infection. However, oral acyclovir, when begun early in the course of either primary or recurrent HSV infection at a dose of 200 mg 5 times a day, significantly shortens or ameliorates the outbreak. Although moderately expensive, side effects are almost nonexistent; in the near future, when this medication becomes available in generic form, the cost should decrease. The medication is generally continued until significant healing has begun, usually about 10 days in primary disease.

More recently, other antiviral agents have become available. Absorption is better with these newer medications, so that less frequent dosing and lower total doses are required, and the cost at this time is comparable. There is no added benefit for the average case of HSV infection, other than a less frequent dosing schedule, making the choice of therapy a matter of personal preference. Choices include famciclovir (Famvir) 125 mg bid for 10 days, or valacyclovir (Valtrex) 500 mg tid for the same duration.

In some patients, supportive care is important. Because a primary HSV infection is often extremely painful, pain control is a major consideration. The pain associated with herpes stomatitis often prevents adequate oral intake. However, systemic analgesia and cold, soothing liquids sometimes obviate the need for intravenous fluids. A topical anesthetic such as diphenhydramine (Benadryl) solution on the oral mucosa can provide some numbing effect, but the initial burning and stinging limit the usefulness of this option.

When occurring in the genital area, pain and edema can produce dysuria, and even urinary retention, especially in women. For those women experiencing extreme dysuria, oral analgesia and urinating while in a sitz bath sometimes produce less burning and can help prevent the need for an indwelling catheter. Cool soaks, compresses, and ice packs can also help alleviate pain. A purulent vaginal discharge often accompanies primary HSV infection; bacterial superinfection is an occasional complication.

Most patients with recurrent HSV infection have short-lived, minimally uncomfortable, outbreaks. However, for the patient who has severe recurrences, or who is bothered psychologically, oral acyclovir at 200 mg 5 times a day begun at the very first sign of an outbreak can significantly ameliorate, and sometimes even abort, recurrent outbreaks. Equally effective are famciclovir 125 mg bid for 5 days[3] and valacyclovir 500 mg tid for the same duration.

Patients plagued with very frequently recurrent HSV infections can be treated safely with long-term suppressant therapy.[4] Acyclovir at a dose of 400 mg bid prevents recurrences in the vast majority of people. Oral acyclovir in these doses is almost entirely without side effects, although the very rare patient experiences some nausea.

An extremely important element in therapy for HSV infection is patient education. For many patients, a diagnosis of HSV infection is a traumatic event. The clinician should have a nonjudgmental, sympathetic attitude. Sometimes, explaining to the patient with a genital HSV infection that this is the same condition as a fever blister, only in a different location, helps a patient feel less stigmatized. However, the examiner should also make the patient fully aware of the infectious nature of HSV infection. The patient with HSV infection of the lip should be advised not to kiss other people and not to share drinking glasses during an outbreak. Patients with genital HSV infection should be cautioned to avoid sexual contact during an outbreak. Some clinicians believe that condoms should be used at all times because of the frequency of asymptomatic viral shedding. Recent evidence confirms the logical assumption that oral acyclovir decreases asymptomatic shedding, revealing a 94% decrease for the number of women shedding when taking acyclovir 400 mg bid.[5]

Women should be advised to report the diagnosis of genital HSV infection to their gynecologists, as a pregnant woman can transmit an HSV infection to her newborn, if the baby is born through the birth canal during an active infection. Nearly always, neonatal HSV infection occurs when the genitalia are affected by a primary outbreak, rather than a recurrence. Also, almost all episodes of neonatal HSV infections are due to HSV-2.

Course and Prognosis

Most patients with HSV infection experience recurrences, with three to four episodes per year the average for those with genital infection.[6] However, this experience ranges from the rare patient with no apparent recurrences to unfortunate individuals with outbreaks once or twice a month. Recurrences generally become less frequent with time.

PRIMARY HERPES SIMPLEX VIRUS INFECTION

Clinical Manifestations

Painful scattered vesicles, pustules, and/or erosions—most often located over the genitalia or around the lips and mouth.

Management in the Emergency Department

1. *Pain control, with narcotic analgesics often required*

(Continues)

(Continued)

2. *Local, supportive care*
   - *Cool tap water soaks for the genitalia*
   - *Cold bland liquids and ice for the mouth*
3. *Acyclovir 5 mg/kg up to 200 mg PO 5 times per day (or famciclovir, valacyclovir) for 10 days*
4. *Patient education (see the patient handouts on p. 343, Fever Blisters and pp. 345-347, Genital Herpes Simplex Virus Infection)*

RECURRENT HERPES SIMPLEX VIRUS INFECTION

Clinical Manifestations

Painful grouped vesicles, pustules, and/or erosions on a pink base.

Management in the Emergency Department

1. *Pain control: cool soaks and acetaminophen or nonsteroidal anti-inflammatory drugs (NSAIDs) usually adequate*
2. *Early, significant disease (first 48 hours): acyclovir 200 mg 5 times per day for 5 days*
3. *Frequently recurrent or severe recurrences: acyclovir 400 mg bid chronically*
4. *Patient education (see patient handouts on p. 343, Fever Blisters and pp. 345-347, Genital Herpes Simplex Virus Infection)*

HERPES ZOSTER INFECTION (SHINGLES)

Herpes zoster is a painful, localized, blistering eruption that represents reactivation of latent varicella zoster virus.

Clinical Manifestations

Although most common in older patients, herpes zoster can occur at any age in a patient with prior varicella infection. Typically, skin lesions are preceded by pain in the affected area. This varies from mild irritation or itching to severe pain. The first visible lesions are red, nonscaling, edematous papules and plaques in a dermatomal distribution. Clustered vesicles form on these plaques and coalesce into slightly larger blisters, until there are scattered plaques of grouped vesicles along the dermatome (Fig. 4.8). Lesions occur in one dermatome and adjacent skin, not crossing the midline. Sometimes, hemorrhage into the vesicles colors the lesions red, purple, or gray. The most common area of involvement is the torso, with the scalp and upper face another common site, although any area of the skin can be affected. When the face is involved, blisters and erosions sometimes occur in the mouth or, particularly if the tip of the nose is involved, in the eye, where scarring can permanently impair vision. In the healing phase, blisters rupture, leaving round or arcuate erosions and crusts.

A diagnosis of herpes zoster can easily be missed in several situations. First, many clinicians do not consider the diagnosis if lesions are not in a classic distribution, such as the face or trunk (Fig. 4.9). Also, herpes zoster can present as pain unaccompanied by typical lesions, most often early in the disease (Fig. 4.10).

Figure 4.8 Herpes zoster, or shingles, is characterized by multiple red plaques in a dermatomal distribution, covered by vesicles. Some of the blisters exhibit a gray color, produced by hemorrhage into the blisters.

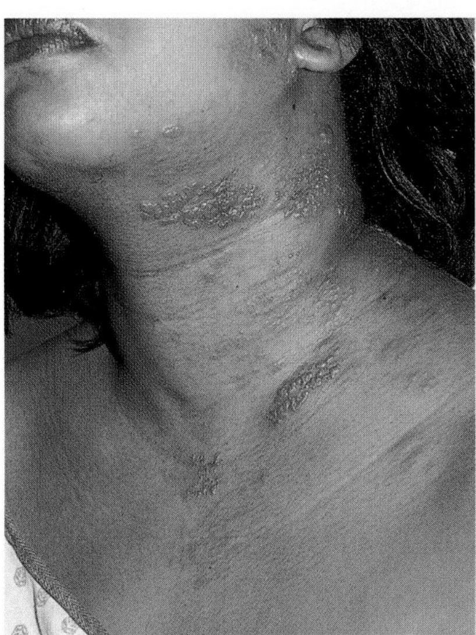

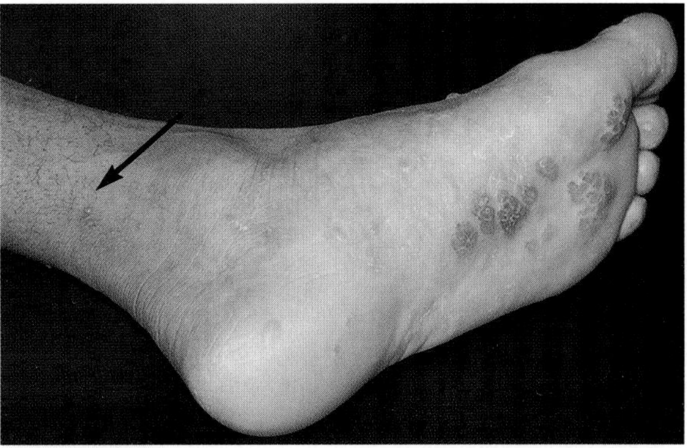

Figure 4.9 A diagnosis of herpes zoster is easy to miss in a patient such as this, in whom an unusual dermatome is involved. Note the vesicles over the ankle (arrow).

Finally, herpes zoster in immunosuppressed patients may be widespread, confluent, or ulcerative (see also Ch. 20). The most well-known variation is disseminated herpes zoster. In this case, typical dermatomal herpes zoster lesions, which may be particularly severe or numerous, are accompanied by nongrouped generalized vesicles that resemble chickenpox (Fig. 4.11). Occasionally, although the herpes zoster infection remains localized to the dermatome, the patient's inadequate immune system is unable to contain the virus locally. The sharply demarcated, circular, or arcuate erosions become chronic, punched-out ulcers.

Figure 4.10 Early herpes zoster is sometimes manifested only by severe pain within a dermatome, with or without associated erythema. Usually, blisters occur in a day or two. This patient exhibited intact vesicles over the right hard palate at presentation.

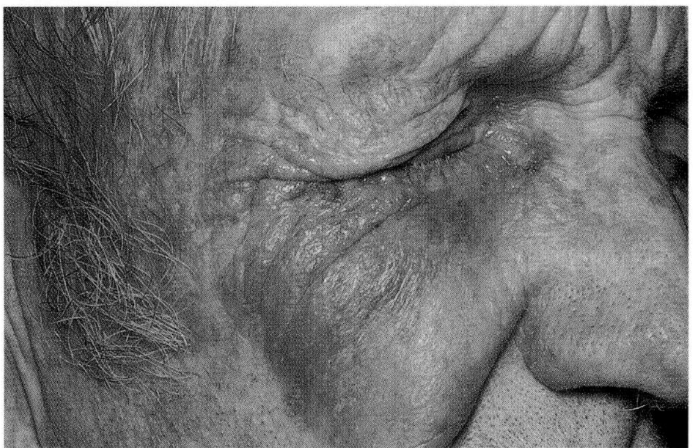

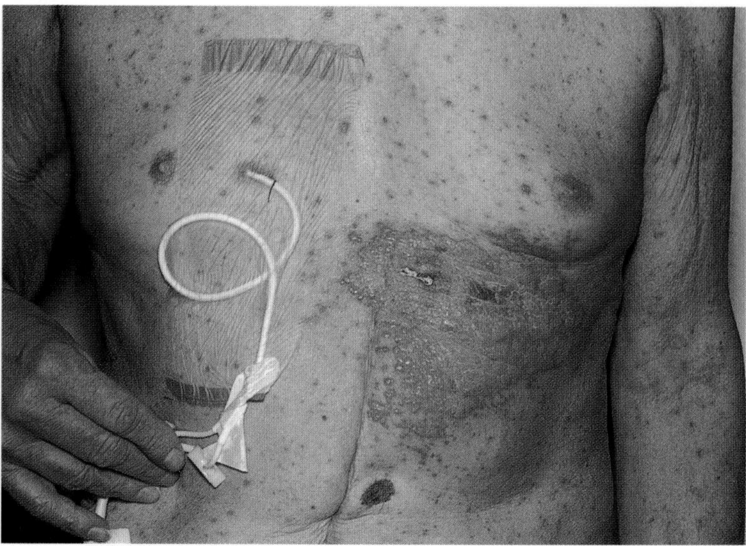

Figure 4.11 Disseminated herpes zoster is a sign of immunosuppression, characterized by typical—or unusually severe—herpes zoster in association with scattered lesions that resemble varicella.

Immunosuppressed patients also can develop confluent plaques of blisters, or even coalescent blisters, leading to large denuded areas. At other times, particularly in patients with the acquired immunodeficiency syndrome (AIDS), the affected area becomes hyperkeratotic and individual lesions are less sharply circumscribed, so that the underlying blistering nature may not be appreciated.

Differential Diagnosis

Although the presentation of clustered vesicles in a dermatomal distribution and the associated pain usually make the diagnosis of herpes zoster obvious, sometimes an atypical location or a lack of pain can be confusing.

The most common disease confused with herpes zoster is HSV infection, as both diseases present with grouped vesicles on an inflammatory base, and both diseases are generally painful. However, patients with herpes zoster tend to be older, and the vesicles are usually larger, more coalescent, and often discolored due to hemorrhage. Although the dermatomal distribution of herpes zoster is generally helpful in making the diagnosis, HSV infections occasionally occur in a dermatome as well. These diseases can be differentiated by a history of recurrence (i.e., only HSV infection recurs), by culture, or by PCR technique. A Tzanck preparation and a skin biopsy, although sensitive evidence for the presence of herpesvirus, do not differentiate between VZV and HSV.

In some locations, such as a foot or leg, the dermatomal distribution is less obvious. In these cases, other blistering diseases, such as bullous pemphigoid, bullous impetigo, vesicular tinea, and trauma, may need to be considered and distinguished by other clinical findings or laboratory tests.

Management

The key aspect in the treatment of herpes zoster in an immunocompetent patient is pain control. For those in significant pain, narcotic analgesia, sometimes for several weeks, is indicated. Topical therapies, including nonspecific measures such as soaks, topical capsaicin (Zostrix), and topical acyclovir (Zovirax) are not indicated for use in patients with active blistering. At best these are not useful, and at worst they are additionally painful.

Acyclovir, famciclovir (Famvir), and valacyclovir (Valtrex) have all been shown to shorten the course of herpes zoster when given within the first 72 hours, and preferably 48 hours, from onset of the rash. However, the decreased duration of pain, viral shedding, and time to crusting are minor, within the range of 1 to 2 days.[7] Although these medications have excellent safety profiles, they are expensive. Because the VZV is less sensitive to these medications than is the HSV, higher doses are required. Acyclovir is given at a dose of 800 mg PO 5 times a day, until healing is well under way, usually 7 to 10 days. Immunosuppressed patients who are ill or who have very severe disease should receive intravenous acyclovir at a dose of 10 mg/kg q8h. This medication should be administered slowly because of the risk of crystallization in the kidneys. Famciclovir and valacyclovir are much better absorbed than acyclovir and, once absorbed, these agents are converted to acyclovir. Valacyclovir is effective at 1,000 mg (two 500-mg caplets) PO tid for 1 week, and famciclovir is given at 500 mg q8h. The main advantage of these medications is the reduced dosing schedule.

Despite the modest effect of oral antiviral agents on the duration of herpes zoster, an important reason for treating patients with acute herpes zoster is the prevention of postherpetic neuralgia.[8–11] Studies have shown a variable effect of the early administration of oral antiviral agents in the prevention of postherpetic neuralgia. Therapy with oral antiviral medications is most clearly indicated in older patients, who are at greatest risk of the development of postherpetic neuralgia, when they present within the first 72 hours. A study that examined the effect of famciclovir on the prevention of postherpetic neuralgia demonstrated no decrease in incidence, but the duration of pain was shortened in patients experiencing chronic pain.[12]

In the past, oral corticosteroids were recommended as effective for the prevention of postherpetic neuralgia. More recent studies have not confirmed this effect, and this medication is no longer indicated for this purpose.[13]

More important than the administration of specific antiviral therapy for acute herpes zoster is the sympathetic and careful management of acute pain and postherpetic neuralgia. When it becomes clear that significant pain of herpes zoster is not resolving as lesions heal, patients should be begun on nighttime tricyclic antidepressants such as amitriptyline or desipramine. Starting at extremely low doses, such as 10 mg, and increasing to as much as 75 mg, will achieve pain control in most patients. Side effects include dryness of the mouth and occasional urinary retention, as occurs with all antihistamines. Drowsiness and occasional palpitations, particularly in patients with pre-existing heart disease, can occur. After the skin has completely healed, topical capsaicin (Zostrix) can produce a significant improvement in the pain associated with postherpetic neuralgia. Because capsaicin is the agent in red pepper that causes burning, it is crucial that this medication not be used on inflamed or eroded skin. Capsaicin is available as a 1% or 5% cream, and it should be applied 3 to 4 times a day. This agent produces its effect by depleting substance P, rather than by a direct analgesic effect on the skin. Patient education and reassurance that postherpetic neuralgia is self-limited are also very beneficial.

Course and Prognosis

The severity and duration of herpes zoster are extremely variable. Some patients develop only a few lesions and others may have nearly confluent blisters. Some have excruciating pain, while others have almost none, and the severity of the pain does not necessarily correlate with the extent or severity of disease. The time from the appearance of the first lesion to healing averages about 3 weeks. However, immunocompromised patients may develop ongoing disease with chronic ulcerations or hyperkeratotic papules and plaques.

Although pain usually abates as lesions begin to heal, occasionally pain continues long after the skin regains its normal appearance. This postherpetic neuralgia is most common in patients over 60 years of age. A recent study that evaluated the risk of postherpetic neuralgia in patients treated with famciclovir, as compared to those treated with placebo, showed no difference in prevalence between these two groups but demonstrated that most postherpetic neuralgia resolves by about 6 months.[12]

Although disseminated herpes zoster was once considered a life-threatening condition, it is now clear that disseminated herpes zoster itself usually does not produce significant systemic disease or death. However, any patient so immunosuppressed as to develop disseminated disease has serious underlying debilitating disease. These patients generally have a poor prognosis due to their underlying disease.

HERPES ZOSTER INFECTION

Clinical Manifestations

Painful grouped vesicles on an inflammatory base in a dermatomal distribution.

Management in the Emergency Department

1. *Pain control, often requiring narcotic analgesics*
2. *Consider oral acyclovir 800 mg 5 times a day if the patient is seen within the first 3 days of illness (famciclovir 500 mg tid and valacyclovir, two 500-mg caplets tid, are alternative therapies).*
3. *Ophthalmic examination in setting of nasal tip lesions*
4. *Consider immunosuppression in young patients, those with atypical lesions, and those with risk factors for AIDS*
5. *Patient education (see the patient handout on p. 349, Herpes Zoster Infection [Shingles])*

POSTHERPETIC NEURALGIA

Clinical Manifestations

Ongoing localized pain following resolution of herpes zoster infection.

Management in the Emergency Department

1. *Short-term narcotic analgesia*
2. *Tricyclic antidepressant medication for neuropathic pain; amitriptyline or desipramine, starting at 10 mg PO at bedtime, increasing until pain is controlled, up to about 75 mg*
3. *Topical capsaicin (Zostrix or Zostrix HP) cream applied to painful healed areas 3 to 4 times a day*
4. *Follow-up evaluation with primary care practitioner or dermatologist in 2 weeks*

VARICELLA

Varicella, or chickenpox, is an extremely contagious viral disease that occurs most often in children. Produced by the varicella zoster-virus (VZV), this disease is most common in the winter and spring.

Clinical Manifestations

Varicella occurring in older children is preceded by fever, malaise, aches, and sometimes cough. Younger children often experience no prodrome, but only malaise and slight fever with the rash.

The skin lesions are usually pruritic, appearing initially as pink, dome-shaped, nonscaling, scattered papules that are indistinguishable from insect bites. Sometimes, these initial lesions are concentrated in a sun-exposed distribution or in areas of inflammation or irritation such as eczema. Very quickly, a small, superficial, clear vesicle appears on the papule; as the vesicle ages, a central crust develops in the middle of the vesicle, generally leaving a peripheral rim of intact blister (Fig. 4.12). Older vesicles become pustular, and eventually a crust covers the entire area of the vesicle before healing occurs. Classically, new lesions continue to appear and evolve, so that lesions in all phases of blistering and crusting are apparent (Fig. 4.13).

Lesions can occur anywhere, but they are usually most concentrated on the trunk and face. The scalp and genital areas are usually prominently involved as well. The oral mucosa and conjunctiva are sometimes affected; lesions in these areas appear erosive, rather than blistering, because of the fragile nature of the epithelium.

Differential Diagnosis

Typical vesicular varicella, with lesions in all phases of blistering and crusting, is generally an obvious diagnosis. However, early papular disease often resembles insect bites. Insect bites can usually be ruled out because bites are rare on scalp and genital areas, and bites do not occur on mucous membranes. Bacterial or irritant folliculitis can sometimes resemble varicella, but the eruption is more chronic and lesions are pustular with no vesicles. A Gram stain of bacterial folliculitis shows gram-positive cocci and white blood cells. Although several other somewhat esoteric diseases can resemble varicella, none is dangerous and none is acute or associated with constitutional symptoms.

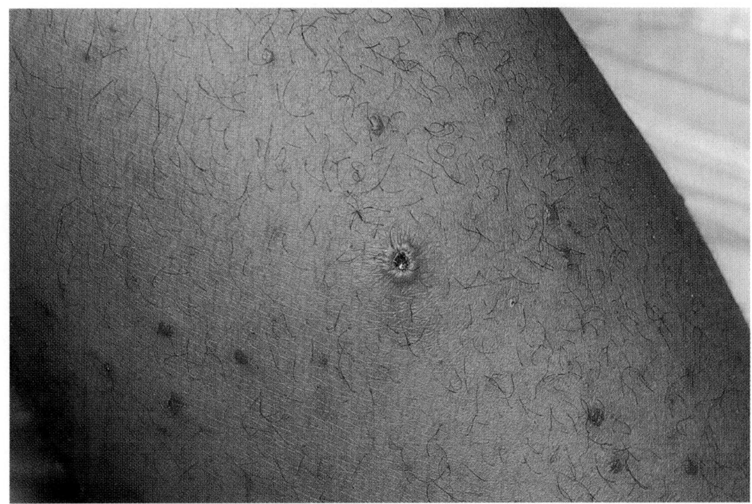

Figure 4.12 Blisters caused by any herpesvirus, including varicella zoster virus, are characteristic, with a central crust and an annular blister as the lesion evolves.

When the diagnosis is unclear but rapid identification is important, a skin biopsy submitted for rush processing as a frozen section or a Tzanck preparation (which is less specific) yields the results typical for herpesvirus. These do not differentiate varicella from HSV infection or herpes zoster. A culture is more specific, but results are delayed and false-negative results can occur.

Management

For most children with varicella, the mainstays of therapy are symptomatic treatment of constitutional symptoms, control of pruritus, and treatment of any secondary bacterial skin infection. Unfortunately, no good medications specific for itching are

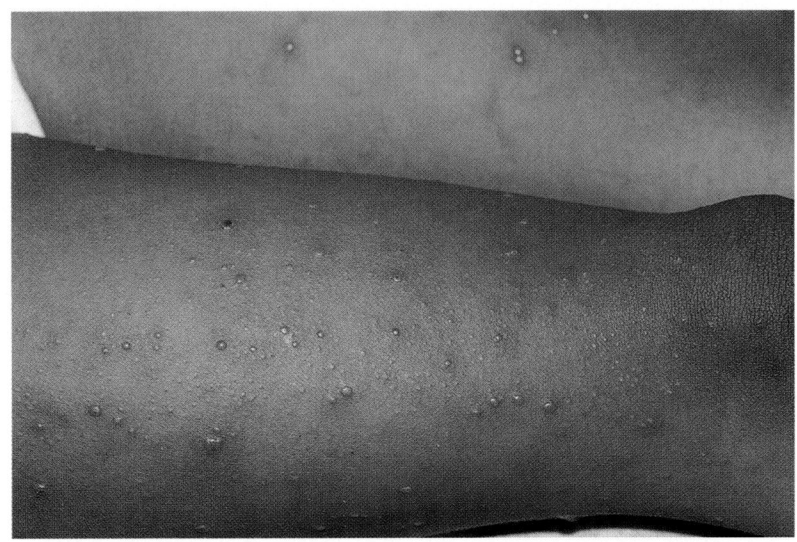

Figure 4.13 Varicella typically exhibits vesicles in all stages of development from tiny edematous papules, to clear vesicles, to crusts.

available. However, sedating doses of diphenhydramine or hydroxyzine HCl allow patients and their parents to sleep at night. Cool baths, especially with colloidal oatmeal (Aveeno) can be soothing and alleviate itching somewhat. Although calamine lotion can help itching briefly by cooling the skin, this very drying preparation should be avoided, as it can ultimately increase itching by producing xerosis. Topical corticosteroids are of no significant benefit for itching in this condition.

If lesions are unusually red or crusted and there is concern about secondary infection, an oral antistaphylococcal agent such as cephalexin (Keflex), dicloxacillin, or erythromycin is indicated. Secondary infection and scratching are the primary causes of scarring from the blisters of varicella.

If begun during the first 24 hours, oral acyclovir at a dose of 20 mg/kg/dose up to 800 mg 5 times a day reduces the severity of the disease and decreases the duration without apparently affecting the development of long-term immunity.[14] This approach is particularly helpful in siblings, as close contact with the index case can produce more severe disease. Because parents are on the alert for the first signs of disease in subsequent children, treatment can be started early enough to make a clinically significant difference. Immunosuppressed patients with varicella should uniformly be treated with acyclovir; usually, these patients require hospital admission for intravenous administration.

Because varicella is more severe and associated with more complications in adults, these patients should also be treated with acyclovir. If ill, adults should also be admitted for intravenous therapy.

Course and Prognosis

The lesions and symptoms of varicella begin about 2 weeks after exposure. The disease can be very mild with few lesions and minimal constitutional symptoms, or much more severe with extreme itching, large numbers of lesions, and significant systemic disease. Rare, but sometimes devastating, complications include varicella encephalitis and pneumonia.

New lesions continue to appear for 3 to 6 days, with crusting of all lesions taking place soon afterward. Children are typically isolated until all lesions are crusted, when they are then believed to no longer be contagious. However, chickenpox is a respiratory-borne disease and infectivity is at its highest 1 to 2 days before the skin lesions appear, until new vesicle formation ceases, when many believe they are no longer infectious.

VARICELLA

Clinical Manifestations

Scattered vesicles, pustules, and crusts in all stages of evolution and usually accompanied by symptoms of an upper respiratory tract infection.

Management in the Emergency Department

1. *Nighttime sedation for control of itching*
2. *Oral cephalexin, dicloxacillin, or erythromycin for those patients displaying signs of secondary bacterial infection*
3. *Specific antiviral medication:*
   - *Consider oral acyclovir at 20 mg/kg up to 800 mg 5 times a day if the child is seen within the first 24 hours*
   - *Systemic acyclovir at above doses should be given especially to adults and to immunosuppressed patients with varicella; hospital admission for intravenous administration if these patients appear ill*
4. *Patient education (see patient handout on p. 370, Varicella [Chicken Pox])*

HAND, FOOT, AND MOUTH DISEASE

Hand, foot, and mouth disease is a vesicular viral disease common during childhood. It is most often caused by coxsackievirus A16 or enterovirus 71, although other coxsackie viruses can also produce this condition. Therefore, hand, foot, and mouth disease can occur more than once in the same patient.

Clinical Manifestations

Hand, foot, and mouth disease is often preceded by mild constitutional symptoms, such as fever, malaise, and a sore mouth. Soon afterward, oral lesions appear. Because of the fragility of mucous

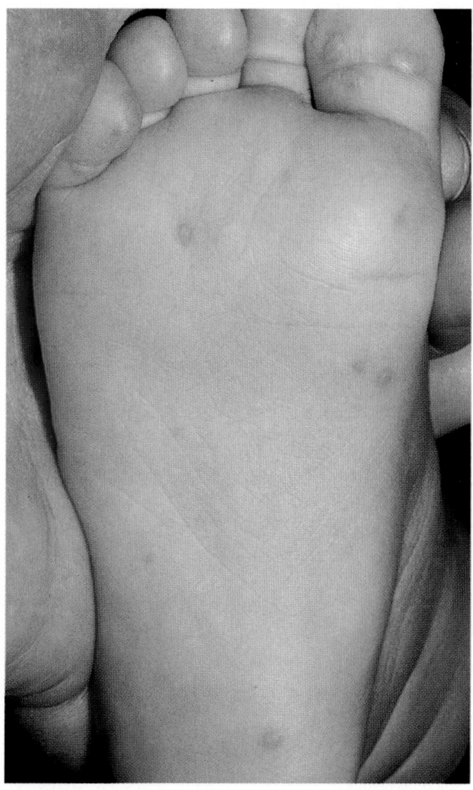

Figure 4.14 Hand, foot, and mouth disease is characterized by oval vesicles, some lying within creases, as seen on the great toe.

membranes, oral vesicles rupture quickly, leaving small, round erosions. Lesions can occur anywhere over the oral mucosa, but the mucosa not overlying bone is the most common site. One to 2 days later, cutaneous lesions appear. Oval vesicles over the hands and feet, with some lying within skin creases, are usual (Fig. 4.14). Genital and buttock papules are also common, especially in young children. Hemorrhage into the vesicles sometimes occurs.

Differential Diagnosis

Although sometimes confused with herpes gingivostomatitis, the lesions of hand, foot, and mouth disease spare the external surface of the lips and the face. The appearance and distribution of cutaneous vesicles usually differentiate this disease from HSV infection. Although varicella regularly affects the mouth and cutaneous surfaces, the wider distribution of varicella and the presence of blisters in all stages of evolution usually clarify differentiation. Aphthae can mimic hand, foot, and mouth disease, but these are usually recurrent, and they are never associated with cutaneous lesions. The diagnosis can be definitively made by viral cultures or serologies when required.

Management

Giving reassurance and suggesting intake of cool, bland liquids and food are usually the only therapy required for hand, foot, and mouth disease. Oral analgesia or topical anesthetics, such as diphenhydramine elixir, can be used for those with especially sore oral lesions.

HAND, FOOT, AND MOUTH DISEASE

Clinical Manifestations

Oral erosions in association with oval vesicles over the hands and feet; erythematous papules common over the buttocks and diaper area of small children.

Management in the Emergency Department

1. *Reassurance*
2. *Pain management for oral lesions, including cool, bland liquids and topical anesthetics*

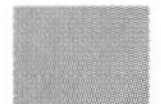

ACUTE ALLERGIC CONTACT DERMATITIS

Allergic contact dermatitis in general is discussed more fully in Chapter 15, Eczematous Diseases. However, several allergens, especially those of plants and topical medications, generate remarkably inflammatory, blistering skin reactions that are mediated by cellular immunity.

An acute allergic contact dermatitis (e.g., rhus dermatitis, poison ivy, poison oak) is a hypersensitivity reaction to a specific allergen that has come into contact with the skin. This never occurs with the first exposure to the allergen because the immune system requires an initial exposure to generate a population of sensitized T cells. Some patients never develop sensitivity, while others develop exquisite sensitivity after only one exposure. The rapidity of sensitization depends on the frequency and degree of exposure, as well as the patient's own genetic makeup and atopic diathesis.

Clinical Manifestations

Edematous papules and clustered, almost confluent, vesicles giving the skin surface a cobblestoned appearance occur over the area that touched the offending substance (Fig. 4.15). This begins 1 to 2 days after exposure to the allergen, so that the patient is often unaware of the offending agent. Rhus (also called plant) dermatitis nearly always shows linear patterns suggestive of allergens being wiped or brushed across the skin (Figs. 4.16 and 4.17). However, other allergens sometimes produce this acute, vesicular reaction, especially topical medications. An acute allergic contact dermatitis to a medication is a not-uncommon cause of apparent worsening of skin disease.

Figure 4.15 Coalescing vesicles and pustules produce a cobblestoned texture to the surface in this patient, who is allergic to neomycin. She was applying medication only to insect bites over her neck but inadvertently spreading it to her leg.

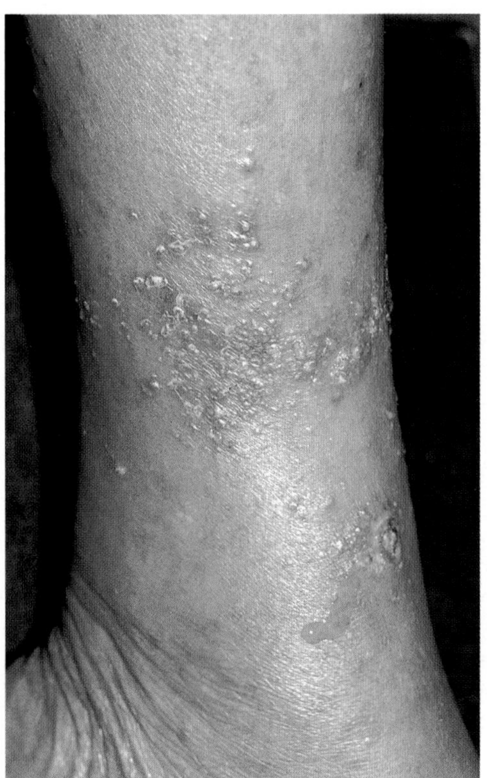

Differential Diagnosis

Diseases in the differential diagnosis include other papulovesicular diseases such as HSV infection and superinfected eczema. In most cases, an allergic contact dermatitis can be differentiated from these other conditions by the history, pattern, and the confluent, cobblestoned, vesicular nature.

Management

The therapy of acutely blistering allergic contact dermatitis is oral prednisone at 40 to 60 mg each morning for 7 to 10 days, with the addition of topical triamcinolone ointment 0.1% as blisters resolve, in lieu of an oral taper. This regimen is often preferred by dermatologists over both intramuscular triamcinolone and a Dosepak, although both provide an automatic taper. Intramuscular triamcinolone gives a suboptimal dose the first few days, and then delivers low doses of corticosteroids for a month (providing exposure to the adrenal glands). In addition, occasional but significant injection site reactions occur, including abscesses and late atrophy. Although a Dosepak avoids injection-site reactions and a full month of systemic exposure to the corticosteroid, it is far more expensive than generic prednisone, and the initial high doses are not continued long enough for the average patient. The last days of a Dosepak deliver doses too low to be of significant benefit, but the adrenal glands are exposed to medication nonetheless.

In addition to corticosteroids, nighttime sedation with hydroxyzine HCl or diphenhydramine and lubrication of the skin as the rash begins to "dry up" are important for optimal improvement. These factors are important in therapy for any dermatitis/eczema (for the specifics of treatment, see Ch. 15, Eczematous Diseases).

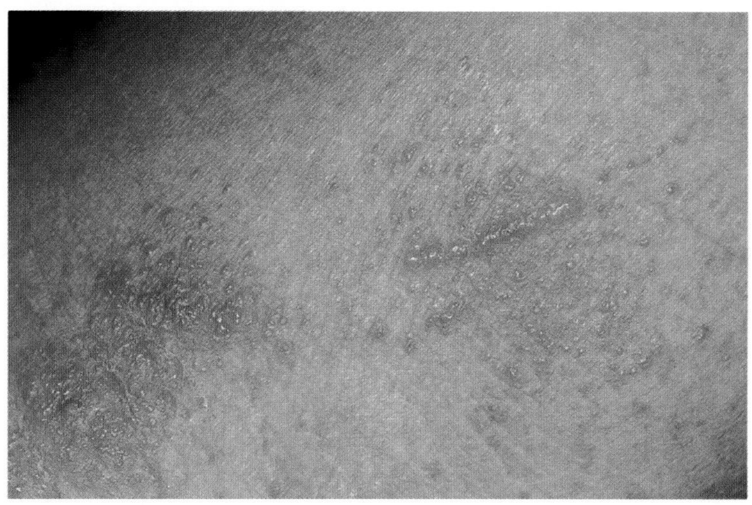

Figure 4.16 Rhus dermatitis. Confluent vesicles are characteristic of acute allergic contact dermatitis, and the linear plaque announces the diagnosis of an allergy to a plant.

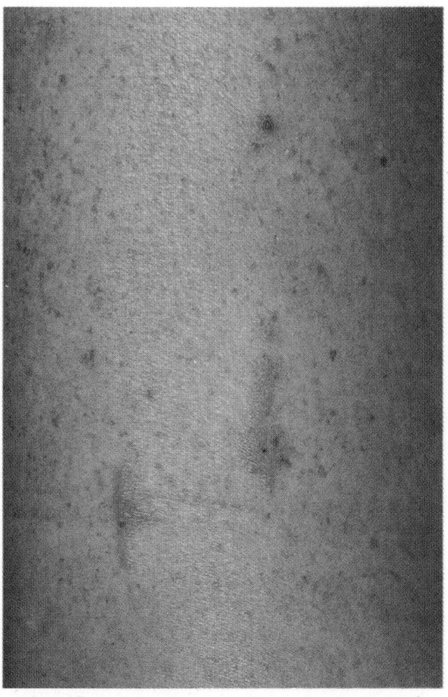

Figure 4.17 Early allergic contact dermatitis exhibits edematous papules and plaques that only blister later, but the linearity of these lesions allows for the diagnosis of plant dermatitis even before blistering occurs.

ACUTE ALLERGIC CONTACT DERMATITIS

Clinical Manifestations

Patchy distribution of edematous papules and plaques with confluent vesicles, some (in the case of plant contact dermatitis) in a linear pattern.

Management in the Emergency Department

1. *Ensure removal of antigen with a shower*
2. *Mild disease: topical triamcinolone ointment 0.1% bid, until clear*

   Moderate to severe disease: prednisone 40 to 60 mg (adult), 1-2 mg/kg (child) for 7-10 days, adding triamcinolone ointment 0.1% as blisters disappear as a taper to prevent rebound, until clear
3. *Eucerin cream (or other cream moisturizer) over corticosteroid twice daily as skin heals*
4. *Nighttime sedation with diphenhydramine 25-75 mg for sleep*
5. *Patient education (see patient handout on p. 356, Poison Ivy)*
6. *Follow-up evaluation with dermatologist if skin not clear in 3-4 weeks, sooner if skin worsens*

DYSHIDROSIS (POMPHYLOX)

Dyshidrosis is a vesiculobullous condition of the hands and feet that derives its name from *dys*, meaning "bad" or "abnormal," and *hidrosis*, meaning "sweating." Originally, the small blisters of dyshidrosis were thought to represent small pockets of sweat trapped within the skin. However, these small blisters are now known to represent edema within the epidermis, most often resulting either from acute atopic dermatitis of the hands and feet or from allergic contact dermatitis. About 20% of all adults exhibit this reaction pattern at times.

Clinical Manifestations

Dyshidrosis is characterized by recurrent crops of small vesicles located predominantly along the lateral digits, with more severe diseases including much of the palms and soles (Figs. 4.18 and 4.19). Occasionally, even the dorsal aspect of the hands and feet exhibits some blistering. When the dorsal aspect of the hands is preferentially affected, an allergic contact dermatitis should be strongly considered, as this dorsal skin is thinner and more sensitive and reacts earlier to allergens than do the palms and soles.

Vesicles in thick skin, especially the palms and soles, may be difficult to recognize. Often, these vesicles appear to be skin-colored papules or deep, light brown, pinpoint macules. Sometimes, the blistering nature of these lesions is not appreciated until collarettes or round, punched-out erosions appear. Long-standing vesicles can sometimes become pustular, but some vesicles are always present.

Atopic patients (those with an allergic diathesis and inherently itchy skin) often report itching that immediately precedes the appearance of vesicles. These patients generally rub and scratch their pruritic hands or feet, producing excoriations, erythema, and scale, resulting in dyshidrotic eczema (see Ch. 15). Patients with more severe disease may experience coalescence of vesicles into larger bullae. Chronic disease occurring near the posterior nail fold can produce dystrophic nails with irregular horizontal ridging.

Differential Diagnosis

Because dyshidrosis and dyshidrotic eczema are descriptive rather than diagnostic terms, the first task of the examiner is to consider whether the underlying cause of inflammation is atopic dermatitis, also called neurodermatitis, for which there is no specific allergen responsible, or whether the inflammation is due to a specific allergen, resulting in acute, vesicular, allergic contact dermatitis. Although the pattern and history can be somewhat helpful, patch testing often is required to help resolve this question. Thus, patients with disease that is not eas-

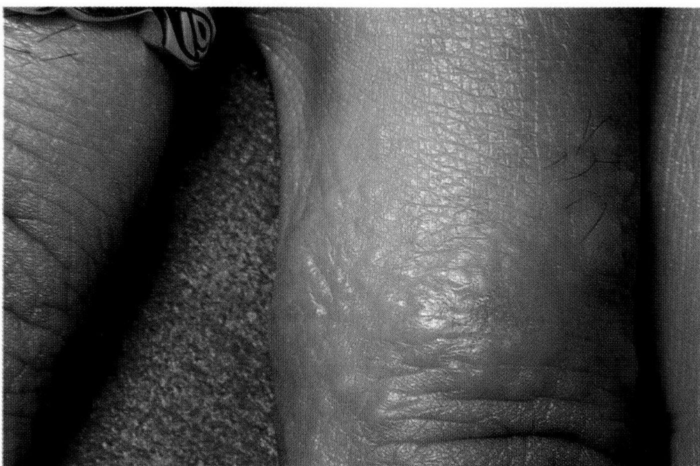

Figure 4.18 This nonspecific clinical picture of dyshidrosis can be produced by inflammatory atopic dermatitis or by acute allergic contact dermatitis; thus, dyshidrosis is more a description than a diagnosis.

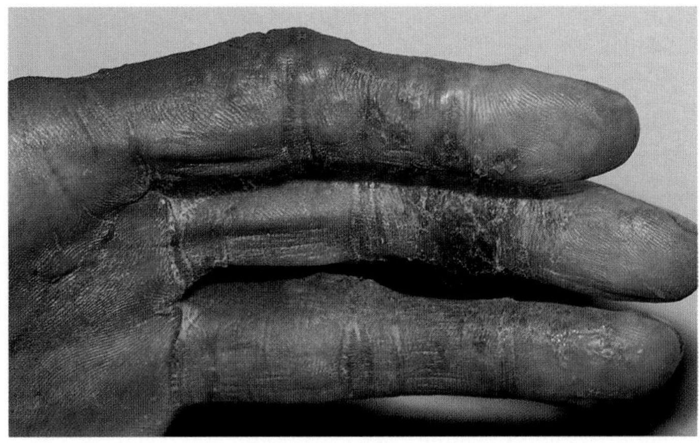

Figure 4.19 An atopic patient often scratches and rubs vesicular hand dermatitis, producing dyshidrotic eczema.

ily controlled with therapy should be advised to seek further evaluation by a dermatologist.

Among other diseases that can produce blistering of the palms or soles is vesicular tinea, which generally occurs on the feet. Although the identification of fungus on a microscopic smear or culture would appear to sort this out, both fungal disease and dyshidrosis are so common that they often coexist. Sometimes, both eczema and the dermatophyte infection require therapy.

Pustular psoriasis sometimes mimics dyshidrosis, but in this case there are no vesicles; only pustules, punched-out erosions, and collarettes are present. In addition, pustular psoriasis is usually manifested by the occurrence of these pustules and erosions within sharply demarcated plaques. Often, but not always, pustular psoriasis is present on skin in areas other than the hands and feet. Nail abnormalities characteristic of psoriasis are usually present, including pitting, "oil-drop" spots, and onycholysis (lifting of the nails) with subungual keratin debris, rather than nonspecific horizontal ridging, as occurs with any local inflammation, including eczema.

In some cases, HSV infection resembles dyshidrosis, but HSV infection is usually localized to one small plaque of vesicles, in contrast to most cases of dyshidrosis, which tend to be more generalized. In addition, HSV infection is usually painful rather than pruritic and much more inflammatory in appearance than dyshidrosis, with surrounding edema and erythema. Finally, dyshidrosis is usually, but not always, bilateral, unlike HSV infection.

Management

The treatment for dyshidrosis and dyshidrotic eczema is the same as for eczema on other parts of the body, only using a slightly higher potency corticosteroid because of the thickness of palmar and plantar skin. Several issues should be addressed simultaneously.

First is patient education regarding the recurrent nature of this condition and exacerbating causes. The patient should be advised to avoid irritants, including frequent handwashing, harsh soaps, irritating chemicals, and trauma to the hands, such as lifting and carrying rough objects. The patient should understand that this is not a curable condition, but is generally controllable with careful skin care.

Second, corticosteroids are the specific medical treatment of choice. Topical corticosteroids are usually sufficient for mild to moderate disease. Generally, a high-potency corticosteroid such as fluocinonide (Lidex) 0.05% is preferred initially, although milder disease usually responds to mid-potency triamcinolone 0.1%. Patients with mild disease prefer creams, whereas those with more erosive disease find ointments less irritating. Patients with multiple erosions, larger blisters, or exudative skin improve more quickly with an initial burst of oral prednisone at 40 to 60 mg each morning. A topical corticosteroid is added to this regimen as blistering and exudation resolve, and within 7 to

10 days, the oral prednisone can be discontinued abruptly without a taper.

A third important aspect of therapy is lubrication. As the skin breaks and cracks, inflammation is perpetuated. A thick emollient such as Eucerin *cream* or Vaseline petroleum jelly should be applied both over the topical corticosteroid and multiple other times during the day as the skin becomes dry and fissured. As skin improves, more cosmetically acceptable but less moisturizing lotions, such as Lubriderm, Vaseline Intensive Care, or Eucerin lotions, can be substituted.

Fourth, those patients who are itchy at night and wake frequently either with pruritus or pain require nighttime sedation to control scratching for maximum improvement. This can usually be achieved with antihistamines such as diphenhydramine (Benadryl) or hydroxyzine HCl (Atarax) in sedating doses of 25 to 100 mg, although some fare better with the longer-acting medications amitriptyline and doxepin at the same doses.

Finally, patients with significant edema and exudation are sometimes superinfected; control of infection will maximize improvement. An oral antistaphylococcal agent such as cephalexin (Keflex) or dicloxacillin for the first 5 to 7 days of therapy also hastens improvement.

Occasionally, the condition fails to be controlled with topical corticosteroids and adjunctive therapy. These patients should be carefully evaluated to investigate the role of allergic contact dermatitis. In addition, other more aggressive therapies, such as ultrapotent topical corticosteroids, topical corticosteroids under nighttime glove occlusion, oral psoralens with ultraviolet A light exposure (PUVA), or immunosuppressive agents, such as azathioprine or methotrexate, are sometimes used by dermatologists.

If there is concern about the presence of vesicular *Tinea pedis* in dyshidrosis, a baseline culture before institution of antifungal therapy is suggested. Because topical antifungal therapy is of limited use with vesicular disease, griseofulvin 500 mg bid is suggested in addition to therapy for dyshidrosis. Therapy without a baseline culture leaves the clinician who follows the patient unable to test for fungus, which will be partially treated.

Course and Prognosis

When dyshidrosis appears as a manifestation of atopic dermatitis, the vesicles usually occur in crops, with some patients experiencing complete healing between occasional outbreaks. Those with more severe dyshidrosis have continual disease that waxes and wanes. In most cases, the condition is controlled with topical skin care, as discussed above. Those with recalcitrant disease deserve referral to a dermatologist for further evaluation and sophisticated therapy.

DYSHIDROSIS

Clinical Manifestations

Characterized by 1- to 2-mm vesicles primarily along the lateral digits, often extending to the palms and soles.

Management in the Emergency Department

1. *Mild to moderate disease: a midpotency (mild disease) topical corticosteroid such as triamcinolone ointment 0.1%, or a high potency (more severe disease) steroid such as fluocinonide ointment 0.05% twice a day*

   Severe bullous or exudative disease: oral prednisone 40 to 60 mg each morning with follow-up in 7 to 10 days in addition to above topical therapy as skin heals
2. *Frequent lubrication with a thick moisturizer such as Eucerin cream should be applied over the medication and prn dryness and cracking*
3. *Patient education regarding chronicity and avoidance of excessive handwashing and other irritants (see patient handout on p. 340, Dyshidrosis)*
4. *Nighttime sedation with antihistamine (diphenhydramine, hydroxyzine HCl, amitriptyline, or doxepin 25 to 75 mg) is important in patients with significant itching or pain*
5. *Obvious infection should be treated with an oral antistaphylococcal medication*
6. *Follow-up evaluation with regular health care provider or dermatologist in 1 month*

VESICULAR TINEA PEDIS

Although tinea pedis is most often an erythematous, scaling condition that follows a clinically obvious fungal infection of the nail, vesicular tinea pedis is a less common, acute blistering infection caused by more inflamogenic strains of dermatophyte (see also Ch. 14, Papulosquamous Diseases).

Clinical Manifestations

Vesicular tinea pedis is characterized by grouped vesicles and bullae, especially common over the instep and medial aspect of one or both feet (Fig. 4.20). The surrounding skin may be scaling.

Differential Diagnosis

The disease most likely to be confused with vesicular tinea pedis is dyshidrosis or an allergic contact dermatitis. If the pattern and history do not allow differentiation, as often happens, a fungal smear performed by a dermatologist or a culture may be required.

Management

Topical antifungal agents are generally not sufficient to treat tinea pedis with significant blistering, since penetration through the vesicles may be poor. First-line oral therapy is griseofulvin, 500 mg bid with meals until the skin heals, usually 1 to 2 weeks. Patients should be warned about the frequent occurrence of nausea, headaches, photosensitivity, and hives with this therapy. Alternative therapies that are not yet approved for tinea pedis by the Food and Drug Administration (FDA), but that are very effective and safe (although expensive) include fluconazole (Diflucan) 100 to 200 mg/day and itraconazole (Sporanox) 200 mg/day. Itraconazole now has indication approval for onychomycosis. Although ketaconazole (Nizoral) is effective, the more frequent occurrence of hepatotoxicity dictates the use of other agents.

For those patients with painful blistering, a few days of oral prednisone at a dose of 40 to 60 mg each morning and abrupt discontinuance hasten symptomatic improvement.

Course and Prognosis

Unlike chronic tinea pedis, acute vesicular tinea pedis usually resolves with adequate therapy, although recurrences are possible. Because both tinea and dyshidrosis are blistering diseases, often coexisting, the end points of therapy can sometimes be difficult to identify. Those patients whose condition does not steadily improve and progress to resolution should consult a dermatologist at a follow-up visit, after having stopped antifungal therapy at least 1 week before the visit, so that an

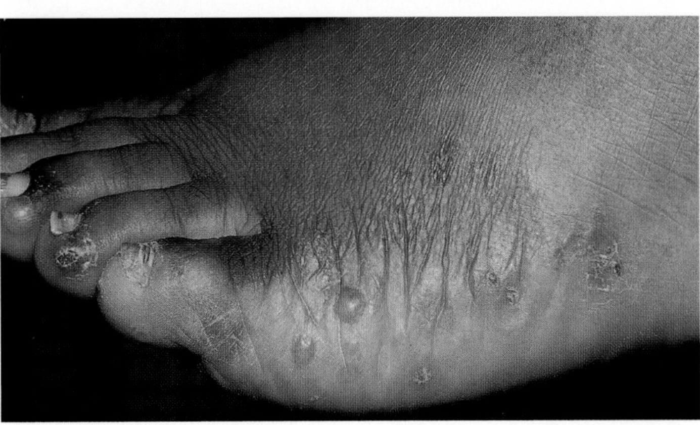

Figure 4.20 Vesicular tinea pedis can be very difficult to differentiate from dyshidrosis—cultures can be important.

evaluation for the presence of remaining fungus yields accurate information.

> **VESICULAR TINEA PEDIS**
>
> ***Clinical Manifestations***
> *Vesicles and inflammation, most often including the medial aspect of feet, with the diagnosis confirmed by a positive fungal preparation or culture.*
>
> ***Management in the Emergency Department***
> 1. *Griseofulvin 500 mg bid with meals for 2 weeks*
> 2. *For unusually painful or severe vesicular disease, add prednisone 40 to 60 mg each morning for 1 week*
> 3. *Follow-up evaluation with a dermatologist in 2 weeks, or sooner if condition worsens*

INSECT BITES

People who are extremely sensitive to some insects develop not only a red papule at the site, but also a central vesicle or, occasionally, even a bulla (See also Ch. 8).

The most common bites to blister are flea bites, which occur in greatest numbers over the lower legs from fleas living in carpets and grass (Figs. 4.21 and 4.22). Children are more likely to have sensitive skin that blisters and are also more likely to be close to the ground and to have more generalized bites.

Mosquito bites blister in some patients as well. These bites are generally seen on the extremities and sometimes on the face. Patients are often aware of mosquito bites, since the bite makes them uncomfortable.

Finally, ant bites, especially fire ant bites, can produce vesicles and pustules. These are also more common on the lower legs and feet, and patients are always aware of the source, since fire ant bites are quite painful.

A primary disease to be differentiated from insect bites is chickenpox, particularly in those who have generalized, scattered bites. However, the trunk is usually spared by insect bites, and the constitutional signs and symptoms of varicella are absent.

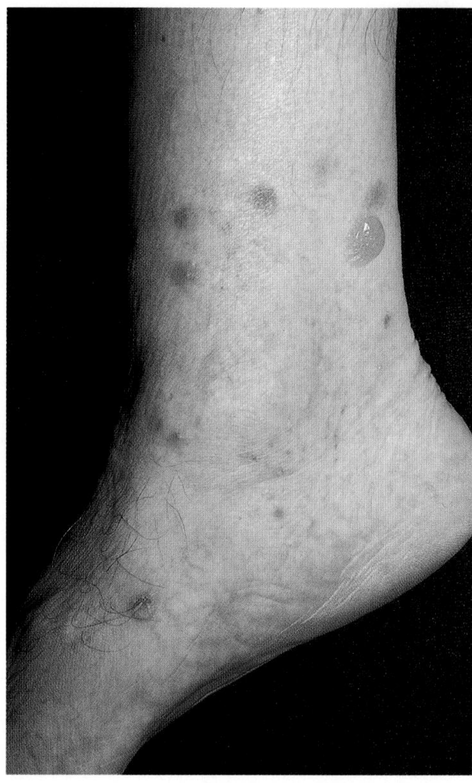

Figure 4.21 Flea bites are usually found on the lower legs; blisters often are accompanied by crusts and edematous papules.

Figure 4.22 Flea bites are often clustered into "breakfast, lunch, and dinner" lesions.

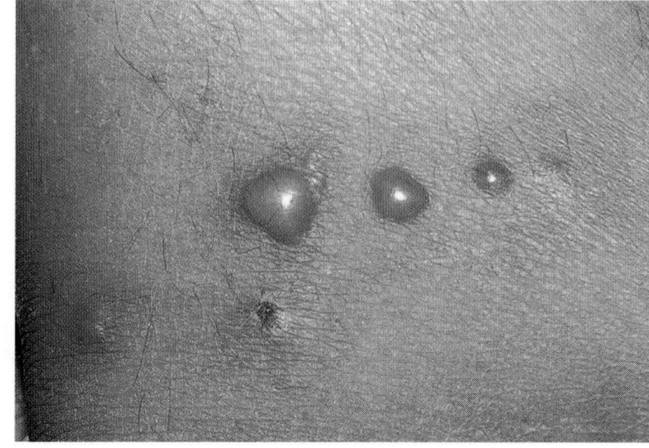

In general, the primary therapy for insect bites is prevention of future bites (see patient handout on p. 351, Insect Bites). Multiple bites with significant blistering can be treated with systemic corticosteroids, using prednisone at 1 mg/kg each morning in children, or 40 mg each morning for adults. The patient is treated until itching and pain are controlled and lesions are beginning to heal, generally from 3 to 5 days. Any secondary infection should be treated with an oral staphylococcal agent such as cephalexin.

> **BULLOUS INSECT BITES**
>
> ***Clinical Manifestations***
>
> *Itchy red papules and nodules with overlying blisters and crusts; most often over lower legs in the case of flea bites and any exposed skin with mosquito bites.*
>
> ***Management in the Emergency Department***
>
> 1. *Mild disease: triamcinolone cream 0.1% bid to bites Severe blistering: prednisone 40 to 60 mg (adults), 1 to 2 mg/kg (children) each morning 3 to 5 days*
> 2. *Patient education regarding pest control (patient handout on p. 351, Insect Bites)*
> 3. *Personal insect repellant (e.g., Off, 6-12)*

UNCOMMON VESICULAR DISEASES

Dermatitis Herpetiformis

Dermatitis herpetiformis is an uncommon, intensely pruritic autoimmune blistering disease. Grouped vesicles occur first over the elbows, knees, and lower back, but patients are so intensely pruritic that rubbing and scratching the area often mechanically remove the blister, making it difficult to appreciate the blistering nature of the condition. Therefore, dermatitis herpetiformis should be considered when intense, recalcitrant pruritus with excoriations occurs, particularly in this distribution. The treatment of choice for this disease is oral dapsone and a gluten-free diet. The disease does not remit, but is usually well controlled with dapsone.

Chronic Bullous Disease of Childhood

Chronic bullous disease of childhood is another uncommon autoimmune blistering disease. This condition occurs in small children between ages 2 and 6 years. Lesions begin in the genital area, and over the hands and feet. Classically, vesicles and small bullae are clustered in an annular configuration. This condition is usually misdiagnosed initially as bullous impetigo or, less often, is attributed to insect bites or to an acute allergic contact dermatitis to poison ivy or poison oak. The chronic and recalcitrant nature of this eruption for these diseases should raise suspicion for chronic bullous disease of childhood. This disease is diagnosed by routine and immunofluorescent biopsies and is treated with oral dapsone, an anti-inflammatory sulfa drug. This disease resolves after several years.

Figure 4.23 Although scabies is a vesicular disease, most patients remove blisters as they scratch almost as quickly as vesicles form. This small, linear vesicle is called a burrow.

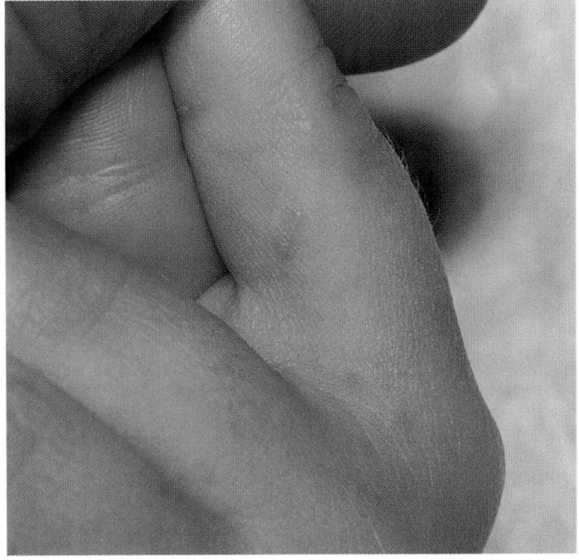

Scabies

Although the primary lesion of scabies is a linear papulovesicle (a burrow), scabies is generally characterized by excoriations and erythema (Fig. 4.23). Occasionally, a very careful search produces two or three typical burrows. This condition should be suspected and patients searched for burrows when there is a sudden onset of eczema with intense pruritus in the characteristic areas of web spaces, skin folds, and the genital area. Pruritic family members provide even more circumstantial evidence for the presence of scabies (for further discussion of this disease, see Ch. 15, Eczematous Diseases).

SCABIES

Clinical Manifestations

Excruciatingly itchy disease characterized by scattered excoriations and papulovesicular lesions distributed especially in skin folds, genital area, finger web spaces, and wrists.

Management in the Emergency Department

1. *Permethrin cream 5% (Elimite) to patient and all family members overnight*
2. *Wash all bedclothes, linens, clothes, etc. in contact with the patient or family members in the previous 24 hours*
3. *Patient education (see patient handout on p. 361, Scabies)*
4. *Triamcinolone 0.1% (adults) or hydrocortisone 1% or 2.5% (children) cream twice daily for scaling, inflamed, and itchy areas*
5. *Nighttime sedation with diphenhydramine, hydroxyzine HCl, or amitriptyline 25 to 75 mg for sleeping if needed*

Please see patient information handouts for this chapter on pages 340, 343, 345–347, 349, 356, and 370–371.

REFERENCES

1. Nahmias AJ et al: Sero-epidemiological and sociological patterns of herpes simplex virus infection in the world. Scand J Infect Dis, suppl. 69:19, 1990
2. Benedetti J, Corey L, Ashley R: Recurrence rates in genital herpes after symptomatic first-episode infection. Ann Intern Med 121:847, 1994
3. Sacks SL, Aoki FY, Diaz-Mitoma F et al, for the Canadian Famciclovir Study Group: Patient-initiated, twice-daily oral famciclovir for early recurrent genital herpes. JAMA 276: 44, 1996
4. Goldberg LH, Kaufman R, Kurtz TO et al: Long-term suppression of recurrent genital herpes with acyclovir: a five year benchmark. Arch Dermatol 129:582, 1993
5. Wald A et al: Suppression of subclinical shedding of herpes simplex virus type 2 with acyclovir. Ann Intern Med 124:8, 1996
6. Memar O, Tyring SK: Cutaneous viral infections. J Am Acad Dermatol 33:279, 1995
7. Huff JC, Bean B, Balfour HH Jr et al: Therapy of herpes zoster with oral acyclovir. Am J Med 85(suppl 2A):84, 1988
8. Wood MJ et al: Efficacy of oral acyclovir treatmet of acute herpes zoster. Am J Med 85(suppl 2A):79, 1988
9. McKendrick MW et al: Oral acyclovir in acute herpes zoster. BMJ 293:1529, 1986
10. Wassilew SW et al: Oral acyclovir for herpes zoster: a double-blind controlled trial in normal subjects. Br J Dermatol 117:495, 1987
11. Huff JC, Drucker JL, Clemmer A et al: Effect of oral acyclovir on pain resolution in herpes zoster: a reanalysis. J Med Virol, suppl 1:93, 1993
12. Tyring S et al: Famciclovir for the treatment of acute herpes zoster: effects on acute disease and postherpetic neuralgia. Ann Intern Med 123:89, 1995
13. Post BT, Philbrick JT: Do corticosteroids prevent post-herpetic neuralgia? A review of the evidence. J Am Acad Dermatol 18:605, 1988

14. Balfour HH Jr, Kelly JM, Suarez CS et al: Acyclovir treatment of varicella in otherwise healthy children. J Pediatr 116:633, 1990

SUGGESTED READINGS

Herpes Simplex Virus Infections

Corey L, Spear PG: Infections with herpes simplex viruses. N Engl J Med 314:686, 749, 1986

Vestey JP, Norval M: Mucocutaneous infections with herpes simplex virus and their management. Clin Exp Dermatol 17:221, 1992

Kinghorn GR: Genital herpes: natural history and treatment of acute episodes. J Med Virol, suppl. 1:33, 1993

Memar O, Tyring SK: Cutaneous viral infections. J Am Acad Dermatol 33:279, 1995

Mooney MA, Janniger CK, Schwartz RA: Kaposi's varicelliform eruption. Cutis 53:243, 1994

Varicella Zoster Virus Infections

Balfour HH Jr: Current management of varicella zoster virus infections. J Med Virol, suppl. 1:74, 1993

Kost RG, Straus SE: Postherpetic neuralgia: pathogenesis, treatment, and prevention. N Engl J Med 335:32, 1996

Tyring SK: Natural history of varicella zoster virus. Semin Dermatol 11:211, 1992

Hand, Foot, and Mouth Disease

Thomas I, Janniger CK: Hand, foot, and mouth disease. Cutis 52:265, 1993

Acute Allergic Contact Dermatitis

Adams RM (ed): Occupational Skin Disease. WB Saunders, Philadelphia, 1990

Marks JG, DeLeo VA: Contact and Occupational Dermatology. Mosby–Year Book, St. Louis, 1992

CHAPTER 5

Bullous Diseases

Bullae are blisters larger than 1 cm that are filled with clear or straw-colored fluid. Although bullae (large blisters) and vesicles (small blisters) are differentiated on the basis of size, bullous diseases sometimes begin as vesicles, so that a differential diagnosis sometimes contains diseases from both groups.

The morphologic appearance of blisters is at least partially dependent on the thickness of the blister roof. Some diseases, such as pemphigus vulgaris and bullous impetigo, have very thin blister roofs. These diseases exhibit either flaccid bullae or, when the blister roof has been totally denuded, round erosions. Other, deeper blisters, such as those of bullous pemphigoid or friction blisters, usually show at least some tense, intact lesions.

A skin biopsy is often required for differentiation among the bullous diseases. Blisters are easily disrupted during the biopsy process, and old lesions often yield nondiagnostic results (see the section on biopsy procedures in Ch. 2.)

BULLOUS PEMPHIGOID

Bullous pemphigoid is an uncommon, autoimmune blistering disease most often seen in elderly patients. Autoantibodies bind to structures in the basement membrane zone. Complement activation probably initiates events that produce separation of the epidermis from the dermis.

Clinical Manifestations

Bullous pemphigoid is often preceded by itching, which is sometimes severe. Blisters ranging from less than 1 cm to several centimeters then appear, arising from both inflamed and noninflamed skin (Fig. 5.1). Blisters show a predilection for the trunk and body folds but gradually spread to cover most of the body. Because even the relatively thick-roofed blisters of bullous pemphigoid are easily ruptured, multiple round erosions and crusts are usual (Fig. 5.2). The skin does not show signs of fragility, so that lateral pressure on the skin does not cause detachment of the epidermis (Nikolsky sign). Most often, mucous membranes are spared, although oral or gingival erosions occasionally occur.

The actual bullae of bullous pemphigoid can be preceded by plaques resembling urticaria or eczema; this phase can sometimes be long-lived, lasting weeks or months. However, unlike urticaria, these plaques are not migratory or transient. Sometimes a very careful examination reveals a small number of vesicles within the plaques.

Differential Diagnosis

Bullous pemphigoid can be confused with blistering forms of erythema multiforme, but erythema multiforme is more explosive in onset and never exhibits blisters arising in noninflamed skin, and oral erosions are nearly always present. Severe acute allergic contact dermatitis sometimes resemble bullous pemphigoid, but the blisters of bullous pemphigoid are usually larger and scattered and have a much more indolent onset. Although pemphigus vulgaris produces large blisters, these blisters are very flaccid, and pemphigus vulgaris occurs in younger patients with predictable, striking, and early oral erosions. Closely related, both clinically and histologically, is cicatricial pemphigoid. This disease occurs in the same age group but differs in its predilection for the oral mucosa and conjunctiva, where it causes severe scarring that sometimes results in blindness.

Figure 5.1 These tense bullae arise from both inflamed and noninflamed skin, unlike blistering forms of erythema multiforme, which always exhibit surrounding erythema.

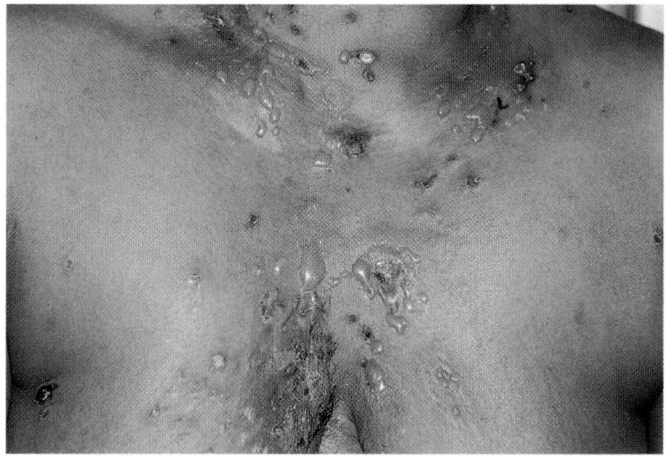

The diagnosis of bullous pemphigoid is made by routine skin biopsy with confirmation by direct immunofluorescent skin biopsy, in which IgG and C3, with or without other immunoglobulins, are deposited at the dermal-epidermal junction.

Figure 5.2 Although relatively thick-roofed, larger blisters often break and form round erosions or crusts that do not necessarily signify superinfection.

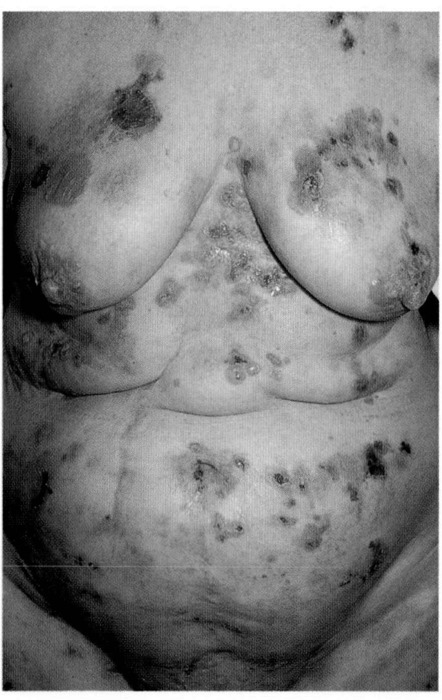

Management

Although bullous pemphigoid is a miserably pruritic and painful disease for the patient, in most cases it is not health-threatening. Beyond the treatment of secondary skin infections and good supportive care, the institution of proper therapy is usually not emergent.

The mainstay of therapy for bullous pemphigoid is corticosteroids. Mild, localized disease occasionally responds somewhat to an ultrapotent topical corticosteroid such as clobetasol propionate cream or ointment.[1] Most often, however, oral prednisone 40 to 80 mg/day is required to control disease. The dose of prednisone is slowly increased every 5 to 7 days if new blisters are appearing. Unfortunately, the older age group most susceptible to bullous pemphigoid also frequently exhibits diseases, such as hypertension and diabetes mellitus, which are complicated by systemic corticosteroid therapy. Patients requiring higher doses of prednisone for control of their disease often benefit from the addition of an antimetabolite such as azathioprine or cyclophosphamide as a steroid-sparing agent, although the action of these medications is delayed by about 1 month. Occasionally, patients respond to other nonspecific nonsteroidal anti-inflammatory drugs (NSAIDs), such as dapsone,[2] and to antibiotics such as tetracycline, with[3] or without[4] nicotinamide.

In the emergency department, the patient can be directed to consult with a dermatologist within a day or so, or an aggressive and confident emergency clinician can do pretherapy skin biopsies to confirm the diagnosis and begin the patient on prednisone, with instructions to follow up with a dermatologist as soon as possible. Routine biopsy for histology should consist of shave removal of a vesicle in toto if possible, or of a shave sample of the edge of a new blister. A biopsy for direct immunofluorescence should be obtained from adjacent, normal skin using a 3-mm punch biopsy. This biopsy can be stored in Michele's solution or transport medium until the results of routine histology are available. Occasionally, routine histology is diagnostic for a different disease, saving the patient several hundred dollars in unnecessary laboratory fees for immunofluorescent studies. The only blistering disease that could be worsened by 1 or 2 days of systemic corticosteroids (or the clinician given credit for a bad outcome) is established severe, blistering erythema multiforme (toxic epidermal necrolysis).

Course and Prognosis

The long-term prognosis of bullous pemphigoid in many patients is one of remission after several months to a year. Once blistering is controlled with oral corticosteroids, and sometimes immunosuppressant agents, a gradual tapering of medications is indicated.

> **BULLOUS PEMPHIGOID**
>
> ***Clinical Manifestations***
>
> *Tense blisters containing straw-colored fluid arising from inflamed and noninflamed skin in older patients, accompanied by erosions and crusts. Usually, no mucous membrane involvement.*
>
> ***Management in the Emergency Department***
>
> 1. *Local wound care and treatment of superinfection*
> 2. *Referral to dermatologist, immediacy dependent on extent of disease*
> 3. *Confirmation of the diagnosis and initiation of therapy are possible for the interested and aggressive emergency department clinician (see text)*

CICATRICIAL PEMPHIGOID

Cicatricial pemphigoid is an autoimmune blistering disorder closely related to, and sometimes clinically and microscopically indistinguishable from, bullous pemphigoid. However, the differentiation can usually be made on the basis of the remarkable predilection for mucous membranes and resulting severe scarring, with little or no involvement of keratinized skin.

Clinical Manifestations

Blisters on mucous membranes quickly rupture to form erosions. These are most common over the gingivae (Fig. 5.3) and the palate and in the eye, although early eye findings can be subtle, appearing only as nonspecific inflammation. Later eye disease reveals scarring consisting of fusion of the palpebral and bulbar conjunctivae, producing symblepharon, and scarring of the cornea from entropion and trichiasis. Less often, the genitalia, esophagus, or nasopharynx are involved. When nonmucous membrane skin is involved, lesions are identical to those of bullous pemphigoid (Figs. 5.1 and 5.2).

Figure 5.3 The primary lesion of cicatricial pemphigoid is a blister, but the mucous membranes are so fragile that the blister roof sloughs almost immediately, resulting in well-demarcated erosions.

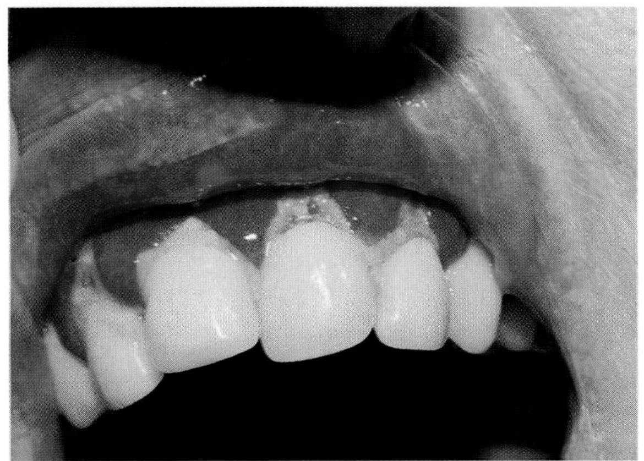

Differential Diagnosis

The diseases most likely to resemble cicatricial pemphigoid are pemphigus vulgaris and erosive lichen planus, both of which produce marked mucous membrane erosions. Blistering erythema multiforme can usually be distinguished by its explosive onset and typical skin lesions. Biopsies are often required for differentiation from pemphigus vulgaris or lichen planus, unless there are pathognomonic signs of oral lichen planus. A biopsy of the edge of an erosion is recommended for routine histology, with a sample from adjacent, noneroded skin saved in transport medium for possible direct immunofluorescence if needed for confirmation.

Management

The management of mild disease consists of careful local care of the mouth and eye, with topical corticosteroids. However, the threat of blindness from progressive scarring of the eye is very real, so that systemic corticosteroids, often with antimetabolites, are generally required. Some patients respond to oral dapsone.

Course and Prognosis

Although some cases of cicatricial pemphigoid are adequately controlled with topical medications, other patients experience recalcitrant, ongoing, scarring disease, which requires systemic medication. Even those who respond to therapy often require ongoing medication or may experience relapse after apparent remission.

CICATRICIAL PEMPHIGOID

Clinical Manifestations

Oral erosions; conjunctival erythema, sensation of dryness, erosions, and/or scarring; sometimes accompanied by cutaneous blisters that are tense and contain straw-colored fluid arising from inflamed and noninflamed skin in older patients

(Continues)

(Continued)

Management in the Emergency Department

1. *Pain control and local wound care*
2. *Referral to dermatologist, with immediacy dependent on extent of disease*
3. *Confirmation of the diagnosis and initiation of therapy are possible for the interested and aggressive emergency department clinician (see text)*

PEMPHIGUS VULGARIS

Pemphigus vulgaris is an uncommon autoimmune blistering disease that usually results in death when untreated.[5–7] This disease can mimic toxic epidermal necrolysis, but the therapy is very different.

Clinical Manifestations

Most common in young and middle-aged adults, pemphigus vulgaris typically begins as erosions in the mouth. The entire mouth may become involved, but the gingiva, posterior palate, and buccal mucosa are areas of predilection. Because these very shallow blisters occur within the epidermis, intact blisters generally are not observed on fragile mucous membranes (Fig. 5.4). Instead, super-

Figure 5.4 Like other blistering diseases that affect mucous membranes, only erosions are generally appreciated with oral pemphigus.

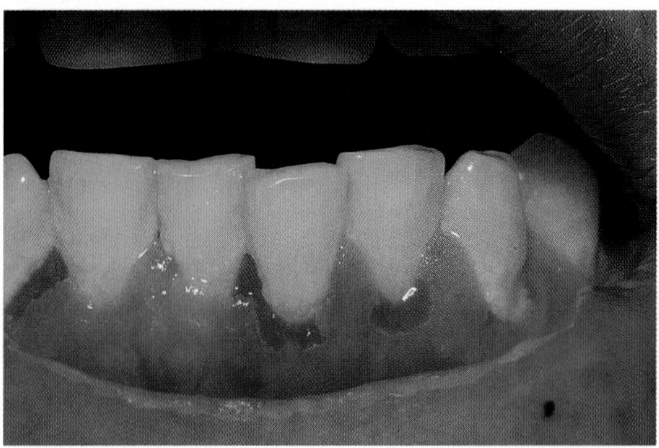

ficial, sharply demarcated erosions that are frequently circular and coalescing are usual. However, extensive disease is less characteristic and mimics the blistering of erythema multiforme (Fig. 5.5). These painful lesions often prevent adequate oral intake. Other squamous epithelial mucous membranes can be affected, including the conjunctiva, pharynx, esophagus, rectal mucosa, vagina, and modified mucous membrane skin of the vulva.

Pemphigus vulgaris ultimately extends to involve nonmucous membrane skin, where flaccid blisters and large, round erosions are present (Figs. 5.6 and 5.7). Skin fragility is demonstrated by the presence of the Nikolsky sign, where a blister or erosion occurs when the skin is rubbed.

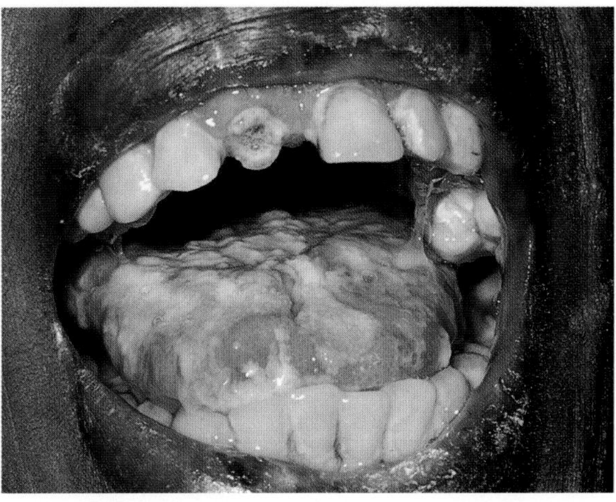

Figure 5.5 Severe oral pemphigus vulgaris is one factor in the high mortality rate associated with untreated cases.

Differential Diagnosis

Pemphigus vulgaris is sometimes confused with other bullous diseases, especially bullous pemphigoid and toxic epidermal necrolysis. However, unlike bullous pemphigoid, pemphigus vulgaris rarely exhibits tense blisters and nearly always exhibits oral erosions. Although both pemphigus vulgaris and toxic epidermal necrolysis are characterized by mucous membrane disease and flaccid blisters with large areas of erosion, pemphigus vulgaris is usually more gradual in onset, has less inflammatory surrounding skin, and patients are less toxic. However, a biopsy is indicated to confirm a diagnosis of pemphigus vulgaris because of the toxic and prolonged therapy required.

Management

Patients who are not ill, and those in whom a diagnosis of toxic epidermal necrolysis is not a consideration, can be discharged with instructions to follow up the next day with a dermatologist. Patients

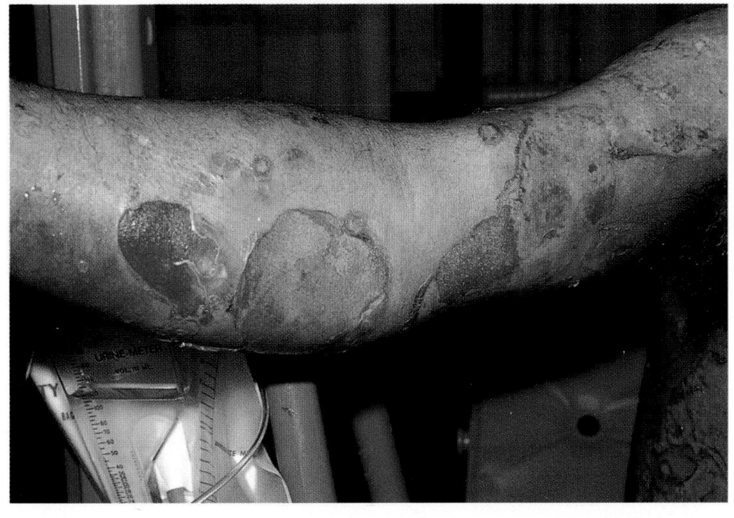

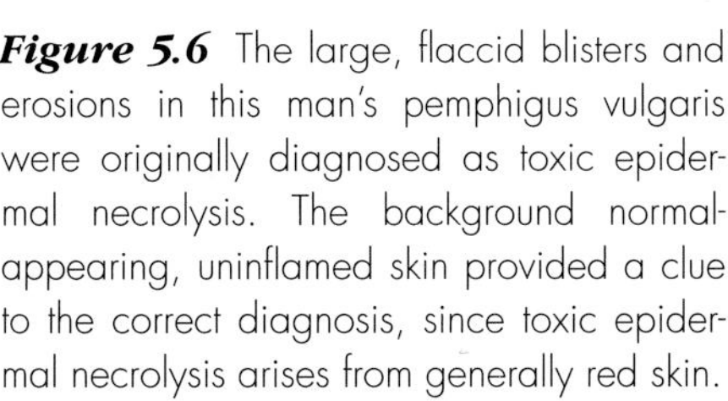

Figure 5.6 The large, flaccid blisters and erosions in this man's pemphigus vulgaris were originally diagnosed as toxic epidermal necrolysis. The background normal-appearing, uninflamed skin provided a clue to the correct diagnosis, since toxic epidermal necrolysis arises from generally red skin.

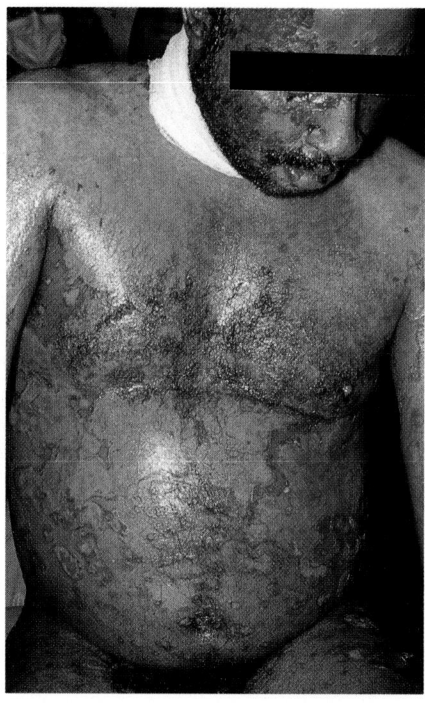

Figure 5.7 Large denuded areas contribute to the high mortality rate in untreated pemphigus vulgaris.

who are ill or who have widespread disease should be admitted for fluid and electrolyte management, infection control, and corticosteroid therapy.

A skin biopsy should be performed before initiation of systemic corticosteroid therapy. A shave biopsy of the edge of a blister or erosion is most helpful, since the rotating motion required for a punch biopsy often removes the blister roof. A second biopsy of adjacent, nonblistered skin should be sampled and stored in transport medium or Michele's solution for later submission for direct immunofluorescence if indicated.

Other than supportive care, first-line therapy for patients with pemphigus vulgaris consists of systemic corticosteroids. Patients with milder disease can be treated with prednisone 60 to 80 mg each morning, with very careful follow-up and an increase in dosage every 4 to 5 days, if new lesions continue to appear. For patients who are ill with extensive disease, hospital admission for intravenous corticosteroid therapy and supportive care is indicated.

Although systemic corticosteroids are the first choice in therapy for phemphigus vulgaris, some patients require prednisone in doses of 150 mg or more for control of their disease. Most of these patients are best treated with steroid-sparing immunosuppressive medications such as azathioprine or cyclophosphamide, as well as corticosteroids. These adjunctive therapies exert their effects slowly, with a month required for improvement. Systemic gold, monthly intravenous cyclophosphamide pulse therapy, and plasmapheresis are all additional treatments used in some patients.

Course and Prognosis

Left untreated, pemphigus vulgaris extends to cover most skin surfaces. Before the advent of corticosteroids, death occurred in up to 80% of patients. Mortality was due to large areas of denuded skin resulting in infection and fluid loss, in combination with severe oral disease limiting adequate intake. With the availability of corticosteroids, patients rarely die from pemphigus vulgaris, but the high and prolonged doses of corticosteroids produce their own morbidity and mortality, most often from infection.

Often, once the disease is under control, medications can be tapered to much more acceptable schedules. In some cases, medications can be entirely discontinued without recurrence.

PEMPHIGUS VULGARIS

Clinical Manifestations

Oral erosions; flaccid cutaneous bullae and erosions with denuded skin. Skin fragility with detachment of epidermis from dermis occurring with minor friction.

Management in the Emergency Department

1. *Pain control and local wound care*
2. *Immediate differentiation from toxic epidermal necrolysis by history (usually) or frozen-section biopsy*
3. *Immediate consultation with dermatologist if ill; otherwise next-day referral*

(Continues)

(Continued)

4. *Confirmation of the diagnosis and initiation of therapy are possible for the interested and aggressive emergency department clinician (see text)*

BULLOUS ERYTHEMA MULTIFORME (STEVENS-JOHNSON SYNDROME, TOXIC EPIDERMAL NECROLYSIS)

Erythema multiforme (Stevens-Johnson syndrome, toxic epidermal necrolysis) is a hypersensitivity reaction that, when sufficiently severe to produce blistering, is usually caused by a medication allergy. Minor blistering is painful but rarely dangerous. Widespread blistering and erosive disease carry a high mortality rate.

Clinical Manifestations

This immunologic reaction exists on an extremely wide spectrum of severity. The mildest and most common forms of erythema multiforme consist of red, nonscaling papules with central dusky or violaceous erythema as a result of more intense inflammation at the center. Individual papules

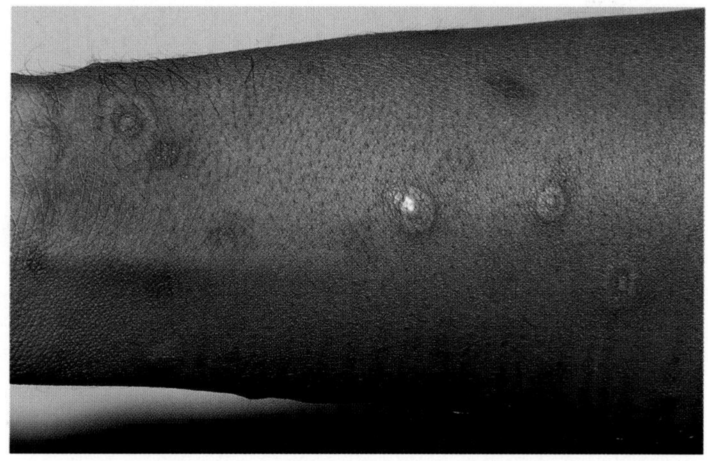

Figure 5.8 This man with erythema multiforme major (Stevens-Johnson syndrome) produced by recurrent herpes labialis exhibits an inflammatory papule with a central blister. As is common in black skin, erythema is not visible in spite of marked edema.

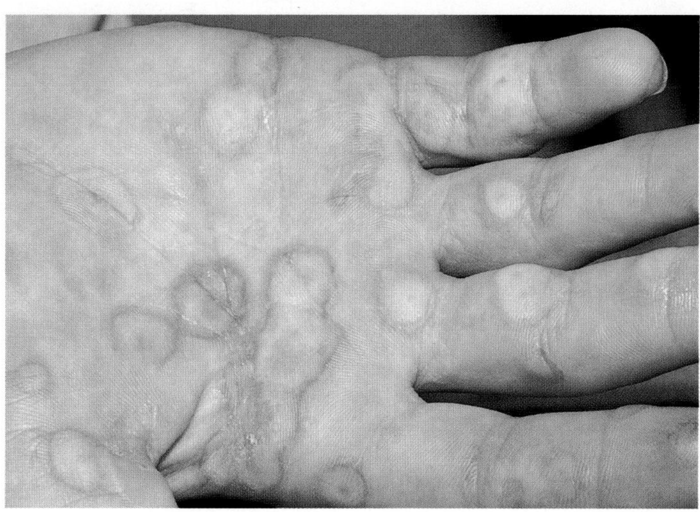

Figure 5.9 The blistering on the palm of this man's hand shows concentric rings that represent different degrees of inflammation and epidermal detachment.

resemble a bull's eye or target in appearance. This eruption, known as erythema multiforme minor, is discussed in Chapter 13. More severe erythema multiforme develops blisters in the most inflammatory center of the papules (Figs. 5.8 and 5.9). This condition, known as bullous erythema multiforme, erythema multiforme major, or Stevens-Johnson syndrome, is associated with erosions of the mucous membranes as well. Toxic epidermal necrolysis (Lyell's type) occurs when erythema multiforme is so extensive that lesions coalesce to produce generalized erythema and large areas of blistering and detached epidermis (Figs. 5.10 and 5.11). Extensive mucous membrane involvement is usual (Fig. 5.12).

Accompanying signs and symptoms largely depend on the severity of blistering. However, the severity of toxicity also depends partly on the patient's baseline status and underlying diseases for which the patient received the allergenic drug.

Differential diagnosis

The differential diagnosis of bullous erythema multiforme includes autoimmune blistering diseases such as pemphigus vulgaris and bullous pemphigoid. However, autoimmune blistering dis-

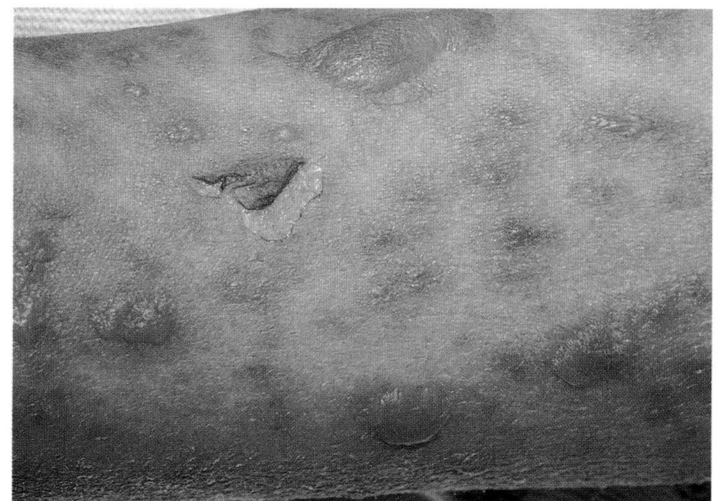

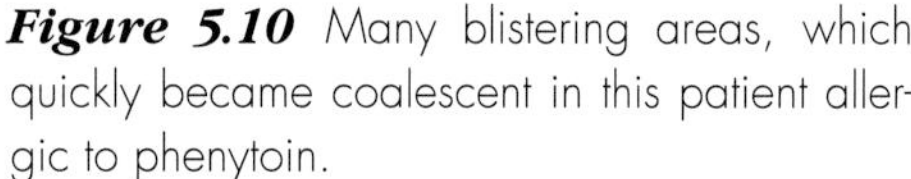

Figure 5.10 Many blistering areas, which quickly became coalescent in this patient allergic to phenytoin.

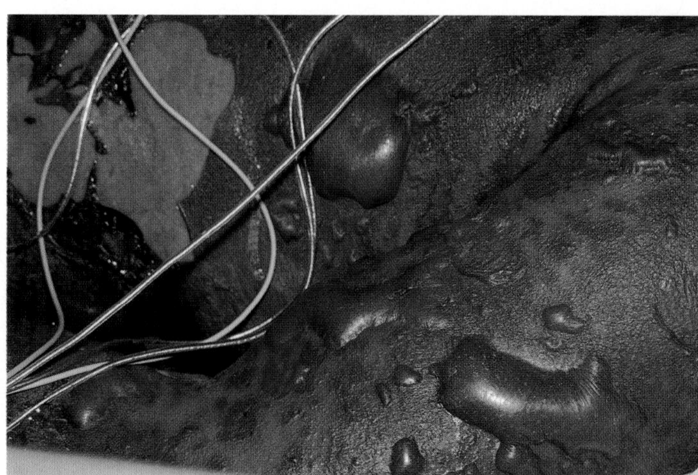

Figure 5.11 Confluent bullae arising from deeply inflamed skin is typical in this 23-year-old man who died from toxic epidermal necrolysis in response to phenytoin and phenobarbital.

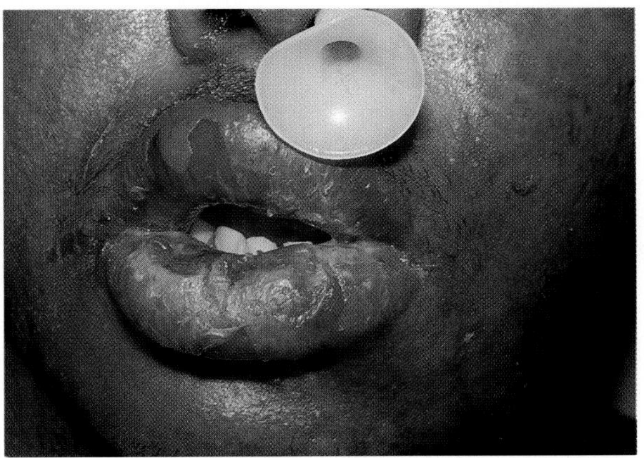

Figure 5.12 Mucous membrane erosions that include both the oral mucosa and the lips are usual in blistering forms of erythema multiforme.

eases are usually slower in onset and lack a history of recent medication exposure. The differentiation of Stevens-Johnson syndrome from bullous pemphigoid can be difficult, since both produce tense blisters and show more well-formed red areas. However, the bullae of bullous pemphigoid are usually larger and arise from both inflamed and noninflamed skin, while the blisters of erythema multiforme major are smaller and are confined to the center of red papules and plaques. Both toxic epidermal necrolysis and pemphigus vulgaris can exhibit large areas of erosion and flaccid blisters, but there are usually areas of normal skin in patients with pemphigus vulgaris, rather than widespread background erythema. Staphylococcal scalded skin syndrome (formerly also called toxic epidermal necrolysis, Ritter type) can resemble drug-induced toxic epidermal necrolysis. However, this occurs almost exclusively in children, mucous membranes are spared, and affected patients usually are not ill. This is primarily because only the most superficial portion of the epidermis is shed.

Even when the diagnosis is relatively secure, patients with toxic epidermal necrolysis should undergo a skin biopsy because of the high mortality associated with this disease and the remarkable difference in management as compared to other blistering diseases.

COMMON MEDICATIONS ASSOCIATED WITH TOXIC EPIDERMAL NECROLYSIS

- Sulfonamides
- Penicillins
- Barbiturates
- Phenytoin
- Carbamazepine
- Allopurinol
- Nonsteroidal anti-inflammatory drugs

Management

The first step in the management of blistering forms of erythema multiforme is the discontinuation of the offending antigen. Although there are uncountable causes of erythema multiforme in general, including infections, Stevens-Johnson syndrome and toxic epidermal necrolysis are usually medication induced, except for the occasional patient who experiences blistering lesions in association with a recurrent herpes simplex virus (HSV) infection.

The medication responsible for the reaction can usually be identified by knowing which medications are especially antigenic, and by examining the time course of the disease in relation to ingestion of the medication. Although nearly every medication is listed in the Physician's Desk Reference having the potential to cause skin rashes, a limited number have a significant association with blistering erythema multiforme.[8] These include the penicillins, cephalosporins, and, especially, sulfa antibiotics. The anticonvulsant drugs phenytoin, carbamazepine, and barbiturates are certainly known to produce bullous erythema multiforme. Allopurinol, hydrochlorothiazide, furosemide, procainamide, quinidine, and NSAIDs should all be considered high-risk medications as well.

Blistering forms of erythema multiforme do not generally occur after many months or years of medication use, but rather within 1 week to 2 months following institution of medication for the first time, or even as early as 1 day for medications that have been previously taken by the patient. Although hypersensitivity reactions do not occur immediately upon the first exposure to an antigen, medications can cross-react, and sometimes patients simply do not remember their first exposure.

Once the causative medication has been discontinued, supportive care becomes the most important therapeutic intervention. Patients with minor blistering generally require only analgesia. However, significant morbidity and mortality due to infection and fluid abnormalities occur with the severe forms of bullous erythema multiforme, just as though these patients had extensive burns. Therefore, scrupulous skin care and attention to infection and fluids are essential. Debridement of necrotic tissue removes this nidus for infection. Many clinicians advocate transferring patients with widespread disease to a burn center.

The use of systemic corticosteroids in these patients is extremely controversial.[9] High-dose intravenous corticosteroid use was once standard therapy for patients with severe blistering as well. However, since infection is a major cause of death in patients with toxic epidermal necrolysis, many now believe that corticosteroids add another, unacceptable, risk factor for infection. Several clinical studies have suggested a poorer outcome in patients treated with corticosteroids.[10,11] However, controlled trials with adequate numbers of patients are impractical and have not been done. The sickest patients are often those who were begun on corticosteroids and, of course, these are the patients with the worst prognosis. Many clinicians, including this author, believe that corticosteroids such as methylprednisolone, 1 g/day, administered very early (within about 48 hours) in the course of the disease can be beneficial.[12,13] Corticosteroids may be useful when the skin is still inflamed, but when many areas have not yet blistered. Because corticosteroids clearly increase complications in late disease, this medication is continued for only 2 or 3 days. Once extensive blistering has occurred, corticosteroids are likely only to add to morbidity.

In addition to general supportive care, local attention to other mucous membrane sites can minimize morbidity in severe disease. For example, careful eye care can often prevent corneal scarring and blindness. Care of the genitalia, particularly the uncircumsized penis and the vagina, can prevent phimosis and vaginal synechiae.

Acute episodes of erythema multiforme major produced by recurrent HSV are often treated with an antiviral medication. Unfortunately, the viral infection precedes the appearance of erythema multiforme, so that the administration of an antiviral agent is generally too delayed to exert a significant beneficial effect. Patients with Stevens-Johnson syndrome associated with recurrent HSV infection should be maintained on a suppressive oral antiviral agent such as chronic acyclovir 400 mg bid, to prevent future episodes.

Other therapies that have been reported, generally as case reports and with variable success, include cyclosporine,[14] plasmapheresis,[15] and hyperbaric oxygen.[16]

BULLOUS ERYTHEMA MULTIFORME (STEVENS-JOHNSON SYNDROME, TOXIC EPIDERMAL NECROLYSIS)

Clinical Manifestations

Sudden onset of painful, red skin with widespread flaccid bullae and erosions; mucosal involvment striking. Patients are often ill, and usually have a history or recent new medication use.

Management in the Emergency Department

1. *Identification and elimination of responsible medication*
2. *Hospital admission; consideration of transfer to burn center*
3. *General supportive care; replacement of fluids, electrolytes, etc.*
4. *Infection control*
5. *Debridement of necrotic skin; wound care*
6. *Careful local care of mucous membranes, especially eyes, genitalia, to prevent late scarring*
7. *Systemic corticosteroids are controversial—read text before using or refusing*

FIXED DRUG ERUPTION

A fixed drug eruption is an interesting and unusual reaction to a medication. One or a few edematous plaques or blisters form in response to a medication. Although individual lesions clinically and histologically resemble erythema multiforme, a fixed drug eruption exhibits many fewer lesions, usually only one or a very few (Fig. 5.13; see also Fig. 13.6). In addition, future challenges with the offending medication produce recurrence of the lesions in the same locations. Deep hyperpigmentation in a sharply demarcated, round shape occurs after multiple episodes of inflammation (see Fig. 11.5). Mucous membrane erosions, including lesions of the oral mucosa, the modified mucous membranes of the vulva, and the glans penis, are common. There are rare reports of generalized disease, with more lesions occurring after each rechallenge of medication.

The most common medications to produce a fixed drug eruption are NSAIDs, salicylates, acetaminophen, barbiturates, penicillins, tetracyclines, sulfas, phenolphthalein, and oral contraceptives. Occasionally, a medication cannot be identified.

In addition to erythema multiforme, a fixed drug eruption can be confused with HSV infection, also characterized by recurrent blistering in the same location. However, HSV infection comprises small, coalescing vesicles and often recurs in the same general rather than exact location. Postinflammatory changes are less dark and well demarcated.

Therapy consists of avoidance of the medication and local care of any erosion.

Figure 5.13 This red papule with a central blister that recurs in this patient repeatedly in the same location in response to tetracycline is typical of a fixed drug eruption. It resembles a lesion of blistering erythema multiforme.

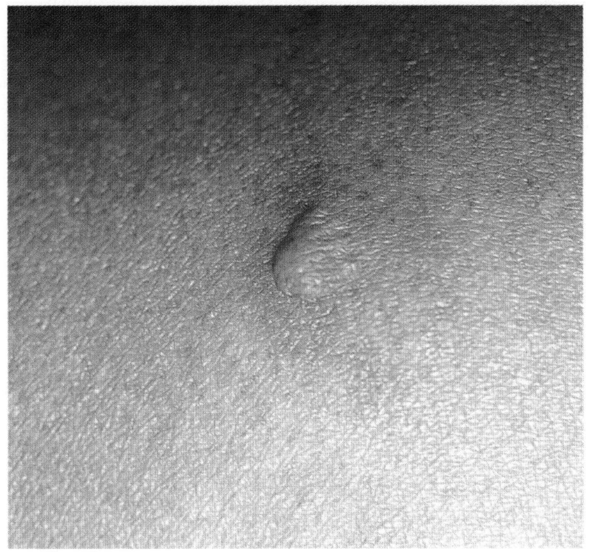

STAPHYLOCOCCAL SCALDED SKIN SYNDROME (SSSS)

Staphylococcal scalded skin syndrome (once also called toxic epidermal necrolysis, Ritter type) produces far less morbidity than occurs with drug-induced toxic epidermal necrolysis. This disease occurs almost exclusively in children and is discussed in Chapter 19.

Detachment of the stratum corneum, the most superficial, dead portion of the epidermis, occurs in response to a toxin produced by some phage types of ***Staphylococcus aureus***. In most cases, the staphylococcal infection is trivial, and the very superficial loss of skin still preserves an epidermis with sufficient barrier function to prevent fluid loss or secondary infection.

Although both staphylococcal scalded skin syndrome and toxic epidermal necrolysis are characterized by large areas of detached skin, patients with the former condition are generally not particularly ill, and they do not have mucous membrane involvement. Also, these patients are nearly always children, and they often lack a history of medication use. Finally, an early, characteristic physical finding in staphylococcal scalded skin syndrome is radial fissuring and crusting around the mouth (Fig. 19.6).

Management consists of identification of the underlying staphylococcal infection, an oral antistaphylococcal antibiotic such as dicloxacillin or cephalexin, and any needed supportive skin care.

STAPHYLOCOCCAL SCALDED SKIN SYNDROME

Clinical Manifestations

Children with radial cracking, crusting around the mouth, and erythematous skin with detachment of very superficial layers. Mucous membrane disease is absent.

Management in the Emergency Department

1. *Oral antistaphylococcal antibiotic*
   - *Cephalexin 50 mg/kg/day, divided qid*
   - *Dicloxacillin 50 mg/kg/day, divided qid*
2. *Local skin care*
3. *If appear ill, admit for fluid therapy and supportive care*

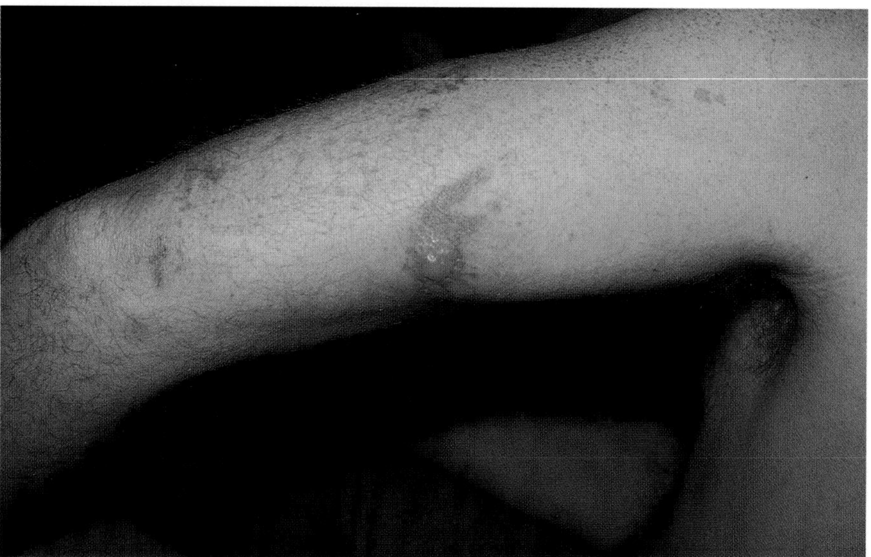

Figure 5.14 The asymmetric and irregular, wiped appearance of the edge of the blister suggest the diagnosis of acute allergic dermatitis to a plant. This pattern of external contact is also suggestive of a chemical or thermal burn.

ACUTE ALLERGIC CONTACT DERMATITIS

Although an acute reaction to a potent allergen such as poison ivy is usually vesicular, the occasional unfortunate patient develops remarkable bullae. This disease is discussed in more detail in Chapter 4.

The most common allergens that produce bullous eruptions are plants such as poison ivy or poison oak. A bullous allergic contact dermatitis is usually manifested clinically by large, intact blisters in the setting of surrounding skin that shows changes more typical of vesicular contact dermatitis (Fig. 5.14). Multiple, small, coalescing vesicles and edematous papules, especially when some are linear, provide clues to the diagnosis.

Management consists of the identification and elimination of the allergen from the skin, as well as avoidance of this allergen in the future. Prednisone at 40 to 60 mg each morning (1 to 2 mg/kg for children) should be given for significant blistering. Those patients with frank bullae should be re-evaluated in 1 week for adjustment of prednisone dosage and institution of a topical corticosteroid—or sooner for signs of infection or extension.

BURNS

A caustic chemical or hot contactant can produce blistering. Generally, patients experience immediate burning and discomfort, so that the diagnosis is often clear. However, children, mentally retarded patients, insensate individuals, and those with altered consiousness due to disease or chemicals may not recognize or be able to relay the history. The clinical appearance usually suggests this diagnosis despite an unhelpful history.

The distribution of burns is usually asymmetric, and the pattern often suggests drips or irregular or characteristic shapes of the contactant (Fig. 19.7). In addition to bullae, erosions are common; sometimes necrotic, but not detached, epithelium produces brown, well-demarcated papules and plaques. Although the clinical appearance of a chemical burn can be identical to that of a thermal burn, a skin biopsy can provide differentiation if important. Therapy consists of local skin care and the prevention of future occurrences.

EDEMA BLISTERS

In the presence of sudden, extreme edema, particularly when the skin is fragile from sun damage or corticosteroid use, noninflammatory bullae may occur. The diagnosis is generally made on the basis of pattern, presence of edema, and, often, other evidence of fragile skin, such as purpura or erosions from adhesive tape. Therapy consists of reduction of edema, often with compression dressings such as an Unna's boot or an elastic wrap, and of local skin care, including keeping the skin moist and free of infection and trauma.

DIABETIC BULLAE

Patients with well-developed diabetes mellitus sometimes develop clear, noninflammatory bullae. These occur primarily over the distal extremities. Some clinicians believe that these occur from injury or pressure in these patients who often exhibit poor sensation due to diabetic neuropathy. Others believe they result from excessive fragility due to damage from microvascular disease.

These blisters can be confused with bullous pemphigoid or porphyria cutanea tarda, another noninflammatory blistering process that occurs over the dorsal hands. The diagnosis can usually be made by the clinical setting but, when necessary, a skin biopsy and a 24-hour urine collection submitted for measurement of uroporphyrins is helpful in ruling out these diseases.

Therapy consists of local skin care, infection control, and protection from future injury.

COMA/PRESSURE BLISTERS

Coma blisters are noninflammatory bullae that occur over areas of pressure, such as the buttocks and heels of patients in a coma, classically but certainly not always induced by barbiturate overdose. These blisters are now believed to be a pressure/ischemia phenomenon. The appearance of noninflammatory blisters over bony prominences in the presence of pressure is a well-known phenomenon, often preceding decubitus ulcers. A skin biopsy of a coma or pressure blister shows detachment of the epidermis from the dermis and characteristic underlying sweat gland necrosis.

The treatment is alleviation of pressure and local care.

REFERENCES

1. Westerhof W: Treatment of bullous pemphigoid with topical clobetasol propionate. J Am Acad Dermatol 20:458, 1989
2. Venning VA, Millard PR, Wojnarowska F: Dapsone as first line therapy for bullous pemphigoid. Br J Dermatol 120:83, 1989
3. Fivenson DP, Breneman DL, Rosen GB, Wander AH: Nicotinamide and tetracycline therapy of bullous pemphigoid. Arch Dermatol 130: 753, 1994
4. Thomas I, Khorenian S, Arbesfeld DN: Treatment of generalized bullous pemphigoid with oral tetracycline. J Am Acad Dermatol 28:74, 1993
5. Lever WF, Talbott JH: Pemphigus. A clinical analysis and follow-up study of sixty-two patients. Arch Dermatol 46:348, 1942
6. Combes FC, Canizares O: Pemphigus vulgaris. A clinicopathological study of one hundred cases. Arch Dermatol 62:786, 1950
7. Gellis S, Glass FA: Pemphigus. A survey of one hundred and seventy six patients admitted to Bellevue Hospital from 1911 to 1941. Arch Dermatol 44:321, 1941
8. Guillaume JC, Roujeau JC, Revuz J et al: The culprit drugs in 87 cases of toxic epidermal necrolysis (Lyell's syndrome). Arch Dermatol 123:1166, 1987
9. Tong P, Mutasim DF: Toxic epidermal necrolysis in the elderly. J Geriatr Dermatol 4:63, 1996
10. Halebian PH, Corder VJ, Madden MR et al: Improved burn center survival of patients with

toxic epidermal necrolysis managed without corticosteroids. Ann Surg 204:503, 1986

11. Nethercott JRF, Choi BCK: Erythema multiforme (Stevens-Johnson syndrome)—chart review of 123 hospitalized patients. Dermatologica 171:597, 1985
12. Fritsch PO, Elias PM: Erythema multiforme and toxic epidermal necrolysis. p. 585. In Fitzpatrick TB, Eisen AZ, Wolff K et al (eds): Dermatology in General Medicine. 4th Ed. McGraw-Hill, New York, 1993
13. Stables GI, Lever RS: Toxic epidermal necrolysis and systemic corticosteroids. Br J Dermatol 128:357, 1993
14. Renfro L, Grant-Kels JM, Daman LA: Drug-induced toxic epidermal necrolysis treated with cyclosporin. Int J Dermatol 28:441, 1989
15. Kamanabroo D, Schmitz-Landgraf W, Czarnetzki BM: Plasmapheresis in severe drug-induced toxic epidermal necrolysis. Arch Dermatol 121: 1548, 1985
16. Ruocco V, Bimonte D, Luongo C et al: Hyperbaric oxygen treatment of toxic epidermal necrolysis. Cutis 38:267, 1986

SUGGESTED READINGS

Bullous and Cicatricial Pemphigoid

Zillikens D, Giudice GJ, Diaz LA: Bullous pemphigoid: an autoimmune blistering disease of the elderly. J Geriatr Dermatol 4:35, 1996

Korman NJ: Bullous pemphigoid. Dermatol Clin 11:483, 1993

Caux FA, Giudice GJ, Diaz LA, Fairley JA: Cicatricial pemphigoid. J Geriatr Dermatol 4:42, 1996

Pemphigus Vulgaris

Korman NJ: Pemphigus vulgaris, pemphigus foliaceus and paraneoplastic pemphigus. J Geriatr Dermatol 4:53, 1996

Toxic Epidermal Necrolysis

Rohrer TE, Ahmed AR: Toxic epidermal necrolysis. Int J Dermatol 30:457, 1991

This detailed review article discusses the causes and differential diagnosis of toxic epidermal necrolysis, including the specifics of supportive and local care.

Tong P, Mutasim DF. Toxic epidermal necrolysis in the elderly. J Geriatr Dermatol 4(2):63, 1996

This article gives an excellent clinical picture of the disease and, especially, a well-researched and -referenced discussion of management of this disease, including the controversy regarding corticosteroid use.

CHAPTER 6

Hemorrhagic Bullous and Necrotic Diseases

Very intense inflammation sometimes damages not only the upper layers of skin but the deep dermis or subcutaneous tissue as well. This can produce overlying blisters with hemorrhage due to ischemia when blood vessels are destroyed, or even from actual necrosis of skin. Several diseases with this deep and intensive inflammation are signs of life-threatening disease.

NECROTIZING FASCIITIS AND OTHER NECROTIZING SUBCUTANEOUS INFECTIONS

Necrotizing soft tissue infections are life-threatening, often rapidly progressive infections characterized by tissue necrosis. Necrotizing fasciitis, gas gangrene, hemolytic streptococcal gangrene, anaerobic gangrene, and necrotizing myositis are common terms, depending on the tissues involved and the causative organisms. However, differentiation among these closely related diseases is often difficult and, when necrosis is present, immediate therapy is imperative and similar. The term *necrotizing fasciitis* is used in this chapter to refer to this group of necrotizing deep soft tissue infections.

Necrotizing fasciitis is a rapidly life-threatening bacterial infection that occurs more often in immunosuppressed patients or after an injury. Most common over extremities, the genitalia are also often involved, in which case the condition is called *Fournier's gangrene*. Abdominal infection sometimes occurs, especially in immunosuppressed patients, apparently as a result of intestinal seeding. Although *Streptococcus pyogenes* often produces this infection, the process usually becomes polymicrobial as necrosis extends. One study of 30 patients found 79% of patients with at least one gram-positive organism, and 73% of patients with gram-negative bacilli.[1]

Clinical Manifestations

Deep bacterial infections can extend along fascial planes, producing not only the erythema, induration, and inflammation characteristic of cellulitis, but also destruction and necrosis of blood vessels. As these vessels are destroyed, blood flow is interrupted, resulting in ischemia of overlying and surrounding structures. The first clinical signs are nonspecific edema and erythema, but extreme pain and pallor or grayish discoloration develop. Anesthesia, purpura, and hemorrhagic bullae are later, grave signs (Figs. 6.1 to 6.3). Because the infection is extending, often rapidly, along fascial planes, overlying skin changes often lag behind the progressing, underlying infection. Thus, serious infection often extends far beyond apparent borders. Also, surface changes may not be contiguous, as bullae filled with blood can be scattered across skin that is apparently otherwise normal.

Patients are generally toxic, often out of proportion to their skin findings. Abnormal body temperatures, hypotension, and confusion are common. The process is often frighteningly rapid, progressing over hours. As deep ischemia progresses, anaerobic bacteria may thrive.

Differential Diagnosis

The diseases most often difficult to differentiate from necrotizing fasciitis are cellulitis and other

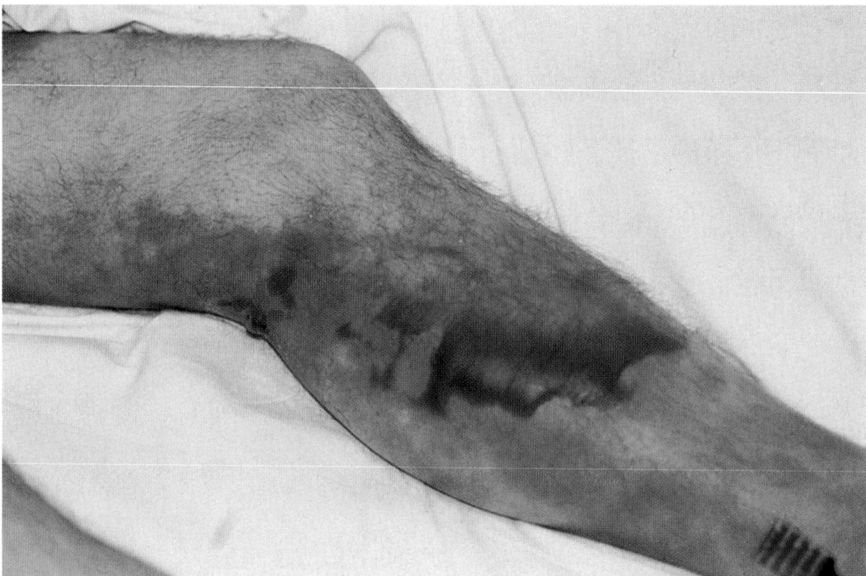

Figure 6.1 Extensive hemorrhagic blistering that progressed over hours in an edematous limb in this hypotensive, toxic patient was typical for necrotizing fasciitis. This patient, who was found to be HIV positive, survived following amputation.

Figure 6.2 Beginning as a painful pustule on the dorsum of the hand one evening, this infection progressed to involve the whole arm within 24 hours. This woman, who was on low doses of prednisone for rheumatoid arthritis, did not survive her necrotizing fasciitis.

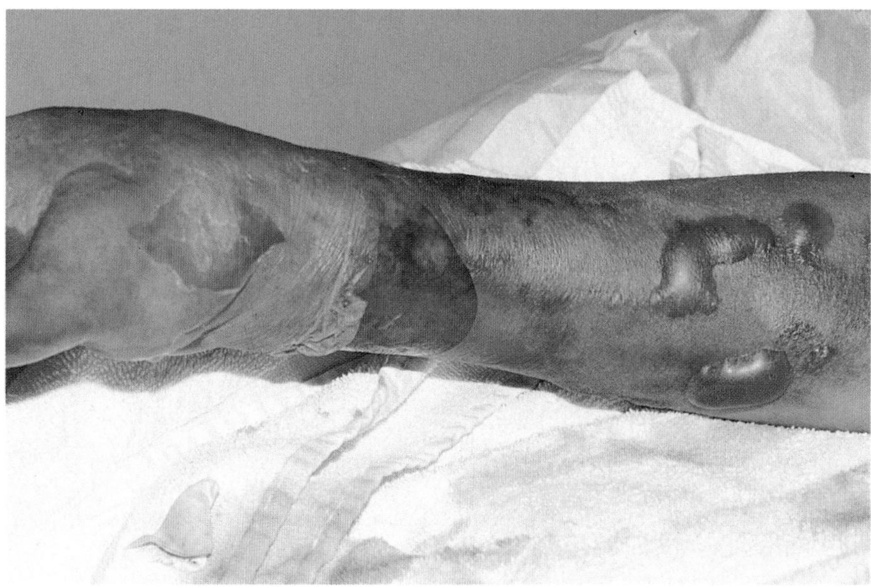

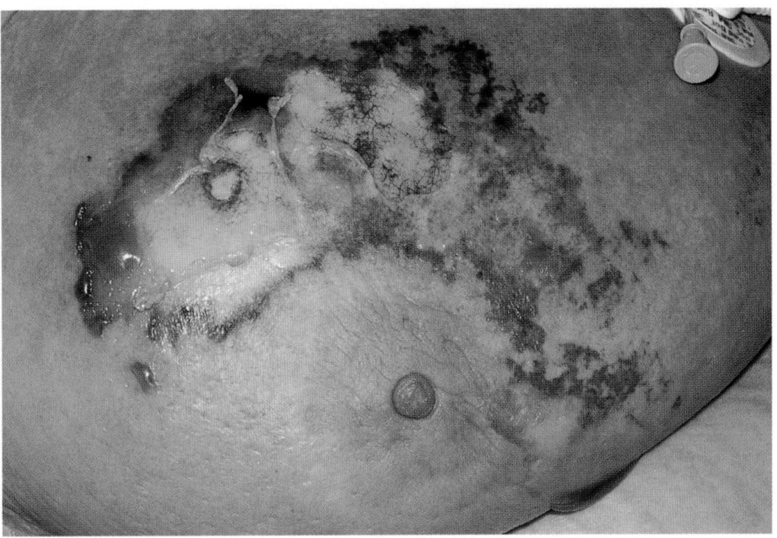

Figure 6.3 This necrotizing fasciitis is manifested by hemorrhage, necrosis, and blistering.

non-necrotizing soft tissue infections. In fact, these tissue infections exist along a spectrum and cannot always be distinguished morphologically. Cellulitis generally lacks blistering and hemorrhage. Patients with these findings should be investigated immediately for the presence of deep necrosis.

Other diseases to be differentiated from necrotizing fasciitis include polyarteritis nodosa, in which similar overlying changes occur after autoimmune destruction of muscular arteries of the upper dermis or subcutaneous fat. However, although this condition can be life-threatening if arteries to other organs are affected, it is rarely rapidly progressive, and patients generally are not toxic. Bullous pyoderma gangrenosum (which is neither gangrene nor a pyoderma) is a necrotic, purpuric eruption that occurs as a response to intense sterile inflammation, usually in association with myeloproliferative processes. This condition is more chronic, and patients are less ill than those with necrotizing fasciitis, unless they are toxic from their underlying disease. Although brown recluse spider bites and rattlesnake bites can sometimes produce similar-appearing lesions, the history is usually helpful—particularly in the case of snake bites—and the relative lack of systemic toxicity usually rules out necrotizing fasciitis in that situation.

Management

Patients with suspected necrotizing fasciitis require emergent evaluation. A soft tissue radiograph of the area to detect gas can be performed, but negative results do not rule out this disease. An immediate incision to visualize the infected area of fascia or muscle should be performed; some investigators believe that this can be done at the bedside.[1] In those with necrotizing fasciitis, a stab incision to fascia reveals soft, necrotic tissue rather than the edematous, inflamed tissue of cellulitis. Another quick approach that has proved useful is an incisional biopsy interpreted immediately by frozen-section technique.[2]

Therapy for necrotizing fasciitis consists of aggressive surgical debridement and antibiotics. Antibiotics alone do not stop this process, because the blood vessels, which have been destroyed, no longer supply the blood that would carry such medications to the affected areas. Therefore, extensive removal of necrotic areas is essential. Because the necrotic area generally extends significantly beyond the areas that appear abnormal from the surface, debridement is often much more extensive than one would expect.

The choice of antibiotics takes into consideration the polymicrobial nature of the infection, as well as the frequent presence of anaerobic organisms. Intravenous penicillin G, 1 to 2 million units, in combination with clindamycin 600 mg every 6 to 8 hours is standard.[1,3,4] Depending on Gram stain results, an aminoglycoside, chloramphenicol, a third-generation cephalosporin, or ciprofloxacin should be added as well.[3,4]

Course and Prognosis

The course of necrotizing fasciitis and other necrotizing subcutaneous infections is variable. Classically, necrosis progresses over a period of hours in a toxic patient, with death occurring quickly in the absence of prompt recognition, surgical intervention, antibiotics, and aggressive supportive care. However, necrotizing fasciitis exists on a spectrum with severe cellulitis. Occasionally, especially when antibiotics are begun very early in the course of infection, necrotizing fasciitis misdiagnosed as cellulitis can be indolent and controlled with antibiotics. It is likely that such cases account for some of those patients with cellulitis who appear to respond poorly to antibiotics. This occasional occurrence should not give the clinician a false sense of security that watching and waiting is an option. The survival of a patient with serious necrotizing fasciitis depends on very early suspicion for the presence of this disease coupled with diagnosis and management. An hour can make the difference between survival and death.

NECROTIZING FASCIITIS

Clinical Manifestations

Toxic patient with sudden onset of pain, and rapid progression of ischemic skin, and blistering with hemorrhage.

Management in the Emergency Department

1. *Immediate surgical exploration and debridement of necrotic tissue*
2. *Intravenous administration of broad specrum antibiotics*
3. *Supportive care with fluids, pressors, and so forth*

VASCULITIS

Vasculitis refers to intense inflammation of blood vessels. When inflammation is sufficient to destroy the vessel, distal ischemia, hemorrhage, and necrosis can occur.

Polyarteritis nodosa

Polyarteritis nodosa is an autoimmune disease that results in neutrophilic destruction of the small and medium arteries of the deep dermis or subcutaneous fat. The inflammation produces one or several large nodules, sometimes with an overlying hemorrhagic blister, or eventually a necrotic, indurated mass as a result of ischemia. With these larger vessels involved, associated livido reticularis is common (Figs. 6.4 and 6.5). This reticulate, netlike dusky erythema is a sign of deep vasculitis. The lacy pattern is produced by alternating areas

Figure 6.4 Hemorrhagic blistering and necrosis of polyarteritis nodosa often occurs in association with surrounding dusky, irregular, and reticulate erythema, known as livido reticularis.

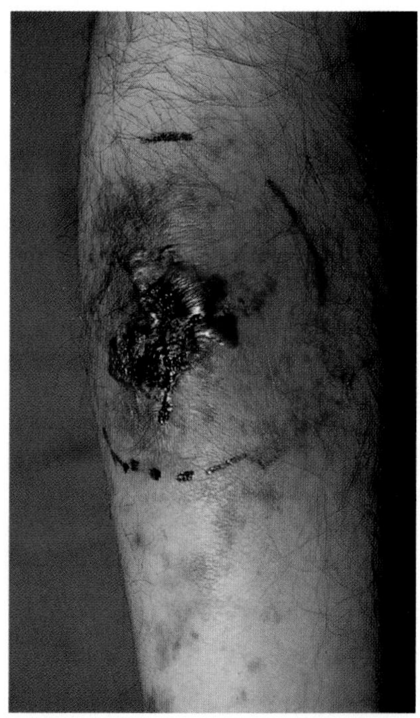

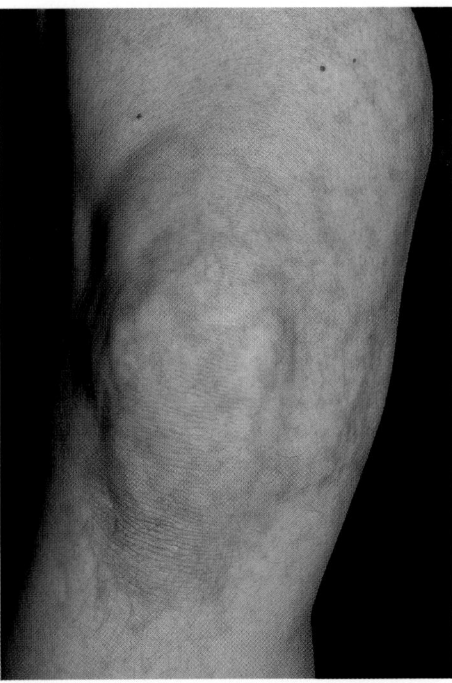

Figure 6.5 Livido reticularis is a nonspecific sign of deep vasculitis; it can be associated with other collagen vascular diseases, as well as polyarteritis nodosa. Physiologic livido, produced by vasomotor instability, can mimic this condition.

of ischemia and normal vascularity, where collateral vessels provide adequate blood supply. Patients often exhibit associated fever, weight loss, and weakness.

Although polyarteritis nodosa is sometimes limited to the skin, most patients experience systemic involvement, with renal disease and peripheral neuropathy most common. However, coronary arteritis, abdominal pain due to gastrointestinal involvement, and joint signs and symptoms are also frequent occurrences.

The differential diagnosis of the hemorrhagic, blistering cutaneous lesions of polyarteritis nodosa includes necrotizing fasciitis, bullous pyoderma gangrenosum, and brown recluse spider bites, as discussed for necrotizing fasciitis. The diagnosis is made by an incisional biopsy well into fat.

Management consists of an evaluation for systemic disease. Systemic corticosteriods, often in combination with immunosuppressive medications such as azathioprine or cyclophosphamide, are required for systemic disease or severe cutaneous disease.[5–7]

Leukocytoclastic Vasculitis

Far more common than polyarteritis nodosa is leukocytoclastic vasculitis of the small vessels. In this case, there are generally multiple, much smaller lesions. Most often, leukocytoclastic vasculitis is manifested by palpable purpura (Figs. 13.9 and 13.10; see Ch. 13: Vascular Reactions and Other Flat-topped, Nonscaling Patches and Plaques). Sometimes, however, more severe disease and larger affected blood vessels produce purpuric papules with overlying blisters or erosions (Figs. 6.6 and 6.7). With more chronic disease, ulcerations with violaceous, sharply demarcated borders appear.

Most often, patients do not appear acutely ill. The lower legs are the most common location for

Figure 6.6 Palpable purpura of leukocytoclastic vasculitis is quickly followed in some patients by superimposed hemorrhagic blisters, especially common over the lower legs.

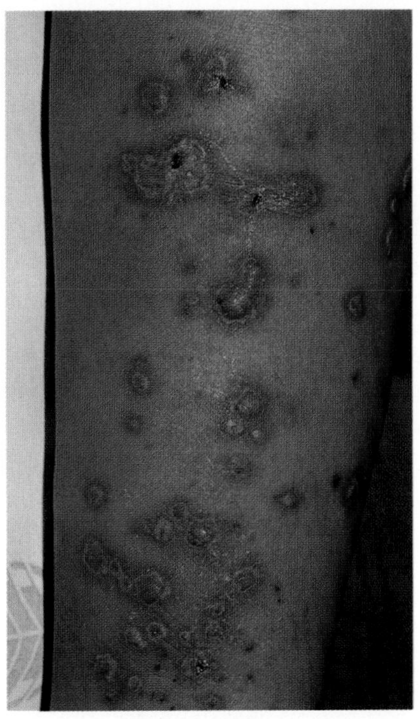

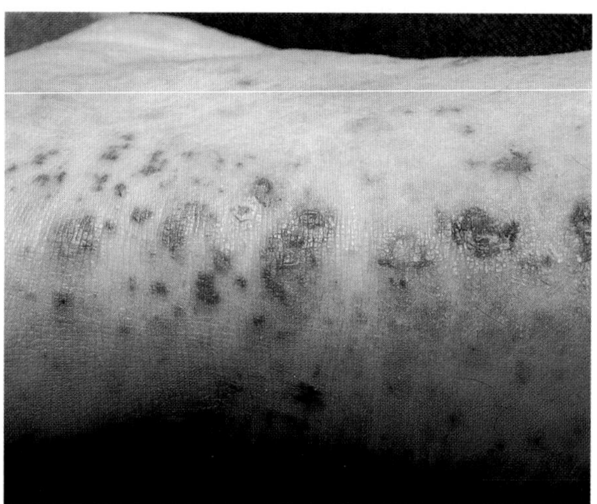

Figure 6.7 Typical hemorrhage and blistering of smaller vessel leukocytoclastic vasculitis.

leukocytoclastic vasculitis, but skin lesions can occur anywhere.

The differential diagnosis for the multiple smaller hemorrhagic blisters of leukocytoclastic vasculitis includes septic vasculitis and, sometimes, emboli. The diagnosis is made by a punch skin biopsy of a fresh lesion and the elimination of sepsis, either clinically or by culture.

Management of this condition includes the identification and elimination of the underlying cause and an evaluation for visceral involvement. Leukocytoclastic vasculitis can occur as an immune response to medication or as a reaction to infection. Other causes include autoimmune diseases such as lupus erythematosus and rheumatoid arthritis. Myelodysplastic diseases and dysproteinemias also generate inappropriate antibodies that may produce leukocytoclastic vasculitis. Often, the underlying cause is not recognized (for a detailed discussion of the causes of vasculitis, see Ch. 13).

An evaluation for systemic involvement includes a survey of those organs that are most often affected: the kidneys, manifested by hematuria and later by an elevated creatinine; the gastrointestinal tract, manifested by abdominal discomfort or hematochezia; and joints, manifested by symptoms or signs of arthritis. Pulmonary, cardiac, or central nervous system involvement can be assessed briefly by a review of systems and physical examination, with radiographs or electrocardiograms if indicated.

The third aspect of management includes treatment of the vasculitis itself. Most patients who have blistering and necrosis on the basis of leukocytoclastic vasculitis require systemic steriods, and this is absolutely true of any patient with systemic involvement. These patients deserve same-day evaluation by a rheumatologist or a dermatologist and institution of oral prednisone 40 to 60 mg each morning, or intravenous therapy at a higher dose for seriously ill patients.

Chronic disease can sometimes be controlled with oral dapsone, colchicine or, for severe disease, immunosuppressive medications.[8,9]

Other Vasculitis

Any form of vasculitis, in which intense inflammation around vessels interrupts blood flow, can produce necrotic, hemorrhagic cutaneous disease. This includes a host of uncommon diseases, classified according to type of inflammation (e.g., granulomatous, neutrophilic) and associated systemic findings.[10]

LEUKOCYTOCLASTIC VASCULITIS

Clinical Manifestations

Palpable purpura, especially over the lower legs; overlying hemorrhagic blisters may occur. The size of the lesions corresponds to the size of the affected vessels.

Management in the Emergency Department

1. *Confirm diagnosis with an incisional biopsy to fat of fresh lesion*
2. *Identify and eliminate antigen when possible (e.g., discontinue drug, treat infection)*
3. *Screen for systemic involvement with a urinalysis, stool guaiac, creatinine, and careful physical examination directed toward joint, gastrointestinal, pulmonary, and neurological abnormalities*
4. *Prednisone 40 to 60 mg/day for systemic involvement or severe skin disease*
5. *Immediate referral to a dermatologist or rheumatologist for further evaluation and ongoing care*

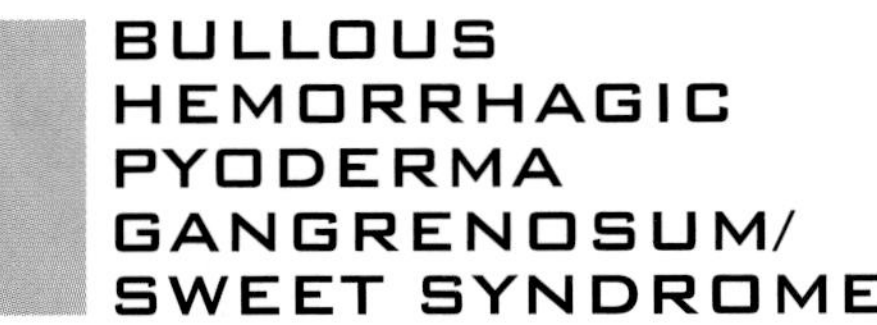

BULLOUS HEMORRHAGIC PYODERMA GANGRENOSUM/ SWEET SYNDROME

Pyoderma gangrenosum (neither a pyoderma nor gangrene) and Sweet syndrome are closely related, noninfectious diseases, exhibited histologically as a dense infiltration of polymorphonuclear leukocytes in the skin. These diseases occur in response to any of several chronic inflammatory diseases or myeloproliferative processes. Although classic pyoderma gangrenosum consists clinically of an undermined ulceration with clean, purple borders (see Ch. 17), and typical Sweet syndrome is manifested by red, edematous papules, both diseases can present as infiltrated, hemorrhagic, and necrotic bullae. This morphology is generally associated with myelodysplastic disease.

Patients exhibit edematous, purpuric plaques or nodules, generally with at least some blistering and, as lesions age, necrosis and ulceration (Fig. 6.8). These often resemble infections ("pyoderma") or even necrotizing fasciitis. Patients with bullous pyoderma gangrenosum and Sweet syndrome may be ill, but these diseases are usually more indolent, with more longlasting skin lesions and much less toxicity. In very ill patients, immediate surgical exploration to rule out necrotizing fasciitis is indicated. Otherwise, a tissue biopsy should be performed both for a histologic examination and for culture. Infection must be eliminated as a cause, especially because therapy for pyoderma gangrenosum and Sweet syndrome consists of systemic corticosteriods. Brown recluse spider bites and hemorrhagic leukocytoclastic vasculitis are other diseases that resemble these conditions.

Therapy consists of an evaluation for myelodysplastic diseases and, when none is found, patient education regarding the likely later development of one of these diseases. Otherwise, systemic corticosteriods, beginning at a dose of 40 to 60 mg/day until healing is established is usual and the only therapy that predictably heals pyoderma gangrenosum/Sweet syndrome.[11] Medication is then tapered. For those with chronic disease, sulfas including dapsone are sometimes useful thereby avoiding the side effects of corticosteriods.[12] Other reported therapies include clofazimine, minocycline, immunosuppressive agents such as azathioprine and cyclophosphamide, and cyclosporine. Plasma exchange, intravenous γ-globulin and hyperbaric oxygen have also been used.[13]

BULLOUS PYODERMA GANGRENOSUM/ SWEET SYNDROME

Clinical Manifestations

Infiltrated, hemorrhagic plaques often with surface blistering, and necrosis and ulceration occurring as surface erodes.

(Continues)

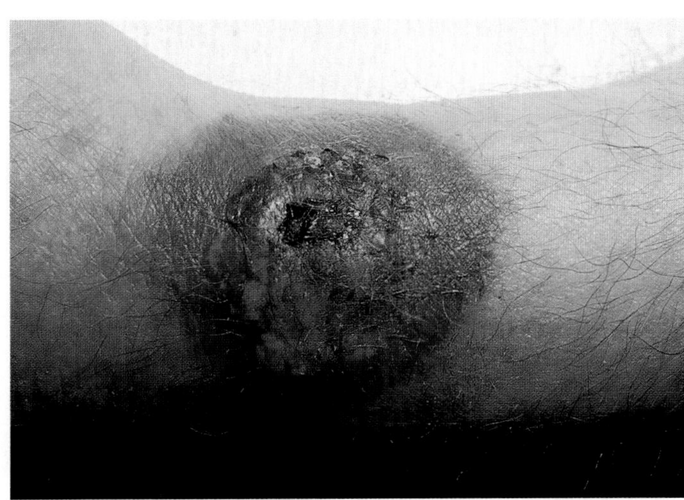

Figure 6.8 Indolent, hemorrhagic blistering and infiltrated, necrotic plaques occur with pyoderma gangrenosum and Sweet syndrome when associated with myeloproliferative diseases.

(Continued)

Management in the Emergency Department

1. *Incisional biopsy for routine histology and for cultures to rule out infection*
2. *If infection is ruled out (which will rarely occur in the emergency department) patients should receive prednisone 40 to 60 mg each morning until healing begins*
3. *Follow-up evaluation, immediately with a dermatologist*

BROWN RECLUSE SPIDER BITE

Occurring primarily in those who have recently been in dusty attics, old garages, or other areas likely to have spiders, brown recluse spider bites are usually single and because the initial bite is painless, there is often no history of a recognized spider bite.

Signs of a spider bite can occur as early as 2 hours after a severe bite, but often symptoms are not noticed until the next day. The skin lesion begins as a painful area of erythema and edema. This is often followed by the development of a small vesicle or pustule that may become hemorrhagic and bullous (Figs. 6.9 and 6.10), after which a necrotic eschar may ensue. The purpura associated with a brown recluse spider bite can occur simply from necrosis or as a result of disseminated intravascular coagulation, which occasionally ensues with these spider bites. Ulcers may occur at the site of the bite, reaching sizes as large as 25 cm in diameter.

Other diseases that can mimic a brown recluse spider bite include a local cellulitis, a localized area of necrotizing fasciitis, and bullous pyoderma gangrenosum. Leukocytoclastic vasculitis and pit viper snake bite can usually be differentiated from brown recluse spider bites by the multiple lesions of the former and the extensive areas involved in some pit viper snake bites.

Therapy for brown recluse spider bites has undergone considerable evolution. Extensive debridement of the involved area was abandoned long ago and, despite some use of systemic corticosteroids, there is no evidence to suggest that this is beneficial. Ice, elevation, analgesia, and treatment of any suspected superinfection can make patients more comfortable. Oral dapsone beginning at 25 mg bid has been reported useful, but this medication must be used with great care because of the usual hemolysis of about 2 g hemoglobin and the uncommon occurrence of bone marrow failure[13] (see Ch. 3). Hyperbaric oxygen has been shown to be beneficial, but this treatment must be instituted early and is quite expensive.

The course and prognosis of a brown recluse spider bite are extremely variable, depending on the variety of spider as well as the size of the inoculum. The aggressiveness of therapy must be individualized according to the known toxic potential of spiders in the area and the appearance of the site. Some bites never ulcerate, and others eventuate in large ulcers that require prolonged healing times.

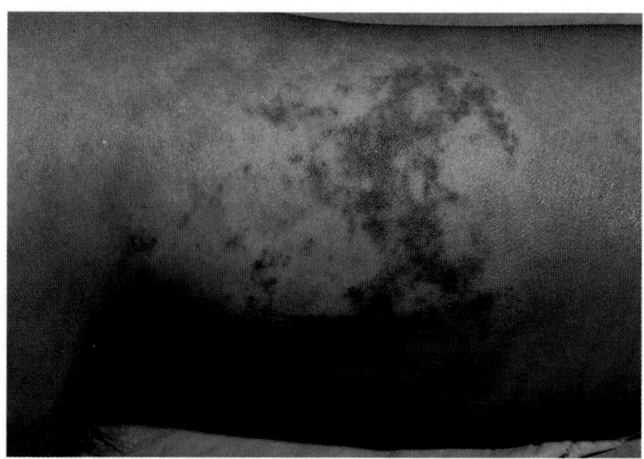

Figure 6.9 Brown recluse spider bites range from erythematous plaques, to small plaques with central ischemia and purpura, to extensive disease.

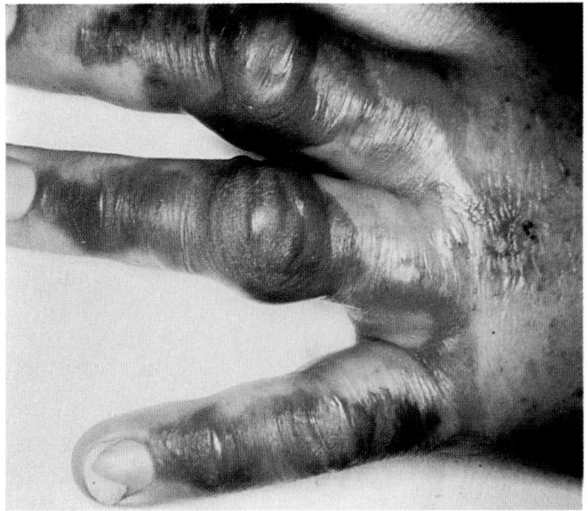

Figure 6.10 Severe brown recluse spider bites produce profound necrosis with resulting hemorrhagic blistering or ulceration, or both. (Courtesy of Charles Reaves, MD)

BROWN RECLUSE SPIDER BITES

Clinical Manifestations

Enlarging red papule or plaque with central punctum or ischemia with hemorrhage; more severe bites developing central necrosis or blistering.

(Continues)

(Continued)

Management in the Emergency Department

1. *Local care and pain control*
2. *Dapsone 25 mg PO bid for significant bites, with baseline complete blood count*
3. *Consider hyperbaric oxygen for severe disease*
4. *Follow-up evaluation in 1 to 2 days, with regular health care provider, to check the site and monitor dapsone if applicable*

PIT VIPER SNAKE BITES

Pit viper snake bites are the most common poisonous snake bite in the United States. Pit vipers include rattlesnakes, copperheads, and water moccasins. Bites from these snakes that result in significant envenomation produce almost immediate pain, edema, purpura, and lymphadenopathy. Bleeding from mucous membrane sites can follow, as well as local edema, hemorrhage, and necrosis, resulting in blistering (Fig. 6.11). Usually, the diagnosis is obvious, since all but the most impaired patients remember having sustained a snake bite, and there are usually marks from the bite. Patients also show local and systemic signs such as paresthesias, numbness, muscle fasciculation, weakness, nausea, hypotension, and a coagulopathy. Severe disease includes renal failure, shock, and death.

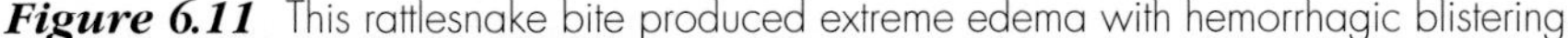

Figure 6.11 This rattlesnake bite produced extreme edema with hemorrhagic blistering.

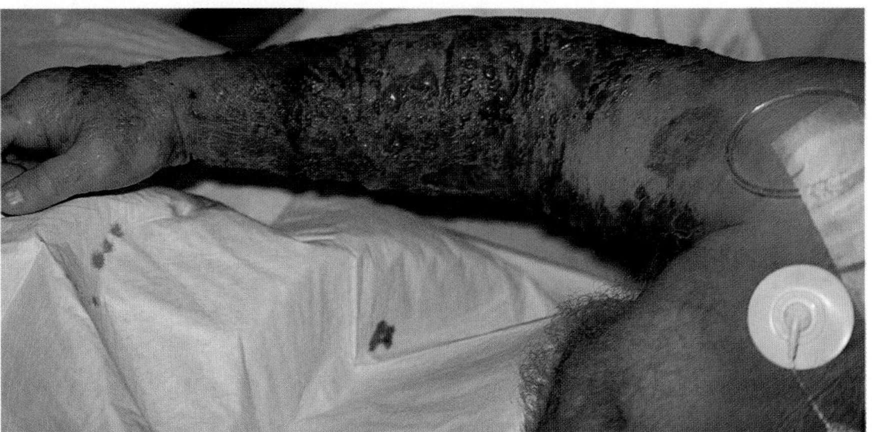

The management of a pit viper snake bite consists of the administration of polyvalent pit viper antivenin in those patients believed to have received significant envenomation. Patients without significant signs within 8 hours can be assumed to be free of envenomation. Otherwise, local wound care is indicated. Fasciotomies are to be avoided, if at all possible. The Antivenin Index, which can be reached at (520) 626–6016, is available 24 hr day to issue advice regarding snake bites.[14]

> **PIT VIPER SNAKE BITES**
>
> ***Clinical Manifestations***
>
> *Pain, edema, purpura, and lymphadenopathy in a patient with a history of a snake bite; with more severe envenomation associated with systemic signs such as paresthesias, numbness, muscle fasciculation, weakness, nausea, hypotension, and a coagulopathy. Usually two fang marks present.*
>
> ***Management in the Emergency Department***
>
> 1. *Local care and observation in the absence of signs of envenomation*
> 2. *Antivenin for those with signs of significant envenomation. For details, call The Antivenin Index, at (520) 626-6016*

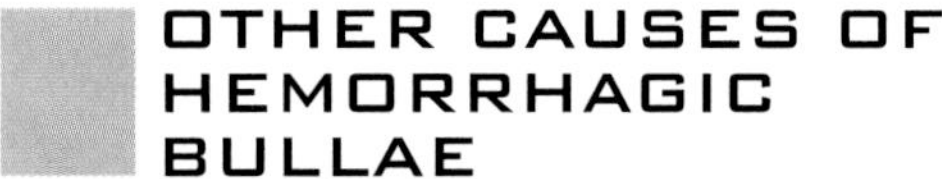

OTHER CAUSES OF HEMORRHAGIC BULLAE

Herpes Zoster

Herpes zoster sometimes exhibits hemorrhage into otherwise typical blisters of shingles. This diagnosis is usually evident by the dermatomal pattern and other typical features of the clinical presentation and setting.

Trauma

Trauma produced by friction, electrical burns, or extreme heat can cause blisters with enough underlying damage to produce hemorrhage. A history of injury and the pattern of the blisters usually makes this diagnosis clear.

REFERENCES

1. Sudarsky LA, Laschinger JC, Coppa GF, Spence FC: Improved results from a standardized approach in treating patients with necrotizing fasciitis. Ann Surg 206:661, 1987
2. Stamenkovic I, Lew DP: Early recognition of potentially fatal necrotizing fasciitis: the use of frozen section biopsy. N Engl J Med 310:1689, 1984
3. Swartz MA: Celllulitis and subcutaneous tissue infections. p. 909. In Mandell GL, Bennett JE, Dolin R (eds): Principles and Practice of Infectious Diseases. 4th Ed. Churchill Livingstone, New York, 1995
4. Stevens DL, Maier KA, Laine BM et al: Comparison of clindamycin, rifampin, tetracycline, and metronidazole, and penicillin for efficacy in prevention of experimental gas gangrene due to *Clostridium perfringens*. J Infect Dis 155:220, 1987
5. Cohen RD, Conn DL, Ilstrup DM: Clinical features, prognosis and response to treatment in polyarteritis nodosa. Mayo Clin Proc 55:146, 1980
6. Fauci AS, Doppman JL, Wolff SM: Cyclophosphamide-induced remissions in advanced polyarteritis nodosa. Am J Med 64:890, 1978
7. Leib ES, Restivo C, Paulus HE: Immunosuppressive and corticosteroid therapy of polyarteritis nodosa. Am J Med 67:941, 1979
8. Callen JP: Colchicine is effective in controlling chronic cutaneous leukocytoclastic vasculitis. J Am Acad Dermatol 13:193, 1985
9. Fauci AS, Katz P, Haynes BF, Wolff SM: Cyclophosphamide therapy of severe systemic necrotizing vasculitis. N Engl J Med 301:235, 1979
10. Hunder GG, Arend WP, Bloch DA et al: The American College of Rheumatology 1990 criteria for the classification of vasculitis. Arthritis Rheum 33:1065, 1990

11. Stingl G et al: Pyoderma gangrenosum. Hautarzt 32:165, 1981
12. Wolff K, Stingl G: Pyoderma gangrenosum. p. 1171. In Fitzpatrick TB, Eisen AZ, Wolff K, Freedberg IM, Austen KF (eds): Dermatology in General Medicine. 4th Ed. McGraw-Hill, New York, 1993
13. Chow RK, Ho VC: Treatment of pyoderma gangrenosum. J Acad Dermatol 36:1047, 1996
14. Skinner RB Jr, Baselski V: Bites, stings, and toxins. p. 189. In Sams WM Jr, Lynch PJ (eds): Principles and Practice of Dermatology. 2nd Ed. Churchill Livingstone, New York, 1996

SUGGESTED READINGS

Necrotizing Infections

Stamenkovic I, Lew DP: Early recognition of potentially fatal necrotizing fasciitis: The use of frozen section biopsy. N Engl J Med 310:1689, 1984

Swartz MA: Cellulitis and subcutaneous tissue infections. p. 909. In Mandell GL, Bennett JE, Dolin R (eds): Principles and Practice of Infectious Diseases. 4th Ed. Churchill Livingstone, New York, 1995

Swartz MA: Myositis. p. 929. In Mandell GL, Bennett JE, Dolin R (eds): Principles and Practice of Infectious Diseases. 4th Ed. Churchill Livingstone, New York, 1995

Vasculitis

Cohen RD, Conn DL, Ilstrup DM: Review of 53 patients with polyarteritis nodosa. Mayo Clin Proc 55:46, 1980

Fauci AS, Haynes BF, Katz P: The spectrum of vasculitis. Ann Intern Med 89:660, 1978

Hunder GG, Arend WP, Bloch DA: The American College of Rheumatology 1990 criteria for the classification of vasculitis. Arthritis Rheum 33:1065, 1990

Pyoderma Gangrenosum/Sweet Syndrome

Chow RK, Ho VC: Treatment of pyoderma gangrenosum. J Acad Dermatol 36:1047, 1996

Koester G, Tarnower A, Levisohn D, Burgdorf W: Bullous pyoderma gangrenosum. J Am Acad Dermatol 29:875–878, 1993

Brown Recluse Spider Bites

Ingber A, Trattner A, Cleper R, Sandbank M: Morbidity of brown recluse spider bites. Acta Derm Venereol (Stockh) 71:337, 1991

King LE, Rees RS: Treatment of brown recluse spider bites. J Am Acad Dermatol 14:691, 1986

Pit Viper Snake Bites

Forks TP: Evaluation and treatment of poisonous snakebites. Am Fam Physician 50:123, 1994

Gold BS, Barish RA: Venomous snakebites. Current concepts in diagnosis, treatment and management. Emerg Med Clin North Am 10:249, 1992

CHAPTER 7

Pustular Diseases

Pustules are blisters filled with inflammatory cells. In general, we think of pustules as being infections, but pustules can also occur as a result of noninfectious inflammation, as with acne or a foreign body (e.g., a splinter).

In addition to true pustules, occasionally skin lesions appear pustular when a substance other than pus is present. For example, molluscum contagiosum and milia, or small epidermal cysts, can appear pustular. These usually have a white appearance rather than yellow (for a detailed discussion, see Ch. 9, White Lesions).

Finally, any blister can become secondarily pustular in appearance after several days, simply from recruitment of white blood cells (WBCs) by the nonspecific inflammation of separation of the skin. Therefore, vesicular diseases should be considered in the differential diagnosis of pustular diseases, but usually at least some vesicles will be present. Also, the fluid in these vesicles cum pustules is usually thin, rather than creamy, thick pus.

FOLLICULITIS

Folliculitis refers to inflammation of the follicle, most often produced by an infection within the follicular epithelium. Folliculitis has a variety of causes.

Staphylococcal Folliculitis

The vast majority of bacterial folliculitis is produced by *Staphylococcus aureus.* Although folliculitis occurs in patients of all ages, both genders, and in people with and without other skin disease, staphylococcal folliculitis is an especially common complication of atopic dermatitis. *S. aureus* is a common colonizer of scaling skin, and the ongoing trauma of rubbing and scratching provides ample opportunity for infection. In addition, folliculitis is often pruritic and can worsen or perpetuate atopic dermatitis. Some patients perceive the inflammation of staphylococcal folliculitis as pain.

Staphylococcal folliculitis presents as red, scattered, follicular papules that later develop into pustules, followed by a crust (Fig. 7.1). The red flare surrounding the central pustule or papule may be relatively large, with the diameter often reaching 1 cm or more, as compared to acne or sterile folliculitis. Patients with staphylococcal folliculitis often exhibit one or more deeper nodules of furunculosis.

The differential diagnosis includes acne, which can usually be differentiated by its distribution over the face, back, and chest, as well as by the presence of comedones (blackheads and whiteheads). Fungal folliculitis normally occurs within a plaque of tinea rather than being evenly scattered over otherwise relatively normal skin. Sterile folliculitis is a more difficult disease to differentiate, but it tends to exhibit less pruritus or pain, a less remarkable surrounding flare of erythema, and cultures are negative except for normal skin organisms. Insect bites often mimic staphylococcal folliculitis, but the distribution, history, and lack of any pustules make differentiation relatively easy.

The treatment of staphylococcal folliculitis is an oral antistaphylococcal agent. Although occasionally mupirocin (Bactroban) ointment can be useful, folliculitis is usually too generalized for this treatment to be practical. Common medications used to treat this disease include cephalexin, dicloxacillin, or erythromycin (in areas where the organism is usually sensitive) at 500 mg bid until the eruption has disappeared, usually about 2 weeks.

Staphylococcal folliculitis usually responds very quickly to medication. However, a significant number of patients exhibit nasopharyngeal carriage, and folliculitis tends to recur when antibiotics are

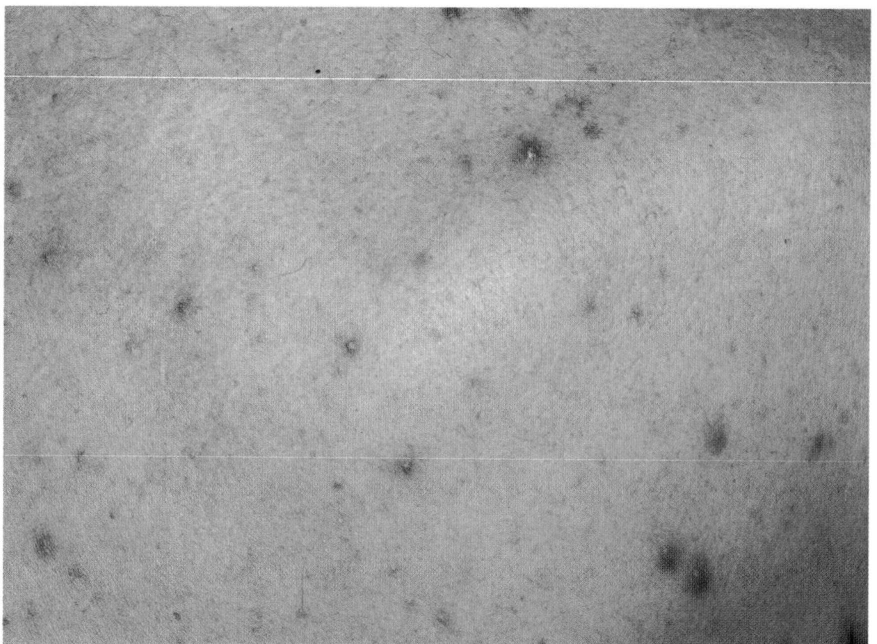

Figure 7.1 Red, scattered papules, some with a central pustule are typical for staphylococcal folliculitis. Because the pustule is very fragile, sometimes lesions show primarily crusts, round erosions, or collarettes.

withdrawn. These patients benefit from intranasal mupirocin ointment 4 times a day for 5 days, as well as from prolonged antibiotic therapy for several months.[1]

Pseudomonas (Hot Tub) Folliculitis

An uncommon but distinctive form of bacterial folliculitis is caused by *Pseudomonas aeruginosa.* The classic presentation of this disease is the patient who has been using an improperly maintained spa, particularly one made of wood. The warm water is an excellent environment for this bacterium, but other sources of *Pseudomonas* have also been reported. These include sponges or loofahs that do not completely dry between use in a bath or in a shower, and even a leaking water bed.

Morphologically, patients exhibit red, usually tender, papules, nodules, and sometimes pustules, distributed primarily in skin folds and under the bathing suit, where contaminated water has been held against the skin (see Fig. 12.9). Sometimes, patients exhibit systemic toxicity, including fever, malaise, nausea, and even earaches.

The differential diagnosis includes insect bites and other forms of folliculitis. Therapy consists of withdrawal of the source of the bacteria. The illness itself is self-limiting and requires no specific treatment. Those patients who are ill may improve more quickly if treated with ciprofloxacin.

STAPHYLOCOCCAL FOLLICULITIS

Clinical Manifestations

Painful or pruritic red papules, some with central pustule or crust, scattered over either relatively normal skin or eczematous skin; differentiated from sterile folliculitis by Gram stain.

Management in the Emergency Department

1. ***Oral antistaphylococcal antibiotic such as cephalexin or dicloxacillin 500 mg bid for 2 weeks***

(Continues)

(Continued)

2. *For longstanding disease, or that associated with eczema, add mupirocin ointment in nares 4 times a day for 5 days*
3. *Patient education regarding the possibility of recurrences*
4. *Follow-up evaluation with a dermatologist if not clear in 2 weeks, or if disease recurs*

Sterile, Inflammatory Folliculitis

At times follicles can become inflamed in the absence of obvious infection. Most often this results from mechanical irritation, such as over the back, under occlusive clothing in the presence of sweating, or from the mild mechanical trauma of leaning against chairbacks. Most commonly occurring over the trunk, sterile folliculitis is usually minimally symptomatic; it presents primarily a cosmetic nuisance.

Sterile folliculitis presents as scattered, very small (1- to 3-mm) red papules that are follicular based. Careful examination usually reveals several red papules with a central small pustule.

The differential diagnosis is the same as for staphylococcal folliculitis discussed above. A bacterial culture is negative. Miliaria (prickly heat) can be confused with, and accompanied by, folliculitis.

The treatment of inflammatory folliculitis includes elimination of irritants when possible. This includes the use of cool, loose clothing. In addition, anti-inflammatory antibiotics as prescribed for acne can be beneficial. These include tetracycline and erythromycin 500 mg bid or, for patients who are intolerant of, or unresponsive to, these medications, doxycycline or minocycline 100 mg bid ongoing.

Fungal Folliculitis

When a dermatophyte (tinea) affects an area with coarse hair, the infection often affects not only the stratum corneum of the surface epithelium, but also this superficial layer of the follicular epithelium. This infection can produce inflammation and pustule formation. Morphologically, fungal folliculitis generally presents as a typical plaque of tinea with scattered papules, nodules, or pustules within the plaque (Fig. 7.2). Occasionally, a very inflammatory form of tinea produces an erythematous, edematous plaque studded with pustules. Follicular involvement with tinea is especially likely in the presence of topical steroid therapy, which allows the infection to behave more aggressively.

Fungal folliculitis also occurs on the lower legs of women with tinea pedis who shave their legs. Tinea is innoculated into hair follicles so that inflammatory papules, pustules, and crust are scattered over the legs, rather than being confined to a well-formed plaque of tinea. This diagnosis requires a high index of suspicion, positive fungal smears or cultures, or a good response to therapy.

Therapy for fungal folliculitis is oral, since topical medications do not penetrate sufficiently for cure. Griseofulvin 500 mg bid (20 to 25 mg/kg/day for children) is the usual therapy, and for those

Figure 7.2 Fungal folliculitis occurs within a plaque of tinea, rather than scattered over relatively normal-appearing skin, as is true of bacterial and sterile folliculitis.

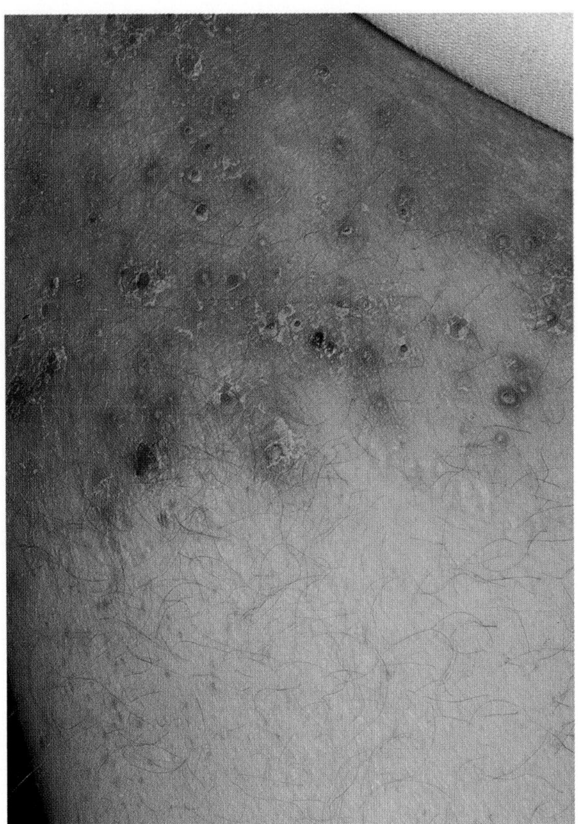

patients who develop side effects such as headache or nausea, fluconazole 100 to 200 mg/day (6 mg/kg for children) or itraconazole at 100 to 200 mg/day (6 mg/kg for children) are better tolerated, although more expensive choices. Most patients require therapy for about one month, and should be re-evaluated at that time. Very mild disease may require a shorter course of medication.

ACNE

Nearly everyone develops acne at some time. This may consist of a very occasional pimple, or severe, draining, scaring cystic acne.

Clinical Manifestations

Acne is a disease of teenagers. However, acne also occurs with regularity in adults, particularly in young and middle-aged women. Sometimes, as in those patients with very severe, cystic cases, acne fails to resolve as teenagers become adults. However, even more often, young and middle-aged women develop acne, but they recall little or no problem with their complexion during their adolescent and teen years.

Lesions are distributed primarily over the face, upper back, and chest. Although often considered a pustular disease, acne is characterized by the presence of polymorphous lesions. Patients with acne exhibit papules, pustules, open and closed comedones, and sometimes cysts and scars (Fig. 7.3). The initial lesion of acne is a hair follicle that becomes blocked with desquamated stratum corneum from the follicular epithelium. When the outlet of the follicle is blocked, the deeper portion of the follicle is distended by additional keratin as stratum corneum is naturally shed, as well as by small amounts of sebaceous material and normal skin flora, including *Propionibacterium acnes*. Open comedones (blackheads) are produced when the follicular plug is superficial and stained dark by melanin. Closed comedones (whiteheads) are produced when the plug is deeper, and the hydrated keratin appears white. As the proximal follicle distends farther, an acne cyst is formed. When a comedone or acne cyst ruptures, keratin and breakdown products from the bacteria are released

Figure 7.3 Acne differs morphologically from folliculitis by the presence of comedones and, sometimes scars, as well as a location limited to the face and upper trunk.

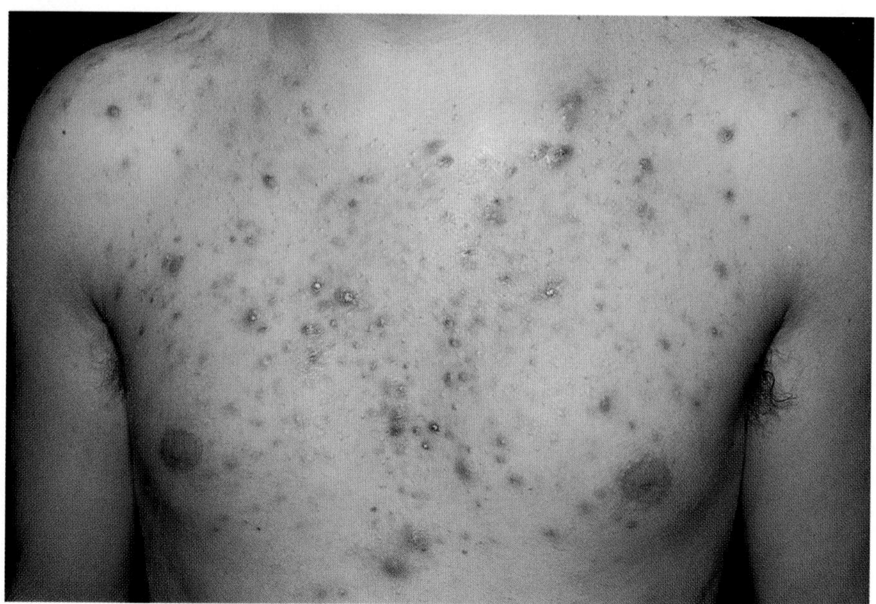

into the surrounding dermis. These contents are extremely inflamogenic, producing a brisk immune response and recruitment of WBCs to form pustules and suppurative cysts. Although bacteria play a role, acne is not an infection.

Differential Diagnosis

Acne is most often confused with sterile or staphylococcal folliculitis. However, the characteristic distribution and the presence of comedones usually make the diagnosis clear.

Management

First-line therapy for acne includes a keratolytic medication to remove follicular plugs. Antibiotics are also standard therapy, used primarily for their anti-inflammatory effect, but also to eliminate *Propionibacterium acnes.*

The primary keratolytic agent used for acne is topical tretinoin 0.025% cream. This medication is applied sparingly at bedtime; patients should be warned about local irritation. A more recent addition to the armamentarium of keratolytics for acne is azelic acid cream.[2] Because keratolytics remove stratum corneum from the surface of the skin, as well as from within the follicles, patients should be careful to wear a sunscreen each day, as the stratum corneum is a significant part of the body's natural sun-protective mechanism.

Patients with inflammatory papules, pustules, and cysts require antibiotics. Those patients with occasional, small pustules can often be treated satisfactorily with a topical antibiotic, such as erythromycin solution 2%, clindamycin, and benzoyl peroxide 5% or 10% bid. For patients with more significant inflammatory disease, oral antibiotics, beginning with tetracycline or erythromycin 500 mg bid, are often effective, but require 2 to 3 months for the full effect to occur. For patients who do not respond to or tolerate these inexpensive antibiotics, doxycycline or minocycline 100 mg bid can be substituted. Clindamycin 150 mg bid is another antibiotic with excellent anti-inflammatory effects.

For those patients who do not derive satisfactory benefit from a keratolytic agent and an anti-inflammatory antibiotic, other therapies are available. For young women without risk factors, high-estrogen birth control pills are often very beneficial. By far the most beneficial therapy for acne, and the only therapy that actually clears the disease, rather than simply controlling it, is isotretinoin (Accutane). Although very effective, this medication is expensive and produces side effects in all patients. Although most of these side effects are simply a nuisance (e.g., extreme dryness), hypertriglyceridemia and extreme teratogenicity are well-known and common occurrences, militating against the use of this medication in the emergency department.

Prognosis and Course

Acne is usually controlled by therapy. The disease usually resolves spontaneously as the patient ages. However, some patients experience chronic disease that continues into middle age. The only therapy that can produce long-lasting remission of acne is oral isotretinoin.

ACNE

Clinical Manifestations

Red papules, comedones, and pustules distributed over the face and/or upper trunk.

Management in the Emergency Department

1. *Comedonal acne: tretinoin (Retin-A) cream 0.025% applied to the area nightly, rinsed off in the morning and replaced by sunscreen with sun protection factor of at least 15*
2. *Inflammatory acne, mild (1 to 3 lesions): tretinoin as above, plus Benzamycin (er thromycin 3%, benzoyl peroxide 5%) or clindamycin solution 10 mg/ml bid*
   Inflammatory acne, moderate or severe: tetracycline or erythromycin 500 mg bid ongoing
3. *Patient education (see patient handout) regarding acne and slow response to therapy*
4. *Follow-up evaluation with personal physician or dermatologist in 2 months*

CUTANEOUS CANDIDA INFECTION

Candida is sometimes characterized by very fragile pustules bordering a red, exudative, or scaling plaque within a skin fold (Fig. 7.4). Usually, the pustules are very short-lived, with multiple collarettes demonstrating their fragility. The diagnosis is based on location, morphology, a positive fungal smear, and response to therapy. This disease is most often confused with a dermatophyte infection. Although dermatophyte infections occur in skin fold areas as well, they are usually annular and lack superficial, peripheral pustules. However, when in doubt, a topical azole usually treats both conditions.

CUTANEOUS CANDIDIASIS

Clinical Manifestations

Red plaque in skin folds with surrounding fragile pustules or collarettes; confirmed with a positive potassium preparation of skin scrapings.

Management in the Emergency Department

1. *Mild disease, without significant inflammation or exudation: topical azole such as clotrimazole qid (over-the-counter) or econazole nitrate 1% bid (by prescription)*
   Disease with significant inflammation or exudation:
   fluconazole 150 mg/d for 4 days, then adding a topical azole as discussed above until clear
2. *For women with vulvar candidiasis, treat the vagina either with fluconazole 150 mg once, or an intravaginal azole*

FIRE ANT BITES

Fire ant bites produce red papules that rapidly become sterile pustules (Fig. 7.5). Patients are generally aware of the diagnosis because the bites are painful. There is no good therapy other than future avoidance of the ants.

PUSTULAR PSORIASIS

Although psoriasis is usually a papulosquamous disease, consisting of well-demarcated, scaling plaques, some patients exhibit severe inflammation sufficient to produce pustules. Patients with pustu-

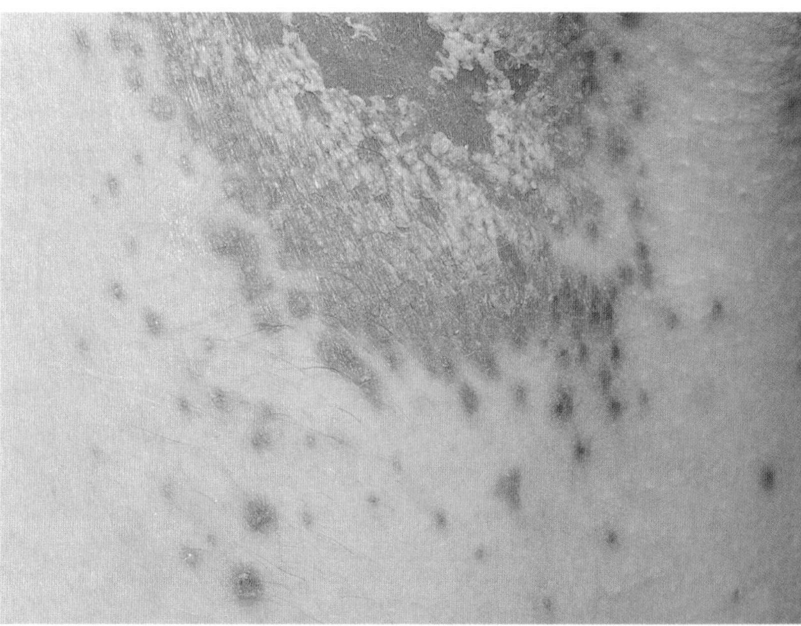

Figure 7.4 Pustules produced by *Candida albicans* surround a red, inflamed plaque. These lesions are extremely fragile, so that sometimes only collarettes are seen, rather than intact pustules.

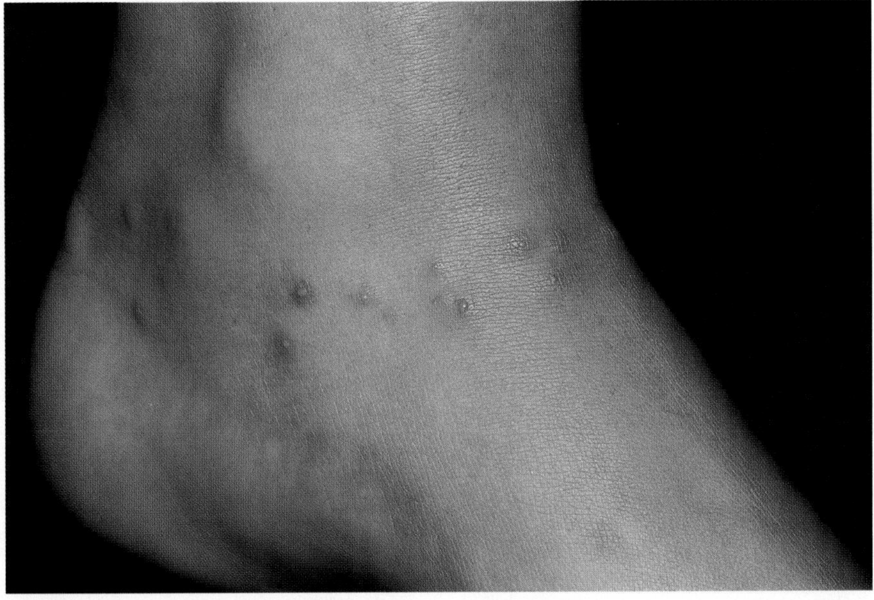

Figure 7.5 Fire ant bites quickly become pustular. The diagnosis is not usually a problem, as patients are aware of the painful sting.

lar psoriasis are sometimes toxic, exhibiting fever, chills, and elevated WBC counts. Pustular psoriasis is often a systemic illness not limited to the skin.

Clinical Manifestations

Pustular psoriasis can arise suddenly, in the absence of a history of pre-existing psoriasis, or common psoriasis can slowly transform into pustular psoriasis. Patient exhibit red plaques that are studded with pustules (Figs. 7.6 and 7.7). These plaques can be generalized, or sometimes limited to the hands or feet, or both. When disease has been present for some time, the pustules evolve into crusts, and the underlying pustular nature may be more difficult to discern. Therefore, pustular psoriasis sometimes presents as sharply demarcated, crusted papules and plaques. A search for pustules is often successful in some areas. When common, plaque-type psoriasis transforms into pustular psoriasis, a yellow color to the scale is often an early sign. This yellow color suggests serum leakage from intense inflammation and rupture of very small pustules.

Patients with pustular psoriasis often have accompanying arthritis. Rarely, these patients can experience mucosal lesions and occasionally inflammatory eye findings such as iritis.

Patients with flaring pustular psoriasis can be extremely ill. Fever and chills from this disease can be difficult to differentiate from those of infection. These skin lesions also put the patient at risk of secondary infection. Because of the cutaneous inflammation, patients experience cutaneous vasodilation and increased cardiac output. There is often shunting of blood from the gastrointestinal tract and kidneys to the skin, resulting in malabsorption. Patients often experience chronic anemia and may show other laboratory abnormalities, such as elevated blood urea nitrogen and a low serum albumin.

Differential Diagnosis

The lesions of pustular psoriasis can be confused with deep superinfected skin disease, most often eczema. However, the plaques of pustular psoriasis are usually sharply demarcated; careful inspec-

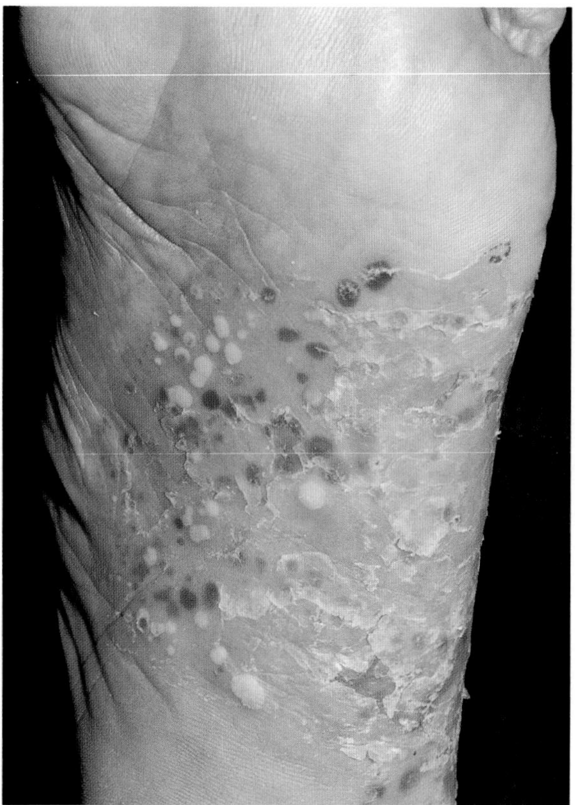

Figure 7.6 Red plaques studded with pustules are typical of pustular psoriasis, and sometimes of Reiter disease.

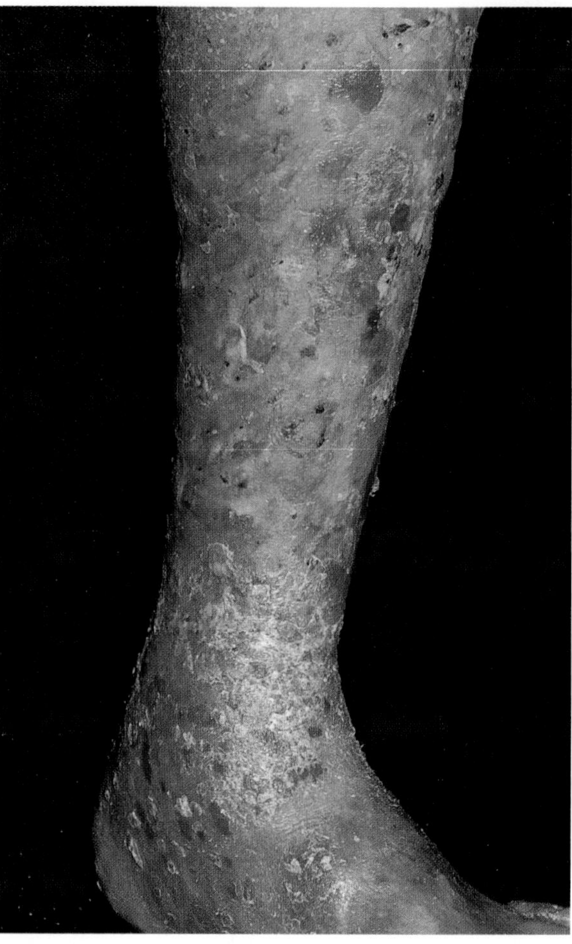

Figure 7.7 The pustules of pustular psoriasis evolve into crusts and erosions; large areas of pustular psoriasis produce health-threatening disease, including fever, loss of fluids, protein, and iron, and an increased risk of infection.

tion of the skin surface will detect the presence of either plaques typical of psoriasis or other findings that suggest this diagnosis, such as scalp lesions or nail pitting. The skin lesions associated with psoriasis are identical to those of Reiter's disease. The lesions of Reiter's disease are more often limited to the genitalia, hands, and feet. Otherwise, these diseases are differentiated by the presence of extra cutaneous findings. Psoriasis is far less likely to exhibit inflammatory eye findings, urethritis, and cervicitis. Although HLA B27 positivity is increased in patients with both diseases, those with Reiter's disease are more likely to show this abnormality. Sometimes these diseases cannot be differentiated, but the diseases are very closely related, and therapy is the same for both entities.

Management

Topical corticosteroids are somewhat beneficial for the skin lesions of pustular psoriasis. Topical steriods are rarely sufficient, but this is the only therapy reasonable in the emergency department. Systemic corticosteroids often improve disease dramatically; unfortunately, in spite of initial improvement with this therapy, systemic corticosteroids sometimes precipitate a worse, occasionally life-threatening, flare of disease. Only under extraordinary circumstances, and in concert with a dermatologist, should systemic corticosteroids be used. Generally, oral etretinate, methotrexate, or ultraviolet light therapy is required.

Obviously, toxic patients may sometimes require hospital admission with supportive care and evaluation for infection. These patients also deserve timely evaluation by a dermatologist.

REITER'S DISEASE

Reiter's disease, which is closely related to pustular psoriasis, exhibits skin lesions identical to those of the latter condition. This reactive disease is most often found in genetically susceptible individuals and it is often associated with an infection. Most patients exhibit HLA B27 positivity. Usually, the precipitating infection (including *Yersinia* and *Salmonella*) has disappeared by the time the patient presents, although *Chlamydia* can play an ongoing role.[3]

By definition, Reiter's disease consists of arthritis, generally asymmetric arthritis of the large joints (e.g., the knees), urethritis, and inflammatory eye changes (e.g., iritis or uveitis). Many patients also exhibit sharply demarcated plaques with overlying scale/crust, and sometimes pustules. These plaques are most prominent over the genitalia (keratoderma blennorrhagica), hands, and feet (Fig. 7.8). Over the uncircumcised glans penis, lesions consist of white annular and arcuate white papules and plaques (balanitis circinata).

The disease most difficult to distinguish from Reiter syndrome is pustular psoriasis. This distinction is not difficult when Reiter's disease presents in its complete form, exhibiting arthritis, urethritis, and iritis. However, most Reiter's disease cases present at the incomplete stage initially. Sometimes, only progression of the disease will permit the correct diagnosis. However, management is the same for these diseases and includes methotrexate, etretinate, and topical corticosteroids.

PUSTULAR PSORIASIS/ REITER'S DISEASE

Clinical Manifestations

Well-demarcated, inflammatory plaques with superimposed pustules or crusting, often associated with

(Continues)

Figure 7.8 Plaques of pustules that evolve into well-demarcated, crusting plaques are characteristic of both Reiter's disease, as shown here, and pustular psoriasis.

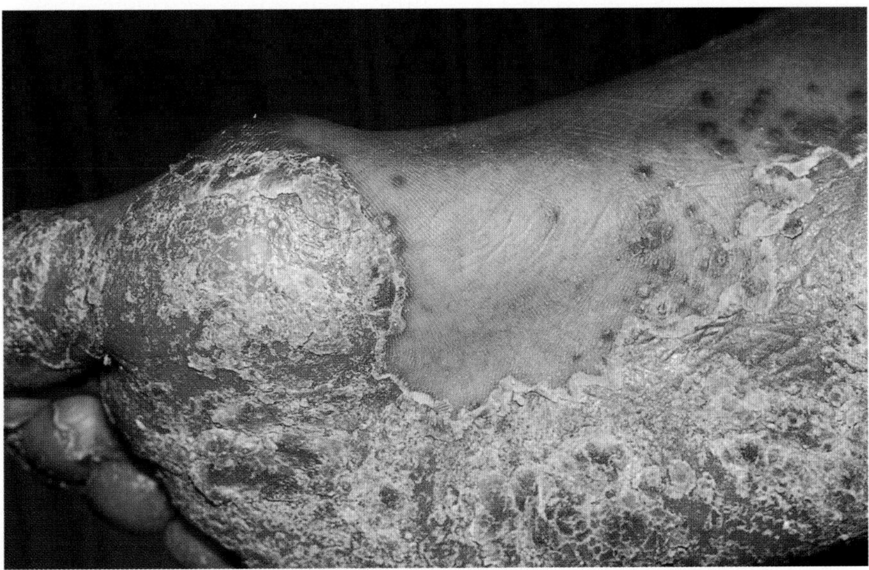

(Continued)

arthritis. Many with constitutional symptoms iand past history of psoriasis.

Management in the Emergency Department

1. *Referral to a dermatologist*
2. *If toxic, rule out infection and admit for supportive care*

INTENSE DERMAL INFLAMMATION OR INFECTION

Any intensely inflammatory disease can produce superficial pustules (see Ch. 14). This includes pyodermas, granulomatous infection as seen with deep fungal infection, parasitic infection, and sometimes atypical mycobacterial infections (Fig. 7.9). Indurated nodules or masses with pustulation require tissue biopsies with special stains and cultures for diagnosis.

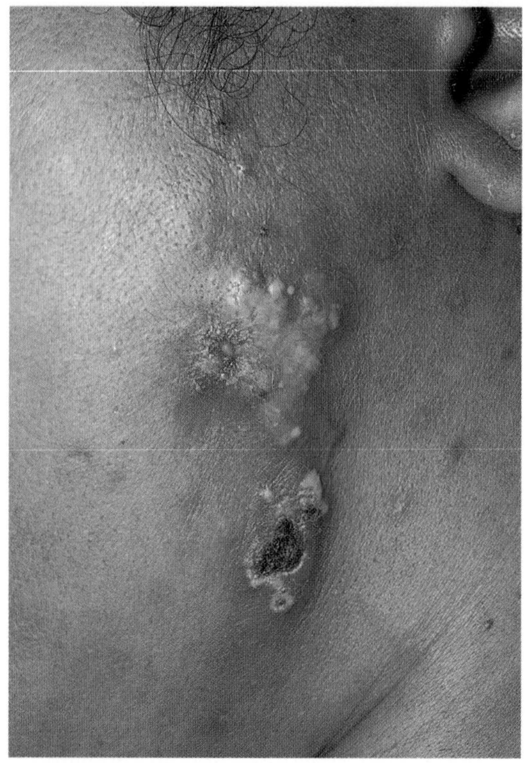

Figure 7.9 Any infection or deep, intense inflammation can produce pustulation, as shown here in a patient with a staphylococcal pyoderma.

DISEASES THAT APPEAR, BUT ARE NOT, PUSTULAR

Any vesicle that has been present for several days typically recruits WBCs and appears pustular (see Fig. 4.15). Therefore, vesicular diseases should be considered in the differential diagnosis of pustules. However, a careful examination usually reveals at least a few clear vesicles. Also, if the lesion is pierced with a needle or No. 11 scalpel blade, the fluid is thin and nearly clear, rather than thick and creamy as occurs in a true pustule.

Mollusca contagiosa (see Ch. 8) are usually skin colored, but sometimes a white core produces a pustular appearance (see Fig. 9.10). Also, when inflamed, these lesions can become pustular secondarily.

Milia, small epidermal inclusion cysts filled with white keratin, can resemble pustules (see Ch. 9). However, these are firm and long-lasting. A small, firm pearly white nodule can be expressed, rather than creamy pus (see Fig. 9.9).

Please see the patient information handout for this chapter on page 324.

REFERENCES

1. Reagan DR, Doebbeling BN, Pfaller MA: Elimination of coincident *Staphylococcus aureus* nasal and hand carriage with intranasal application of mupirocin calcium ointment. Ann Intern Med 114: 101, 1991
2. Cunliffe WJ, Holland KT: Clinical and laboratory studies on treatment with 20% azelic acid cream for acne. Acta Derm Venereol (Stockh), suppl. 69:31, 1989

3. Rahman MU, Hudson AP, Schumacher HR: *Chlamydia* and Reiter's syndrome (reactive arthritis). Rheum Dis Clin North Am 18: 67, 1992

SUGGESTED READINGS

Folliculitis

Gregory DW, Schaffner W: *Pseudomonas* infection associated with hot tubs and other environments. Infect Dis Clin North Am 1:635, 1987

Wortman PD: Bacterial infections of the skin. Curr Probl Dermatol 5:193, 1993

Acne

Lever L, Marks R: Current views on the etiology, pathogenesis and treatment of acne vulgaris. Drugs 39:681, 1990

Pustular Psoriasis/Reiter's Disease

Baker H: Pustular psoriasis. Dermatol Clin 2:455, 1994

Rothe MJ, Derdel FA: Reiter syndrome. Int J Dermatol 30:173, 1991

Zelickson BD, Muller SA: Generalized pustular psoriasis. A review of 63 cases. Arch Dermatol 127: 1339, 1991

CHAPTER 8

Skin-Colored Lesions

Most tumors are inherently skin colored. However, most tumors also can become red due to increased vascularity or inflammation from trauma or rapid growth that produces necrosis with an inflammatory reaction. Therefore, a solitary inflamed, normally skin-colored tumor can sometimes appear as a red nodule; skin-colored lesions should sometimes be considered in the differential diagnosis of the solitary inflamed nodule.

Skin-colored lesions are divided into two main groups: those with a keratotic (rough, extremely scaly, or hard) surface, and those that are nonkeratotic, with a smooth or soft surface.

SKIN-COLORED, KERATOTIC PAPULES

Keratotic papules and nodules are scaly tumors that often feel hard or crusty because of the buildup of scale and thickened epidermis.

Warts

Warts (common warts and plantar warts) are extraordinarily common tumors produced by many different types of human papillomavirus (HPV), with morphology and location dependent primarily on HPV type.

Clinical Manifestations

Common Warts Most often found in children, common warts are skin-colored, sharply demarcated papules that have a firm and rough surface (Fig. 8.1). Sometimes warts have a verrucous (papillomatous) surface; occasionally, the verrucous nature is so marked that the entire lesion is composed of a cluster of keratotic, filiform papules whose tips curve toward the center of the lesion. Although most often located over dorsal fingers and hands, common warts are also frequently found over the knees and can actually be seen over any area of keratinized skin. These lesions are most often multiple.

Flat Warts Usually located on the face, dorsal hands, or lower legs, flat warts are minimally raised, flat-topped, smooth, skin-colored papules.

Plantar Warts Plantar warts are located on the plantar surface of the foot and palmar surface of the hand. Plantar warts are relatively well-demarcated, firm papules and plaques with little or no elevation, as compared to the surrounding skin (Fig. 8.2). The keratotic nature of these plaques can be recognized by the hard surface, even though obvious scale or a verrucous surface are absent.

Differential Diagnosis The primary disease in the differential diagnosis of common and flat warts is seborrheic keratosis. Seborrheic keratoses are found almost exclusively in adults and are usually brown in color, as well as broader and flatter than most warts. Sometimes seborrheic keratoses can be indistinguishable from common warts. Occasionally, keratotic squamous cell carcinomas can resemble irritated common warts. However, these malignant tumors usually differ by a surface and border that are irregular and asymmetric. Rarely, prurigo nodules (picker's nodules), callus-like thickening of the skin from chronic picking, can resemble an irritated wart. Once again, these are usually not flat-topped, and they show evidence of excoriation over the surface.

Calluses and corns are the major diseases to be differentiated from plantar warts. There are

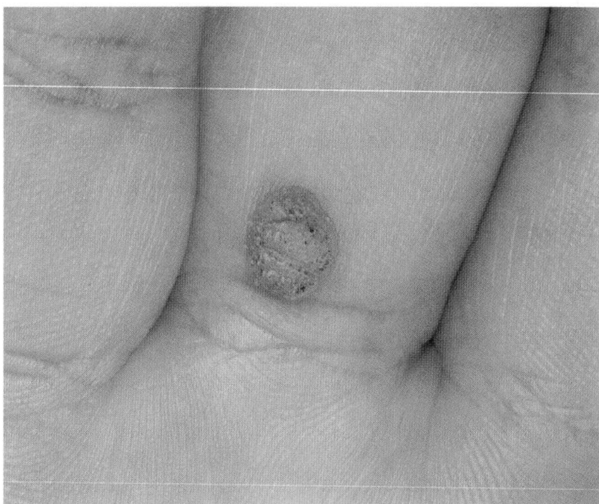

Figure 8.1 This keratotic surface with black spots is typical of a common wart. These black spots are responsible for the name *seed warts,* and these represent thrombosed vessels.

Figure 8.2 This plantar wart shows interruption of normal skin lines and dark dots that represent thrombosed vessels, both hallmarks that differentiate warts from calluses.

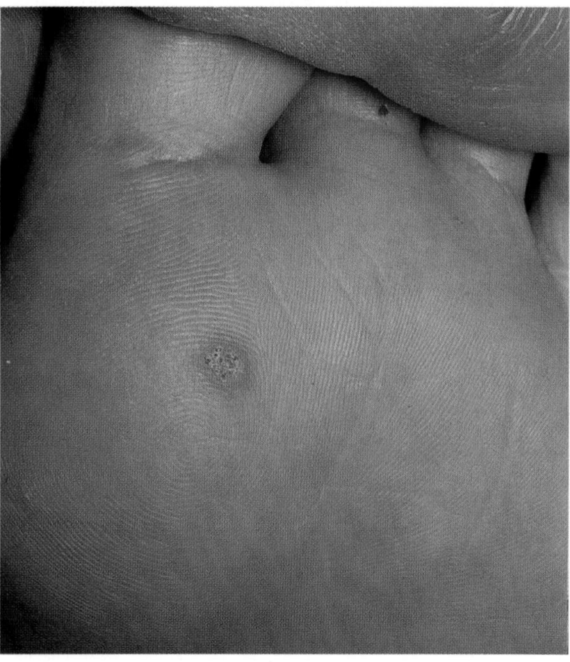

several distinguishing morphologic features, although sometimes differentiating the two can be very difficult. Unlike calluses, plantar warts do not preferentially affect areas of pressure. Plantar warts are often more sharply demarcated, and normal skin markings do not extend through the lesion.

Management Because no specific antiviral medications demonstrate sufficient activity against warts to be effective, all means of eliminating keratotic warts require destruction of the skin harboring this virus. There are several means of destroying common warts.

Cryotherapy (treatment with liquid nitrogen) is the fastest, nonscarring, widely available means of removal, when warts are few in number and the patient is stoic. Blisters form in the treated area, and part or all of the wart is shed with the blister roof. Several treatments at 3- to 4-week intervals may be required for larger lesions. Hypopigmentation is an occasional long-lasting complication; underlying nerve damage can occur when lateral digits are treated overly aggressively.

When liquid nitrogen is not available or when patients are unable to tolerate the pain of cryotherapy, caustic topical agents can be used at home. Salicylic acid preparations are most common (e.g., Duofilm, Occlusal HP) (for directions on application, see the patient handout on p. 374, Warts). The wart is soaked in water until the surface softens. The keratotic surface and old medication are then removed with an emery board or pumice stone, and medication is reapplied. This is repeated nightly until the warts have disappeared, usually several months. Cantharidin, formerly available in the United States as Cantherone or Cantherone Plus, is too caustic for home use, but it can be applied in the office painlessly. A blister forms the next day and the process is repeated every 2 to 3 weeks. This therapy is especially useful in children who have large numbers of warts. However, this medication must now be compounded by pharmacists or ordered from distributors in other countries, such as Canada.

Warts can also be removed by hyfrecation (electrocautery), which usually produces scarring. Laser therapy is effective and produces minimal scarring, but it is extraordinarily expensive and is not uniformly available. High doses of oral cimetadine have been reported to clear common warts, but a more recent controlled trial failed to show a beneficial effect with this medication.[1,2] Finally, the clinician should remember that common warts found on a child almost always eventually disappear spontaneously, so that very aggressive and scarring therapy should be avoided. Reassurance and observation are a viable option in some of these children.

The treatment of plantar warts is more difficult than that for common warts, since destructive therapy can produce pain that interferes with normal walking for days to weeks after treatment. For this reason, a 15% (Trans-Ver-Sa) or 40% salicylic acid (Sal-Acid) plaster trimmed to cover the precise area of the wart is useful therapy that can maintain the patient's mobility during treatment. The plaster can be removed every few days; necrotic, white wart is removed with an emery board or pumice stone and a new plaster applied. Sometimes, the plaster should be secured with tape, to ensure that it remains securely in place. Other treatments include the application of salicylic acid liquids at home or destructive treatments in the office, to include a series of light liquid nitrogen treatments, laser therapy, curettage, and the intralesional administration of bleomycin.[3]

Course and Prognosis Prepubertal children usually experience resolution of their warts with or without therapy, but this process often takes several years. Because warts are infectious, new warts often continue to appear as old warts disappear. Adults rarely experience resolution of warts without therapy. Immunosuppressed individuals are unlikely to undergo successful definitive treatment of their warts, although intermittent therapy may control the size and extent of warts.

Calluses and Corns

Calluses consist of thickened epidermis and hyperkeratosis that occur primarily on the feet in response to pressure and serve to protect the integrity of the skin. These poorly demarcated, firm plaques overlie deep bony prominences, such as the metatarsal heads. Although sometimes difficult to distinguish from plantar warts, the prominent skin markings of the plantar surface of the foot usually traverse a callus uninterrupted. *Corns* are similar protective lesions that are produced by pressure on bony prominences just under the skin, such as over toes.

Treatment for a callus or corn includes the alleviation of pressure by changing to carefully fitted shoes or inserts when possible. In addition, the lesion can be pared with a No. 15 scalpel blade after the area has been soaked with water and softened. Finally, a plaster impregnated with salicylic acid, as discussed for plantar warts, can be applied to the corn or callus. This will slowly dissolve the thickened, hard surface.

Actinic Keratoses

Actinic keratoses are areas of cytologic dysplasia within the epidermis, produced by chronic exposure to ultraviolet light. Although these lesions are sometimes referred to as "precancers," transformation into squamous cell carcinoma occurs in only about 0.001% of actinic keratoses.[4] However, actinic keratoses serve as an important marker for significant ultraviolet radiation damage, with many affected patients developing either basal cell or squamous cell carcinoma.[5]

Actinic keratoses occur as skin-colored, inflamed, brown, or yellowish scaling papules or plaques located most often over the face, ears, bald scalp, and dorsal hands and forearms. These areas are generally poorly demarcated and are usually multiple.

When skin colored, there are few diseases in the differential diagnosis unless the lesions are hyperkeratotic, in which case they can resemble irritated warts, seborrheic keratoses, and squamous cell carcinomas. The diagnosis is made on the basis of the setting and any surrounding typical lesions. Sometimes, when pink and scaling, actinic keratoses can appear eczematous, mimicking atopic dermatitis or seborrheic dermatitis. Also, the scaling nature over the lateral face resembles chronic cutaneous discoid lupus erythematosus.

Because the primary significance of actinic keratosis is that sufficient sun exposure to cause epidermal malignant changes has occurred, the management of actinic keratoses consists of careful patient education. Patients should understand that sun protection and regular skin examinations for early identification of skin cancers is important. For thin, asymptomatic actinic keratoses, observation is a reasonable course. For those that are thickened or rapidly enlarging, or that have underlying induration, removal or biopsy is indicated to prevent or rule out the possibility of early malignant change. The most common therapy is the office application of liquid nitrogen. Second is the home application of fluorouracil twice daily for about 4 months. Treated areas—both actinic keratoses and any areas with even microscopic dysplastic changes—become red, crusted, and exudative before healing. Dermabrasion and chemical peels also treat the keratoses as well as improve the appearance and texture of the skin.

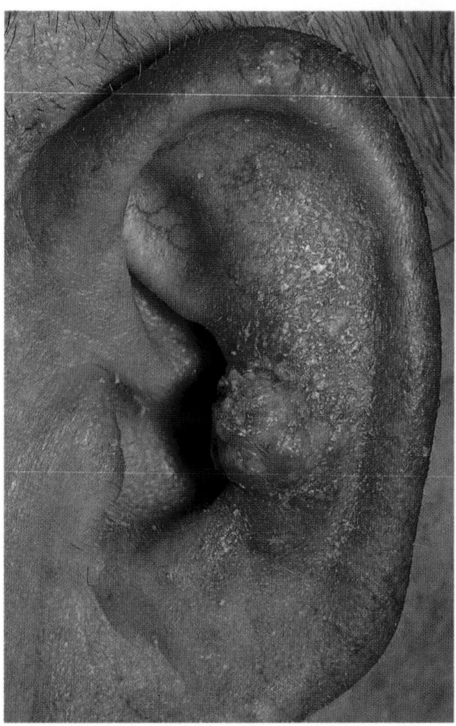

Figure 8.3 This sunlight-induced, irregular, solid-appearing hyperkeratotic squamous cell carcinoma is located over clinically dyspigmented, actinically damaged skin.

Squamous Cell Carcinoma

Squamous cell carcinomas are malignant tumors of the epithelium produced by various chronic irritants, such as sun damage, human papillomavirus (HPV) infection, and chronic inflammation of any cause, such as that associated with leg ulcers and chronic cutaneous (discoid) lupus erythematosus.

Clinical Manifestations Squamous cell carcinomas, particularly when induced by chronic sun exposure, often appear as keratotic, infiltrated papules, plaques, or nodules. Unlike a basal cell carcinoma, the lesion is generally not pearly in character but rather solid-appearing. The surface can be dome-shaped or irregular, and the borders may or may not be well demarcated (Fig. 8.3). Most common in light-complexioned men, actinically induced squamous carcinomas occur most often on the bald scalp, face, and dorsal hands and forearms, surrounded by significantly sun-damaged skin. Squamous cell carcinomas of the lip are usually located over the lower lip and present as a persistent erosion or firm nodule, with or without overlying hyperkeratosis. Surrounding actinic damage of the lip is usual, consisting of scale and loss of the sharp demarcation of the vermilion border.

Differential Diagnosis The differential diagnosis includes all keratotic, skin-colored lesions, particularly when they have been irritated, so that the surface and borders are more irregular. The diagnosis can be made with a shave biopsy that extends into the dermis, but the biopsy need not include normal skin and need not attempt to remove the entire tumor. A shave is preferable to a punch biopsy for actinically induced squamous cell carcinomas, so that choices for later definitive therapy are not limited and curettage and electrodesiccation can be performed if desired.

Management Management in the emergency department consists essentially of referral. Although many providers are qualified to excise lesions, only dermatologists have the in-depth training needed for visual evaluation of lesions. Therefore, referral to a dermatologist sometimes results in a clinical diagnosis, such as an irritated seborrheic keratosis, obviating the need for a biopsy.

Course and Prognosis Unless treated, actinically induced squamous cell carcinomas continue to grow. There is a low (0.3 to 5.0%) metastatic rate for most actinally induced squamous cell carcinomas,[6] but rates are higher for larger tumors, in immunosuppressed patients, and for tumors on the lip or other modified mucous membrane surfaces. In these high-risk cases, and when a squamous cell carcinoma is not induced by sunlight, but rather by HPV infection, ionizing radiation, or chronic inflammation, the metastatic rate is as high as 30%, and the patient should be referred promptly for excision with suture closure.

SQUAMOUS CELL CARCINOMA

Clinical Manifestations
Skin-colored or pink irregular nodule, papule or plaque, that is usually hyperkeratotic and located over the scalp, face, ears, or backs of hands and forearms when induced by chronic sunlight; when occurring as a result of chronic inflammation as on an ulcer, the lesions are often eroded without hyperkeratosis.

Management in the Emergency Department
1. *Referral to a dermatologist for further clinical evaluation and possible biopsy and removal, or to a surgeon for biopsy and removal*
2. *If there is marked concern about patient compliance, a shave biopsy can be performed in the emergency department, or the lesion can even be removed with excision and suture closure*

Cutaneous Horns

A cutaneous horn is a column of keratin that protrudes from the skin (Fig. 8.4). These usually occur over a papule or nodule. Cutaneous horns can be produced by an underlying wart, seborrheic keratosis, squamous cell carcinoma, actinic keratosis, or basal cell carcinoma.

Because some of these lesions are malignant, a deep shave removal that includes a generous piece of underlying skin should be performed for biopsy. A common biopsy mistake is removal of the keratotic column without sufficient associated skin to allow for adequate diagnosis. Occasionally, the morphology of the underlying skin or surrounding typical lesions allows for a diagnosis of wart or seborrheic keratosis without biopsy.

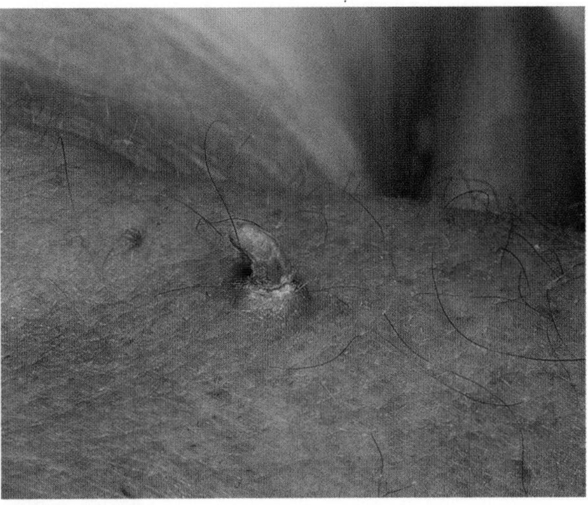

Figure 8.4 A cutaneous horn represents extreme hyperkeratosis and can result from abnormal keratin formation from a squamous cell carcinoma, as occurred here, or from a wart, actinic keratosis, or seborrheic keratosis.

Seborrheic Keratoses

Seborrheic keratoses are well-demarcated, flat-topped, keratotic papules found most often on patients over the age of 40 years. These are usually brown, but occasionally they can be skin colored or, when irritated, pink (for an in-depth discussion, see Ch. 11).

Prurigo Nodules

A prurigo nodule (Picker's nodule) is a dome-shaped, firm, hyperkeratotic callus produced by picking. Lesions can be skin-colored, inflamed, or brown from postinflammatory hyperpigmentation, especially in patients with naturally dark complexions. These are often multiple, and usually have an excoriation overlying the center of the lesion (Fig. 8.5). Some patients are resistant to this diagnosis and deny manipulation, but the characteristic appearance and locations are pathognomonic.

Prurigo nodules are most common in areas that frequently itch, such as the upper back, and in

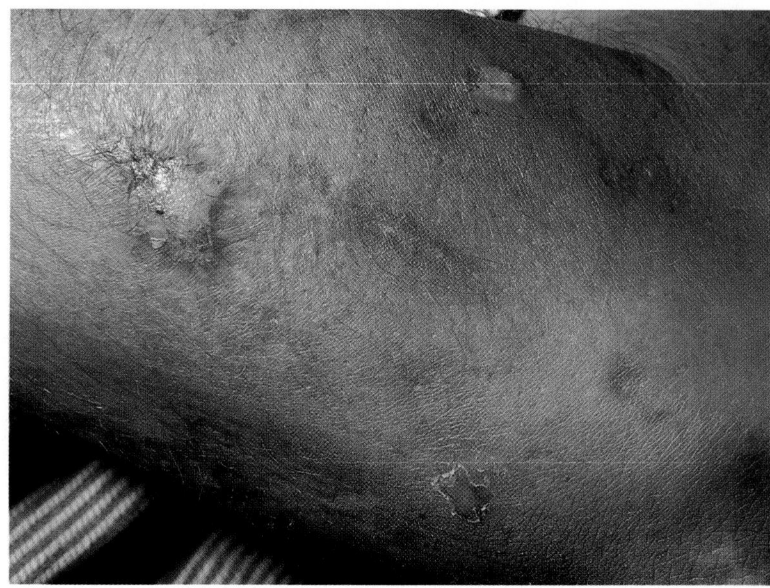

Figure 8.5 Prurigo nodules (picker's nodules) are calluses produced by chronic picking. These lesions are thickened and scaling, usually with a central excoriation and are only found in areas that the patient can reach.

areas that are easily accessible to fingernails, such as the upper arms. However, dexterous patients can produce these lesions nearly anywhere on the body, except for the very center of the back.

Management consists of delicate patient education and of an examination for a correctable cause of pruritus, with folliculitis being a common underlying association. Sometimes, an empirical trial of oral antistaphylococcal antibiotics, such as cephalexin, can be beneficial if folliculitis is suspected. Otherwise, a high-potency topical steroid such as fluocinonide (Lidex 0.05% cream) applied twice a day may help pruritus somewhat and, because habit and stress play prominent roles, nighttime amitriptyline can be useful. These patients should be followed up with a dermatologist about 1 month after institution of therapy.

NONKERATOTIC PAPULES, NODULES, AND PLAQUES

Nonkeratotic papules and nodules have smooth surfaces and are usually relatively soft.

Intradermal Nevi

Intradermal nevi are common, soft, well-demarcated papules that are usually less than 7 mm in diameter (Fig. 8.6). Although these can occur anywhere on the body, they are most common on the face, trunk, and upper arms.

Skin lesions to be differentiated from intradermal nevi include neurofibromas, which are often slightly larger and even softer, and tend to be single, whereas intradermal nevi are more likely to be multiple. On the face, some intradermal nevi exhibit a slightly pearly texture that can mimic that of a basal cell carcinoma. Although basal cell carcinomas are usually slightly firm to the touch, a shave biopsy is sometimes required to differentiate these two skin lesions.

The only management required for a typical intradermal nevus is reassurance and, because single neurofibromas also have no medical significance, differentiation is unimportant and does not affect therapy. These lesions can be excised for cosmetic purposes, and they can often be shaved flush with the surface with a nice cosmetic result.

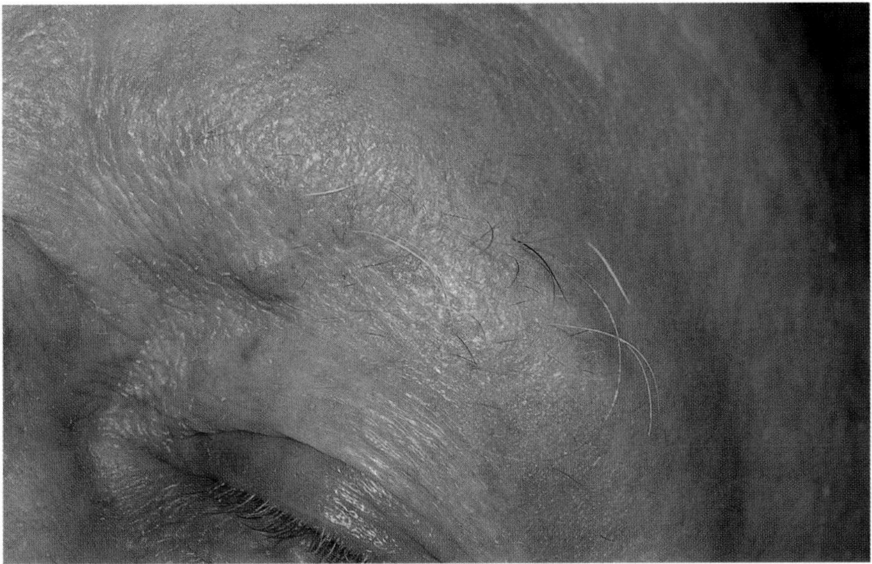

Figure 8.6 An intradermal nevus is soft, skin colored, and sometimes indistinguishable from a neurofibroma.

Neurofibromas

Neurofibromas are innocuous, benign tumors of neural origin. When solitary, they are not a marker for neurofibromatosis. However, large numbers of neurofibromas and multiple café-au-lait spots are pathognomonic for that disease.

Neurofibromas are dome-shaped or pedunculated, extremely soft, skin-colored nodules (Fig. 8.7). They are sometimes indistinguishable from intradermal nevi, but are often softer and larger.

When single or few in number, these lesions have no medical significance and require no therapy other than reassurance.

Epidermal Cysts

Most epidermal cysts (epidermoid cysts, "sebaceous cysts") are formed from hair follicles that become blocked by a keratin plug or inflammation in a superficial scar over the surface. As follicular epithelium continues to turn over, desquamated stratum corneum remains trapped in the follicle and keratin distends the follicle, forming the cyst. Even though the damp keratin is white, this color is usually not appreciated in larger, deeper cysts. Occasionally, if the cyst is large so that the follicular epithelium is stretched thin around its contents, or if the cyst is traumatized, the cyst ruptures and contents leak into surrounding dermis. This can produce a brisk inflammatory response that is often misdiagnosed as an infected cyst or furuncle (see Ch. 12).

The differential diagnosis includes any dermal tumor, but usually the texture and smooth, well-demarcated borders of an epidermal cyst allow diagnosis without a biopsy. Sometimes, the differentiation of an epidermal cyst from a lipoma can be difficult. However, a lipoma is usually softer and less well demarcated. Also, a lipoma is usually more obvious on palpation, while a cyst is easily seen.

Therapy is generally unnecessary, but for those patients who desire treatment, surgical removal is required. These cysts are often much larger than initially appreciated, and removal sometimes leaves

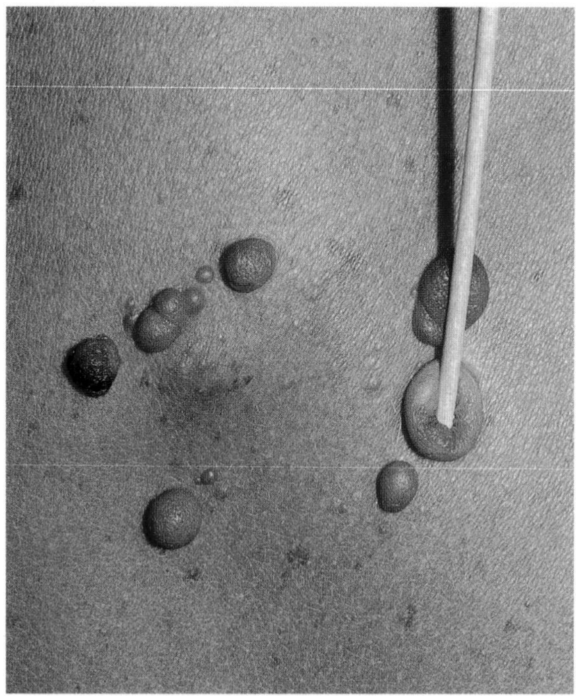

Figure 8.7 A neurofibroma is distinguished by its extremely soft texture; although one or a very few neurofibromas are medically inconsequential, multiple lesions, as shown here, are associated with neurofibromatosis.

an impressive defect. Excision with sac removal should not be attempted if the cysts are inflamed.

Lipoma

A lipoma is a very common hamartoma of fatty tissue. Most often located on the trunk or proximal extremities, this tumor has a characteristic soft, mushy texture.

Except for the occasional lipoma that is painful, these require no therapy. Removal requires surgical excision, and the tumor is often larger and deeper than expected. Lipomas over the forehead can be especially and unexpectedly deep.

Genital Warts

Genital warts (condylomata acuminata) are soft, usually skin-colored, papules produced by certain HPV types. Generally transmitted sexually, this disease derives its primary importance from its association with cervical carcinoma.

HPV is extremely common in people between the ages of 18 and 45 years. An estimated 2% of sexually active people are reported to have clinically visible anogenital warts, although far more have evidence of HPV with more sophisticated testing.[7]

Genital warts can exhibit any of several morphologies. Filiform warts are tubular with acuminate tips that often appear white, whereas other warts can be pedunculated and cauliflower-shaped (Fig. 8.8). Some genital warts are flat. These are especially likely to be pigmented and exhibit dysplasia histologically. Verrucous papules are also common.

Usually, the diagnosis can be made clinically, but sometimes intradermal nevi, skin tags, enlarged sebaceous glands, or seborrheic keratoses can make the diagnosis difficult. Because of both the

Figure 8.8 Genital warts exhibit several different morphologies, including verrucous papules, cauliflower shapes, filiform warts, and flat lesions.

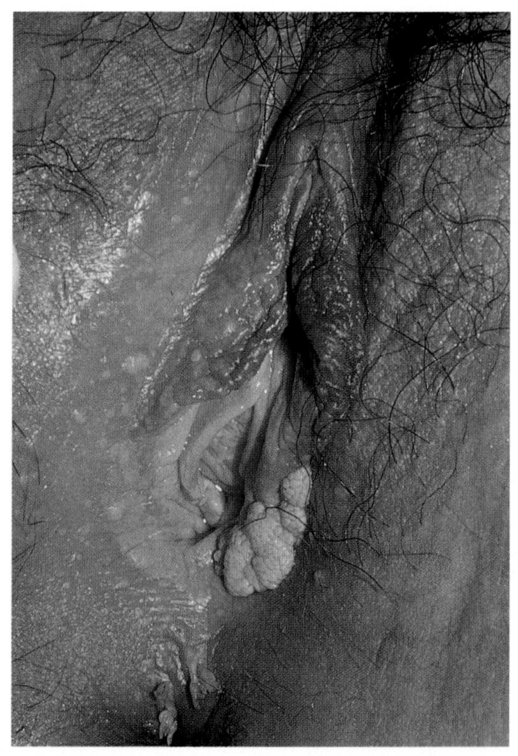

psychological and medical implications of this diagnosis, a biopsy is indicated in unclear cases. Even a biopsy does not give absolute answers at times, since the genital area is susceptible to normal histologic findings suggestive of wart virus, and some pathologists have a low index of suspicion. Flat warts especially should be biopsied because of the increased risk of dysplasia.

The management of genital warts requires careful patient education. This disease is usually—but not always—sexually transmitted; the long incubation period and common occurrence of latency make contact tracing very difficult. However and whenever the warts were acquired, the patient should know that they can sexually transmit this infection to others. Because some wart infections are associated with cervical dysplasia and carcinoma,[8] women and female sexual partners should be evaluated by a gynecologist with a Papanicolaou smear and ongoing follow-up evaluation. Also, the virus generally cannot be eliminated, even though the wart tumors are eventually successfully treated. Therefore, patients should be advised that recurrences are common and that therapy is often prolonged.

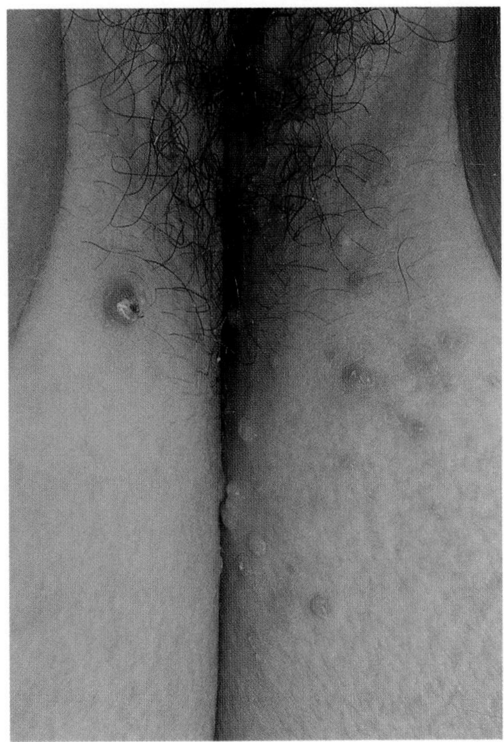

Figure 8.9 Molluscum contagiosum consists of dome-shaped, skin colored or white viral lesions. The classic central depression is often absent.

Molluscum Contagiosum

Molluscum contagiosum (water warts) is a virus-induced skin lesion. These occur most often anywhere over the skin surface in small children, over the genital area of adults as a sexually transmitted disease, and particularly on the face in patients with the acquired immunodeficiency syndrome.

Although generally skin colored, mollusca contagiosa can appear white, pink, or pustular. The lesions are dome-shaped and are often shiny; usually at least some of the lesions will have a central depression (Fig. 8.9). They tend to be clustered.

Removal of these lesions requires destruction. Unlike true warts, molluscum contagiosum always resolve in the immunocompetent patient, although this can take months to years. Also, unlike genital warts, no significant medical consequences result from these lesions. Therefore, therapy is not crucial. They can be curetted, treated lightly with liquid nitrogen (even a superficial blister usually results in eradication of the lesions), or treated with topical cantharidin, a painless substance which produces a blister the following day.[9] Dyspigmentation frequently follows, and several treatments are generally required to eliminate new or recurring lesions.

Skin Tags

Skin tags are soft, pedunculated papules that are extremely common in adults, particularly in association with obesity (Fig. 8.10). They are most often seen in skin folds, such as the axillae, around the neck, under the breast, and in the groin. Although usually skin colored, they are occasionally brown.

Skin tags represent a pedunculated form of any of several different skin lesions. Most common are nevi, seborrheic keratoses, neurofibromas, and acrochordons. Acrochordons are skin tags that histologically show normal epidermis overlying loose connective tissue.

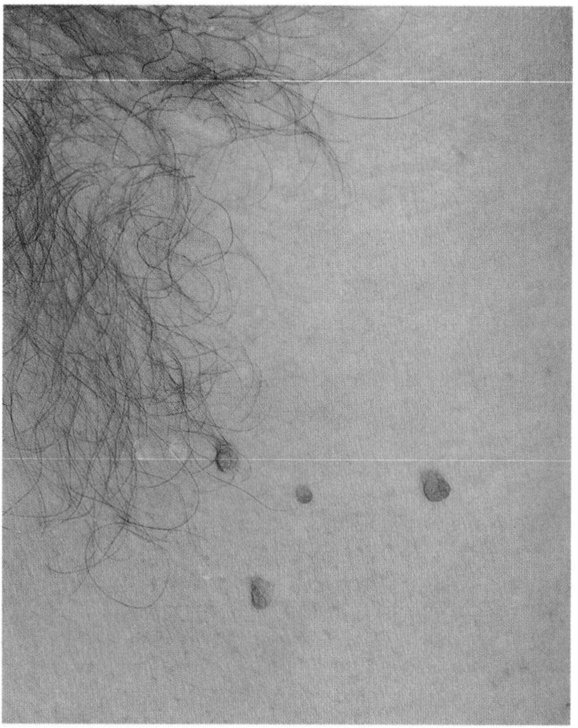

Figure 8.10 Skin tags are outpouchings of skin, often produced by intradermal nevi, neurofibromas, seborrheic keratoses, or simply friction in a skin fold. Unlike cutaneous horns, they are not associated with malignant skin lesions.

Skin tags have no medical significance, but they can be removed easily for cosmetic purposes or if friction causes irritation. Occasionally, a skin tag will twist, resulting in infarction, pain, and inflammation.

Skin tags can be removed by anesthetizing the base with lidocaine 1% with epinephrine, followed by snip removal with curved iris scissors and hemostasis achieved by ferric chloride or ferrous subsulfate.

Unlike cutaneous horns, skin tags that have been removed can be discarded, rather than submitted for pathology, since there are no dangerous diseases to be excluded.

Basal Cell Carcinomas

Basal cell carcinomas are the most common of all cancers in white patients.

Clinical Manifestations These tumors are induced primarily by chronic sun exposure, and they are therefore most often located on the head, neck, upper trunk, and, less often, over the dorsal hands and forearms. Basal cell carcinomas often, but not always, appear on skin with surrounding actinic keratoses, actinically induced dyspigmentation, and wrinkling. Occasionally, the skin can be remarkably undamaged; sometimes basal cell carcinomas can be found even in sun-protected areas such as the axilla, a scalp well shielded by abundant hair, or the genitalia.

There are four main morphologic variants of the basal cell carcinomas.

Nodular Most common is the nodular basal cell carcinoma, consisting of a pearly, skin-colored, well-demarcated papule (Fig. 8.11). Classically, the borders are elevated with a central depression, and telangiectasias are prominent.

Superficial A second very common variant is composed of superficial basal cell carcinomas, which are sharply demarcated, pink, flat papules or plaques (see Fig. 14.21). The surface can be slightly scaling or thinned and without scale. These occur primarily over the upper arms and upper trunk.

Pigmented Both nodular basal cell carcinomas and superficial basal cell carcinomas occasionally exhibit a brown or blue-black color that can be uniform or speckled. These tumors are called pigmented basal cell carcinomas.

Morpheaform The morpheaform basal cell carcinoma is a poorly demarcated, depressed, skin-colored papule or plaque that often resembles scar. Fairly often it is slightly hypopigmented.

Differential Diagnosis Nodular basal cell carcinomas often resemble intradermal nevi, but they usually differ by their pearly, almost translucent appearance. Superficial basal cell carcinomas may mimic small spots of eczema, papulosquamous diseases, actinic keratoses, or Bowen's disease (squamous cell carcinoma confined to the epidermis). Suspicion of a superficial basal cell carcinoma is usually enhanced by chronicity and relative stability of the lesion, a setting of sun damage, and a

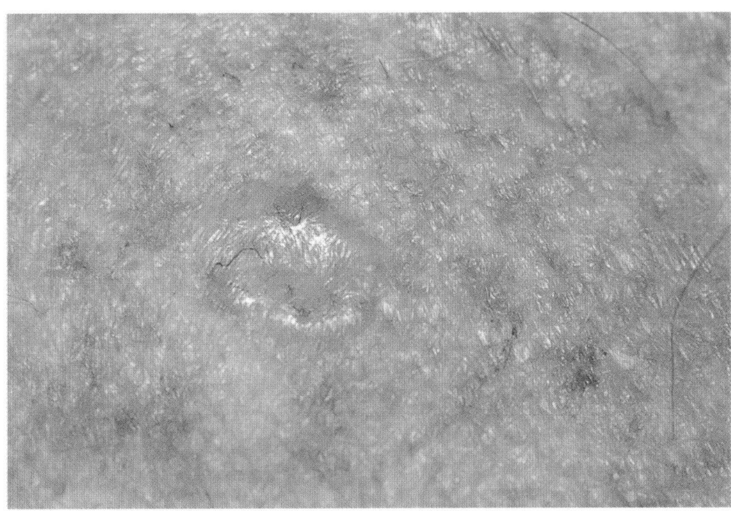

Figure 8.11 The pearly, translucent texture of a nodular basal cell carcinoma is characteristic, as are the slightly firm, waxy feel to the touch and the rolled borders.

poor response to medical therapy. The diagnosis is confirmed by biopsy. Pigmented tumors often require biopsy differentiation from nevi or melanoma. Morpheaform cancers most often resemble scar, requiring a high index of suspicion and biopsy for diagnosis.

Management Management in the emergency department consists primarily of recognition and referral. If the skin cancer is to be biopsied for confirmation, a shave biopsy is generally preferred, so that curettage and electrodesiccation remain a choice for definitive therapy. Because the tumor is so characteristic histologically, only a very small piece of the tumor is required for diagnosis. Normal surrounding skin need not be included on the biopsy, and it is often preferable to avoid removal of the entire surface of the tumor, so that the dermatologist or surgeon responsible for later therapy can more easily identify the site. Patients with suspected skin cancers on the nose, central face, and around the eyes and nose should be advised to see a dermatologist, ideally one with training in Moh's surgery (particularly if the diagnosis is not obvious) within several weeks. If this is not possible, a plastic surgeon can be consulted. For those with small lesions in other areas, the patient can see a physician at their earliest convenience, but preferably within several months.

Course and Prognosis Basal cell carcinomas do not metastasize. However, they continue to enlarge until they are removed or destroyed, with some skin cancers enlarging fairly rapidly and others growing so slowly that patients insist the lesion has been present and unchanged for years. The medical significance of basal cell carcinomas depends on their location. Skin cancers near eyes, over the nose, or around the ears can cause enormous destruction; their removal can be very difficult, even when the tumor appears innocuous on a superficial examination.

BASAL CELL CARCINOMA

Clinical Manifestations

Skin-colored or pink pearly nodule, papule or plaque, classically with telangiectasias and rolled borders often around a central depression; located most often on the face and ears. Superficial basal cell carcinomas are red, scaling or thinned, well-demarcated papules or plaques that often appear inflammatory, rather than neoplastic.

Management in the Emergency Department

1. *Referral to a dermatologist for further clinical evaluation and possible biopsy and removal or to a surgeon for biopsy and removal*
2. *If there is marked concern about patient compliance, a shave biopsy can be performed in the emergency department, or the lesion can even be removed with excision and suture closure*

Sebaceous Hyperplasia

Sebaceous hyperplasia, characterized by 2- to 5-mm skin-colored or yellowish lobular papules, occur on the face in response to sun damage. They are discussed in more detail in the section on yellow lesions.

Squamous Cell Carcinomas

Some squamous cell carcinomas, especially those unassociated with sun damage, are not keratotic (see earlier section on keratotic squamous cell carcinomas, p. 106). These solid-appearing tumors often have irregular, soft surfaces, and sometimes exhibit erosion or ulceration. The diagnosis is made on the basis of the morphology of the lesion, the clinical setting of sun damage or chronic inflammation, and a biopsy. Treatment generally consists of excision or radiation therapy.

Please see patient information handouts for this chapter on pages 341, 348, 363, and 374.

REFERENCES

1. Orlow SJ, Paller A: Cimetidine therapy for multiple viral warts in children. J Am Acad Dermatol 28:794, 1993
2. Yilmaz E, Alpsoy E, Basaran E: Cimetadine therapy for warts: a placebo-controlled, double-blind study. J Am Acad Dermatol 34:1005, 1996
3. Shumer SM, O'Keefe CJ: Bleomycin in the treatment of recalcitrant warts. J Am Acad Dermatol 9:91, 1983
4. Marks R, Rennie G, Selwood T: Malignant transformation of solar keratoses to squamous cell carcinoma. Lancet 1:795, 1988
5. Marks R, Rennie G, Selwood T et al: The relationship of basal cell carcinomas and squamous cell carcinomas to solar keratoses. Arch Dermatol 124:1039, 1988
6. Moller R: Metastases in dermatological patients with squamous cell carcinoma. Arch Dermatol 115:703, 1979
7. Ferenczy A: Epidemiology and clinical pathophysiology of condylomata acuminata. Am J Obstet Gynecol 172:1331, 1995
8. Quan MB, Moy L: The role of human papillomavirus in carcinoma. J Am Acad Dermatol 25: 698, 1991
9. Epstein E: Cantharidin treatment of molluscum contagiosum. Acta Derm Venereol (Stockh) 69: 91, 1989

SUGGESTED READINGS

Warts

Goldfarb MT, Reid R (eds): Human papillomavirus infection. Dermatol Clin 9:2, 1991

Actinic Keratoses

Schwartz RA: Therapeutic perspectives in actinic and other keratoses. Int J Dermatol 35:533, 1996

Squamous Cell Carcinoma

Marks R: Squamous cell carcinoma. Lancet 347:735, 1996

Genital Warts

Bauer HM, Ting Y, Greet CE et al: Genital human papillomavirus infection in female university students as determined by a PCR-based method. JAMA 265:472, 1991

Heaton CL: Clinical manifestations and modern management of condylomata acuminata: a dermatologic perspective. Am J Obstet Gynecol 172:1345, 1995

Stone KM: Human papillomavirus infection and genital warts: update on epidemiology and treatment. Clin Infect Dis, suppl 1. 20:S91, 1995

Molluscum Contagiosum

Epstein WL: Molluscum contagiosum. Semin Dermatol 11:184, 1992

Basal Cell Carcinoma

Goldberg LH: Basal cell carcinoma. Lancet 347:663, 1996

CHAPTER 9

White Lesions

Most white lesions are produced by a decrease or absence of melanin. However, white papules or nodules occasionally occur from light-colored substances contained in the skin, such as calcium or the hydrated keratin that fills an epidermal cyst. This chapter is divided into 2 major sections: white macules and patches, representing a lack of pigment, and white papules and nodules, primarily representing light-colored deposits in the skin.

WHITE MACULES AND PATCHES

Light-colored macules and patches can either be totally devoid of pigment (depigmented) or simply lighter than surrounding skin, but not totally lacking in color (hypopigmented). Usually, depigmented skin appears milk-white, in striking contrast to surrounding, normal skin. However, particularly in patients whose natural color is very pale, differentiation of depigmentation from hypopigmentation may be difficult. An examination of the skin in a dark room with a Wood's light can be useful. Depigmented skin illuminated with a Wood's lamp in a dark room shows a brilliant white color, whereas hypopigmented skin appears almost the same color as the patient's normal skin.

Another important distinction that can sometimes be surprisingly difficult is the judgment as to which skin change is normal—the light area or the pigmented area (Fig. 9.1). When large areas of hypopigmentation are present, normal skin may be mistaken to represent hyperpigmentation. Even the patient is often mistaken or unsure. A general examination of the body can usually help judge correctly which skin is abnormal.

Vitiligo

Vitiligo is a disease of depigmentation that is incompletely understood but that probably results, at least in part, from the autoimmune destruction of melanocytes. This common disease occurs in 1% to 2% of the population,[1] and 20% to 30% of patients report a family history of vitiligo.[2] Vitiligo affects women more often than men at a ratio of about 2 : 1, with pigment loss usually beginning in childhood or early adult life.

Clinical Manifestations Vitiligo consists of color change only. There is no scale, surface texture change, induration, or evidence of old scarring. Most often, vitiligo begins as sharply demarcated, completely white macules over the extensor surface of joints and around orifices, such as the eyes, nose, and ears. The vulva is often affected in women, with the glans penis frequently involved in men. These areas are preferentially affected because vitiligo exhibits the Koebner phenomenon, wherein skin disease is precipitated by trauma or inflammation. The extensor surfaces of joints are preferentially affected because these areas tend to be bumped, and orifices may be common sites because they are irritated by body fluids or rubbing.

Vitiligo is generally progressive, beginning as small macules that coalesce into larger patches. Occasionally, skin can be slightly pink from the very mild inflammation of the underlying process or, more often, from sunlight exposure to skin that no longer has protection against ultraviolet light. Rarely, in addition to normal skin and depigmented skin, there are intermediate areas of hypopigmentation or peripheral hyperpigmenta-

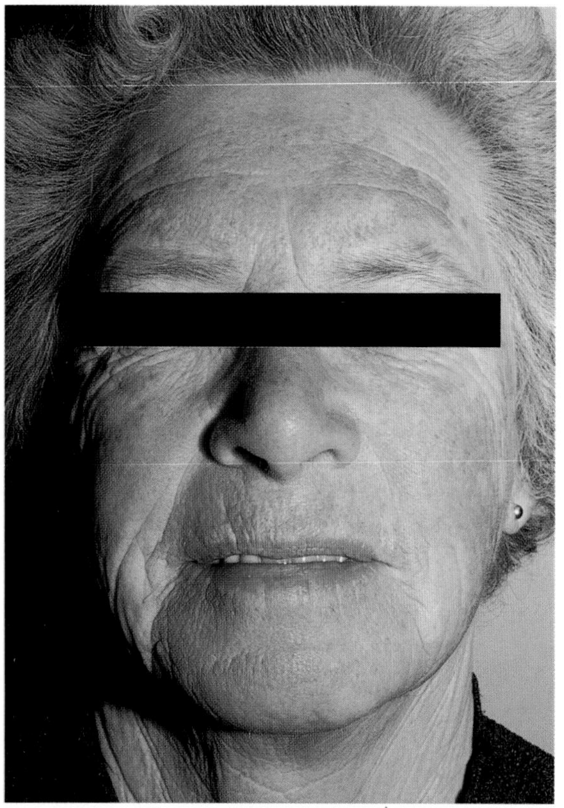

Figure 9.1 This patient presented to her dermatologist with a complaint of brown spots on her face. Careful examination showed the brown color to be her normal skin, and the lighter areas to represent new onset of vitiligo.

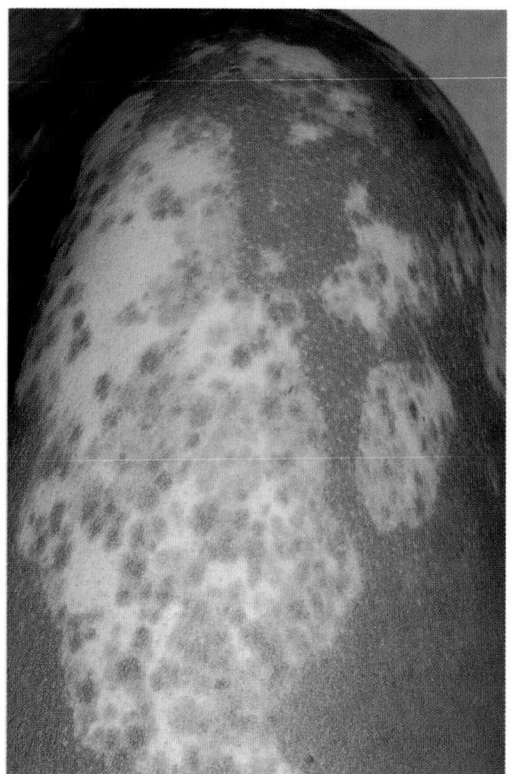

Figure 9.2 Trichrome vitiligo exhibits depigmented skin, hypopigmented skin, and normal color.

tion, producing trichrome vitiligo with three or more colors (Fig. 9.2)

Vitiligo ranges from small macules in light-complexioned patients that are extremely subtle because of the lack of contrast, to extensive, severely disfiguring disease that can be cosmetically devastating in darkly pigmented patients (Fig. 9.3). In addition, vitiligo is a life-ruining disease in patients from some countries where hypopigmentation is a strong social stigma. Also, because early lesions of leprosy sometimes present as hypopigmented patches, fear makes some people with vitiligo outcasts in these endemic areas.

Like patients with other autoimmune diseases, those with vitiligo have a slightly increased risk of additional autoimmune conditions and autoantibodies.[3] This increased incidence is negligible, although thyroid disease is the most likely association. Some physicians routinely obtain thyroid function tests, and patients should be at least briefly questioned and examined for findings suggestive of thyroid disease. Choroidal depigmentation can also occur, and some patients exhibit iritis on an eye examination.[4] However, visual acuity is generally unaffected, and eye examinations are not performed routinely.

Differential Diagnosis The primary disease to be differentiated from vitiligo is postinflammatory hypopigmentation. A Wood's light examination that demonstrates the depigmented nature of the affected skin confirms a diagnosis of vitiligo.

Management Therapy for vitiligo is very slow, with unpredictable results. Many dermatologists are fatalistic and tell their patients that there is no good therapy, suggesting cosmetic coverup only. Other dermatologists are quite aggressive and find

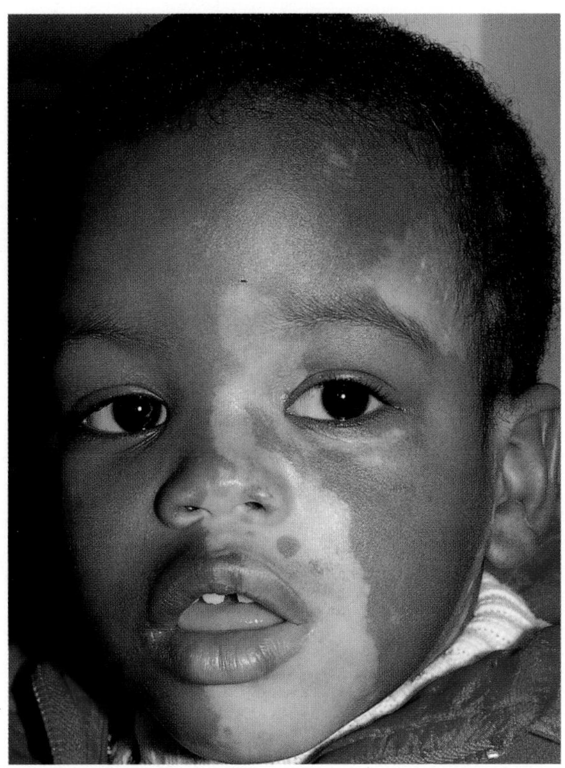

Figure 9.3 The darker the natural complexion of the patient, the more obvious these milk-white patches appear.

that some patients, although certainly not all, do very well.

Sun protection of depigmented areas in all patients is extremely important. Patients should be counseled to use a sunscreen with a high sun-protection factor (SPF) daily over depigmented skin. This not only prevents sunburn but helps prevent chronic sun damage and skin cancer in the future. In addition, sunscreen use on surrounding skin minimizes tanning, decreasing the contrast of vitiligo with surrounding skin.

The easiest specific therapy, and the only one suitable for the emergency department, is topical corticosteroids.[5] A midpotency topical corticosteroid such as triamcinolone cream 0.1% applied twice daily is a reasonable first choice, with follow-up evaluation in a dermatologist's office after about 1 month of therapy. Patients, particularly children and patients with facial or skin fold involvement, should be given limited amounts of medication. Patients should be counseled that repigmentation is extremely slow and that follow-up evaluation in 1 month is very important, because local thinning of the skin and steroid dermatitis can occur as a result of chronic corticosteroid use.

Other methods of treating vitiligo include oral or topical psoralens (a photosensitizing medication) followed by exposure to ultraviolet A light (PUVA),[6] and skin grafting.[7] For very light-complexioned patients, simply wearing a sunscreen so that surrounding skin remains as pale as possible sometimes makes vitiligo nearly invisible and therapy unimportant. A mainstay in the treatment of vitiligo is cosmetic camouflage. The skilled application of an opaque makeup, such as Dermablend or Lydia O'Leary's Covermark, can totally hide the disfigurement of vitiligo.

VITILIGO

Clinical Manifestations

Depigmented macules and patches most often located around orifices and over dorsal aspect of joints.

Management in the Emergency Department

1. *Triamcinolone cream 0.1% (hydrocortisone cream 1% or 2.5% for face and skin folds) applied sparingly twice a day, and give limited quantity*
2. *Daily sunscreen with a SPF of 15 or higher*
3. *Cosmetic coverups (Dermablend, Lydia O'Leary's Covermark)*
4. *Patient education (see the patient handout on p. 373, Vitiligo)*
5. *Follow-up evaluation with a dermatologist in 1 month*

Piebaldism

Piebaldism consists of congenital depigmented, stable patches, generally including a white forelock. Occasionally they are associated with hyperpigmented macules and patches as well. Generally, children are otherwise normal. This condition consists of an absence of melanocytes within white skin. This condition is differentiated from vitiligo by its congenital, stable nature, and from hypochromic nevi by virtue of its total depigmentation.

Management consists of the early recognition of any associated abnormalities. However, repigmentation in piebaldism is not possible.

Albinism

Albinism constitutes a group of genetic disorders characterized by generalized loss of pigment. This loss of pigment can be total (tyrosinase-negative albinism), in which the skin is milk-white, the blue eyes produce a remarkable red reflex due to loss of pigmentation of the iris and retina, and the hair is white. These patients also have extremely poor vision due in part to pigment loss, but also because of neurologic abnormalities. Other forms of albinism produce varying amounts of partial pigmentation, so that the hair may be blond, some pigment occurs in the eyes, and pigmented nevi are present. These patients often have very poor vision.

Management consists of genetic counseling, sun protection, and the early recognition and management of visual abnormalities.

Postinflammatory Hypopigmentation and Depigmentation

Injury to the skin, either traumatic or inflammatory, often increases or decreases the production of melanin. Depending on the natural tendency of the patient and the nature and severity of injury, this can result in hyperpigmentation, varying degrees of hypopigmentation, and, rarely, depigmentation.

Clinical Manifestations The pattern of the light areas of the skin corresponds to the area of injury or inflammation. Often the patient recalls the preexisting condition, although sometimes either the preceding event was very minor or subtle, or the patient is simply unobservant, making the history unhelpful. In spite of a negative history, the diagnosis can often be made on the basis of the pattern and distribution of the hypopigmentation, as well as the history of recent onset (Fig. 9.4).

Morphologically, unless the underlying inflammation is ongoing, postinflammatory hypopigmentation consists of color change only, without scale, texture change, or other surface characteristics. In addition, postinflammatory hypopigmentation is not associated with itching or pain.

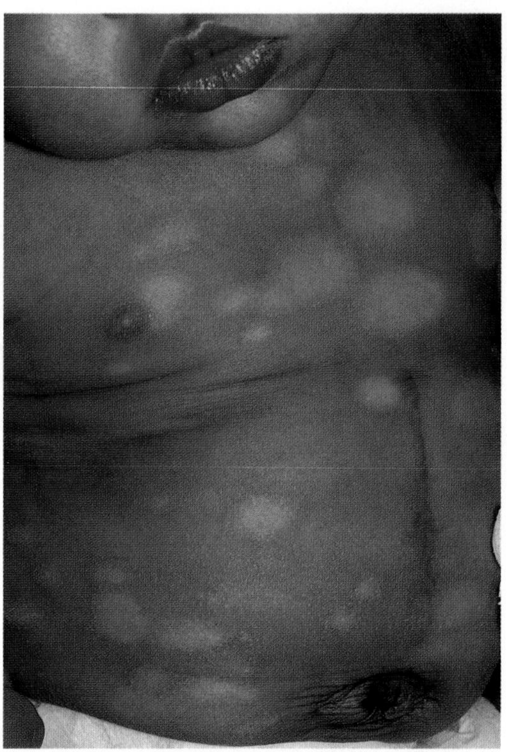

Figure 9.4 Postinflammatory hypopigmentation differs from vitiligo by its lighter, rather than totally white, color, and by a pattern or history consistent with previous inflammation. This baby has seborrheic dermatitis, and continuing inflammation can be seen at the borders of the hypopigmented patches.

Differential Diagnosis The primary condition to be considered in the differential diagnosis of postinflammatory hypopigmentation and depigmentation is vitiligo. However, the distribution of vitiligo is usually characteristic, the borders are more sharply demarcated, and the skin is uniformly depigmented. Mild postinflammatory hypopigmentation associated with low-grade, ongoing eczema located primarily over the lateral arms, cheeks, and anterior thighs is called *pityriasis alba* (Fig. 9.5). Hypopigmented macules and patches associated with various neurocutaneous syndromes (e.g., tuberous sclerosis, neurofibromatosis, and incontinentia pigmentia achromians) are more longstanding and stable than postinflammatory hypopigmentation. The differentiation of these diseases sometimes rests entirely on the clinical presentation, since biopsies may be nonspecific.

Management Therapy for postinflammatory hypopigmentation consists of the elimination of any ongoing inflammation, such as eczema or repetitive trauma. In addition, a sunscreen with a high SPF over the entire area helps prevent tanning of surrounding skin, minimizing the contrast of the hypopigmented area with normal skin. Otherwise, there is no specific treatment to hasten repigmentation of postinflammatory hypopigmentation.

The natural course of postinflammatory hypopigmentation is slow repigmentation. However, extreme inflammation or trauma may actually obliterate melanocytes, resulting in permanent depigmentation, especially in black patients.

POSTINFLAMMATORY HYPOPIGMENTATION AND DEPIGMENTATION, PITYRIASIS ALBA

Clinical Manifestations

Light or white skin that corresponds in location to previous inflammation or injury, either by history or

(Continues)

(Continued)

pattern. Pityriasis alba represents poorly demarcated postinflammatory hypopigmentation due to mild eczema, most often of the lateral arm and cheeks.

Management in the Emergency Department

1. *Treat any ongoing inflammation, using hydrocortisone cream 1% or 2.5% for pityriasis alba*
2. *Reassurance*
3. *Sunscreen with a SPF of 15 or higher, to prevent tanning of surrounding skin that increases contrast with light skin*

Achromic Nevus

Occasionally, hypopigmented macules or patches occur during childhood or infancy, remaining stable throughout life or gradually fading in adult years. Also called hypochromic nevus, hypomelanosis of Ito, and incontinentia pigmenti achromians, these light spots are most often located on the trunk and usually have no medical significance. However, when these are multiple or large, associated neuroectodermal abnormalities may be present, and the patient should be referred for further evaluation.

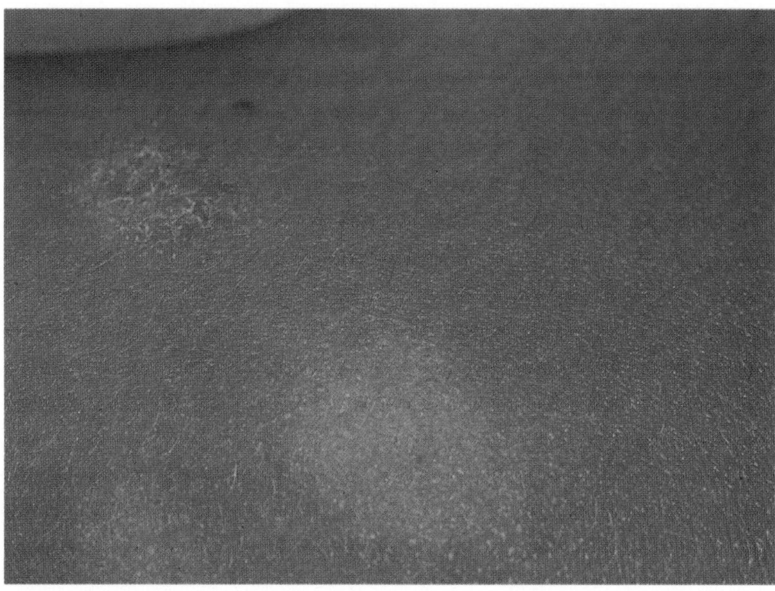

Figure 9.5 Pityriasis alba represents postinflammatory hypopigmentation produced by mild eczema.

Pityriasis "Tinea" Versicolor

Pityriasis "tinea" versicolor is a yeast infection that can present with hypopigmented, hyperpigmented, and/or pink skin lesions (for detailed discussion, see Ch. 11, Brown Lesions). More common in young men, hypopigmented lesions are most obvious in the summer because sunlight tans surrounding, but not affected, skin, increasing the contrast with abnormal skin.

Usually the lesions of pityriasis versicolor first occur and are most concentrated over the upper central back and chest (Fig. 9.6). Flat, small, lightly scaling papules that appear macular due to the very subtle surface change coalesce into larger plaques.

The definitive diagnosis of a typical tinea versicolor can be made with a potassium hydroxide preparation, by culture, or by response to therapy. Therapy consists of topical medications such as selenium sulfide 2.5% (Selsun) lotion applied overnight weekly, any topical azole cream (e.g., clotrimazole or miconazole) applied twice a day, or 50% propylene glycol in water, which is very easy to apply and cosmetically well accepted. Oral therapies include fluconazole 400 mg once[8] or ketoconazole 200 mg each morning for 3 to 5 days.[9] The risk of hepatotoxicity with this dose is low but present. In addition, itraconazole has been shown to be beneficial at a dose of 200 mg/day for 1 week.[10] Oral griseofulvin is not beneficial. Prophylactic topical therapy every 1 to 3 months should be advised because of the high relapse rate.

Lichen Sclerosus (et Atrophicus)

Lichen sclerosus (et atrophicus) is a disease most often located over the vulva of women and girls. Probably of autoimmune etiology, this disease can be asymptomatic, or it can produce extreme pruritus.

Lichen sclerosus typically presents as a white, well-demarcated plaque that begins around the clitoral area and eventually encompasses the entire vulva and perianal area (Fig. 9.7). Shininess, crinkling of the skin, a cellophane paper appearance, or a waxy appearance are all common, specific findings. Often, purpura and erosions are present due to fragility of the skin and the effects of

Figure 9.6 Pityriasis "tinea" versicolor can be diagnosed by the location and presence of fine scale on sharply demarcated papules that coalesce into plaques. Confirmation by an examination of a fungal smear can be obtained when needed.

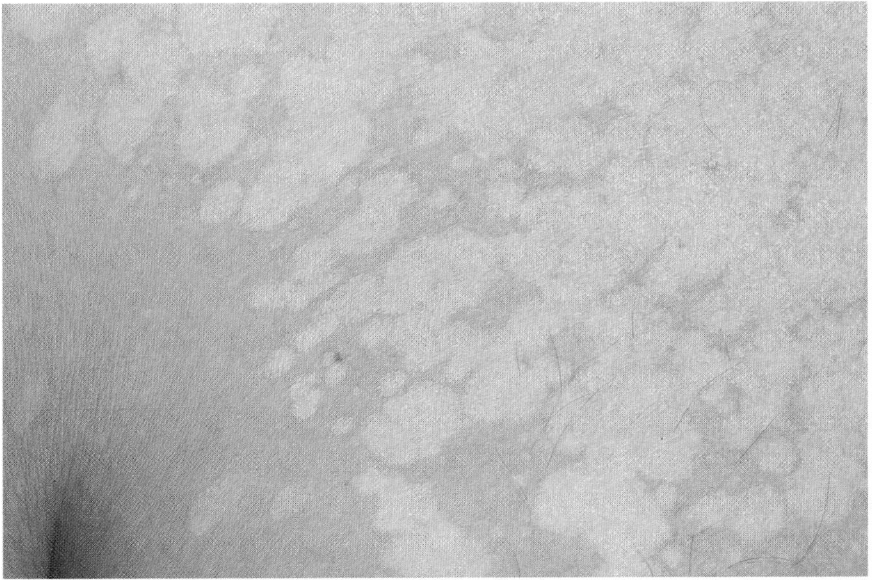

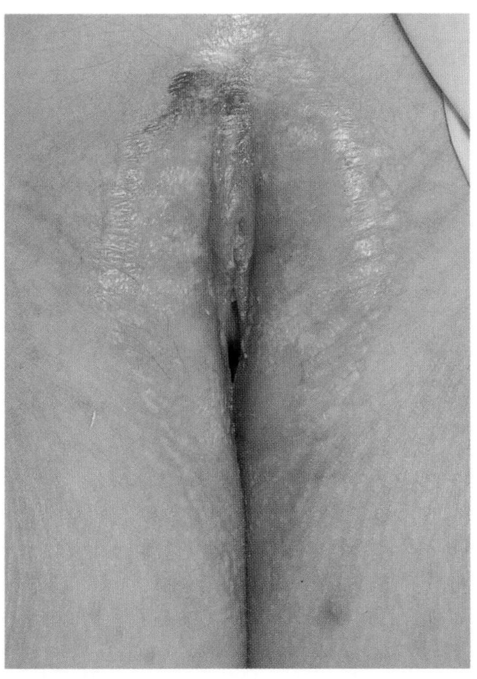

Figure 9.7 Lichen sclerosus (et atrophicus) presents as a white, well-demarcated plaque. Fragility is manifested by crusts and erosions, and shininess can be seen in the small follicular papules at the border.

scratching. As the disease progresses, the labia minora are resorbed, and the clitoral hood scars to the underlying structures, completely burying the clitoris. Eventually, the introitus is narrowed.

The main diseases in the differential diagnosis are vitiligo, which also preferentially affects this location. However, vitiligo consists of depigmentation only, without any surface texture changes, scale, or purpura. Postinflammatory hypopigmentation from neurodermatitis can be very difficult to distinguish, especially since lichenification can obscure lichen sclerosus in some patients who rub and scratch. Usually, a biopsy differentiates these two diseases.

Therapy for lichen sclerosus consists of an ultrapotent topical corticosteroid, although the prescribing clinician should be very aware of the adverse reactions of a highly potent medication in the genital area. The patient should seek immediate follow-up evaluation with a dermatologist. This will give the dermatologist the opportunity to record a baseline evaluation before significant healing occurs.

Most patients improve rapidly with this therapy. However, this disease is chronic and requires ongoing topical corticosteroid therapy. The appropriate potency and frequency of application must be individualized and discovered by trial and error. Patients should be aware that about 5% of untreated women with lichen sclerosus develop an associated squamous cell carcinoma.

Mucosal Lichen Planus

Lichen planus, an autoimmune skin disease, appears white when it occurs on a wet surface, such as the oral mucosa or the modified mucous membrane of the vulva or uncircumcised penis. Most often, lichen planus presents as white, lacey, reticulate, or fern-like striae (Fig. 9.8), although

Figure 9.8 When occurring on a mucous membrane or modified mucous membrane, lichen planus most often presents as white, fern-like, reticulate, or lacey papules and plaques.

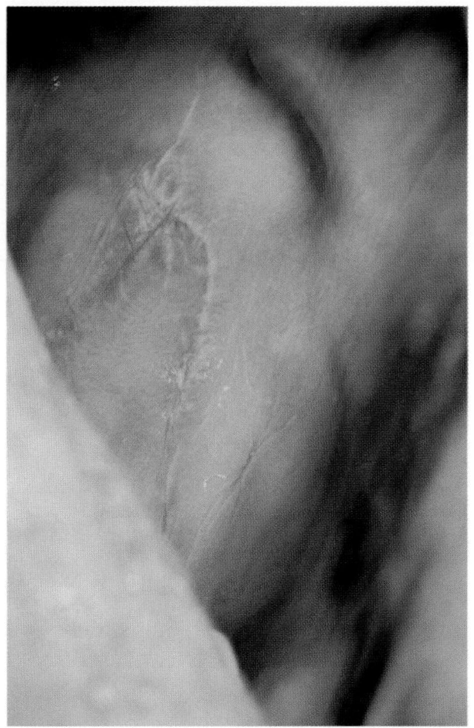

more solid-appearing white epithelium or erosions with surrounding white epithelium, are common as well (Fig. 17.9). The posterior buccal mucosa is the most often affected epithelial surface, but the gingiva and tongue can be involved as well (for further discussion, see Chs. 14 and 17).

WHITE PAPULES AND NODULES

Epidermal Inclusion Cyst

Hydrated keratin appears white. Therefore, keratin-filled cysts that are close to the surface of the skin appear white (Fig. 9.9). Most epidermal inclusion cysts (milia, epidermoid cyst, epidermal cyst, "sebaceous" cyst) are formed from hair follicles that become blocked by a keratin plug or inflammation in a superficial scar over the surface. Very small (about 1 mm) superficial cysts are called milia, whereas larger ones are called epidermal or epidermoid cysts (for detailed discussion, see Ch. 8, Skin-Colored Lesions). Larger cysts are more often deep, and the white contents are not appreciated. Therapy is generally unnecessary but, for those patients who desire treatment, surgical removal is required. Small milia can often be teased from the skin with an 18-gauge needle or a No. 11 scalpel.

Molluscum Contagiosum

Molluscum contagiosum (water warts) is a virus-induced skin lesion that occasionally appears white. Lesions are most often skin-colored (these are discussed primarily in Ch. 8). They occur most often anywhere over the skin surface in small children, over the genital area of adults as a sexually transmitted disease, and particularly on the face in patients with the acquired immunodeficiency syndrome (AIDS).

Although generally skin colored, mollusca can appear white, pink, or pustular (Fig. 9.10; see also Fig. 8.9). Lesions are dome-shaped and often

Figure 9.9 These milia, which are small epidermal inclusion cysts, occurred when erosions of bullous pemphigoid healed, obstructing the orifices of hair follicles. Blocked follicles become distended with white keratin shed from the follicular epithelium.

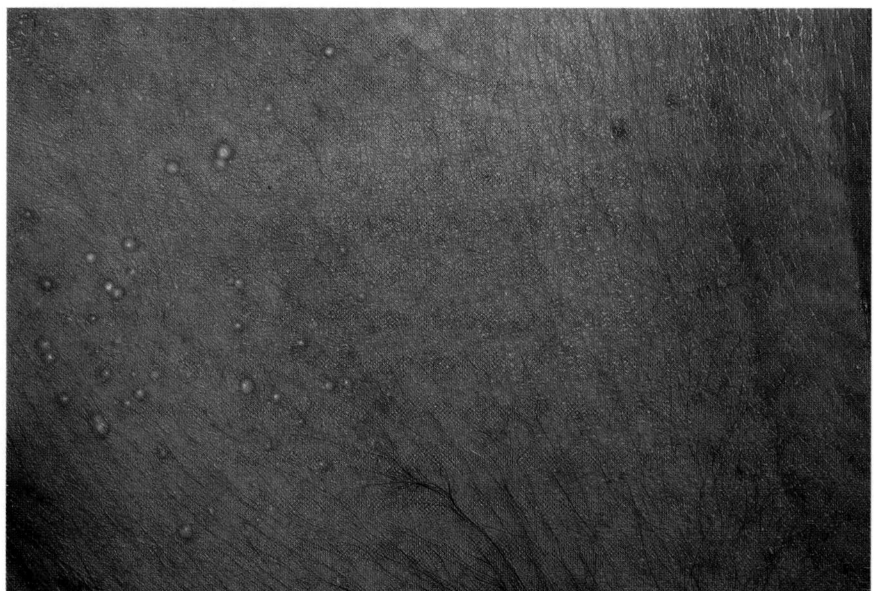

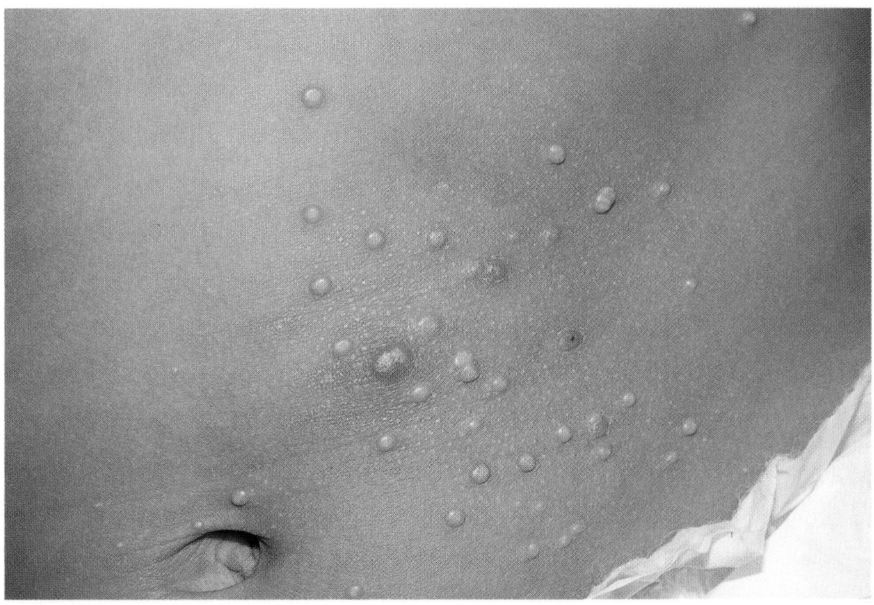

Figure 9.10 Molluscum contagiosum often appears white, because of mollusca bodies (consisting of viral protein) within the epidermis.

shiny; usually at least some of the lesions will have a central depression. They tend to be clustered.

Removal of these lesions requires destruction. They can be curetted, treated lightly with liquid nitrogen (even a superficial blister usually results in eradication of the lesions), or treated with topical cantharidin, a painless substance that produces a blister the next day.[11] Dyspigmentation frequently follows, and several treatments are generally required to eliminate new or recurring lesions.

Calcinosis Cutis

Calcinosis cutis, the deposition of calcium in the upper dermis, can produce white papules, nodules, or plaques. This occurs most often as a result of local injury or inflammation, but conditions such as hypercalcemia, and extravasated intravenous solutions containing calcium can produce this condition as well. The papules are usually very firm, and the diagnosis is made either by history or on biopsy. There is no specific therapy.

Chronic Cutaneous (Discoid) Lupus Erythematosus

In patients with chronic cutaneous (discoid) lupus erythematosus, depigmentation develops within very inflammatory plaques as the disease progresses. The depigmented areas are scarred and firm, and surrounding skin is inflammatory or hyperpigmented, with scale or crust (see Fig. 14.4). The location is most often over the lateral face or scalp, but any area can be involved.

The diagnosis is made on the basis of the morphology of the individual lesions and a confirmatory biopsy. Patients should be evaluated with a history and physical examination to detect early abnormalities consistent with systemic lupus erythematosus. In addition, screening laboratory tests should be performed to include measurements of antinuclear antibody, erythrocyte sedimentation rate, complement, complete blood count, and renal function. A urinalysis to detect early proteinuria is also indicated. However, most patients with chronic cutaneous lupus erythematosus do not have significant systemic disease.

Please see the patient information handout for this chapter on page 373.

REFERENCES

1. Grimes PE: Diseases of hypopigmentation. p. 843. In Sams WM Jr, Lynch PJ (eds): Principles and Practice of Dermatology. 2nd Ed. Churchill Livingstone, New York, 1996
2. Mosher DB, Fitzpatrick TB, Hori Y, Ortonne JP: Disorders of melanocytes. p. 901. In Fitzpatrick TB, Eisen AZ, Wolff K et al (eds): Dermatology in General Medicine. 4th Ed. McGraw-Hill, New York, 1993
3. Brostoff J: Autoantibodies in patients with vitiligo. Lancet 2:117, 1969
4. Cowan CL, Halder RM, Grimes PE: Ocular disturbances in vitiligo. J Am Acad Dermatol 5:17, 1986
5. Lui XQ, Shao CG, Jin PV et al: Treatment of localized vitiligo with clobetasol cream. Int J Dermatol 29:295, 1990
6. Honig B, Moreson WL, Karp D: Photochemotherapy beyond psoriasis. J Am Acad Dermatol 31:775, 1994
7. Koga M: Epidermal grafting using the tops of suction blisters in the treatment of vitiligo. Arch Dermatol 124:1656, 1988
8. Faergemann J: Treatment of pityriasis versicolor with a single dose of fluconazole. Acta Derm Venereol (Stockh) 72:74, 1992
9. Elgart ML, Warren NG: The superficial and subcutaneous mycoses. p. 869. In Moschella SL, Hurley HJ (eds): Dermatology. 3rd Ed. WB Saunders, Philadelphia, 1992
10. Hickman JG: A double-blind, randomized, placebo-controlled evaluation of short-term treatment with oral itraconazole in patients with tinea versicolor. J Am Acad Dermatol 34: 785, 1996
11. Epstein E: Cantharidin treatment of molluscum contagiosum. Acta Derm Venereol (Stockh) 69: 91, 1989

SUGGESTED READINGS

Vitiligo

Grimes PE: Vitiligo: an overview of therapeutic approaches. Dermatol Clin 11:325, 1993

Grimes PE: Diseases of hypopigmentation. p. 843. In Sams WM Jr, Lynch PJ (eds): Principles and Practice of Dermatology. 2nd Ed. Churchill Livingstone, New York, 1996

Pityriasis "Tinea" Versicolor

Faergemann J, Gothenburg S: *Pityrosporum* infections. J Am Acad Dermatol 31:S18, 1994

Lichen Sclerosus (et Atrophicus)

Ridley MC: Lichen sclerosus. Dermatol Clin 10:309, 1992

Mucosal Lichen Planus

Bricker SL. Oral lichen planus: a review. Semin Dermatol 13:87, 1994

Molluscum Contagiosum

Epstein WL: Molluscum contagiosum. Semin Dermatol 11:184, 1992

CHAPTER 10

Yellow Lesions

Yellow lesions are divided into two primary groups. The first includes lesions that are smooth surfaced with a slightly yellowish color due to lipid or the deposition of substances that are slightly yellowish in color, such as amyloid. The second group comprises lesions that are not inherently yellow but that are covered with a yellow crust; these can occur with any erosion that allows serum to collect and dry.

SMOOTH-SURFACED YELLOW LESIONS

Necrobiosis Lipoidica

Necrobiosis lipoidica (diabeticorum) is an uncommon, inflammatory plaque that occurs most often over the anterior lower legs. About two-thirds of patients with necrobiosis lipoidica have diabetes mellitus.

These plaques are red or pink, with central yellowish discoloration (Fig. 10.1). The overlying skin is atrophic (thinned) and often anesthetic. This atrophy can be detected by the shiny, smooth character of the surface. When the plaques are well developed, the blood vessels are easily seen through thin epidermis. Occasionally, scale is present as a result of the ongoing inflammation, and the borders of the lesions are sometimes slightly thickened due to granulomatous inflammation within the dermis.

The cause of this condition is unknown, and therapy is difficult. All patients with necrobiosis lipoidica should be evaluated for diabetes mellitus. First-line therapy consists of a topical corticosteroid, such as triamcinolone cream 0.1% applied twice a day. Another therapy used by some dermatologists is intralesionally administered corticosteroids.[1] Steroid therapy is a double-edged sword; although corticosteroids can decrease the granulomatous inflammation, atrophy is a side effect of corticosteroids.

Most patients have one or two lesions that eventually stabilize spontaneously. In rare cases, there are multiple lesions or very aggressive lesions that ulcerate. These patients should be referred to a dermatologist for long-term follow-up management.

Xanthomas

Xanthomas are yellow as a result of yellow lipid within the skin. This deposition occurs in several settings, some important and others not.

Xanthelasma Xanthelasma are common papules or plaques that consist of lipid-filled macrophages. These flat-topped, well-demarcated lesions occur over the eyelids.

About 40% of patients with xanthelasma exhibit an associated lipid disorder that places them at an increased risk of cardiovascular disease. Therefore, a fasting lipid profile should be obtained for all patients with xanthelasma.

Therapy is unnecessary, except for cosmetic reasons. There is no medical therapy; destruction is required. This can be achieved by surgical excision of small lesions. Occasionally, laser vaporization, light electrocautery, and chemical peels are reported as effective in some patients. However, lesions recur.

Eruptive Xanthomas An uncommon but urgent sign of hypertriglyceridemia is eruptive xanthomas. These multiple lesions appear as red, dome-shaped, nonscaling papules with a yellowish center (Fig. 10.2). Since trauma can precipitate forma-

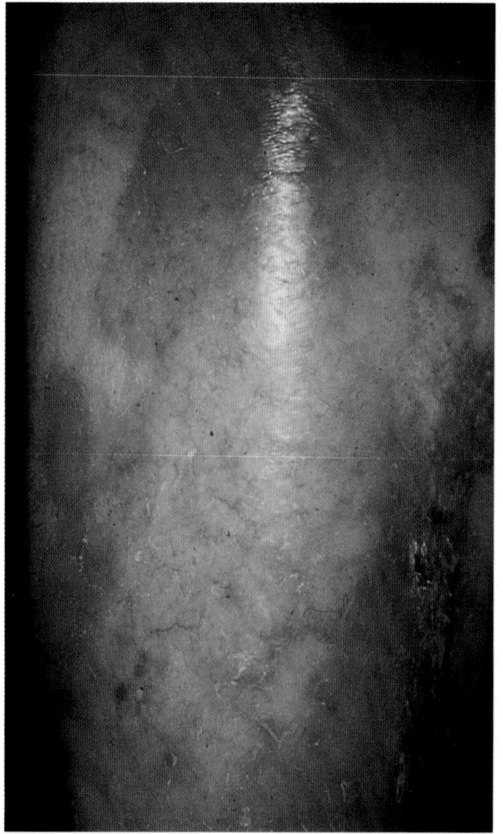

Figure 10.1 Necrobiosis lipoidica is most often located over the lower leg. It is characterized by a yellow color and by thinned, shiny skin with telangiectasias.

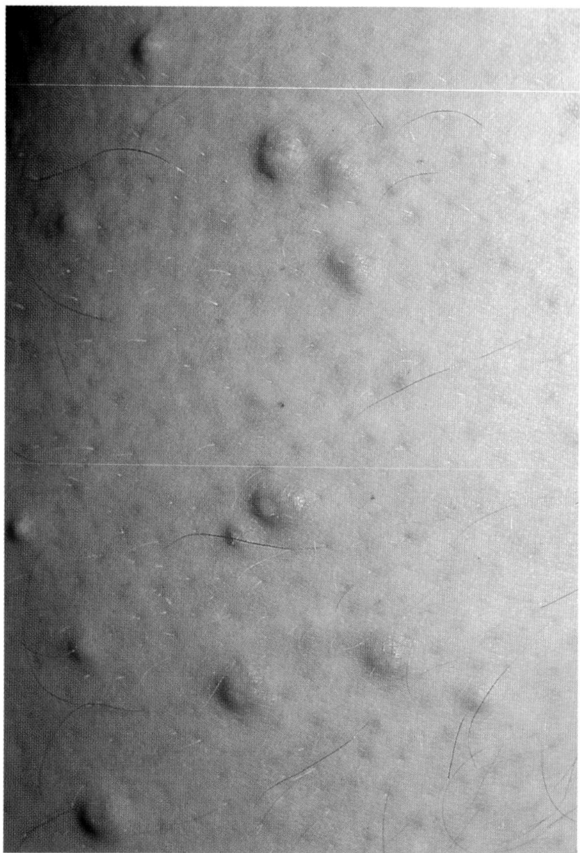

Figure 10.2 Eruptive xanthomas present as multiple papules that often appear inflamed, but a yellowish "pseudo-pustular" character and the pattern of lesions in scars and scratches suggest the correct diagnosis.

tion of these papules, lesions form lines in some areas. Usually asymptomatic, eruptive xanthomas appear rather rapidly, over days to weeks.

The diagnosis is generally made on clinical grounds, with confirmation by high serum triglyceride levels. An occasional, serious, associated medical complication is acute pancreatitis. Patients should be counseled to avoid consumption of alcoholic beverages and referred immediately to an internist or family physician for therapy to decrease triglyceride levels, to prevent pancreatitis. Eruptive xanthomas resolve with control of triglyceride levels.

Other Xanthomas Other xanthomas occasionally occur, always as a result of hyperlipidemia. These occur around tendons, over the palms, and over joints as infiltrated yellowish plaques with a smooth surface. The diagnosis is made on the basis of abnormal findings on testing for lipids. Improvement in these xanthomas occurs with improvement of hyperlipidemia.

Amyloidosis

Amyloidosis consists of deposition of amyloid in the skin and sometimes in other tissues. Amyloid is composed of portions of immunoglobulins that can be produced in response to several unrelated conditions and then deposited locally in the skin or systemically, including the viscera. Therefore, some forms of amyloidosis are innocuous with no medical implications, whereas those forms of amyloidosis associated with visceral involvement often result in organ dysfunction and death.

Systemic amyloidosis secondary to chronic inflammatory diseases such as rheumatoid arthritis is generally unaccompanied by skin findings. However, systemic disease that is primary or produced by myeloma is more often accompanied by skin findings. With significant deposition of amyloid around blood vessels, the vessels become fragile, and purpura appears after minor trauma, such as rubbing or scratching the eyes or after increased venous pressure from coughing, sneezing, or vomiting. With greater deposition, the skin may develop a yellowish, infiltrated appearance, particularly in the thin skin around the eyes (Fig. 10.3). *Localized cutaneous amyloidosis* does not appear yellow, but rather hyperpigmented or skin colored.

There are few diseases in the differential diagnosis of the yellow and purpuric lesions of amyloidosis. Xanthelasma are much more sharply demarcated, stable, and without purpura. The diagnosis can be confirmed by skin biopsy.

There is no treatment for the skin disease associated with systemic amyloidosis. Appropriate management includes referral to a rheumatologist or general internist to evaluate the patient for an underlying rheumatologic etiology, multiple myeloma, or other systemic involvement.

Sebaceous Hyperplasia

Sebaceous hyperplasia consists of sun-induced, small, benign lesions that occur primarily over the face. They are enlarged (2- to 5-mm), lobular sebaceous glands encircling a hair follicle. They are smooth-surfaced, and skin-colored to yellowish. A central depression formed by the follicle sometimes mimics that of a basal cell carcinoma.

These lesions are innocuous and asymptomatic, and their significance is limited to their role as a marker for chronic sun damage. They can be destroyed by hyfrecation or curettage, but a scar results.

Colloid Milium

Colloid milium is generally seen in adults as a degenerative finding caused by chronic sun damage. Multiple small, yellow, translucent, dome-shaped papules cover the dorsal hands or lateral neck or face. The diagnosis can be made by the distinctive morphologic appearance. Dermabrasion

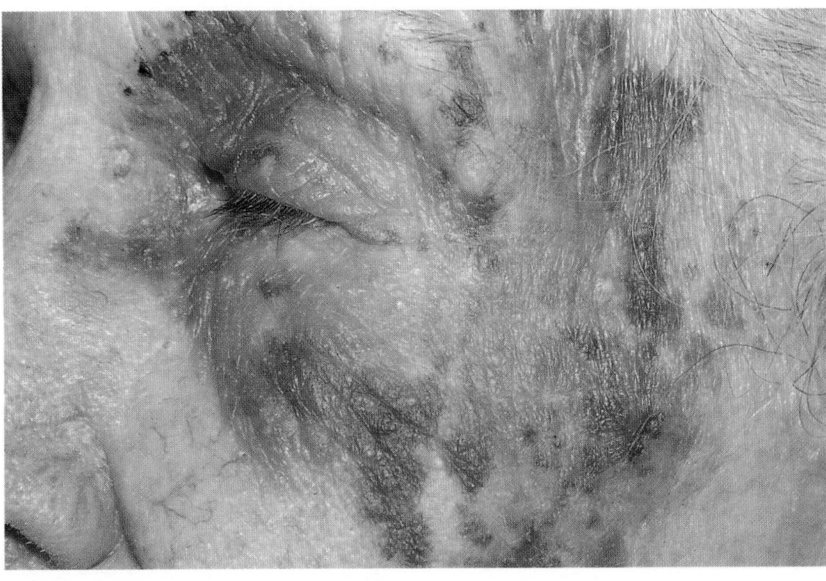

Figure 10.3 Systemic amyloidosis results in infiltration of the skin with amyloid, giving a yellowish color to the skin and producing fragility of blood vessels, so that purpura is common.

and destruction by liquid nitrogen can improve the appearance.

LESIONS THAT APPEAR YELLOW DUE TO CRUSTED SURFACE

Although any eroded lesions can crust, several are more likely to exhibit abundant yellow crust. These diseases are usually primarily blistering diseases that form a crust when the overlying blister roof is denuded.

Impetigo

Impetigo is a bacterial infection affecting the very uppermost portion of the epidermis. The organisms responsible are predominantly *Staphylococcus aureus* and, less often, group A α-hemolytic streptococcus. When *S. aureus* is present, there is often superficial blistering. In either case, the involved skin quickly develops a honey-crusted appearance (Fig. 10.4). Although most common over the face and around the nares, impetigo often complicates insect bites over the extremities as well.

The disease most often confused with impetigo is herpes simplex virus (HSV) infection, particularly when occurring on the face. In fact, HSV infection is a common preceding event, and both bacteria and virus may be present in lesions around the mouth or nose. Other erosive diseases that sometimes exhibit obvious crusting include very inflammatory forms of tinea infection and bullous pemphigoid.

The treatment of impetigo involves the use of an antibiotic. Any antistaphylococcal antibiotic, such as cephalexin or dicloxacillin, is nearly always effective and, in some areas of the United States, most *S. aureus* is also sensitive to oral erythromycin. For limited disease, topical mupirocin (Bactroban) ointment applied four times a day is as effective as oral therapy.[2] Because many patients are carriers of *S. aureus*, recurrence is common. Mupirocin ointment applied in the nares four times a day for 5 days decreases the carrier state and the risk of recurrence.[3]

Bullous Pemphigoid

The erosions left by unroofed bullae of bullous pemphigoid are often covered with yellow crust. However, because the blisters of pemphigoid are

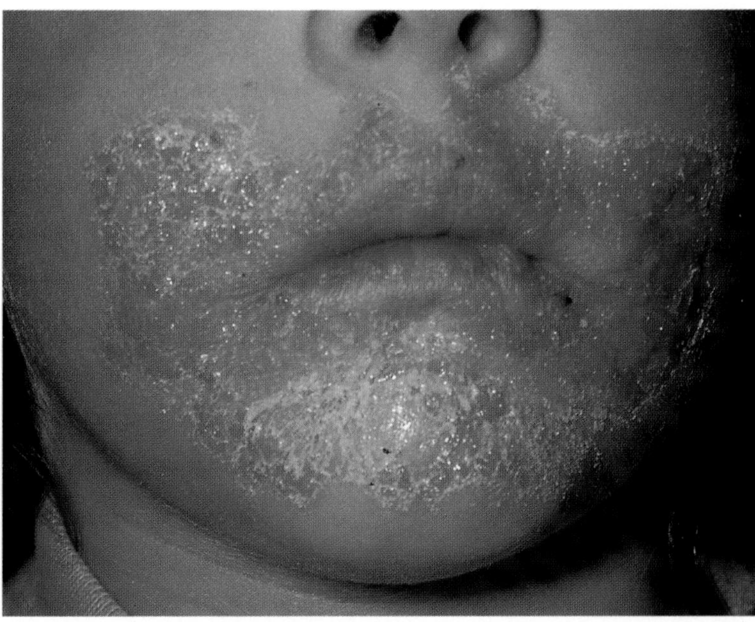

Figure 10.4 Crusting of any cause can appear yellow, but this is a classic presentation for impetigo.

relatively thick, bullae are usually present, facilitating their recognition as a primarily blistering disease, with crust appearing only secondarily (for further discussion, see Ch. 5, Bullous Diseases).

Actinic Keratoses

Actinic keratoses are poorly demarcated, scaling papules that arise in response to chronic solar radiation. Although these lesions are most often skin colored or pink, the scale of these lesions is sometimes yellowish in color or crusted (see also Ch. 8, Skin-Colored Lesions).

REFERENCE

1. Boulton AJM, Cutfield RG, Abouganem D et al: Necrobiosis lipoidica diabeticorum: a clinicopathologic study. J Am Acad Dermatol 18:530, 1988
2. McLinn S: A bacteriologically controlled, randomized study comparing the efficacy of 2% mupirocin ointment (Bactroban) with oral erythromyacin in the treatment of patients with impetigo. J Am Acad Dermatol 22:883, 1990
3. Reagen DR et al: Elimination of coincident *Staphylococcal aureus* nasal and hand carriage with intranasal application of mupirocin calcium ointment. Ann Intern Med 114:101, 1991

SUGGESTED READINGS

Necrobiosis lipoidica

Boulton AJM, Cutfield RG, Abouganem D et al: Necrobiosis lipoidica diabeticorum: a clinicopathologic study. J Am Acad Dermatol 18:530, 1988

Lowitt MH, Dover JJ: Necrosis lipoidica. J Am Acad Dermatol 25:735, 1991

Xanthomas

Hu CH: Xanthoma and lipid metabolism. p. 725. In Sams WM Jr, Lynch PJ (eds): Principles and Practice of Dermatology. 2nd Ed. Churchill Livingstone, New York, 1996

Amyloidosis

Breathnach SM: Amyloid and amyloidosis. J Am Acad Dermatol 18:1, 1988

CHAPTER 11

Brown Lesions

Melanin is the pigment most often responsible for brown color. Heavy deposition of melanin may appear black and, due to refractive properties in the skin, melanin within the dermis often produces a blue color. Therefore, brown, black, and blue lesions are grouped together within the brown lesion category. Also, hemosiderin can produce brown pigment, particularly as petechiae resolve.

The brown lesions are divided into two main subdivisions: flat lesions, which generally consist of increased pigment; and papules, which are tumors.

BROWN MACULES

Ephelides

Ephelides (freckles) are multiple, tan, sharply demarcated, small macules that occur in sun-exposed areas. These are most common on the face of light-complexioned children. Freckles appear and darken rapidly after sun exposure, but they fade and may become barely noticeable in winter. Freckles tend to become less prominent in adulthood.

Frequently confused with freckles are solar lentigines (see below). However, those sun-induced lesions are often larger and more stellate in shape, and the color is stable rather than fading in winter. The lentigo simplex and junctional nevus are also pigmented macules, but they are usually easily differentiated from freckles by their darker brown color, fewer numbers, and lack of clustering.

Freckles serve as a marker of both susceptibility for sun damage and of significant past sun exposure. Therapy consists of education regarding avoidance of sun exposure to prevent long-term damage.

Solar Lentigo

Solar lentigines are sun-induced, well-marginated brown macules that often exhibit a stellate configuration, especially over the shoulders (Fig. 11.1). Although normally tan in color, there is often some irregularity of color within the lesion, and sometimes lesions are quite dark. Solar lentigines are multiple and are generally distributed over the upper back and shoulders. In older individuals, lentigines are very common on the backs of the hands, where they represent so-called "liver spots."

The only important disease in the differential diagnosis is the lentigo maligna or malignant melanoma. These conditions are differentiated by their larger size, greater irregularity of color, and lack of surrounding similar lesions. A biopsy is indicated for larger and more irregular solar lentigines.

Management in the emergency department consists of reassurance, application of sunscreen, and patient education regarding sun avoidance. A fade cream such as topical hydroquinone 2%, 3% (Melanex solution), or 4% (Solaquin Forte cream or gel, Eldoquin Forte cream) applied twice daily is useful.

Lentigo Simplex

The lentigo simplex is a small, brown, sharply demarcated, evenly pigmented macule that can be impossible to differentiate from a benign, junctional melanocytic nevus (Fig. 11.2). However, differentiation is unimportant, since these lesions are of cosmetic importance only.

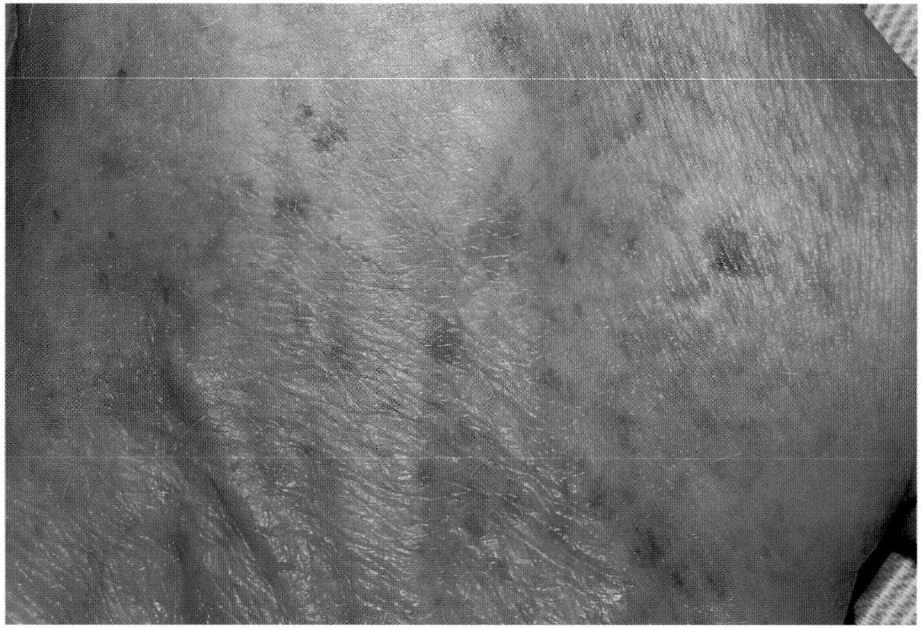

Figure 11.1 Solar lentigines, most common on the backs of hands and the shoulders, are brown, stellate macules.

"Tinea" (Pityriasis) Versicolor

Pityriasis versicolor is an extremely common yeast infection caused by *Pityrosporum ovale*, also called *Malasezzia furfur*. In this case, "tinea" is a misnomer, since this term otherwise refers to fungal dermatophyte infections that lack budding yeast, such as tinea pedis and tinea capitis.

Most common in young men, pityriasis versicolor begins as 5- to 10-mm, sharply demarcated, round papules, generally in the central upper chest

Figure 11.2 The lentigo simplex and the junctional nevus are often indistinguishable. Both are evenly pigmented, small, brown, regular macules.

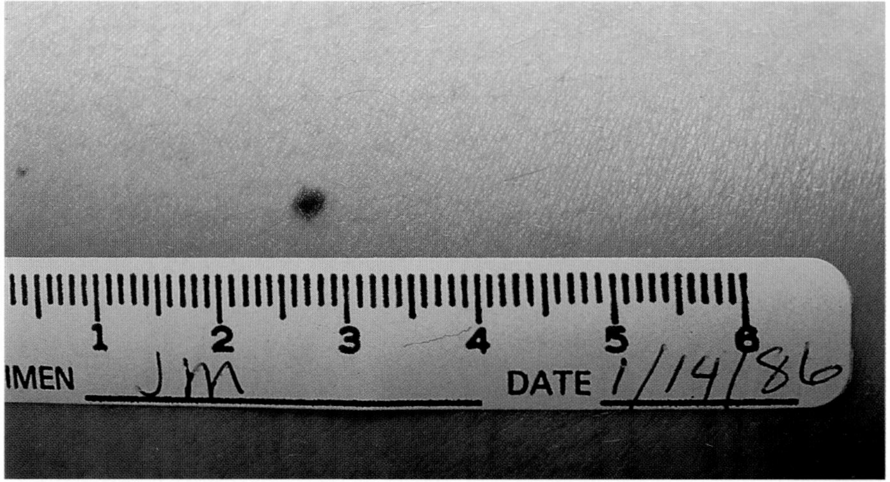

and back, and occasionally over the antecubital fossae as well. These papules become coalescent, producing patches with a characteristic arcuate border. The color is most often light tan or pinkish tan, with black patients sometimes exhibiting extremely dark brown lesions (Fig. 11.3; see also Fig. 9.6). Although present, scale is often so subtle that it is easily missed (see Fig. 1.2). Some patients, particularly those with significant tanning, may have hypopigmented erythematous lesions.

The diagnosis is made on the grounds of the characteristic appearance. When scaling is not appreciated, there are no other common diseases in the differential diagnosis. In the occasional patient with more prominent scale, pityriasis rosea, secondary syphilis, and tinea corporis may rarely require consideration. The diagnosis can be established with a positive microscopic fungal preparation, but this generally requires skill outside the expertise of a nondermatologist. The interpretation of fungal preparations for pityriasis versicolor is more difficult than that of a dermatophyte infection because hyphae tend to be short and curved. Fortunately, microscopic confirmation is rarely required.

Treatment is simple and effective, although recurrence is common. When pityriasis versicolor is extensive, oral therapy is most practical. Ketoconazole (Nizoral) 200 mg each morning for 3 to 5 days is a common regimen.[1] Although hepatotoxicity is possible, it is extremely rare in this dosing schedule. Fluconazole (Diflucan) 400 mg once and itraconazole (Sporanox) 200 mg/day for 1 week have also been suggested.[2,3] Griseofulvin is ineffective for yeast infections such as pityriasis versicolor and *Candida*. For more limited disease, topical azoles such as miconazole, clotrimazole, and ketoconazole applied twice daily, are practical. A classic but tiresome alternative is selenium sulfide 2.5% (Selsun) lotion applied overnight every other day for 2 weeks, or nightly for 1 week. Patients should be warned that selenium sulfide can be irritating.

Patients should be advised that recurrence is common. Some people are susceptible to this ubiquitous organism; for these patients, monthly prophylactic therapy can help prevent recurrences. This can be achieved by a monthly application of a mixture of propylene glycol and water mixed in equal proportions, selenium sulfide lotion, or an azole cream.

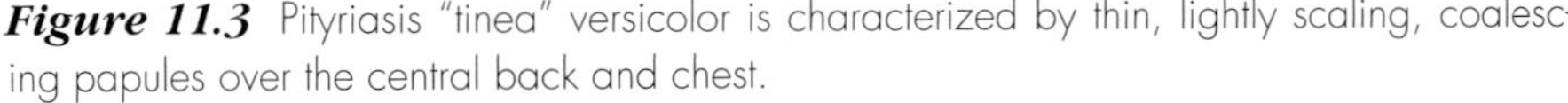

Figure 11.3 Pityriasis "tinea" versicolor is characterized by thin, lightly scaling, coalescing papules over the central back and chest.

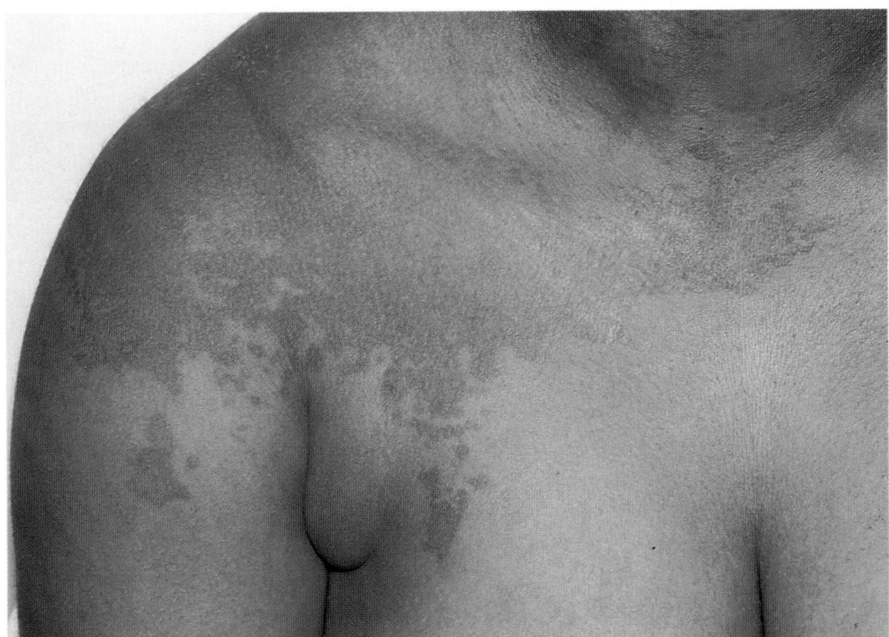

PITYRIASIS "TINEA" VERSICOLOR

Clinical Presentation

Tan, hypopigmented, or pink round, coalescing, lightly scaling papules over central chest, back, and shoulders.

Management in the Emergency Department

1. *Ketoconazole 200 mg PO each day for 5 days*
2. *Propylene glycol and water 50%*
   - *Dispense 16 ounces*
   - *Apply to the affected area once a month to prevent recurrence*
3. *Patient education regarding recurring nature (see the patient handout on p. 355, Pityriasis "Tinea" Versicolor)*

BROWN PATCHES

Café-au-Lait Spots

Café-au-lait spots are tan (although often dark brown in black patients), sharply demarcated patches most often located over the trunk (Fig. 11.4). These can be present at birth or may develop during childhood. They range widely from less than 2 cm to patches that cover much of the trunk, with an average dimension being palm-sized.

When single, these are a normal finding. When multiple, they are associated with several neurocutaneous syndromes. Neurofibromatosis is the most common, with five or more café-au-lait spots 5 cm or more in size representing a pathognomonic sign. Albright syndrome (polyostotic fibrous dysplasia) is also associated with large or numerous café-au-lait spots. Café-au-lait spots are more common in black patients and more numerous, without necessarily indicating associated disease.

The only important disease that could be confused with a café-au-lait spot is a congenital nevus, but this latter condition should be palpable and is usually darker in color. Mongolian spots are bluish in color, with poorly demarcated borders.

Therapy consists of reassurance when the patient has one or two lesions, and referral to a primary care physician or a dermatologist for greater numbers.

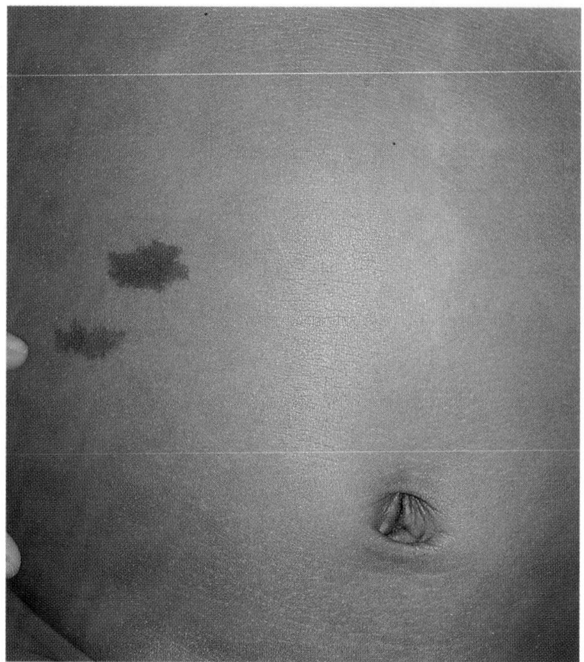

Figure 11.4 Café-au-lait spots are evenly colored, light brown (but may be much darker in black patients), well-demarcated patches without any surface change.

Postinflammatory Hyperpigmentation

Postinflammatory hyperpigmentation results from a temporary increase in melanin production as a result of injury. This is especially common in patients with a darker natural skin color. The area of hyperpigmentation corresponds to the area of injury, with location, size, and borders depending on the nature of the original insult (Fig. 11.5). The color varies from light brown to nearly black, with the darker colors occurring in patients with darker natural complexion. Darker colors are also characteristic of some inflammatory diseases, particularly lichen planus, fixed drug eruption, and lupus erythematosus. Sometimes the patient does not remember preceding injury or inflammation, but in most cases the diagnosis can still be made with confidence because of the pattern of hyperpigmentation.

Although postinflammatory hyperpigmentation fades naturally, this can sometimes be a slow process. Therapy therefore consists of reassurance, and of topical hydroquinone 2%, 3% (Melanex solution), or 4% (Solaquin Forte cream or gel, Eldoquin Forte cream) applied twice daily, to hasten resolution. A potent sunscreen minimizes the additional darkening from ultraviolet light.

Fixed Drug Eruption

The fixed drug eruption is a peculiar, recurrent reaction to medication that results in deep postinflammatory hyperpigmentation (see Chs. 5 and 13). Exposure to a medication produces one or a few red, round, edematous, or blistering plaques (see Figs. 5.13 and 13.6). With each exposure, the lesions recur in the same place, and postinflammatory changes ensue. Clinically, sharply demarcated, round, dark brown patches are seen, and the patient usually gives a history of recurrent inflammation in that area (Fig. 11.5).

Therapy consists of avoidance of the medication, and topical hydroquinone 2%, 3% (Melanex solution), or 4% (Solaquin Forte cream or gel, Eldoquin Forte cream) applied twice daily.

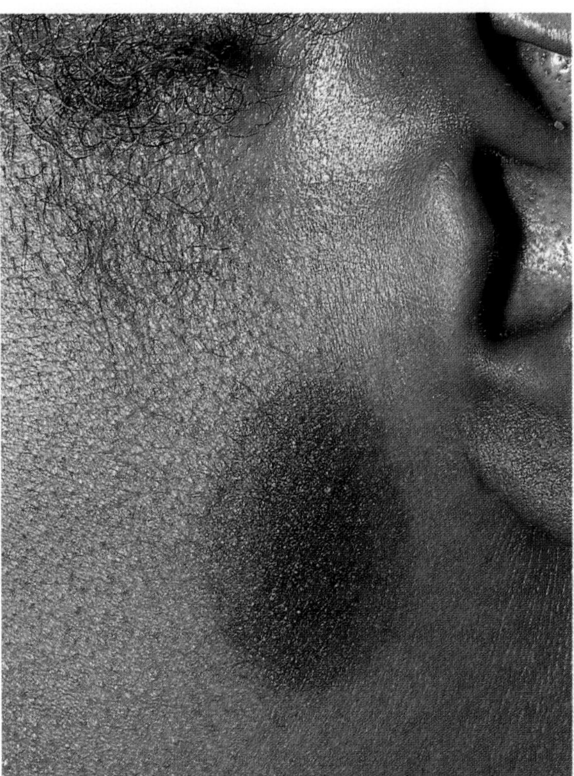

Figure 11.5 Postinflammatory hyperpigmentation consists of brown patches that correspond to areas of previous or ongoing inflammation. This deeply pigmented, round patch is typical of a fixed drug eruption, and the patient confirms the occurrence of a recurrent "puffy spot."

Becker's nevus

Becker's nevus is located most often over the shoulder, upper back, or thighs of men, usually occurring around puberty. This innocuous lesion consists of a large, light brown, well-demarcated patch with associated coarse hair, roughly corresponding to the area of hyperpigmentation. Therapy consists of reassurance.

Melasma

Occurring most often in women over the lateral face, melasma (chloasma) appears as light brown, often reticulate, patches (Fig. 11.6). Sometimes called the "mask of pregnancy," melasma appears to be hormonally influenced and often precipitated by oral contraceptives or pregnancy. However, this condition occasionally occurs in men and in women who are neither pregnant nor taking oral contraceptives. Melasma occasionally occurs over the dorsal arms as well, underscoring a role for sunlight.

Therapy consists of removal of hormonal influences if possible, as well as daily sunscreen use and twice daily topical hydroquinone 2%, 3% (Melanex solution), or 4% (Solaquin Forte cream or gel, Eldoquin Forte cream).

Futcher's lines

A common, normal finding in black patients is Futcher's lines. These occur over the anteromedial upper arms and posteromedial upper legs. They occur as a sharp line of demarcation, running longitudinally with slight hyperpigmentation on the lateral aspect, and of a lighter skin color medially.

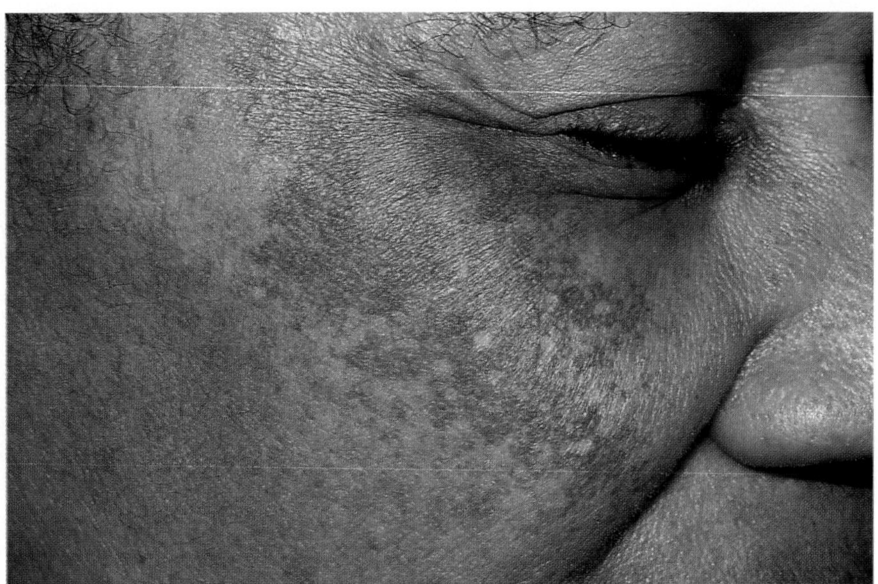

Figure 11.6 Melasma is most common in women, occurring over the lateral face as well-demarcated, irregular, reticulate patches.

BROWN PAPULES

Seborrheic Keratoses

Seborrheic keratoses are extraordinarily common brown papules, often referred to erroneously as "moles" by patients who identify nearly all brown papules as such. Classically, these are oval, well-demarcated, flat-topped, keratotic papules (Fig. 11.7). They often have a "stuck-on" appearance and can be peeled off with fingernails, only to recur. A common variant is slightly more dome-shaped with a more waxy texture to the touch. Almost all people except blacks have developed at least one of these innocuous tumors by the age of 40 years. The tendency to develop very large numbers is inherited and is common.

Seborrheic keratoses occur on any surface except the palms, soles, and mucous membranes, but they are most common over the trunk and, sometimes, the lateral face. They are also relatively common over the dorsal aspect of the feet and ankle, where they may be skin-colored or hypopigmented, and over the dorsal hands, where they are sometimes unusually flat. Extremely dark seborrheic keratoses are relatively common over the cheeks of black patients, where these inherited lesions are called *dermatosis papulosa nigra* (Fig. 11.8).

When irritated, seborrheic keratoses can lose their brown color and sometimes their characteristic flat-topped and uniform, symmetric configuration, mimicking a squamous cell carcinoma or a wart. Otherwise, the primary lesion in the differential diagnosis is a benign compound nevus or, when irregular, a malignant melanoma.

Seborrheic keratoses have no malignant potential, so when their appearance is characteristic, reassurance is the only therapy needed. For patients who are experiencing irritation or pain from rubbing, or for those who want them removed for cosmetic reasons, this can be achieved with nonscarring destructive techniques, since the lesion is a very superficial one. Common therapies include cryotherapy, light hyfrecation and curettage, and shave removal flush with the skin.

Melanocytic Nevi

Melanocytic nevi (pigmented nevi, nevocellular nevi) are benign hamartomas of melanocytes.

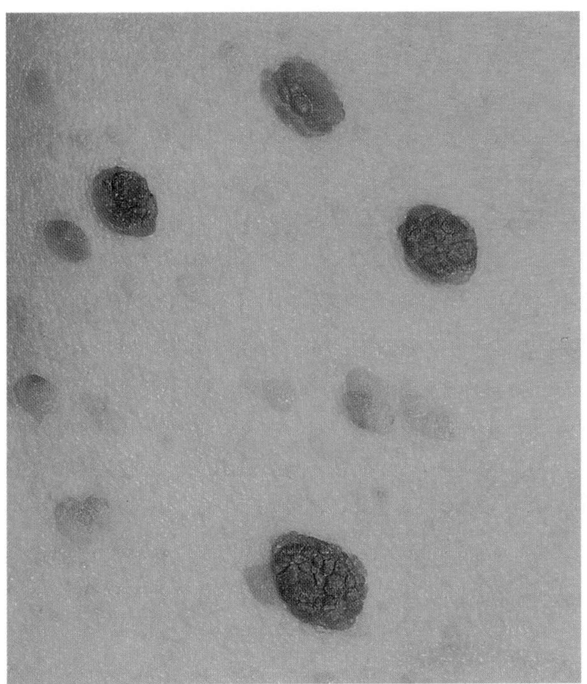

Figure 11.7 Seborrheic keratoses are usually flat-topped, keratotic, well-demarcated papules that feel "stuck on." However, some varieties are smooth surfaced and dome-shaped, strongly resembling a nevus.

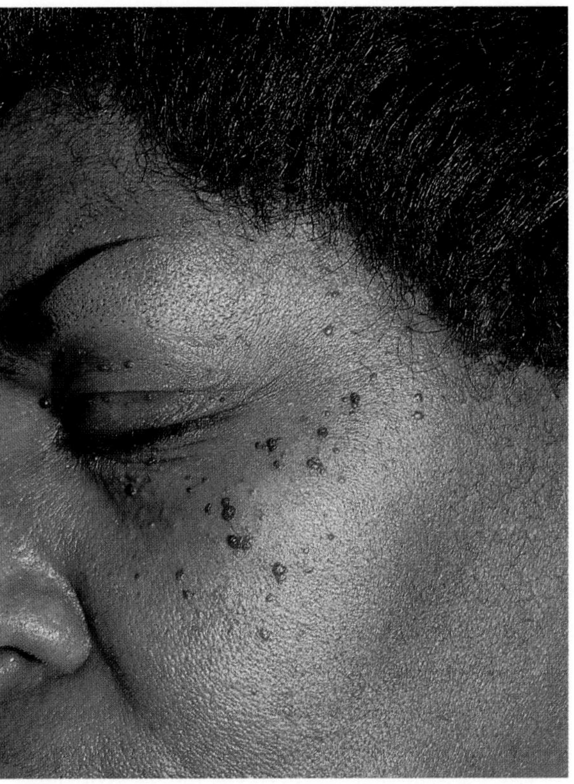

Figure 11.8 Dermatosis papulosa nigra are histologically identical to seborrheic keratoses but occur over the central face of black patients.

These are extremely common, with nearly every nonblack patient having up to 40 lesions. Melanocytic nevi generally first start to appear in infancy, with the greatest number developing at puberty. The appearance of new nevi after the mid-20s is uncommon, and nevi begin to disappear at about 40 years of age. By the age of 70 years, most people have few or no nevi but instead they usually manifest many age-related "barnacles," such as seborrheic and actinic keratoses. Although nevi can occur anywhere on the body, they are concentrated over sun-exposed areas.

A benign nevus is an evenly pigmented brown (ranging from light to very dark brown) lesion. When flat, these represent junctional nevi (Fig. 11.2) and when papular, these are compound or intradermal nevi (Fig. 11.9). These nevi tend to lose their brown color as the patient ages, and many intradermal nevi are skin colored. Benign nevi typically are small (less than 7 mm in diameter, or less than the diameter of a pencil eraser), with sharply demarcated, regular borders. Most benign nevi have at least one mildly atypical feature, such as large size or a slightly irregular border. One mildly atypical feature should not concern the examiner.

Because bland-appearing nevi are normal and ubiquitous, therapy is unnecessary for cosmetic reasons or for discomfort, except when lesions are located in an area that is subject to friction. Pigmented nevi are best removed by excision with suture closure.

Congenital Melanocytic Nevi

About 1% of infants are born with a congenital melanocytic nevus. These are usually larger than acquired nevi and, in rare instances, they can be

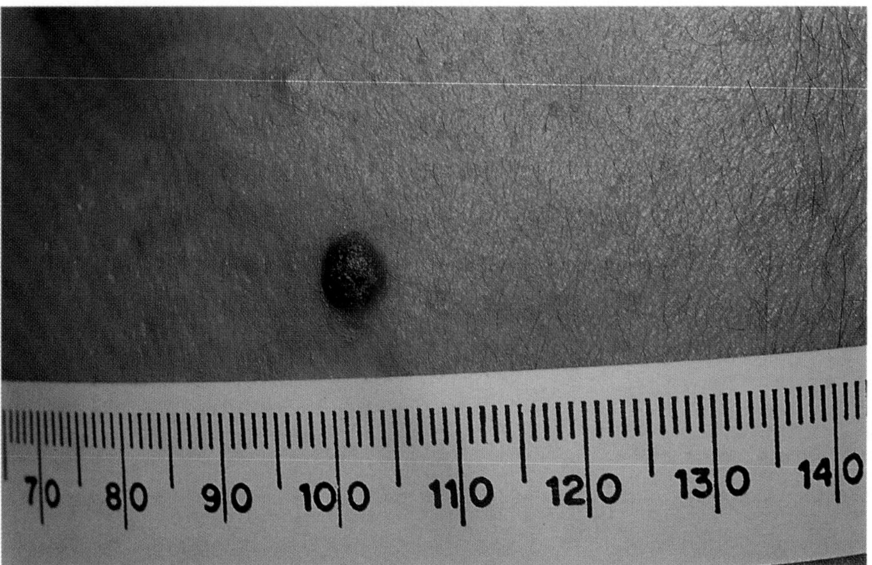

Figure 11.9 A benign compound nevus is smaller than 7 mm in diameter with regular, well-demarcated borders and even pigmentation.

very large (sometimes called "bathing trunk" nevi, or giant congenital melanocytic nevi). The larger the nevus the more likely it is to have atypical features such as irregular or poorly demarcated borders, satellite lesions, or variegate pigmentation (Fig. 19.1).

The significance of congenital nevi is several fold. First is their increased risk of malignant transformation into malignant melanoma. Whereas small congenital nevi have only a slightly increased risk, the risk of malignant melanoma increases dramatically with the largest lesions.[4,5] In addition, melanocytes as well as benign or malignant melanocytic tumors are sometimes identified in underlying tissue such as leptomeninges, primarily when nevi are located over the head and spine.[6] Underlying bony abnormalities can occur and dysfunction due to bony changes or neural involvement is possible.[6]

Management in the emergency department entails advising patients or parents of the increased risk of melanoma, which is slight in small nevi and higher in large nevi, and referral to a dermatologist or a pediatrician for more specific education and recommendations.

Atypical Moles

Relatively recently recognized is the existence of melanocytic nevi whose morphologic appearance is intermediate between malignant melanoma and benign nevi. Their prevalence, significance, and prognosis are hotly debated, but nearly all dermatologists agree that these lesions do exist and at least at times are associated with a significant increase in the development of malignant melanoma.[7,8]

Atypical moles (dysplastic nevi) are most common over the back and chest, but they can be located anywhere on the skin surface. These lesions exhibit at least one, and usually more, of the following features: large size, irregular borders, poor demarcation of the borders, and variegate pigmentation, often with reddish tones (Fig. 11.10). The differentiation of an atypical mole from malignant melanoma usually can be made by the more pronounced abnormalities of a melanoma, but a biopsy is often required.

The prognosis of this condition is related to the number of total nevi, the number of atypical moles,

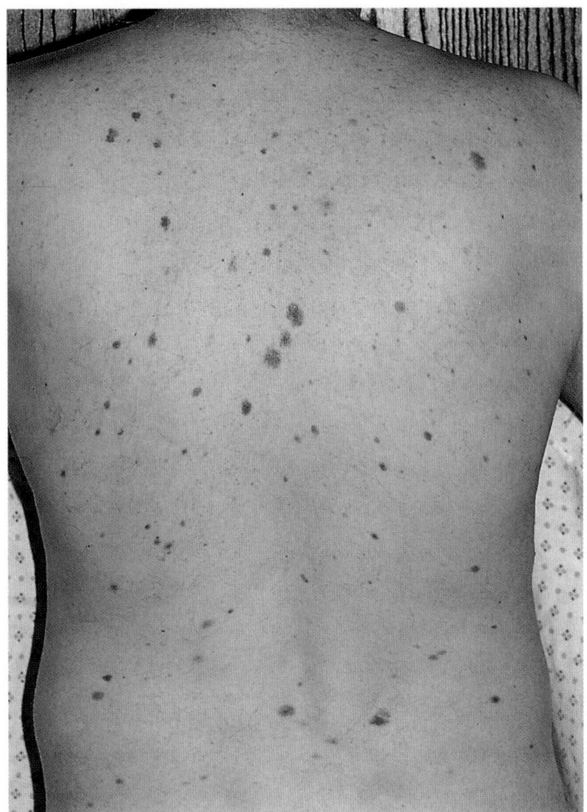

Figure 11.10 Atypical moles (dysplastic nevi) are often larger than 7 mm, with irregular or poorly demarcated borders, and a color that is irregular or that has reddish hues. These abnormalities are less remarkable than those found in a malignant melanoma, but a biopsy may be required to differentiate the two lesions.

and possibly the degree of abnormalities of the clinical and histologic features. In addition, a family history of atypical moles and, even more so, of malignant melanoma, remarkably increases an individual patient's risk of the development of melanoma.

Management in the emergency department includes a brief overall skin examination for any obviously extremely atypical lesions that might represent a malignant melanoma and referral to a dermatologist for reevaluation and ongoing surveillance.

Cutaneous Malignant Melanoma

A malignant melanoma is a malignant tumor of melanocytes. These can arise from pre-existing nevi or de novo from normal-appearing skin. Although most common on the upper back of men or the lower legs of women, these tumors can occur anywhere, including the palms and soles, under nails, and on mucous membranes. Cutaneous melanoma in black patients usually occurs only on the palms and soles, under nails, or on mucous membranes.

Very early melanoma is nearly macular and is generally greater than 7 mm in diameter. The borders are irregular or blurred, or both, with one of the most striking features being the variegate pattern of pigmentation. Colors often include differing hues of brown, blue, gray, or black, sometimes with associated erythema (Figs. 11.11 and 11.12). As the melanoma progresses, it becomes slightly raised with an irregular surface. Malignant melanomas rarely exhibit all these morphologic characteristics. However, this diagnosis should be suspected and aggressively investigated when two or more prominent features are present.

In general, the best emergency department management of a suspected melanoma is referral to a dermatologist within the next few days. Irritated seborrheic keratoses, dermatofibromas, pigmented basal cells, and angiokeratomas can sometimes show an extraordinary resemblance to melanoma, and an experienced dermatologist can sometimes either differentiate these tumors without a biopsy or perform a less aggressive excisional biopsy than would normally be recommended (Fig. 11.13). Occasionally, the clinician maintains a high index of suspicion that the patient will not seek follow-up evaluation as directed. An excisional biopsy to fat, using 1- or 2-mm borders with suture closure, is indicated in these patients while they are "captive." If the lesion is too large to excise comfortably, punch biopsy of representative areas usually gives reliable, although not definitive, information on the diagnosis and the thickness of the tumor, so that definitive therapy can be planned. Except under extraordinary social circumstances, a suspected melanoma should not be treated definitively without a biopsy, since the margins to be

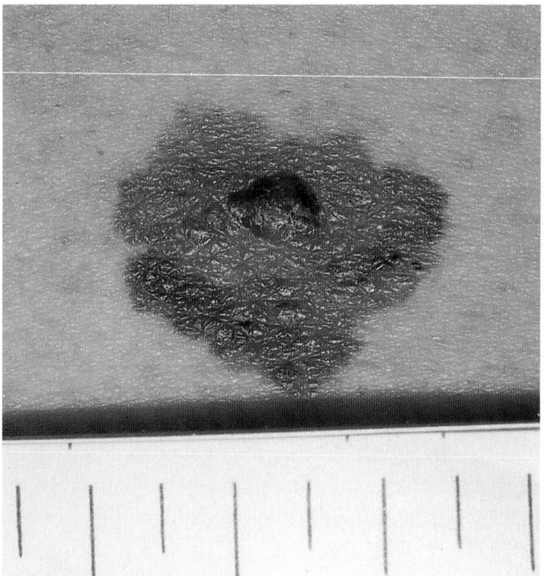

Figure 11.11 This patient presented to the emergency department with an upper respiratory infection, but this lesion was noted during an examination of his lungs. The large size, and the irregular borders, surface, and color predict the diagnosis of melanoma.

Figure 11.12 This patient was seen in the emergency department because she was rightly worried about this large lesion with irregular, gray color and irregular borders. This was a thin melanoma.

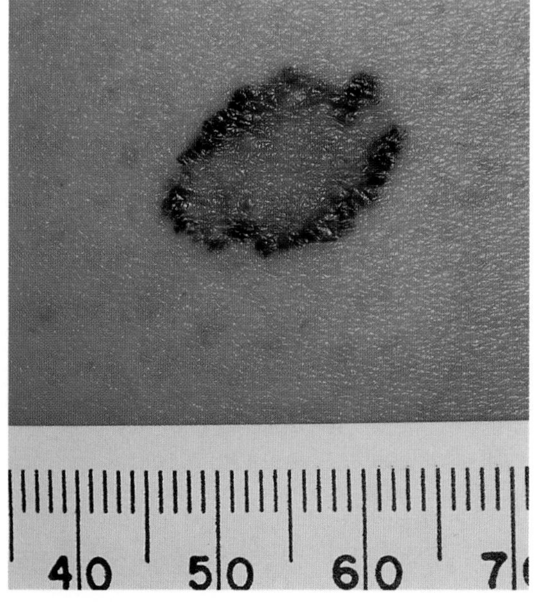

included depend on the tumor thickness, the single most important prognostic indicator for metastasis and long-term survival.

Therapy for melanoma consists of definitive surgical excision. Excision with very wide margins, as was standard therapy in the past, is no longer indicated. Generally, 1-cm margins are removed with tumors that are less than 1 mm thick, 2-cm margins are removed with tumors 1 to 2 mm thick, and 3-cm margins are removed with tumors 2 mm or thicker. However, some are more conservative, taking even smaller margins.[9] Generally, lymph node dissection is not indicated for very thin tumors (less than 1 mm) or thick tumors, because the prognosis of the former is very good, and the prognosis of the latter is very poor, with the outcome not appreciably changed.[10] Other studies have found no benefit from node dissection.[11] No chemotherapeutic regimens have been found that significantly prolong life, except for α-interferon (IFN-α) given as adjunctive therapy for prevention of metastases.[12] However, the benefit is marginal, and the therapy is toxic. Although some follow patients carefully with periodic laboratory and radiographic screening, most recurrences are discovered by a history or by physical examination.[13] Therefore, these expensive and anxiety-producing tests are probably largely unnecessary.

The prognosis associated with melanoma is dependent primarily on the thickness of the tumor from the surface to its deepest area. Generally, patients with tumors less than 1 mm thick have a 5-year survival rate of 90 to 93%, those patients with tumors of 1 to 1.5 mm have a survival rate of 85%, people with melanomas 1.5 to 4 mm thick have a survival rate of 70 to 77%, and those with thicker melanomas have a survival rate of 35 to 40%.[14] These are 5-year survival rates—not cures—they are not disease-free survival rates. Melanomas can recur many years later, and cure rates are significantly lower.

MALIGNANT MELANOMA

Clinical Manifestations

Asymmetry of the lesion

Borders are often irregular or indistinct

Color is usually irregular and variegate

Diameter is usually 7 mm or greater

(Continues)

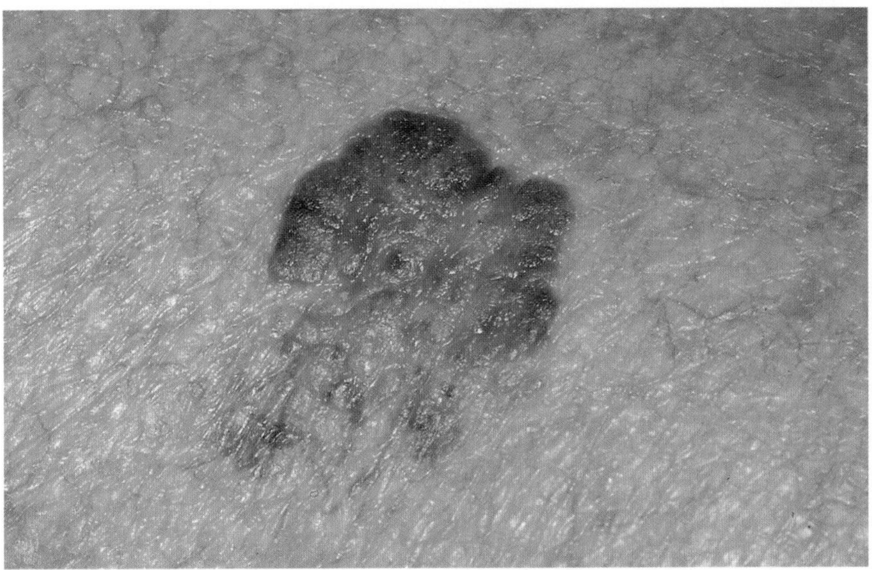

Figure 11.13 Not all irregular, pigmented lesions represent melanomas. A seborrheic keratosis, as shown here, as well as pigmented basal cell carcinomas and lentigines, can also resemble a melanoma. For this reason, lesions should be biopsied before definitive therapy is planned.

(Continued)

Management in the Emergency Department

1. *Referral to a dermatologist*
2. *If compliance is questionable, consider excisional biopsy with suture closure, taking margins of 2 mm*

Dermatofibroma

The dermatofibroma is a benign tumor that resembles scar tissue microscopically. This very common lesion is found most often on the lower leg or upper arms and shoulders of women, but it is sometimes seen in other locations in either sex.

A dermatofibroma usually appears flat and brown with poorly demarcated borders. Sometimes, a reddish component to the color and variegation of pigment are present (Fig. 11.14). Although the lesion superficially resembles an atypical mole, when it is palpated a firm dermal nodule underlying the pigmented change is easily appreciated and is simply not found with nevi.

Treatment consists of reassurance. Although these lesions can be removed with very aggressive cryotherapy or with excision with suture closure, both procedures can produce scarring.

Prurigo Nodules

Prurigo nodules (Picker's nodules) (see Ch. 8) are nodules produced by chronic picking that produces protective thickening of the skin, similar to a callus. Usually, there is an excoriation over the surface. Although these are often skin colored, the chronic nature often results in postinflammatory hyperpigmentation that secondarily colors them brown. This is particularly true in patients with naturally dark complexions.

Bowenoid Papulosis

Genital warts produced by certain types of human papillomavirus (HPV) are likely to exhibit hyperpigmentation. These HPV types are also those most often associated with epithelial dysplasia and cervi-

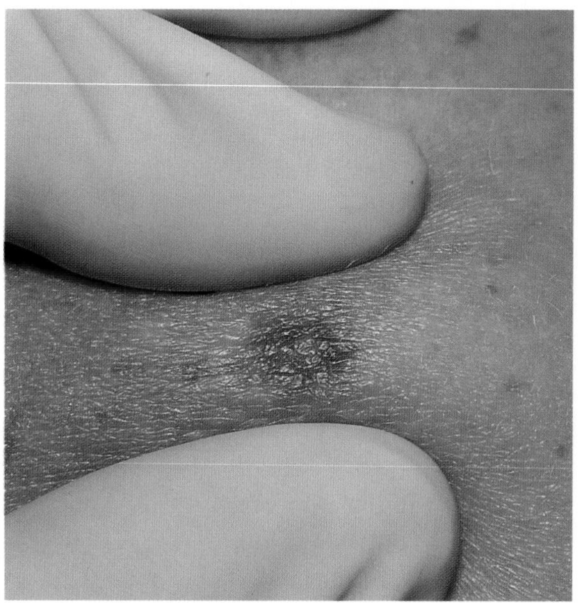

Figure 11.14 A dermatofibroma is a common tumor that is usually brown, poorly demarcated, and easily palpated as a firm dermal nodule, unlike nevi and melanoma.

cal carcinoma. There are many names for these cutaneous dysplastic lesions (e.g., pigmented squamous cell carcinoma in situ, pigmented Bowen's disease, pigmented vulvar or penile intraepithelial neoplasia). Whereas dermatologists generally call them bowenoid papulosis, gynecologists use a classification stratified by degree of atypia.

Pigmented warts with cellular dysplasia are usually flat, and they are sometimes associated with other, more typical warts (Fig. 11.15). These lesions can be indistinguishable from seborrheic keratoses and nevi. However, flat, brown warts characteristic of dysplastic warts sometimes exhibit histologic findings of benign warts on biopsy. In spite of this, any pigmented genital lesion should be biopsied, unless the diagnosis is obvious, since even banal lesions may represent precancerous change.

Women with bowenoid papulosis, and female partners of any patient with this condition, should be referred to a gynecologist for evaluation of the cervix. Because podophylin is a theoretical carcinogen, these warts should be treated more destructively, such as by laser, cryotherapy, excision, or hyfrecation.

Figure 11.15 These pigmented papules of squamous cell carcinoma in situ associated with genital wart infection resemble seborrheic keratoses, pigmented nevi, melanoma, or postinflammatory changes.

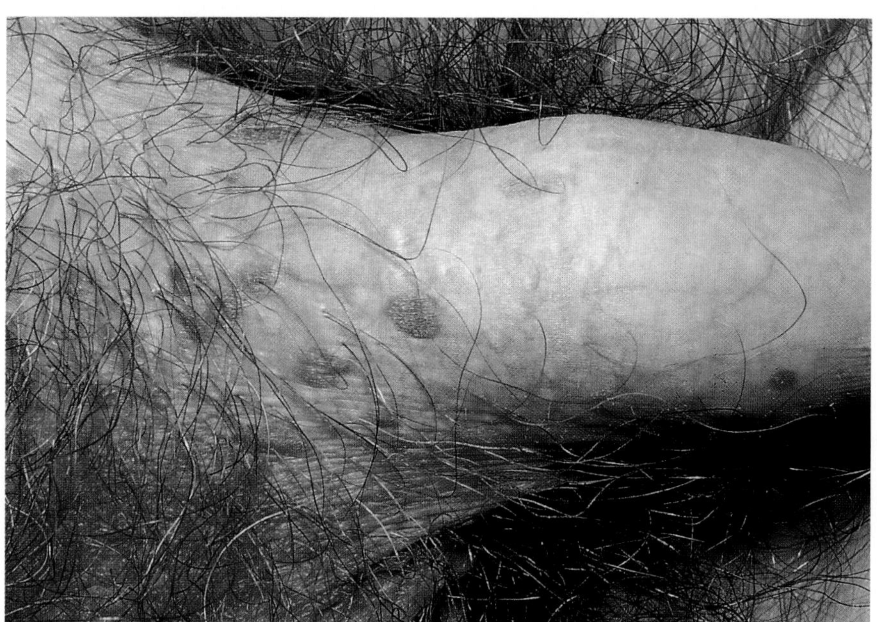

Please see patient information handouts for this chapter on pages 334 and 355.

REFERENCES

1. Elgart ML, Warren NG: The superficial and subcutaneous mycoses. p. 869. In Moschella SL, Hurley HJ (eds): Dermatology. 3rd Ed. WB Saunders, Philadelphia, 1992
2. Faergemann J: Treatment of pityriasis versicolor with a single dose of fluconazole. Acta Derm Venereol (Stockh) 72:74, 1992
3. Hickman JG: A double-blind, randomized, placebo-controlled evaluation of short-term treatment with oral itraconazole in patients with tinea versicolor. J Am Acad Dermatol 34:785, 1996
4. Dawson HA, Atherton DJ, Mayou B: A prospective study of congenital melanocytic naevi: progress report and evaluation after 6 years. Br J Dermatol 134:617, 1996
5. Gari LM, Rivers JK, Kopf AW: Melanomas arising in large congenital melanocytic nevi: a prospective study. Pediatr Dermatol 5:151, 1988
6. Wagner AM, Hansen RC: Neonatal skin and skin disorders. p. 263. In Schachner LA, Hansen RC (eds): Pediatric Dermatology. 2nd Ed. Churchill Livingstone, New York, 1996
7. Kang S, Barnhill RL, Mihm MC Jr et al: Melanoma risk in individuals with clinically atypical nevi. Arch Dermatol 130:999, 1994
8. Schneider JS, Moore DH II, Sagebiel RW: Risk factors for melanoma incidence in prospective follow-up: the importance of atypical (dysplastic) nevi. Arch Dermatol 130:1002, 1994
9. Rivers JK: Melanoma. Lancet 347:803-07, 1996
10. Balch CM: Surgical management of regional lymph nodes in cutaneous melanoma. J Am Acad Dermatol 3:511, 1980
11. Veronesi U, Adamus J, Gandiera DC et al: Delayed regional lymph node dissection in stage I melanoma of the skin of the lower extremity. Cancer 49:2420, 1982
12. Kirkwood JM, Strawderman MH, Ernstoff MS et al: Interferon alfa-2b adjuvant therapy of high-risk resected cutaneous melanoma: the Eastern Cooperative Oncology Group Trial EST 1684. J Clin Oncol 14:7, 1996
13. Weiss M, Loprinzi CL, Creagan ET et al: Utility of follow-up tests for detecting recurrent disease in patients with malignant melanomas. JAMA 274:1703, 1995
14. Levine N: Pigmentary abnormalities. p. 539. In Schachner LA, Hansen RC (eds): Pediatric Dermatology. 2nd Ed. Churchill Livingstone, New York, 1996

SUGGESTED READINGS

Atypical Moles (Dysplastic Nevi)

Consensus Development Panel on Early Melanoma: Diagnosis and treatment of early melanoma. JAMA 268:1314, 1992

Slade J, Marghoob AA, Salopek TG et al: Atypical mole syndrome: risk factor for cutaneous malignant melanoma and implications for management. J Am Acad Dermatol 32:479, 1995

Malignant Melanoma

Marshall MU: Surgical management of primary cutaneous melanoma. CA Cancer J Clin 46:217, 1996

Rigel DS: Malignant melanoma: perspectives on incidence and its effects on awareness, diagnosis, and treatment. CA Cancer J Clin 46:195, 1996

Rivers JK: Melanoma. Lancet 347:803, 1996

Piepkorn M, Barnhill RL: A factual, not arbitrary, basis for choice of resection margins in melanoma. Arch Dermatol 132:811, 1996

Bowenoid Papulosis

Schwartz RA, Fanniger CK: Bowenoid papulosis. J Am Acad Dermatol 24:261, 1991

Wilkinson EJ: The 1989 Presidential address. International Society for the Study of Vulvar Disease. J Reprod Med 35:981, 1990

CHAPTER 12

Red Papules and Nodules

Most of the conditions that present as *red papules* or *nodules* are inflammatory. However, tumors of blood vessel origin, such as cherry angiomas, fit into this category as well. Generally, vascular tumors are bright, cherry red or purple with very sharply demarcated borders, whereas inflammatory papules and nodules are deeper red in the center, fading out to a pinker color at the edges.

Many skin-colored lesions appear red at times due to secondary inflammation or increased vascularity visible in a light-complexioned patient. Therefore, when faced with an inflamed papule or nodule, the clinician should sometimes consider lesions in the skin-colored group.

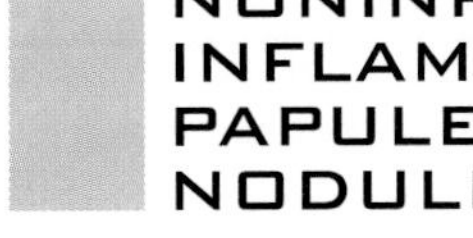

NONINFECTIOUS INFLAMMATORY PAPULES AND NODULES

Insect Bites

Susceptible people develop hypersensitivity reactions to insect bites, particularly flea and mosquito bites. Many patients resist the suggestion of a diagnosis of insects bites because only one or two members of the family exhibit the lesions. However, most people are not sensitive to insect bites, so the bites leave no lasting visible reminder. Insect bites occur primarily during warm weather.

Clinical Manifestations Flea bites are usually distributed over the lower legs, from fleas jumping up from the floor, except in small children, who spend more time closer to the floor, and to flea-bearing pets. Although flea bites are usually dome-shaped, red or pink papules (Fig. 12.1), very sensitive individuals sometimes exhibit blistering, ranging from a very small vesicle to a bulla as large as several centimeters, obscuring the original nature of the lesion (see Fig. 4.21 and 4.22).

Mosquito bites occur on exposed areas such as the face and arms, as well as the legs. Blistering is much less common. Pruritus of both flea and mosquito bites often results in scratching with excoriation and sometimes secondary infection, changing the surface character of the lesions. Usually, one or two primary, untouched papules can be found upon careful examination.

Fire ants and stinging insects also produce inflammatory papules and nodules, but the remarkable pain with the bite or sting usually clues the patient to the diagnosis. In addition, fire ant stings are often pustular (see Fig. 7.5), and stinging insects produce fewer but larger lesions. However, the kissing bug, a resident of the Southwest United States, bites painlessly in the night to produce a very large red nodule or urticarial plaque in sensitive individuals. As usual, redness can be difficult to appreciate in black skin, and these lesions may simply appear hyperpigmented in those individuals.

Differential Diagnosis Skin diseases that can be confused with insect bites include folliculitis, before a well-formed pustule occurs, and early lesions of varicella. Usually, at least one lesion typical of these diseases can be found by a careful search, but sometimes a biopsy is required for a definitive diagnosis. The diagnosis is usually not important enough to perform a biopsy, since the diagnosis of varicella generally becomes clear within a day or so. More important diseases to differentiate from insect bites are the red papules of septic emboli or septic vasculitis, but these nearly always occur in ill, usually hospitalized, patients. Finally, lesions of leukocytoclastic vasculitis can resemble

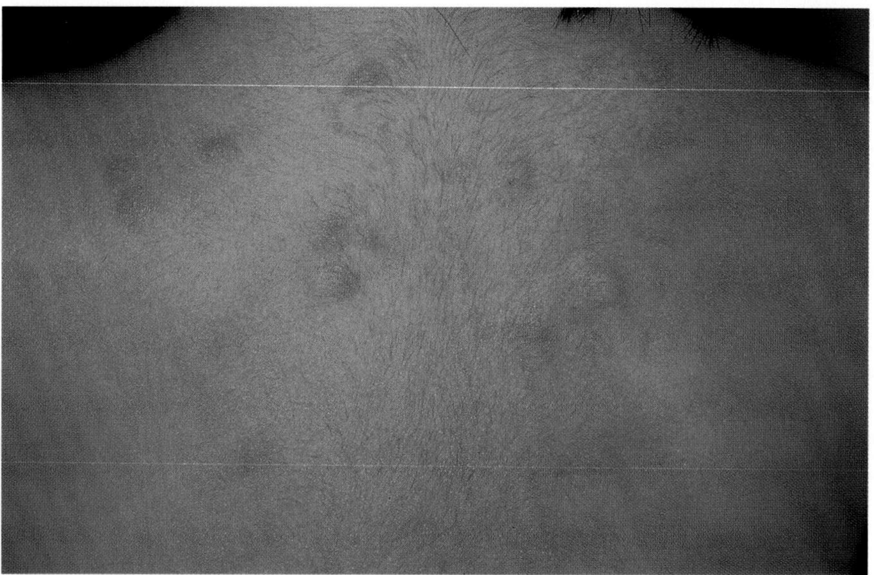

Figure 12.1 Insect bites are generally multiple, inflamed, dome-shaped papules. Often, crusts due to scratching or small vesicles are present.

bites, but these are purpuric (i.e., they do not blanch when pressed with a finger or glass slide) and are usually far too numerous to be insect bites.

Management The primary management of insect bites is avoidance of the insect. This often requires very careful patient education and a nonjudgmental attitude, since many patients and families erroneously believe that insect bites, especially flea bites, only occur in a home with poor hygiene. First, a personal insect repellent such as Off, Cutter, or 6–12 can be useful. Simply defleaing a pet does not eliminate fleas and, in fact, can increase the attractiveness of human skin from the perspective of hungry fleas living in a carpet or in the yard. Therefore, the home and surrounding yard must often be treated at the same time as the pet. This can be accomplished with the use of flea bombs purchased at drug stores; even more effective are the professional services that specialize in the elimination of fleas. In addition to the use of an insect repellent, mosquito bites can be minimized by avoiding the outdoors in the evening, when mosquitoes are most active. Wearing long sleeves and long pants can also help protect the skin. Any areas of standing water, where mosquitoes breed, should be eliminated if possible.

A topical corticosteroid such as hydrocortisone 1% or 2.5% cream (for children) or triamcinolone 0.1% cream (for adults) can sometimes relieve itching and slightly hasten resolution. Patients with multiple lesions or severe blistering benefit from prednisone 1 to 2 mg/kg (for children) or 40 to 60 mg (for adults) each morning for 5 to 7 days. Ice cubes held to pruritic lesions can provide short-term anesthesia, as can a commercial mixture of the anesthetic pramoxine HCl and hydrocortisone (Pramosone cream) or topical lidocaine ointment 5%. The local anesthetics available in most over-the-counter products (e.g., diphenhydramine) are potent sensitizers and are best avoided. Nighttime sedation improves the overall comfort of patients, and the prompt treatment of secondary infections with an oral antistaphylococcal antibiotic minimizes scarring.

Course and Prognosis Itching of individual lesions usually resolves after 2 or 3 days, and the lesions fade over 1 or 2 weeks. Often, brown macules of postinflammatory hyperpigmentation linger

INSECT BITES

Clinical Manifestations

Pink and red, pruritic, dome-shaped, discrete papules over lower legs (fleas) or exposed skin such as the face and extremities (mosquitoes); often accompanied by crusts and postinflammatory hyperpigmentation, and occasionally associated with some vesicles.

Management in the Emergency Department

1. *Tactful patient education regarding the etiology and necessity of eliminating exposure by defleaing pet, house, and yard, or by avoiding areas with insects*
2. *Personal insect repellent such as Off, Cutter, 6–12*
3. *For minor itching, triamcinolone cream 0.1% applied twice a day and nighttime sedation with diphenhydramine (Benadryl)*
4. *For the unusual patient with recalcitrant symptoms associated with severe bites, prednisone 1 to 2 mg/kg/day (children) or 40 to 60 mg/day (adults) for 2 to 3 days can hasten resolution*
5. *Treat secondary infection with an oral antistaphylococcal antibiotic (e.g., cephalexin, dicloxacillin)*
6. *Patient should seek follow-up attention with regular health care provider in 1 week if not improved, and in 1 month if not clear*

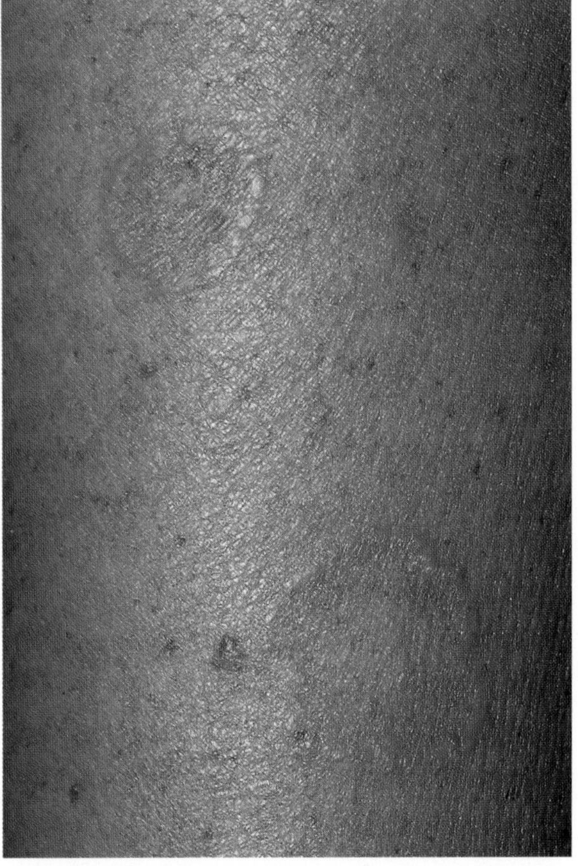

Figure 12.2 Granuloma annulare is often confused with tinea corporis, or ringworm, because the small, pink papules are usually arranged in an annulus; however, there is no scaling.

for several weeks, especially in darker-complexioned individuals. Occasionally, the inflammatory papules can last several weeks.

Granuloma Annulare

Clinical Manifestations Granuloma annulare is an inflammatory, granulomatous disease of unknown origin. Most often located on the dorsal hands and wrists, this condition can occur anywhere on the body. Usually, these small, dome-shaped, light pink papules are arranged in a confluent, annular pattern (Fig. 12.2). Sometimes, however, they can be scattered and generalized; this generalized pattern is referred to as *disseminated granuloma annulare.* In rare cases, granuloma annulare, especially when occurring over the dorsal feet, can appear as a macular pink flush that resembles a nevus flammeus, a so-called *vascular pattern* of granuloma annulare.

Differential Diagnosis The classic, annular form of granuloma annulare is sometimes confused with tinea corporis by generalists because of the annular appearance. However, granuloma annulare is stable and nonscaling. Disseminated granuloma annulare can sometimes be confused with insect bites, lichen planus, or multiple dermal tumors; often a biopsy is required to make this diagnosis.

"Vascular" granuloma annulare is occasionally confused with a vascular reaction (see Ch. 13, Vascular Reactions and Other Flat-Topped, Nonscaling Patches and Plaques) a nevus flammeus, or a superficial cellulitis. The history usually differentiates these diseases. If a biopsy is performed, the clinician should be aware that histologically, granuloma annulare is sometimes indistinguishable from both rheumatoid nodules and necrobiosis lipoidica. However, these three diseases are usually clinically distinct.

Management There is no good therapy for granuloma annulare. Granuloma annulare is slightly corticosteroid responsive, so that a topical corticosteroid such as triamcinolone cream 0.1% applied twice a day is a reasonable therapeutic option. Often, a much higher potency preparation must be used, but this should be done only with careful follow-up evaluation with an experienced clinician because surrounding atrophy is a real threat. There are other anecdotal reports of therapies not believed by many dermatologists to be beneficial, including oral niacinamide, retinoids,[1,2] dapsone,[3] and potassium iodide. A chart review suggested some benefits with ultraviolet light, intralesional corticosteroids (undoubtedly effective, but not practical for a multitude of lesions), and liquid nitrogen therapy.[4] Controlled trials have not been performed using these therapies.

Course and Prognosis Usually, granuloma annulare gradually resolves over several years. Occasionally, patients with disseminated granuloma annulare have associated diabetes mellitus. A fasting blood sugar is indicated in those patients.

Sarcoidosis

Another granulomatous disease that produces dome-shaped papules and nodules is sarcoidosis.

Clinical Manifestations Most common over the face of black patients in the Southeastern United States, classic lesions of sarcoidosis are infiltrated, shiny, inflammatory nodules with an almost vesicular appearance (Fig. 12.3). However, cutaneous sarcoidosis can have many different, less common morphologies, including scaling plaques, ichthyosis, ulcers, and cutaneous atrophy. Although usually red or violaceous, individual papules may be skin-colored, hyperpigmented, hypopigmented in black patients, or yellowish brown in lighter-complex-

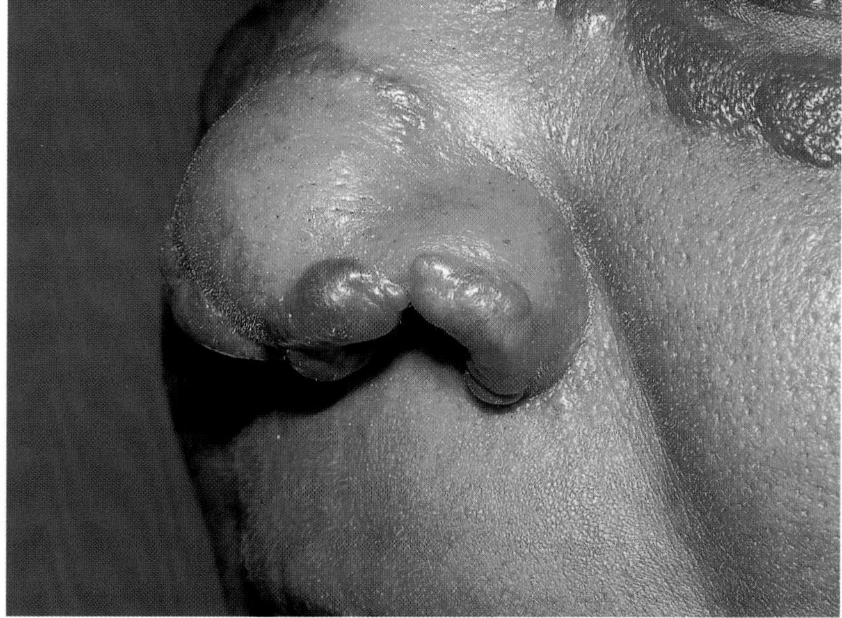

Figure 12.3 The lesions of sarcoidosis can exhibit widely variable morphology, but this patient exhibits the classic facial, dome-shaped, smooth papules and nodules. Although inflammatory, lesions can appear red, skin colored, or hyperpigmented, especially in dark-complexioned patients.

ioned individuals. When lesions cluster around the edges of the nares and mouth, upper airway disease is likely.[5]

Often, these asymptomatic lesions have no discernible associated systemic disease. However, all patients should be evaluated for visceral involvement, especially pulmonary and eye disease.

A classic but nonspecific skin finding in some patients with sarcoidosis is erythema nodosum. This is a good prognostic sign.

Differential Diagnosis Although the appearance of sarcoidosis is very characteristic, it cannot be absolutely distinguished clinically from granulomatous infections, and sometimes from lupus erythematosus. Biopsy confirmation is indicated.

Management The first step in management is an evaluation for systemic involvement. A chest radiograph and an ophthalmologic examination are essential.

The only therapy that predictably resolves cutaneous sarcoidosis is oral prednisone. Unfortunately, as soon as prednisone is withdrawn, lesions reappear. For that reason, systemic steroids are generally avoided unless visceral involvement is present and causing disease, or mucocutaneous lesions are extremely severe and disfiguring.

Some patients improve with topical corticosteroids. A reasonable starting medication is a midpotency preparation such as triamcinolone cream 0.1% applied twice a day. Although not appropriate for institution in the emergency department, oral hydroxychloroquine (Plaquenil) 200 mg bid and low-dose weekly methotrexate have also been reported beneficial in the hands of clinicians experienced with these medications and their side effects.[6,7]

Course and Prognosis The course of sarcoidosis is extremely variable. Some patients have scattered, relatively subtle lesions and others have large, cosmetically disfiguring nodules over the face. Some patients develop systemic disease, requiring aggressive systemic therapy. Hilar adenopathy and pulmonary infiltrates are common, sometimes resulting in severe pulmonary dysfunction. Iridocyclitis, keratoconjunctivitis, and chorioretinitis are often seen as well. Neurologic disease, parotid gland enlargement, and polyarthritis can also occur. Liver and spleen involvement are relatively common as well.

SARCOIDOSIS

Clinical Manifestations

Most common skin presentation is inflammatory, firm, edematous, translucent papules, plaques, and nodules over the face. Individual lesions can be skin colored or hyperpigmented, especially in blacks, or yellowish in lighter complexioned patients. Other morphologies include red, scaling infiltrated plaques, hypopigmented papules and plaques, and atrophic areas. Lesions often found in scars.

Management in the Emergency Department

1. *If no immediate danger from systemic disease, refer to dermatologist*
2. *If patient is insistent on therapy, small tube of triamcinolone cream 0.1% applied twice daily, with follow-up evaluation by a dermatologist at patient's earliest convenience.*

Rosacea

Although sometimes referred to as "adult acne," rosacea is unrelated to acne vulgaris. Whereas the primary lesion of acne vulgaris is the comedone, or blocked hair follicle, the inflammation of rosacea is not always follicular. Comedones are not part of this process. The cause of rosacea is unknown.

Rosacea encompasses several morphologies that somewhat represent different stages of the disease. Most common in light-complexioned patients, the first stage is flushing, and then a stable red flush to the skin with telangiectases occurs. Later, patients develop red papules and papulopustules. Last, some patients develop enlargement of the nose (rhinophyma).

The differential diagnosis includes seborrhea, with its central facial erythema, and true adult acne. The red nodules of lupus erythematosus can resemble rosacea, as can an uncommon condition called polymorphous light eruption. In some cases, a biopsy is required to sort out these diagnoses because of either atypical morphology or poor response to therapy.

Treatment consists of topical metronidazole cream or gel (Metrogel) applied twice daily. More recalcitrant patients require oral tetracycline 500 mg bid. Avoidance of heat, hot beverages, and spicy foods can minimize rosacea, especially the flushing phase.

> **ROSACEA**
>
> ***Clinical Manifestations***
>
> *Red papules, often with pustules, over central face, usually accompanied by ruddy complexion and telangiectasias; late disease may also be manifested by rhinophyma.*
>
> ***Management in the Emergency Department***
>
> 1. *Metronidazole gel (Metrogel) applied twice a day to affected areas*
> 2. *Patient education regarding the chronic nature of the problem and the delay of 1 to 2 months to respond to therapy (see the patient handout on p. 360, Rosacea)*

Inflamed Epidermal Cysts ("Infected Sebaceous Cysts")

Epidermal, or epidermoid, cysts are dermal sacs of keratin lined with epithelium. Epidermal cysts usually result from occlusion of a follicle, with subsequent distention of the follicle by keratin produced by the follicular epithelium and by small amounts of sebaceous secretions. As the cysts enlarge and the epithelial lining stretches and flattens, the cysts become more subject to trauma and possible rupture. Subsequent leakage of this debris into the dermis is extremely inflammogenic, resulting in exquisite pain, erythema, and fluctuance (Fig. 12.4). This inflammation is nearly always sterile. However, a wide zone of erythema and edema that extends beyond the borders of the cyst itself suggest a superimposed bacterial infection, generally with *Staphylococcus aureus* (Fig. 12.5).

The diagnosis is made by the clinical presentation and the usual history of a preexisting, smaller, painless lesion. Rarely, a culture is required to rule out a staphylococcal abscess.

Initially, an inflamed epidermal cyst has a firm consistency. At this stage, therapy consists of the injection of 0.1 to 0.5 ml of triamcinolone acetonide 3.0 to 3.3 mg/ml into the cyst and cyst wall. This can be purchased as TAC-3, or easily mixed by adding triamcinolone acetonide 10 mg/ml (Kenalog 10), 0.3 ml with 0.6 ml of injectable saline. This generally produces extraordinarily fast resolution of the inflammation, with the patient becoming much more comfortable by the next day.

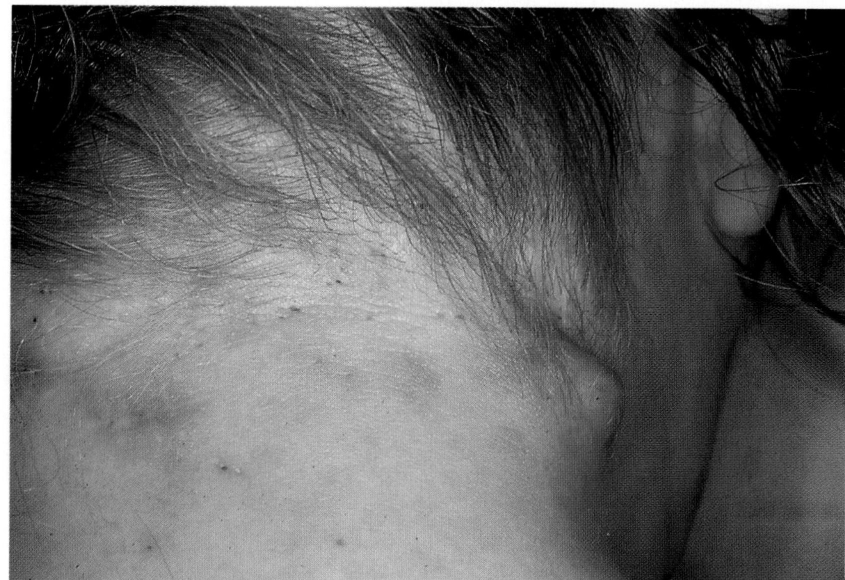

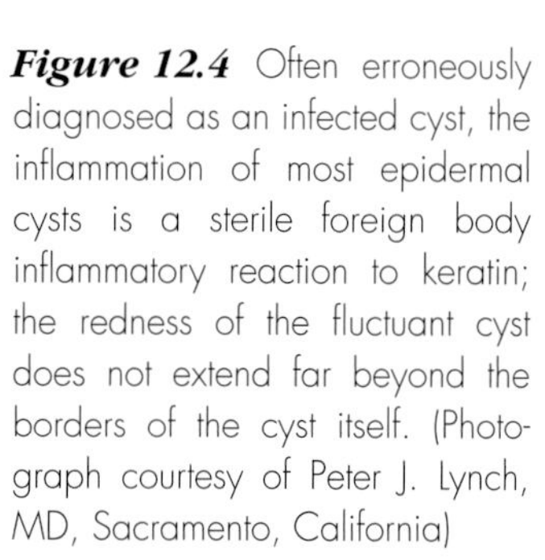

Figure 12.4 Often erroneously diagnosed as an infected cyst, the inflammation of most epidermal cysts is a sterile foreign body inflammatory reaction to keratin; the redness of the fluctuant cyst does not extend far beyond the borders of the cyst itself. (Photograph courtesy of Peter J. Lynch, MD, Sacramento, California)

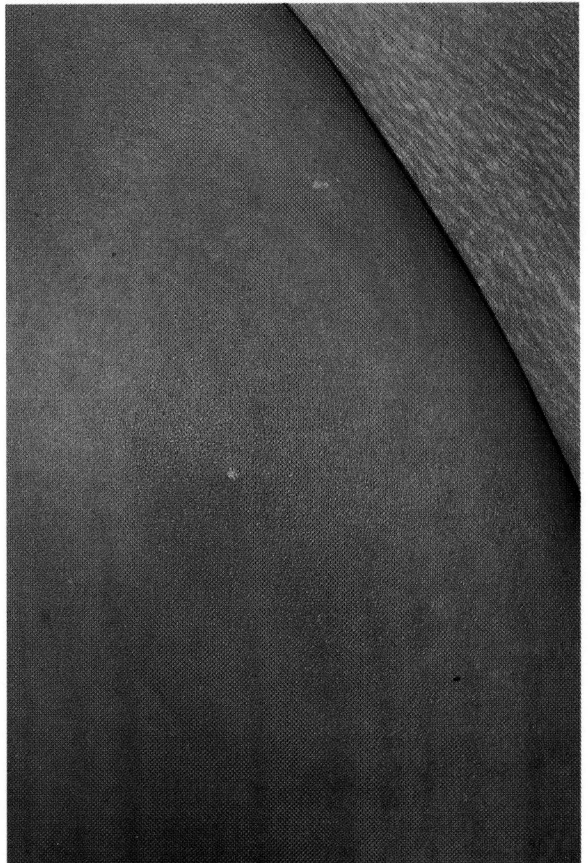

Figure 12.5 A furuncle, a deep staphylococcal abscess, differs from an inflamed (but not infected) cyst by the wide zone of erythema and edema, frequent spontaneous rupture, and often a patient who is febrile or ill. Compare this photograph to Figure 12.4.

As inflammation progresses, the nodule becomes fluctuant. At this point, the cyst benefits from a small stab incision with a No. 11 scalpel blade and gentle drainage of the cyst contents, followed by intralesional triamcinolone. The cyst should not be surgically excised, nor should sac removal be attempted while inflammation is present, since the edema and inflammation make the borders difficult to appreciate. A more conservative procedure can be accomplished after inflammation has resolved, with much less scarring. Antibiotics are rarely needed, but in case of a concern about infection, any antistaphylococcal medication including cephalexin or dicloxacillin can be used.

Hidradenitis Suppurativa (Apocrine acne)

Hidradenitis suppurativa is most often misdiagnosed as recurrent bacterial furuncles but actually represents cystic acne of the axillae or groin, or both.

Clinical Manifestations Usually occurring after puberty, and both more common and more severe in black patients, hidradenitis suppurativa presents with tender, recurrent, red nodules within areas of skin containing apocrine glands. This includes the axillae and the genital area, sometimes extending to the mons and lower abdomen, inner thighs, and buttocks. The red nodules often become fluctuant and drain, producing chronic sinus tracts. Comedones are often present, and as the disease progresses scarring becomes prominent (Fig. 12.6).

Differential Diagnosis Although hidradenitis suppurativa superficially resembles staphylococcal furunculosis, the localization to the axillae and genital area, the recurring nature, scarring, and the lack of cure with antibiotics all differentiate these two diseases. Cultures performed of drainage from these nodules show variable quantities and types of bacteria, as these lesions are found in areas favorable to superinfection and colonization.

Management Chronic anti-inflammatory antibiotics of the same type used for acne are the mainstay in medical therapy; these are appropriate for initiating in the emergency department. These antibiotics include oral tetracycline and erythromycin 500 mg bid, doxycycline and minocycline 100 mg bid, and clindamycin 150 mg bid. The anti-inflammatory effects often are not obvious until after 1 to 2 months of therapy.

Other therapies available, if antibiotics fail to produce acceptable improvement, include antiandrogen therapy, because hidradenitis suppurativa is androgen-driven. In women, high estrogen oral contraceptives that contain at least 50 μg of estrogen can improve disease, and the antiandrogen effects of spironolactone are helpful for some. Dermatologists also use oral retinoids, which only provide short-term improvement,[8] as well as intralesional triamcinolone to abort early lesions.

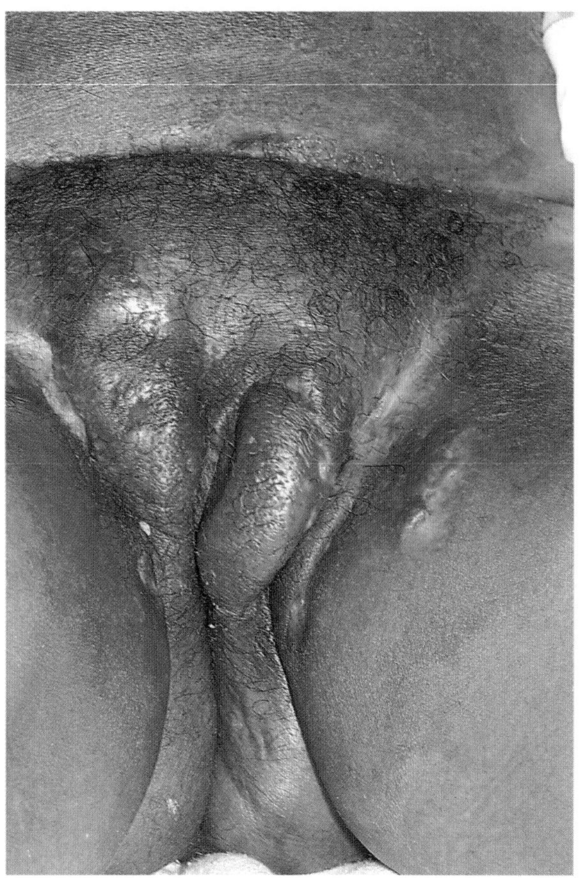

Figure 12.6 Hidradenitis suppurativa exhibits painful red nodules in the axillae or groin, or both. Later disease shows draining sinus tracts and scarring.

For severe disease, or for disease not controlled with reasonable medical therapy, surgery is not only an option, but an excellent alternative for the axillae.[9,10] When skin containing the apocrine glands is removed, the disease resolves. Unfortunately, apocrine glands are not as well localized in the genital area and, unless unreasonably large areas of skin are removed, recurrence at the edges is common.

Course and Prognosis Although mild to moderate disease is often controlled by chronic anti-inflammatory antibiotics, severe disease can be a therapeutic nightmare, particularly in the genital region. Hidradenitis suppurativa remains active and produces progressive scarring and draining sinus tracts.

HIDRADENITIS SUPPURATIVA

Clinical Manifestations

Recurrent tender nodules in the axillae or groin, or both, not cleared (although perhaps improved) by oral antistaphylococcal antibiotics. Comedones are common. Draining sinus tracts and scarring occur in late disease.

Management in the Emergency Department

1. *Begin anti-inflammatory antibiotic such as tetracycline 500 mg bid chronically*
2. *Incision and drainage of any acutely inflamed, fluctuant nodules*
3. *Injection into acutely inflamed lesion walls with triamcinolone acetonide (0.1 ml of triamcinolone 10 mg/ml mixed with 0.2 ml of injectable saline)*
4. *Patient education regarding similarity of this condition with acne, its chronic nature, and delay in response to therapy*
5. *Follow-up evaluation with personal health care provider or dermatologist in 2 months*

Cystic Acne

Inflamed acne cysts, which represent plugged hair follicles distended by keratin debris from desquamated follicular epithelium, sometimes rupture and become inflamed. This condition is differentiated from inflamed epidermal cysts of other origins and staphylococcal furunculosis by the location and the association with other acne lesions, including open and closed comedones, red papules, and frequent scarring (see Fig. 7.3; for more discussion of acne, see Ch. 7, Pustular Diseases). Acute therapy for acne cysts is the same as for inflamed epidermal cysts (see above).

Dissecting Cellulitis of the Scalp

Dissecting cellulitis of the scalp, or perifolliculitis capitis abscedens et suffodiens, is a misnomer that refers to cystic acne of the scalp. This is not a bacterial disease, although secondary infection can occur. Dissecting cellulitis of the scalp is a painful, disfiguring, and usually recalcitrant disease that occurs most often in black men. Like cystic acne and hidradenitis suppurativa, dissecting cellulitis of the scalp begins as plugged hair follicles that become distended by keratin debris, normal skin flora, and small amounts of sebaceous and apocrine secretions. If these inflamogenic contents leak into the surrounding dermis, red nodules occur. In late disease, draining sinus tracts, scarring, and new evolving lesions coexist, producing scarring hair loss (Fig. 12.7).

The treatment is the same as for cystic acne and hidradenitis suppurativa. Chronic anti-inflammatory antibiotics such as tetracycline or erythromycin at 500 mg bid, doxycycline or minocycline at 100 mg bid, and clindamycin at 150 mg bid generally improve the skin over 2 to 3 months. For very fluctuant lesions, incision and drainage can temporarily make patients more comfortable, and early lesions can be improved with intralesional triamcinolone injections (TAC-3, or triamcinolone acetonide 10 mg/ml [Kenalog 10], 0.1 ml with 0.2 ml of injectable saline). Although oral isotretinoin temporarily improves disease, it does not clear this condition permanently as it does acne.[11]

DISSECTING CELLULITIS OF THE SCALP

Clinical Manifestations

Red nodules, some fluctuant, in the scalp of black men; late diseases characterized by chronic draining sinuses from confluent sterile abscesses, with scarring and hair loss.

Management in the Emergency Department

1. *Begin anti-inflammatory antibiotic such as tetracycline 500 mg bid chronically*
2. *Incision and drainage of any acutely inflamed, fluctuant nodules*
3. *Injection into acutely inflamed lesion walls with triamcinolone acetonide (0.1 ml of triamcinolone 10 mg/ml mixed with 0.2 ml of injectable saline)*
4. *Patient education regarding similarity of this condition with acne, its chronic nature, and delay in response to therapy*
5. *Follow-up evaluation with personal health care provider or dermatologist in 2 months*

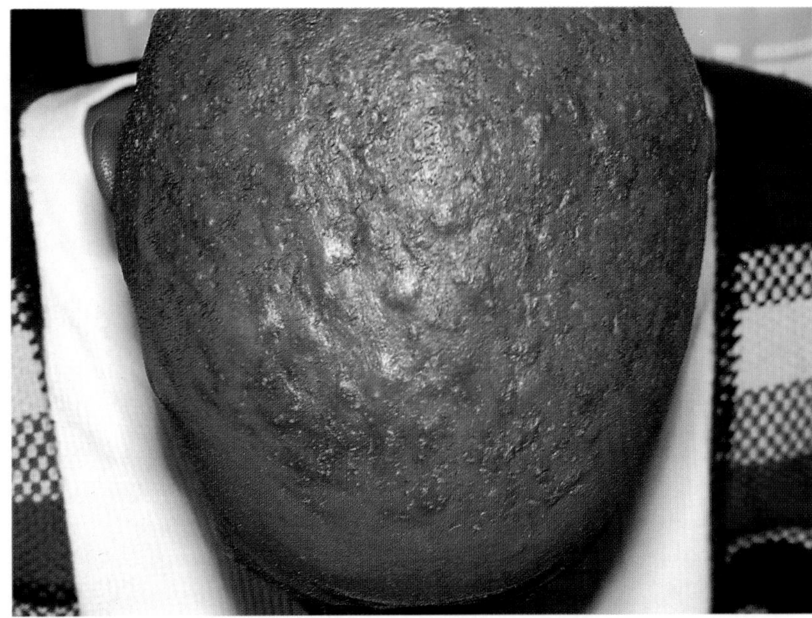

Figure 12.7 Dissecting cellulitis of the scalp is manifested by suppurative nodules that coalesce and drain, producing hair loss and scarring. (Photograph courtesy of Jennifer Helton, MD, Charlotte, North Carolina)

INFECTIOUS NODULES

Cutaneous infections are often manifested by inflammatory nodules. These lesions are either granulomatous or neutrophilic and can generally be differentiated from noninfectious red nodules by their more inflammatory nature. A boggy texture and areas of crusting or pustulation, or both, on the surface are common.

Granulomatous Infections

Deep Fungal Infections Deep fungal infections are well-known causes of granulomatous dermal and subcutaneous infections. Sporotrichosis classically presents as inflammatory nodules distributed in a linear pattern along lymphatic channels proximal to the site of inoculation (Fig. 12.8). Most common on the hand and arm, these nodules are not usually associated with constitutional symptoms, although regional lymphadenopathy is usual. Therapy consists of saturated solution of potassium iodide, although itraconazole appears to be effective with fewer side effects. Cutaneous coccidioidomycosis (Valley fever) is a relatively common finding in the southwestern United States. Because cutaneous involvement with this fungus usually results from systemic disease acquired by respiratory exposure, cough, fever, and malaise are often associated with the skin lesions. Skin lesions are usually few in number, and there is no particular pattern. Therapy entails the use of oral antifungal agents. Skin lesions from histoplasmosis are seen primarily in immunosuppressed patients, and lesions can have widely variable morphology. Red papules and pustules are most common. Patients are generally ill with systemic symptoms that include cough and fever. Blastomycosis is a serious pulmonary disease occurring primarily in patients with exposure to soil. Associated skin lesions are often hyperkeratotic, verrucous, and characteristically progress in some areas, while healing occurs in other areas.

Parasites Parasites can also cause granulomatous cutaneous nodules, but these are not common in the United States. Cutaneous amebiasis and leishmaniasis are occasionally seen, but generally these diseases are contracted in other countries.

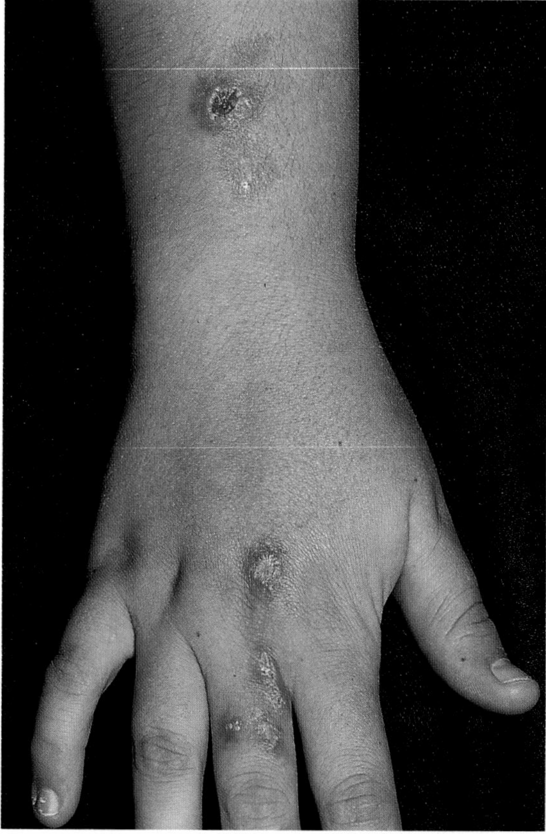

Figure 12.8 Sporotrichosis can be suspected when red, indurated nodules occur in a linear pattern in a path of lymphatic drainage.

Mycobacterial Infections Mycobacterial infections also cause red nodules as well as ulcers. Most common is *Mycobacterium marinum*, the causative organism of a fish tank granuloma. This water-borne organism becomes implanted in broken skin. Red nodules are generally indolent and single and occur most often on the hands. The nodules may become warty and may ulcerate. Patients are not usually ill, and the diagnosis is made on tissue biopsy for routine histology and specific culture for mycobacteria. This infection generally responds to oral minocycline or doxycycline 100 mg bid or to trimethoprim/sulfamethoxazole 160/800 bid.

Furuncle

A furuncle is a deep lesion of bacterial folliculitis. This painful, erythematous, indurated nodule may be single or occur in crops. It is often associated with a superficial folliculitis characterized by small follicular papules and pustules. Furunculosis is usually a nodule associated with a surrounding red flare; as the lesion matures, a central pustule develops and ruptures with drainage of contents (Fig. 12.5).

The primary disease in the differential diagnosis is an inflamed epidermal cyst. The lack of a preceding lesion, greater surrounding inflammation, the presence of several lesions, and the development of a central pustule with drainage all suggest bacterial infection.

First-line therapy for early, nonfluctuant lesions is an oral antistaphylococcal agent such as cephalexin or dicloxacillin at 250 mg qid. Once the lesion has become fluctuant, incision and drainage also become important aspects of therapy.

Hot Tub Folliculitis (Pseudomonas Folliculitis)

Although folliculitis is generally classified as a pustular disease, early lesions of folliculitis, no matter what the cause, are usually red papules. Patients with folliculitis caused by *Pseudomonas aeruginosa* generally exhibit primarily red or pink, dome-shaped, fairly superficial papules, and pustules may be subtle or absent (Fig. 12.9).

These patients usually have a history of exposure to stagnant, warm water. Although inadequately disinfected hot tubs are the most well-known source of this condition, situations as varied as leaking water beds and chronically wet, reused washcloths can serve as a reservoir for the organism. Sometimes, even in patients with recurrent *Pseudomonas* folliculitis, no source is identified after careful patient questioning.

These pink papules are concentrated in body folds and over skin that has been occluded by clothing or swim suits soaked by the contaminated

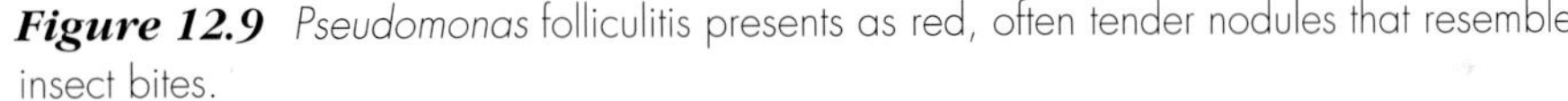
Figure 12.9 *Pseudomonas* folliculitis presents as red, often tender nodules that resemble insect bites.

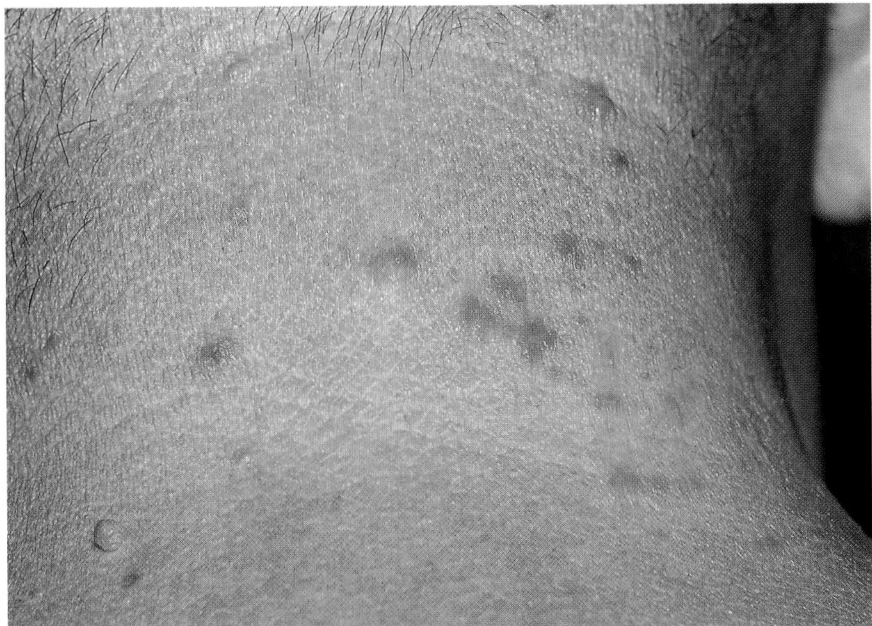

water. Lesions are often painful and some patients have associated constitutional symptoms including sore throat, fever, malaise, and occasionally ear pain, but patients are not usually particularly toxic.

The differential diagnosis includes insect bites, cutaneous lesions of sepsis, and sterile and staphylococcal folliculitis. The diagnosis can usually be made on clinical and historical grounds, although immunosuppressed patients or very ill patients should have further evaluation by a punch biopsy.

Therapy consists of removing the source of infection because lesions and symptoms resolve spontaneously. Patients who are particularly uncomfortable can be treated with oral ciprofloxacin.

HOT TUB FOLLICULITIS

Clinical Manifestations

Tender red papules, sometimes with pustules concentrated primarily over skin folds or where wet clothing has occluded skin. Sometimes associated with constitutional symptoms including sore throat, fever, malaise, and earache.

Management in the Emergency Department

1. *Remove source of Pseudomonas (e.g., clean spa, discontinue use of wet washcloths that have not been given a chance to dry out*
2. *Reassurance and observation*

Sepsis

Patients who are septic sometimes develop inflammation of vessels from local invasion of organisms, especially yeast forms but also bacteria. This septic vasculitis presents initially as red, cutaneous papules that resemble insect bites. Often, intense inflammation produces necrosis of vessels with resulting ischemia, resulting in extravasation of red blood cells with clinical purpura and/or necrosis of overlying skin, as can occur with meningococcemia.

The lesions of sepsis often present as widely scattered, pink, dome-shaped papules in an immunosuppressed, toxic patient. Sometimes, a pustule or local ischemia, ulceration, and cellulitis can occur. When the organism is *Pseudomonas aeruginosa*, the process is called ecthyma gangrenosum. Unless the patient is known to be septic with a specific organism, these lesions should be punch-biopsied immediately so that the causative pathogen can be identified quickly and specific therapy instituted. The biopsy often reveals nonspecific results or an unrelated or nonemergent condition. However, the survival of those patients whose lesions do represent sepsis may depend on early recognition of, and therapy for, the causative organism.

These lesions most often resemble insect bites or the papules of folliculitis. However, in the setting of an ill patient, the clinician should consider this more significant diagnosis. An early biopsy of inflammatory papules in an immunosuppressed patient to facilitate diagnosis and therapy is indicated, unless the underlying disease process is already known.

VASCULAR TUMORS

Tumors of blood vessel origin are understandably red. When vessels are larger and, when these tumors are not located on lower extremities, the color is often a very bright, cherry red, as opposed to the pink or violaceous erythema of inflammation. However, blood vessel tumors over lower legs or those with very small blood vessels with a slow blood flow tend to be more purple in color due to oxygen desaturation.

Cherry Angiomas (Senile Angiomas)

Cherry angiomas are small blood vessel tumors that are ubiquitous in white patients over 45 years of age, and almost never seen in black patients. These 1- to 4-mm bright red, sharply demarcated papules are most concentrated over the trunk and proximal extremities. Occasionally, the red color may take on a more purple hue.

These small tumors do not regress spontaneously, and patients tend to develop more lesions as they age. Because there is a strong genetic predisposition for these angiomas, some patients only have a very small number, whereas other patients have several hundred.

These lesions are of cosmetic importance only, and therapy is not essential. If the patient wishes to have them removed, destruction by laser or electrocautery, or shave excision is required.

Capillary Hemangiomas

Capillary hemangiomas are aggressive blood vessel tumors that occur in infancy (see Fig. 19.2). These rapidly enlarge for several months, and then usually resolve spontaneously during childhood (for further discussion, see Ch. 19, Pediatric Dermatology).

Kaposi Sarcoma

Kaposi sarcoma is a tumor of vascular proliferation and inflammation that occurs most often in the United States in association with sexually contracted acquired immunodeficiency syndrome (for more discussion of this form of Kaposi sarcoma, see Ch. 20, Cutaneous Signs of Immunosuppression and AIDS).

However, Kaposi sarcoma is also seen occasionally as an indolent, multicentric, violaceous to hyperpigmented eruption found primarily in men of Mediterranean extraction, particularly if immunosuppressed by virtue of medication or disease. Classic Kaposi sarcoma occurs most often over the lower extremities in association with stasis changes. The lesions are generally asymptomatic until and unless the eruption becomes widespread and infiltrative, when edema and ulceration can occur.

The primary findings to be differentiated from Kaposi sarcoma are the hyperpigmentation and varicosities associated with venous stasis on the lower legs. However, the purple areas of Kaposi sarcoma are not compressible, and the diagnosis can be made on the basis of biopsy.

Therapy often is not required. In progressive disease, patients can be referred to an oncologist for evaluation for low-dose vinca alkaloids or radiotherapy.

Pyogenic Granuloma

This tumor of vascular proliferation and inflammation often occurs after minor trauma. In addition, it is particularly common in young women during pregnancy and is sometimes called the "tumor of pregnancy." The term "pyogenic granuloma" is a misnomer, because this lesion is neither pyogenic (infected) nor a granuloma.

These red-purple, exophytic nodules are usually singular but occasionally occur in crops (Fig. 12.10). The surface epithelium is either very thin or eroded and glistening. Common locations include the gingivae, the fingertips and hands, and the face.

The primary disease to be differentiated from a pyogenic granuloma is a nodular amelanotic melanoma. For this reason, even very typical pyogenic granulomas should be submitted for pathologic confirmation after removal.

The treatment of a pyogenic granuloma is surgical removal. This can be accomplished by shave removal with curettage of the base and light hyfrecation. Alternatively but requiring more time, the lesion can be excised with suture closure. Although these lesions occasionally recur, therapy is generally curative.

LYMPHOCYTIC INFILTRATES

Lymphocytes within the skin produce a violaceous color. Not only can the clinical differentiation of skin diseases characterized by lymphocytes be difficult, but even a biopsy may not yield a definitive diagnosis. Lymphocytic infiltrates can occur as a result of infection, malignancy, or inflammation of autoimmune or unknown cause.

Leukemia and Lymphoma

Leukemia and lymphoma can sometimes affect the skin. These generally consist of multiple, scattered, infiltrated dusky or violaceous nodules. Although these are generally late findings in leukemia or lymphoma, occasionally skin findings precede obvious systemic disease. These patients warrant referral to a dermatologist for evaluation and a skin biopsy if the diagnosis is unclear; otherwise, a direct referral to an oncologist is reasonable. Cutaneous T-cell lymphoma (*Mycosis fungoides*) initially appears as a papulosquamous disease (see Ch. 14, Papulosquamous Diseases: Red, Scaling,

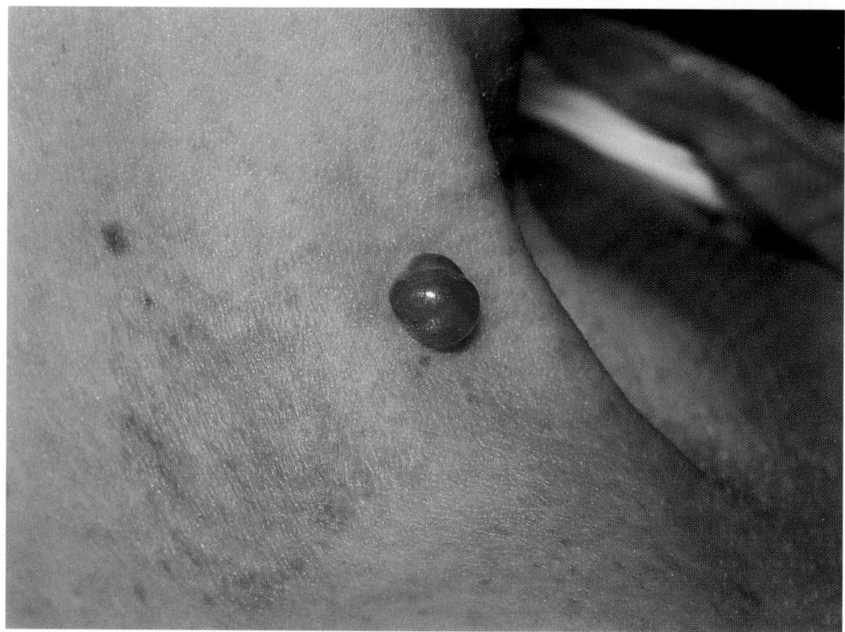

Figure 12.10 Pyogenic granulomas are usually pedunculated, red, glistening tumors of recent origin.

Well-Demarcated Papules and Plaques) but later tumor-stage disease shows infiltrated nodules that are often superimposed over plaques. However, this indolent disease is generally diagnosed long before actual tumors form, and the patient is aware of the diagnosis.

Cutaneous Lupus Erythematosus

Systemic lupus erythematosus is occasionally associated with dermal lymphocytic infiltrates. These dusky red nodules are usually multiple and are located over the face and occasionally upper trunk. This diagnosis is generally made on biopsy except in patients with known lupus erythematosus, when patients should be referred to a rheumatologist or a dermatologist for further workup and treatment.

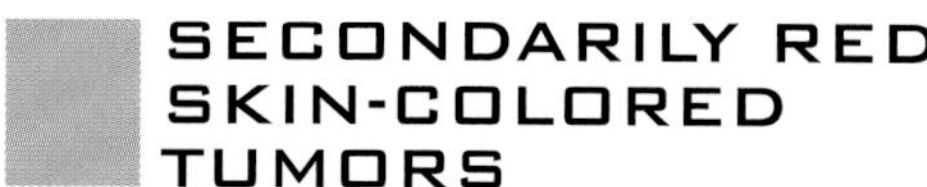

SECONDARILY RED SKIN-COLORED TUMORS

Any tumors that are normally skin colored can, particularly in a light-complexioned patient, appear red due to secondary inflammation or increased vascularity seen through pale skin (for further discussion of these tumors, see Ch. 8, Skin-Colored Lesions). Several common tumors are especially likely to appear pink.

Intradermal Nevi

Intradermal nevi often appear quite pink and may appear to be inflammatory papules, rather than tumors. Usually, there are surrounding typical nevi that allow the examiner to make a diagnosis. Nevi are soft, nontender, well-demarcated macules or papules distributed primarily over the upper back and arms.

Basal and Squamous Cell Carcinomas

Basal cell carcinomas are frequently secondarily inflamed due to minor trauma to these fragile lesions and because of the body's immunologic response to the tumors. Generally, pink basal cell carcinomas appear typical otherwise. Squamous cell carcinomas may be inflamed as well. These tumors are usually either scaly and keratotic or more solid-appearing than basal cell carcinomas. Both basal and squamous cell carcinomas are generally found in a sun-exposed distribution.

Seborrheic Keratoses

Seborrheic keratoses sometimes become secondarily inflamed due to trauma. The normal brown color can disappear, and the lesion simply becomes scaly and pink. The diagnosis can often be made presumptively because there are usually surrounding, typical seborrheic keratoses. Occasionally, a biopsy must be performed to rule out the presence of a squamous cell carcinoma.

Please see patient information handouts for this chapter on pages 339, 350, 351, and 360.

REFERENCES

1. Schleicher SM, Milstein HJ, Sim SHM: Resolution of disseminated granuloma annulare with isotretinoin. Int J Dermatol 31:371, 1992
2. Botella-Estrada R, Guillen C, Sanmartin O, Aliaga A: Disseminated granuloma annulare: resolution with etretinate therapy. J Am Acad Dermatol 26:777, 1992
3. Steiner A, Pehamberger H, Wolff K: Sulfone treatment of granuloma annulare. J Am Acad Dermatol 13:1004, 1985
4. Dabski K, Winkelmann RK: Generalized granuloma annulare: clinical and laboratory findings in 100 patients. J Am Acad Dermatol 20:39, 1989
5. Zax RH, Callen JP. Granulomatous reactions. p. 629. In Sams WM Jr, Lynch PJ (eds): Principles and Practice of Dermatology. 2nd Ed. Churchill Livingstone, New York, 1996
6. Jones E, Callen JP: Hydroxychloroquine is effective therapy for control of cutaneous sarcoidal granulomas. J Am Acad Dermatol 23:487, 1990
7. Webster G, Razsi LK, Sanchez M, Shupack JL: Weekly low-dose methotrexate therapy for cutaneous sarcoidosis. J Am Acad Dermatol 24:451, 1991
8. Dicken CH, Powell ST, Spear ST et al: Evaluation of isotretinoin treatment of hidradenitis suppurativa. J Am Acad Dermatol 11:500, 1984
9. Finley EM, Ratz JL: Treatment of hidradenitis suppurativa with carbon dioxide laser excision and second-intention healing. J Am Acad Dermatol 34:465, 1996
10. Banerjee AK: Surgical treatment of hidradenitis suppurativa. Br J Surg 79:863, 1992
11. Bjellerup M, Wallengren J: Familial perifolliculitis capitis abscedens et suffodiens in two brothers successfully treated with isotretinoin. J Am Acad Dermatol 23:752, 1990

SUGGESTED READINGS

Insect Bites

Howard R, Frieden IJ: Papular urticaria in children. Pediatr Dermatol 13:246, 1996

Granuloma annulare

Muhgauer JE: Granuloma annulare. J Am Acad Dermatol 3:217, 1980

Sarcoidosis

Samstov AV: Cutaneous sarcoidosis. Int J Dermatol 31:385, 1992

Zax RH, Callen JP: Sarcoidosis. Dermatol Clin 7:505, 1989

Acne and Rosacea

Plewig G, Kligman AM: Acne and Rosacea. Springer-Verlag, Berlin, 1993

Hidradenitis Suppurativa

Ebling FJG: Apocrine glands in health and disorder. Int J Dermatol 28:508, 1989

Hot Tub Folliculitis

Gregory DW, Schaffner W: *Pseudomonas* infection associated with hot tubs and other environments. Infect Dis Clin North Am 1:635, 1987

Kaposi Sarcoma

Geddes M, Francheschi S, Barchielli A et al: Kaposi's sarcoma in Italy before and after the AIDS epidemic. Br J Cancer 69:333, 1994

CHAPTER 13

Vascular Reactions and Other Flat-Topped, Nonscaling Patches and Plaques

Unlike most morphologic groups that comprise skin diseases based on morphologic appearance, the vascular reaction group comprises diseases that both share clinical appearance and that have related pathogeneses. These diseases are all hypersensitivity reactions. Included in this morphologic group are a few diseases that are unrelated except for appearance—sunburn, cellulitis, erysipelas, and actinic/steroid purpura—but these rarely pose diagnostic difficulties because of the settings in which they occur.

Vascular reactions are red, nonscaling, flat-topped eruptions, with a tendency for individual lesions to become confluent. This group includes urticaria, erythema multiforme, leukocytoclastic vasculitis, erythema nodosum, and the majority of those red rashes found when patients arrive with a chief complaint of fever and rash. The differential diagnosis of potentially dangerous causes of fever and rash is seen in Table 13.1, although these diseases are discussed individually in other parts of this book that correspond to the morphologic appearances of the rashes. Although these specific eruptions are vascular reactions, very often the eruptions are more nonspecific, lacking the migratory nature of urticaria or the target-patterned lesions of erythema multiforme, for example. Or, a patient may have several different vascular reactions along the spectrum at the same time.

The vascular reaction group comprises the childhood viral exanthems, which generally do not exhibit specific eruptions (see Table 19.1). These diagnoses must be made on the basis of minor variations in the distribution of the eruption, the accompanying signs and symptoms, serologic studies, and knowledge of patterns of infections in the community during that time (for an in-depth discussion, see Ch. 19, Pediatric Diseases).

The vascular reaction group also encompasses the nonspecific, morbilliform eruptions sometimes associated with an allergy to medications (a "drug rash") and with rashes often associated with a "viral syndrome."

The schema of vascular reactions discussed in this chapter is, by simplifying this group of hypersensitivity reactions, quite overly simplified. However, for the purposes of patient care as well as an understanding of the medical implications, workup, and therapy in an emergency department, this schema is certainly sufficient. Generally, the differentiation of one vascular reaction from another is not crucial, as these are all hyperimmune eruptions with the same underlying allergens. However, each disease within this group does present possible unique complications that must be considered. When present, these complications can produce considerable morbidity or even death. For example, urticaria is occasionally associated with anaphylaxis, erythema multiforme with widespread blistering, and leukocytoclastic vasculitis with end-organ damage from ischemia due to systemic vasculitis.

Vascular reactions are a response to systemic exposure to allergens, rather than to an external contactant. Therefore, except for the uncommon case of contact urticaria, there is no need to worry about which detergent is used, or what perfumes and medications are being applied to the skin.

Vascular reactions can occur in response to almost any antigenic stimulus or chronic inflammation. Obviously, this covers an enormous range of possibilities. Although a skin biopsy differentiates between urticaria and erythema multiforme, a biopsy does not elucidate the cause of the hypersensitivity reaction producing either eruption. Therefore, detective work is needed. Fortunately, of the almost infinite number of possible offending allergens, some are far more likely to produce a vascular reaction.[1–5]

Young people, particularly children, most often develop a vascular reaction on the basis of an infection, since children especially tend to have frequent, minor infections. Any infection can induce a vascular reaction by precipitating an immune response. Viral infections are the most common infections to produce a rash. Recurrent erythema multiforme is nearly always produced by recurrent herpes simplex virus (HSV) infection.[6] Other viruses, such as hepatitis B, induce vascular reactions in most infected patients. However, the most common infection to cause a vascular reaction is whichever virus is "going around" at that time. Even if a relatively small percentage of patients with a particular infection develop a rash, sheer numbers of infected patients will produce a few who experience a hypersensitivity reaction to that virus. Measles, rubella, rubeola, and fifth disease (subitum infantum) are regularly associated with vascular reactions (see Ch. 19, for a discussion of pediatric diseases). Other viruses with a known association with vascular reactions include Epstein-Barr virus (EBV) (particularly when the patient receives an antibiotic) and cytomegalovirus (CMV).

Bacteria are sometimes associated with vascular reactions. More common offending bacteria include *Streptococcus* and *Staphylococcus aureus*. *Mycoplasma* and *Mycobacteria* also produce vascular reactions in some patients. Bacterial infections responsible for vascular reactions are usually symptomatic; therefore, laboratory screening and cultures are not indicated in the absence of symptoms and signs. With the exception of some cases of chronic sinusitis and dental abscesses, patients have a suspicious pertinent review of systems.

Other infections can produce vascular reactions. Deep fungus infections that can produce vascular reactions include coccidioidomycosis (Valley fever), which is especially likely to cause erythema nodosum, and histoplasmosis. In addition, rickettsia (e.g., Rocky Mountain spotted fever) and spirochetes (Lyme disease) can cause vascular reactions.

For older patients, medications are the most common cause of vascular reactions. Although nearly every medication available has been reported to cause a rash, many, if not most, are coincidental and only reported because the skin is so visible and patients and clinicians so ready to ascribe rashes to medications. Most vascular reactions due to medications are found with a small number of medications.[2,3] A good working knowledge of this relatively small list as well as attention to the timing of the development of vascular reactions help the clinician to sort through possible causes of rashes in those patients who are taking a multitude of medications. Extremely common and well-known medications that cause vascular reac-

CAUSES OF VASCULAR REACTIONS

- *Infections*
- *Medications*
- *Autoimmune diseases*
- *Lymphoreticular malignancies*
- *Blood dyscrasias*
- *Other*

MORE COMMON INFECTIONS CAUSING VASCULAR REACTIONS

Viruses

- *Herpes simplex virus*
- *Epstein-Barr virus*
- *Cytomegalovirus*
- *Hepatitis viruses, especially B*
- *Many acute viral syndromes*

Bacteria

- *Streptococcus*
- *Staphylococcus*
- *Yersinia*
- *Mycobacterium (tuberculosis)*

Fungus

- *Coccidioidomycosis*
- *Histoplasmosis*

Other

- *Rickettsia*
- *Mycoplasma*
- *Spirochete (Lyme disease)*

Table 13.1 Dangerous Causes of Rash in a Sick Patient[a]

DISEASE	SKIN FINDINGS	ASSOCIATED SIGNS	DIAGNOSIS
Discrete red papules/plaques			
Acute meningococcemia (see Figs. 16.4 and 16.6)	Scattered pink papules, often ot large numbers; may become purpuric, vesiculopustular. Purpura fulminans with severe disease	Abrupt onset of headache, malaise, fever, myalgias, nausea, vomiting. Severe disease: hypotension, disseminated intravascular coagulation	Organisms identified in spinal fluid, smears from skin lesions
Rocky Mountain Spotted Fever (see Fig. 16.3)	Pinpoint pink macules beginning on hands, feet, extending centripetally; lesions becoming petechial. Conjunctival hyperemia. Purpura fulminans with severe disease	Periorbital edema, fever, chills, frontal headache, photophobia, myalgias, arthralgias, vomiting, diarrhea	Clinical suspicion; direct immunofluorescent skin biopsy for organism (many false negatives)
Sepsis, bacterial or fungal (see Fig 16.2)	Scattered pink papules resembling insect bites, sometimes becoming purpuric	Fever, septic shock when severe. Other findings depend upon etiology and site of infection	Clinical suspicion; skin biopsy for routine histology and culture, blood cultures
Erythema migrans (see Fig. 13.7)	Red nonscaling papule, plaque, macule or patch either solid or annular; sometimes multiple lesions	Low grade fever, malaise, myalgias, arthralgias, ausea, headache, local lymphadenopathy	Clinical presentation, rule out other causes when atypical
Juvenile rheumatoid arthritis	Small, pink, nonscaling, blanchable papules, often with peripheral pallor, evanescent. Beginning over trunk and proximal extremities	Arthritis, sometimes fever, malaise, serositis	Clinical case definition (see Ch. 19)
Systemic lupus erythematosus (see Fig. 13.14)	Erythematous flushing over malar area, lid margins, posterior ailfold, sometimes with scale	Arthritis, serositis; kidney, central nervous system disease with dysfunction; leukopenia, thrombocytopenia, photosensitivity	Clinical case definition, positive serologies

(Continues)

Table 13.1 (Continued)

DISEASE	SKIN FINDINGS	ASSOCIATED SIGNS	DIAGNOSIS
Generalized erythema			
Toxic shock syndrome	Generalized erythema beginning over the trunk, sandpapery texture, accentuation of skin folds; prominent oral and conjunctival erythema. Late peeling of fingertips	Hypotension, diarrhea, headache, sore throat, periorbital and joint edema (see Table 13.7)	Clinical case definition (see boxed list, p. 184)
Scarlet fever	Pink, sandpapery eruption, with accentuation in skin folds, Pastia's lines. Flushed face, circumoral pallor. Red (sometimes exudative) oropharynx, white then red strawberry tongue. Late desquamation	Preceding fever, rigors, sore throat, headache, abdominal pain	Throat culture positive for group A streptococcus
Early staphylococcal scalded skin syndrome (see Fig. 19.6)	Early red macular erythema around mouth, becoming generalized and painful, but sparing mucous membranes. A sandpapery texture develops before the upper epidermis wrinkles and detaches; radial fissuring around the mouth	Fever, skin pain, irritability, anorexia; found in children under 5 yrs. of age	Clinical presentation, culture that yields *Staphylococcus aureus* from nasopharynx, eye, or a site of infection
Early toxic epidermal ecrolysis (drug induced; see Figs 5-10, 5-11, and 5-12)	Generalized erythema with detachment of the epidermis producing bullae, erosions, and large areas of unattached skin. Mucous membranes with erosions	Early: skin pain. Late: secondary sepsis is common	Clinical onset, consistent medication history, and characteristic skin lesions; skin biopsy for frozen section when in doubt, especially to rule out pemphigus vulgaris
Exfoliative erythroderma (see Fig. 3.1)	Generalized, usually chronic, erythema and scale, with mucous membranes generally unaffected	Chills, fever, leukocytosis, elevated blood urea nitrogen, anemia, dependent edema	Clinical presentation. A history of a preexisting skin disease that worsened usually provides underlying cause. Otherwise, referral to a dermatologist for evaluation

(Continues)

Table 13.1 (Continued)

DISEASE	SKIN FINDINGS	ASSOCIATED SIGNS	DIAGNOSIS
Purpuric lesions (see Ch. 16)			
Purpura fulminans (skin finding produced by several infections when severe; see Fig. 16.4)	Irregular, stellate plaques of purpura with central necrosis manifested by gray or black discoloration initially, and later by erosion or ulceration	Hypotension, disseminated intravascular coagulation, multiorgan failure	Clinical presentation. The etiology of the sepsis should be investigated, with special attention to the possibilities of group A streptococcal, pneumococcal, and meningococcal infection. Also postvaricella, Rocky Mountain Spotted Fever, and gram egative enteric organisms can produce this condition
Rocky Mountain Spotted Fever (see Fig. 16.3)	See above, under *Discrete red papules*	See above, under *Discrete red papules*	See above, under *Discrete red papules*
Acute meningococcemia	See above, under *Discrete red papules*	See above, under *Discrete red papules*	See above, under *Discrete red papules*
Leukocytoclastic vasculitis (hyper-sensitivity to a medication, infection, or autoimmune disease; see Figs. 13.11,13.12, 6.6, and 6.7)	Purpuric papules, plaques or nodules, usually beginning over the lower extremities. Sometimes associated with hemorrhagic vesicles or bullae	Associated findings depend upon the etiology of the LCV. Also, if LCV is cutaneous only, there are no associated findings. If involvement is systemic, signs of organ dysfunction or inflammation are present	Skin biopsy. However, the cause of the LCV should be investigated
Disseminated gonococcemia	Few, scattered, small purpuric pustules primarily over joints, most often in women	Fever, chills, arthralgias, arthritis, tenosynovitis	Clinical presentation. Confirmation sometimes made with a blood culture, and rarely on joint effusion

(Continues)

Table 13.1 (Continued)

DISEASE	SKIN FINDINGS	ASSOCIATED SIGNS	DIAGNOSIS
Other			
Kawasaki disease	Polymorphous; generally red or pink, nonscaling macules, papules, plaques or patches occurring anywhere; face, hands, and feet prominently affected. Erythema of the oropharynx, lips usual. Late peeling of the genital area, palms, and soles	Fever, acute nonpurulent cervical lymphadenopathy, edema of hands and feet, coronary artery aneurysms (see Table 19.2)	Clinical case definition (see Table 19.2)
Pustular psoriasis (see Figs. 7.6 and 7.7)	Red plaques or pustules, or crusted plaques	Fever, leukocytosis, chills, arthritis	History of worsening psoriasis; skin biopsy. Typical psoriatic lesions and distribution often absent

[a]Any infection or autoimmune disease can produce a nonspecific erythematous, nonscaling macular or papular eruption that is no more helpful diagnostically than fever.

tions include some antibiotics, particularly sulfas and penicillins. Included in the penicillins are newer medications, such as Augmentin, which contain a penicillin, although that is not necessarily reflected in the name. In addition, some medications can cause reactions in patients allergic to a similar medication, such as crossreactivity of penicillin and imipenem or cephalosporin. This is generally reported in books such as the *American Medical Association Manual of Medical Therapeutics* or the *Physician's Desk Reference.* However, innocuous antibiotics are frequently blamed for vascular reactions, since most patients who receive these have signs or symptoms of an infection as well, so that sorting out whether the rash is due to the antibiotic, the infection, or the unique combination of the two can be very difficult. The mislabeling of a patient as allergic to an antibiotic is a perennial problem for which there is often no good answer.

The anticonvulsants phenytoin (Dilantin), carbamazepine (Tegretol), and phenobarbital are frequent offenders that can either crossreact with or potentiate the effects of each other. Phenytoin in particular can produce long-lasting eruptions due to its long serum half-life.

The diuretics hydrochlorothiazide and furosemide produce vascular reactions, as do the antiarrhythmic drugs procainamide and quinidine. Nonsteroidal anti-inflammatory drugs (NSAIDs) and phenothiazines are medications that regularly produce vascular reactions as well. Finally, allopurinol is a common offender that is not only quite allergenic but that is also likely to cause severe disease including a life-threatening form of erythema multiforme, toxic epidermal necrolysis.

Other conditions associated with vascular reactions include lymphoreticular malignancies and blood dyscrasias, and autoimmune diseases. These diseases may produce rashes by the production of

COMMON MEDICATIONS CAUSING VASCULAR REACTIONS

Antibiotics
- *Sulfas*
- *Penicillins*
- *Cephalosporins*

Anticonvulsants
- *Phenytoin*
- *Carbamazepine*
- *Phenobarbital*

Diuretics
- *Hydrochlorothiazide*
- *Furosemide*

Antiarrhythmic medications
- *Quinidine*
- *Procainamide*

Other
- *Allopurinol*
- *Phenothiazines*
- *Nonsteroidal anti-inflammatory drugs (NSAIDs)*
- *Vaccinations*
- *Radiocontrast dyes*

inappropriate antibodies rather than providing antigenic stimuli. Food (generally in children, since adults have already learned their food allergies from multiple exposures), dyes, envenomation, blood products, and vaccinations are other examples of allergens that can produce vascular reactions.

AUTOIMMUNE DISEASES CAUSING VASCULAR REACTIONS
- *Lupus erythematosus*
- *Rheumatoid arthritis*
- *Dermatomyositis*
- *Inflammatory bowel disease*
- *Polyarteritis nodosa*
- *Sarcoidosis*

OTHER CAUSES OF VASCULAR REACTIONS

Malignancies
- *Leukemias*
- *Lymphomas*
- *Myeloma*

Dysproteinemias
- *Gammopathies*
- *Cryoglobulinemia*

Foods
- *Eggs, milk, shellfish, nuts, berries*
- *Food dyes—tartrazine, azo dyes*
- *Preservatives—monosodium glutamate*

Envenomation

Blood products

URTICARIA

Patients often find the excruciating itching of urticaria (hives) intolerable: these are the patients most likely to present to the emergency department. Skin lesions are produced by cutaneous edema occurring at least partly as a result of degranulation of mast cells. Although a type I hypersensitivity reaction is the most common underlying mechanism, other immunologic and nonimmunologic reactions can produce this end result.

The causes of urticaria are the same as those listed in the boxed list on page 162. Although these causes are shared by other vascular reactions, some allergens are more likely to cause urticaria, rather than other hypersensitivity patterns. More common causes of an urticarial reaction pattern include penicillin, sulfa, food allergies, envenomation (insect bites and stings), and infections. Often, there is no obvious cause of the patient's urticaria, but a history of fairly recent fever, malaise, upper respiratory tract symptoms, or diarrhea can be elicited, suggesting a viral etiology. Psychological factors sometimes play a precipitating and exacerbating role in this condition. NSAIDs, including aspirin, as well as narcotics, can both cause urticaria by hypersensitivity mechanisms and worsen outbreaks because they are obligate mast cell degranulators.

Interestingly, physical environmental factors can produce urticaria in some. Water, cold, pressure, and sunlight have all been shown to cause hives. The most common of these is *dermographism*, in which a firm stroke on the skin produces a linear wheal.

Finally, some chemicals produce urticaria as a result of contact with the skin. These can occur as a result of specific allergy (as to Latex), or by direct, nonimmunologic actions, as occurs with sorbic acid and cinnamic acid. This type of contact urticaria occurs in anyone exposed to the agent, although some people are more sensitive to lower concentrations.

Clinical Manifestations

Morphologically, urticaria consists of edematous, usually coalescing papules and plaques. These wheals are pink, nonscaling, and flat-topped (Fig. 13.1). They are also rapidly migratory, so that a specific urticarial wheal outlined with a pen no longer corresponds to these borders several hours later. Rather, some of the areas become uninvolved, while other edges advance. Coalescing papules and plaques often produce larger arcuate plaques; sometimes the centers of the lesions are paler than the borders due to edema fluid.

Urticaria is often accentuated in areas of heat or after trauma or friction, as occurs in dermographism. Many otherwise normal patients exhibit dermographism, which probably represents subclinical urticaria. Obviously, itchy patients with urticaria who scratch will produce new wheals as a dermographic response to their scratching.

Despite the intensely pruritic nature of urticaria, visible excoriations and secondary eczematous change are uncommon, perhaps because of the migratory nature of hives.

Occasionally, urticaria is associated with similar, deeper, less well demarcated edema referred to as *angioedema*. Angioedema is more often associated with systemic signs of anaphylaxis, including life-threatening bronchoconstriction and hypotension.

Figure 13.1 Pink, coalescing wheals of urticaria. The center is blanched due to greater edema, giving the plaques an annular appearance.

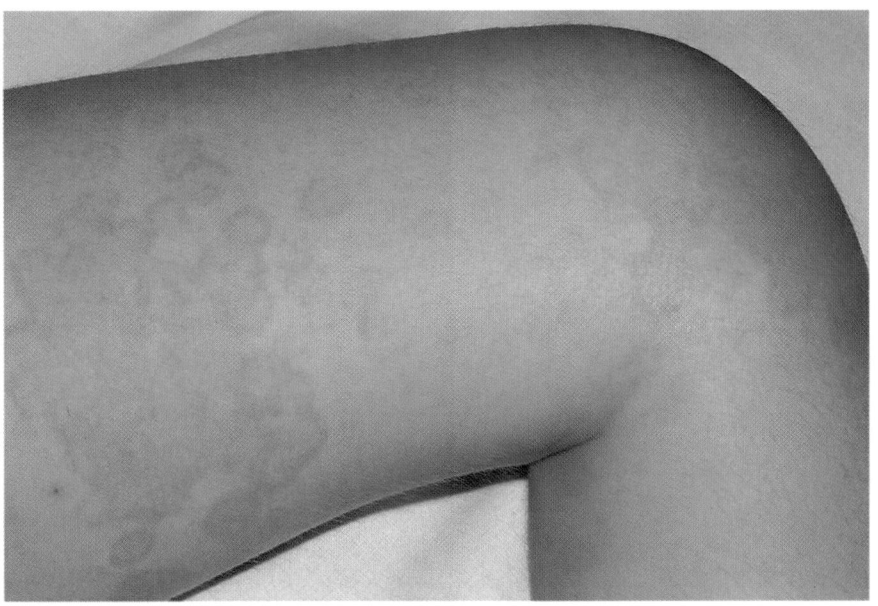

An uncommon variant of urticaria is urticarial vasculitis, which is associated with an underlying leukocytoclastic vasculitis that produces pale purpura within the region. Therefore, the urticarial plaques leave dusky staining of the skin as they migrate, and they migrate much more slowly, over several days, rather than over several hours. Urticarial vasculitis often is less itchy but tends to produce burning sensations. A biopsy is required to differentiate this disease from common urticaria.

Differential Diagnosis

The typical morphology and short-lived nature of individual skin lesions in association with intense pruritus usually make this diagnosis easy even when skin lesions are currently not present. Almost no other skin eruption occurs so quickly and can disappear in less than 1 day without a trace. However, sometimes patients are rather unobservant and the duration of individual lesions is unclear. Insect bites can sometimes resemble smaller lesions of urticaria and, in fact, one name for insect bites is *papular urticaria*.

Atypical erythema multiforme, which lacks the classic concentric rings of erythema, can sometimes be difficult to differentiate, although urticaria is usually less red and far itchier. Differentiation of atypical erythema multiforme or other vascular reactions, except for leukocytoclastic vasculitis, is not particularly important, as these diseases exist on a spectrum, have the same underlying causes, and have essentially the same medical implications. Urticaria can be differentiated from leukocytoclastic vasculitis by the more stable and purpuric (nonblanching) nature of the latter.

Finally, very early allergic contact dermatitis (e.g., poison ivy) and very early bullous pemphigoid can appear urticarial before the epidermal edema has formed blisters. Occasionally a biopsy is indicated when the differentiation of urticaria from any of the above diseases is important.

Management

When possible, withdrawal of the offending antigen is the first step in treatment. A directed history and physical examination designed to uncover likely medications and infections responsible for the eruption are indicated. A cause is usually found in those patients with acute urticaria, but patients with chronic urticaria are best investigated and managed by a dermatologist. When urticaria has been present for about 6 weeks or longer without an obvious underlying etiology, the cause of the urticaria is almost never found, even with extensive and expensive laboratory testing. In these patients, the clinician's and patient's energies should be directed toward the control of symptoms rather than to an exhaustive diagnostic workup. In general, laboratory testing is useful only for investigation of symptoms or abnormality on a history or physical examination.[7] Asymptomatic dental infections and chronic sinusitis are exceptions, and radiographs of these areas should be considered in patients with unremitting and unresponsive disease.[7]

Obviously, the rare patient with angioedema, bronchospasm, and particularly signs of anaphylaxis, should receive immediate epinephrine and systemic corticosteroids in addition to discontinuing the antigen when possible. In those patients without an obvious etiology, referral to an allergist is warranted.

Far more often, the problem is simply extreme pruritus. First-line therapy for most patients with acute urticaria, and all patients with chronic urticaria, is an oral antihistamine. Some patients with urticaria are exquisitely sensitive to even very low doses of any H_1 blocker, including diphenhydramine (Benadryl), which is over the counter, and hydroxyzine HCl (Atarax) which is available by a prescription but very inexpensive.[8–10] Antihistamines are much more effective at preventing new urticarial wheals than at eliminating existing wheals, so that it is extremely important for patients to take antihistamines around the clock, rather than only when they are especially bothered. Patients who do not respond to these antihistamines can then be switched empirically to other H_1 blockers on a trial-and-error basis. Common typical choices from each of the original major groups of antihistamines include cyproheptadine (Periactin), which exerts antiserotonin as well as antihistamine effects, chlorpheniramine (Chlor-trimeton), pyralamine (Triaminic), promethazine

(Vistaril), and doxepin (Sinequan). Doxepin is sometimes a superior choice because it exhibits H_1 and H_2 blocking effects.[11] Patient who are either unresponsive to these older antihistamines or who are too sedated while taking them can be treated with newer, nonsedating medications that have been shown in clinical trials to exert similar beneficial effects on urticaria compared to older drugs with fewer side effects.[8–10] Other studies have shown superior efficacy.[12] These include terfenadine (Seldane), loratadine (Claritin), astemizole (Hismanal), and cetirizine (Zyrtec). These also share the advantages of less frequent dosing and much less sedation, but the disadvantages include higher cost and, especially with terfenadine and astemizole, drug interactions.

Patients not adequately treated with an H_1 blocker sometimes improve with the addition of an H_2 blocker such as cimetidine (Tagamet) 300 mg qid or ranitidine HCl (Zantac).[13] Terbutaline and ephedrine sulfate can be useful as well in patients without contraindications, although side effects are limiting.[14]

Those patients who have severe, poorly tolerated acute urticaria on the basis of a known factor can be treated with prednisone at a dose of 40 to 60 mg each morning for 5 to 7 days to suppress the hives while waiting for the process to resolve spontaneously. However, all patients, especially those without a clear etiology, should be warned that prednisone is suppressive only and, because of its potentially dangerous side effects, is not a long-term option. Urticaria can be so miserable for some patients that once they have experienced the dramatic improvement afforded by prednisone, they are unhappy with any other therapy. Corticosteroids are to be avoided in patients with chronic urticaria.

Patient education is crucial in the management of urticaria. Patients with acute urticaria should be reassured that this condition is nearly always self-limited, even when an underlying etiology cannot be identified. Those unfortunate few with chronic urticaria should be sympathetically counseled that extensive laboratory testing is very unlikely to reveal the underlying etiology and that a cure is not possible. These patients should be advised that control of symptoms is considered success and usually, urticaria eventually improves spontaneously, although this may require months to years.

Course and Prognosis

Acute urticaria is most often due to a medication or infection and, once the cause is eliminated, the urticaria resolves. The complete time course is generally from one to three weeks. These patients are often atopic, that is, susceptible to the development of allergies; therefore, they are at slightly increased risk of future vascular reactions to medications or to infections.

Those few patients with chronic urticaria who have had the eruption for 6 weeks or longer without an identifiable underlying cause are likely to have recurrent or ongoing urticaria that can last years. These are the patients for whom trial-and-error therapy is indicated and systemic corticosteroids are to be avoided. Over months to years, most patients with urticaria experience significant improvement or remission.

ACUTE URTICARIA

Clinical Manifestations

Pink, coalescing, nonscaling, migratory papules and arcuate plaques, often with central pallor.

Management in the Emergency Department

1. *Identification and elimination of allergen when possible*
2. *Antihistamine (H_1 blocker) such as hydroxyzine HCl 25 mg q6h around the clock*
3. *Prednisone 40 to 60 mg po each morning for severe, acute urticaria with a known, temporary cause*
4. *Addition of an H_2 blocker such as cimetidine 300 mg q6h for those uncontrolled with H_1 blockers alone*
5. *Patient education (see the patient handout on p. 326, Acute Urticaria)*

CHRONIC URTICARIA

Clinical Manifestations

Pink, coalescing, nonscaling, migratory papules and arcuate plaques, often with central pallor.

(Continues)

(Continued)

Clinical Manifestations

Pink, coalescing, nonscaling, migratory papules and arcuate plaques, often with central pallor.

Management in the Emergency Department

1. *Careful patient education regarding incurability (see the patient handout on p. 335, Chronic Urticaria)*
2. *Empiric trials with various H_1 blockers, such as hydroxyzine HCl 25 mg q6h round the clock, switching to newer nonsedating antihistamines, such as cetirizine 10 mg/day if needed*
3. *Addition of H_2 blocker cimetidine 300 mg q6h if needed*
4. *Avoidance of systemic corticosteroids*

ERYTHEMA MULTIFORME

Erythema multiforme is an extremely common hypersensitivity reaction that is polymorphous. The more common and milder form of erythema multiforme, erythema multiforme minor, is short-lived and relatively asymptomatic, while very severe blistering forms of erythema multiforme (erythema multiforme major, Stevens-Johnson syndrome, toxic epidermal necrolysis) are painful and sometimes life-threatening (for a discussion of these variants, see Ch. 5, Bullous Diseases).

The causes of erythema multiforme are the same as those listed for vascular reactions in general in the boxed list on page 162. However, some allergens are more likely to produce vascular reactions with an erythema multiforme morphology than are others. These allergens include HSV infection, which accounts for almost all cases of recurrent erythema multiforme, and the related herpesvirus EBV. Streptococcal and *Mycoplasma* infections as well as tuberculosis, coccidioidomycosis, and histoplasmosis are all known to produce this reaction pattern. Medications most likely to generate erythema multiforme include sulfas, penicillins, tetracyclines, anticonvulsants, NSAIDs, and allopurinol.[1,2]

Clinical Manifestations

Classic erythema multiforme consists of the abrupt onset of red, nonpruritic, nonscaling, flat-topped papules. The centers of the lesions exhibit the greatest inflammation, producing violaceous, dusky, brown, or gray epithelium in the center, producing the classic bull's-eye or target-shaped appearance (Fig. 13.2). The lesions are fixed, and whereas the patient may develop more lesions over hours or days, existing lesions cannot resolve in hours or in 1 or 2 days. In milder disease, the lesions remain more discrete and range from 1 to 3 cm in size. More severe disease is characterized by coalescence of individual lesions.

More common than classic erythema multiforme is atypical erythema multiforme, where the target appearance of the lesion is not appreciated (Fig. 13.3). The papules and small plaques are an even red color, but again are flat topped, and without scale. Mucous membranes are usually not affected.

Although erythema multiforme is usually generalized, lesions often occur early on hands and feet, extending proximally. Palms and soles are often preferentially involved, and patients with intense involvement of the centers of lesions can experience blistering of the central portion (Fig. 13-4). When blistering occurs, it is often accompanied by mucous membrane erosions that represent blisters whose fragile blister roofs have sloughed (see Fig. 5-12). This form of erythema multiforme is called erythema multiforme major, or Stevens-Johnson syndrome (see Ch. 5, Bullous Diseases).

Occasionally, patients have associated fever or malaise, which can be related either to the erythema multiforme itself or to an underlying infection that precipitated the skin disease.

Differential Diagnosis

Classic, target-shaped erythema multiforme is sometimes confused with annular skin lesions that exhibit central clearing, rather than a discolored center due to more intense inflammation. Tinea corporis, granuloma annulare, and annular subacute cutaneous lupus erythematosus are all possi-

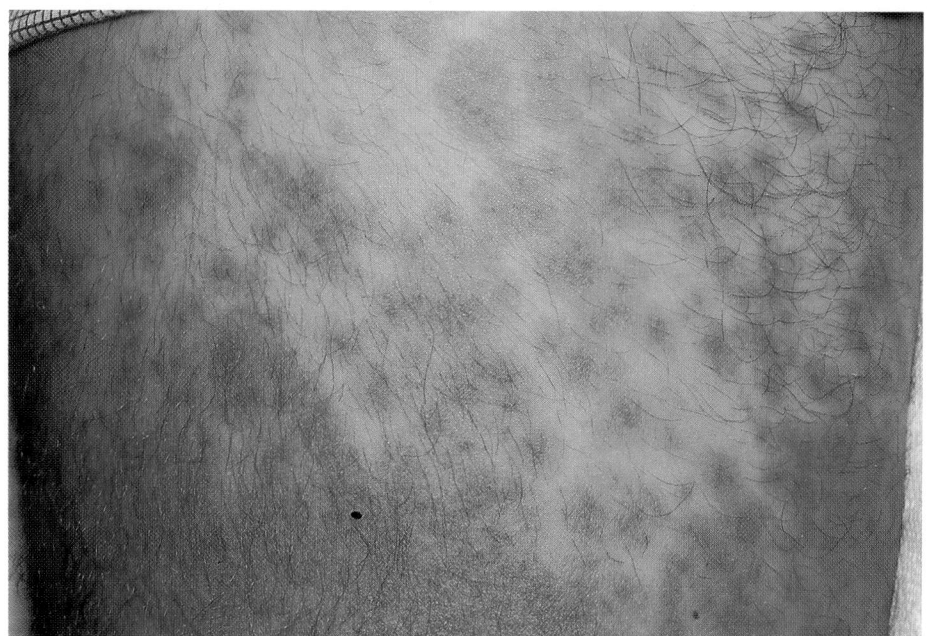

Figure 13.2 Typical erythema multiforme, showing red, flat-topped papules with darker centers due to more intense inflammation or even epidermal necrosis.

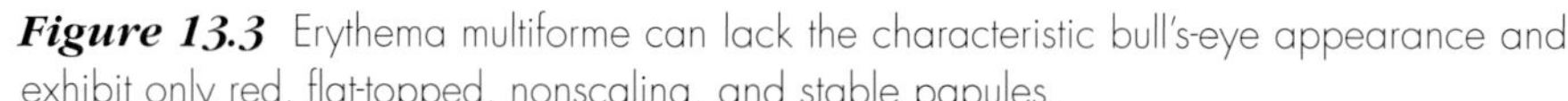

Figure 13.3 Erythema multiforme can lack the characteristic bull's-eye appearance and exhibit only red, flat-topped, nonscaling, and stable papules.

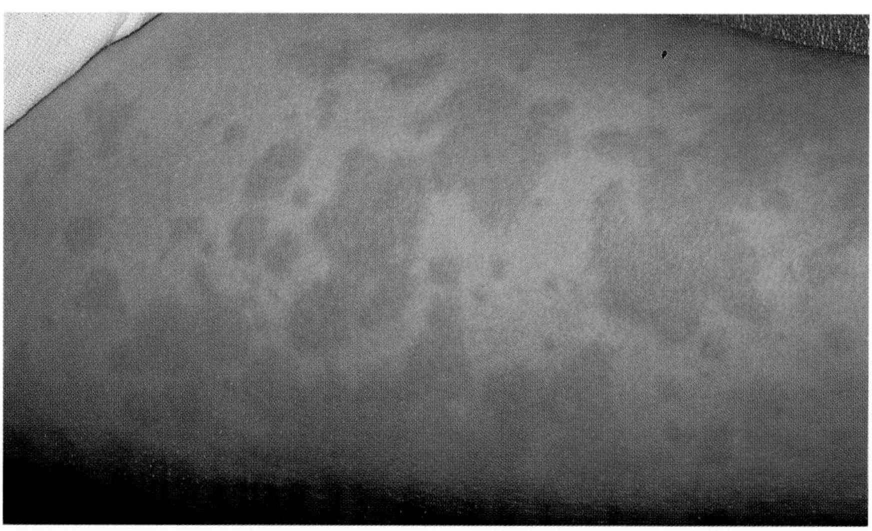

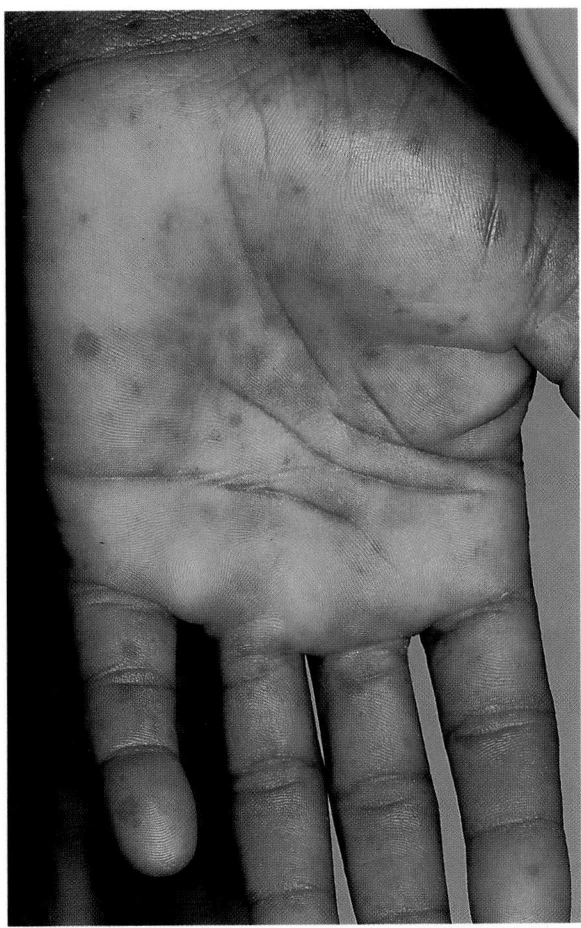

Figure 13.4 Palms and soles are common areas of involvement, and they may show blistering in addition to papules. Palm and sole lesions in association with oral erosions can be the only sign of erythema multiforme.

ble confusing conditions. Urticaria with central pallor due to edema can sometimes mimic erythema multiforme as well. Atypical erythema multiforme, which lacks the target-shaped morphology, can be confused with urticaria, leukocytoclastic vasculitis, insect bites, and small plaques of papulosquamous diseases when the scale is subtle, such as pityriasis rosea or secondary syphilis.

Management The elimination of the offending allergen is the first step in the management of erythema multiforme. A directed history and physical examination to uncover the cause of the eruption is indicated. Specific questions about medications and symptoms of recent infections should be asked, after which a physical examination with particular attention to common infectious diseases should be performed. Autoimmune diseases, lymphoreticular diseases, food allergies, and insect bites and stings are possible causes, but these are uncommon in patients with acute erythema multiforme, as compared to those infections and medications discussed in the introduction to this section. Patients with recurrent erythema multiforme can be assumed to have HSV infection, unless they are taking a medication episodically, and those with chronic erythema multiforme warrant referral to a dermatologist.

After elimination of the underlying etiology when possible, reassurance is the primary therapy needed for common erythema multiforme minor. Erythema multiforme is generally not pruritic or painful, except when blistering occurs (see Ch. 5, Bullous Diseases). Therefore, most patients can simply be counseled that the eruption is temporary and that it will resolve spontaneously. These patients can be reassured that, although some peeling may occur during the healing phase, this is not a reason for concern. Most patients are bothered primarily by the appearance of erythema multiforme, but for those who also report significant symptoms, many physicians believe that oral prednisone 40 to 60 mg/day (in children, 1 to 2 mg/kg/day) ameliorates itching and soreness if begun early. However, systemic corticosteroids are very rarely indicated, and there is no place in the treatment of erythema multiforme for topical corticosteroids.

Patients with frequently recurrent erythema multiforme benefit from empirical therapy with ongoing oral acyclovir, 400 mg bid, to prevent recurrent HSV infection.[15] Although oral antihistamines are frequently used for nearly any rash, they have little, or no effect, on erythema multiforme other than the benefit of nighttime sedation.

Course and Prognosis Those patients who have an identified etiology for their erythema multiforme generally begin to improve several days after the discontinuation of the allergen. Allergens associated with an infection may be more long lasting, with the eruption continuing for up to 6 weeks. Patients in whom erythema multiforme develops are at higher risk than the general population for another episode of this condition.

ERYTHEMA MULTIFORME MINOR

Clinical Manifestations

Scattered red, nonscaling, flat-topped papules, often with target shape due to more intense central inflammation.

Management in the Emergency Department

1. *Identification and elimination of allergen*
2. *Reassurance*
3. *Acyclovir 400 mg bid if erythema multiforme is recurrent and there is no appropriate medication history*
4. *For symptomatic disease: nighttime sedation with diphenhydramine 25 to 50 mg for symptomatic disease*
5. *For very symptomatic disease: consider prednisone 40 to 60 mg AM for early disease (The use of systemic corticosteroids is controversial in the presence of significant blistering. For this form of erythema multiforme, see the section regarding therapy for blistering forms of erythema multiforme in Ch. 5, Bullous Diseases)*
6. *Patient education (see the patient handout on p. 372, Vascular Reactions)*

ERYTHEMA NODOSUM

Erythema nodosum is a vascular hypersensitivity reaction that occurs in the subcutaneous fat. Although the usual causes of any vascular reaction can produce erythema nodosum, some etiologies are more likely to produce this phenomenon, and no obvious cause is found in about one-half of cases. Infections, especially streptococcal disease in children, coccidioidomycosis, histoplasmosis, tuberculosis, and *Yersinia* are known causes. Medications, including oral contraceptives, oral estrogens, and sulfas, are particularly well-known causes. Chronic inflammatory diseases such as sarcoidosis and inflammatory bowel disease are also classic associations (see the discussion in the Introduction and in the boxed list on p. 162).

Clinical Manifestations

Although most often located over the shins, erythema nodosum can occasionally occur in other areas. This condition appears as dusky red, discrete but poorly demarcated, red plaques (Fig. 13.5). These are rather long lasting, and older lesions frequently resemble bruises. In addition, they are often tender and, when occurring over joints such as the ankle, erythema nodosum can mimic an inflammatory arthritis.

Figure 13.5 Erythema nodosum typically shows poorly demarcated red plaques over the anterior lower legs.

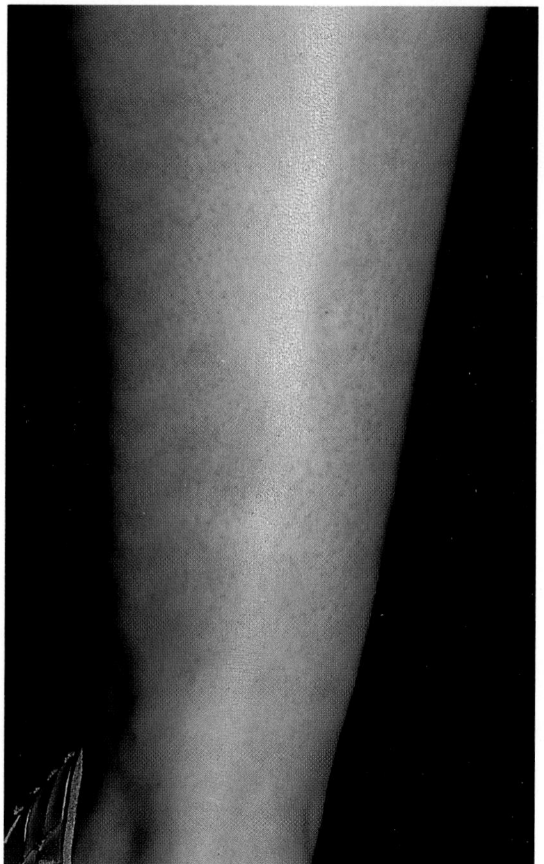

Differential Diagnosis Erythema nodosum can sometimes be difficult to distinguish from other causes of inflammation of the fat (panniculitis). These include pancreatic fat necrosis, cold panniculitis, lupus panniculitis, bacterial cellulitis, erythema induratum, Weber-Christian disease (idiopathic lobular panniculitis), and thrombophlebitis. The location of the lesions, the lack of significant systemic toxicity, and the nondraining nature of the lesions usually differentiate erythema nodosum from these other diseases. When any doubt exists, a deep incisional biopsy to fat is helpful in differentiating these diseases.

Management

Therapy for erythema nodosum includes the elimination of any precipitating causes, the institution of an NSAID, and the use of elastic wraps to minimize discomfort. Patients who do not respond well to therapy within 1 to 2 weeks should seek follow-up evaluation with a dermatologist. Other second-line therapies include oral potassium iodide or a short burst of prednisone.

Course and Prognosis

Most patients with erythema nodosum experience resolution within one to two months, although some experience chronic disease.

> ERYTHEMA NODOSUM
>
> ***Clinical Manifestations***
>
> *Red, often dusky or violaceous, tender nodules occurring primarily over the shins.*
>
> ***Management in the Emergency Department***
>
> 1. *Identification and elimination of cause*
> 2. *Use of NSAIDs*
> 3. *Elastic wraps and elevation*
> 4. *Patient education (see the patient handout on p. 372, Vascular Reactions)*

FIXED DRUG REACTION

The fixed drug reaction (see Ch. 5, Bullous Diseases) is an interesting and very characteristic reaction to certain medications. With each challenge of the medication, an edematous plaque, sometimes with a central or overlying blister, occurs in exactly the same location on the skin (Fig. 13.6; see also Fig. 5.13). With each recurrence, deeper postinflammatory hyperpigmentation occurs (see Fig. 11.5). One or a few recurring plaques are usual, and lesions in the mouth or on the genitalia are common. Often, there are additional affected sites with each recurrence.

Figure 13.6 A fixed drug reaction can be blistering or, as seen here, a round, edematous, nonscaling plaque that recurs. The central ulcer is a biopsy site.

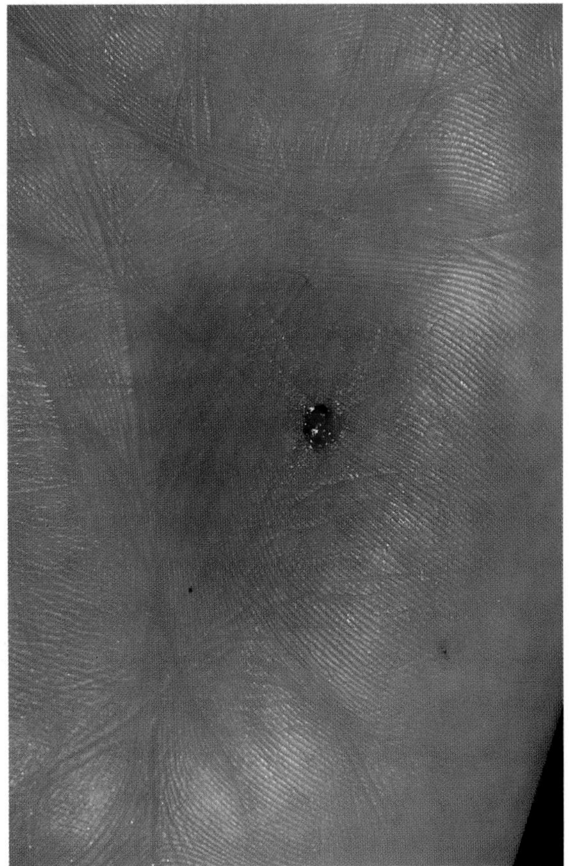

Medications well known to produce a fixed drug eruption are NSAIDs, salicylates, acetaminophen, barbiturates, penicillins, tetracyclines, sulfas, phenolphthalein, and oral contraceptives. Occasionally, no medication is identified.

The primary diseases in the differential diagnosis are HSV infection, because of its recurring nature, and erythema multiforme, when there are large numbers of lesions, because of the morphology.

Therapy consists of identification and avoidance of the offending medication, as well as reassurance.

FIXED GYRATE ERYTHEMAS

The gyrate erythemas are a group of vascular reactions that show annular, coalescing, red, nonscaling papules and plaques. Unlike urticaria, which can also exhibit a gyrate morphology, these fixed gyrate erythemas are relatively stable, with individual plaques progressing over days. These are usually asymptomatic.

Erythema Annulare Centrifugum

Erythema annulare centrifugum consists of one or a few annular, red plaques. These gradually enlarge centrifugally, and over the inner border there is often, but not always, a rim of postinflammatory scale. The classic etiology of erythema annulare centrifugum is a dermatophyte infection, but other implicated causes include medications, chronic infections such as tinea, autoimmune diseases, and blood dyscrasias. Erythema annulare centrifugum is most often confused with tinea corporis, because of the red annular plaques with scale. However, the scale of erythema annulare centrifugum is located over the inner, trailing edge of the erythema, rather than the leading, outer border, as occurs with ringworm. Also, a microscopic examination or culture of scale for fungus is negative in the case of erythema annulare centrifugum. Annular subacute lupus erythematosus and some lesions of annular psoriasis can be very difficult to differentiate from erythema annulare centrifugum.

Erythema Gyratum Repens

Erythema gyratum repens is a peculiar and characteristic, fairly rapidly migratory eruption, consisting of concentric and parallel gyrate red plaques with peripheral scale, giving the skin the appearance of wood grain, with its concentric circles. Sparing the palms and soles, this vascular reaction is usually a sign of internal malignancy, especially of the lung.

Erythema (Chronicum) Migrans

Erythema (chronicum) migrans is the hypersensitivity lesion associated with Lyme disease. Although the classic lesion is a red, nonscaling annulis that occurs around the tick bite in the center, there are sometimes multiple lesions, not all of which represent tick bites (Fig. 13-7). At times, these lesions are not annular, but rather are solid, red, nonscaling plaques. The diagnosis of erythema migrans is made by the setting, accompanying signs and symptoms, and the results of assays, most often enzyme-linked immunoabsorbent assays (ELISAs), for the organism. Therapy must be individualized for the age of the patient. Adults and children over 8 years of age are normally treated with doxycycline 100 mg bid or amoxicillin 500 mg qid to 1,000 mg tid, with doses of amoxicillin 20 to 40 mg/kg/day for small children. Erythromycin at a dose of 30 to 50 mg/kg/day is also appropriate for children. Therapy should be continued for 10 days to 4 weeks.

Erythema Marginatum

Erythema marginatum is the classic and characteristic, but not specific, rash that accompanies rheumatic fever. The eruption consists of annular, coalescing, and often serpiginous or arcuate, red plaques (Fig. 13.8). The plaques are evanescent, lasting a few hours and then recurring. The rapid evolution of the skin findings makes urticaria a consideration in the differential diagnosis, but the diagnosis is made on the basis of other signs and symptoms of the disease. Treatment of the rash consists of treatment of the underlying rheumatic fever with penicillin.

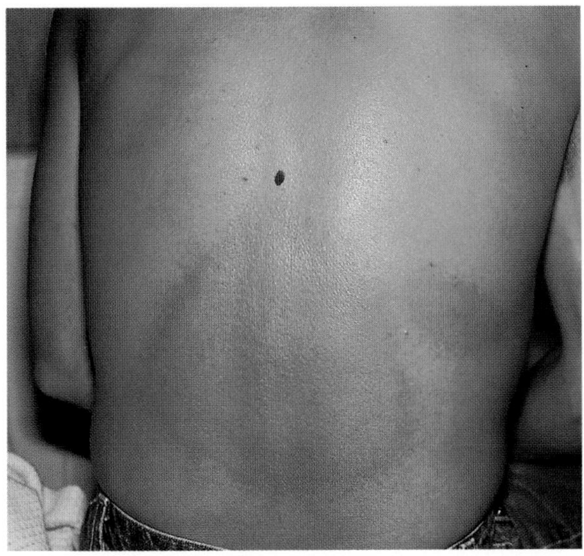

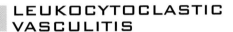

Figure 13.7 This patient has a large, nonscaling, round lesion of erythema migrans without the classic central clearing. (Photograph courtesy of John C. Wiles, M.D.)

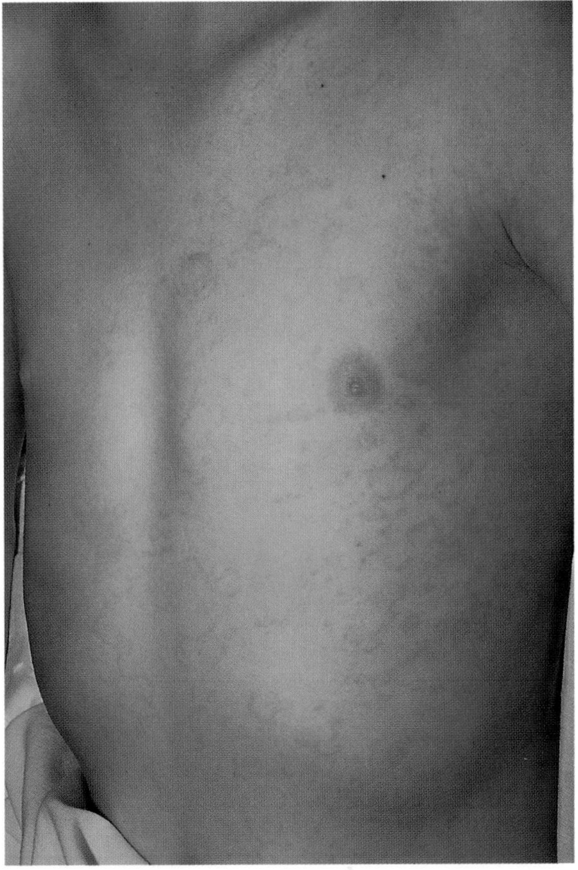

Figure 13.8 These pink, annular, coalescing papules of erythema marginatum concentrated over the trunk of this young man with rheumatic fever reappeared every afternoon. Although this is a characteristic morphology for this disease, it is not specific.

LEUKOCYTOCLASTIC VASCULITIS

Leukocytoclastic vasculitis is a hypersensitivity reaction that occurs when blood vessels are infiltrated and destroyed by polymorphonuclear leukocytes. As the blood vessels are damaged, red blood cells leak out of the vessels into the surrounding tissue, producing purpura. Most other causes of purpura, including trauma or coagulopathies, are clinically manifested by flat, nonpalpable ecchymoses or bruising. However, leukocytoclastic vasculitis is papable because of the initial intense inflammatory reaction consisting of white blood cells and edema. Therefore, palpable purpura should be considered leukocytoclastic vasculitis until proved otherwise.

The causes of leukocytoclastic vasculitis are the same as causes for other vascular reactions, and about one-half of patients have no identifiable cause.[16] Medications, infections, and autoimmune diseases lead the list. The medications most often associated with leukocytoclastic vasculitis include penicillins and sulfas, aspirin, quinidine, and allopurinol. The most common infections are streptococcus B, hepatitis B, the herpesviruses EBV and CMV, influenza, and tuberculosis. The possible causative autoimmune diseases include lupus erythematosus, rheumatoid arthritis, and polyarteritis nodosum, and several lymphomas and leukemias.

Clinical Manifestations

Leukocytoclastic vasculitis most often begins over the feet and lower legs, as 1-mm to 2-cm deep red or purple, nonblanching papules (Fig. 13-9). When larger vessels are involved, larger lesions occur,

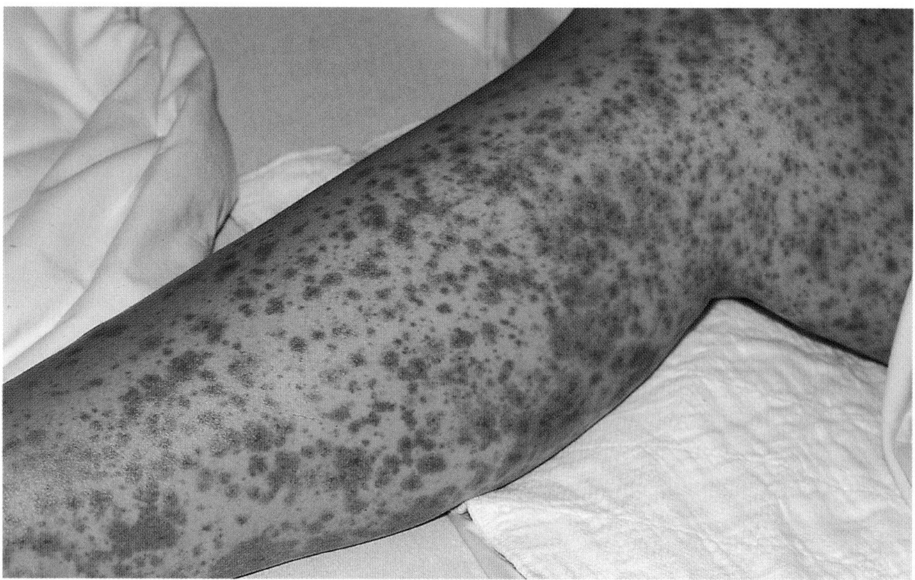

Figure 13.9 Although these deep red, nonblanching, nonscaling, flat-topped papules are classic for leukocytoclastic vasculitis, some patients present with pink lesions that superficially do not appear to be purpuric until the nonblanching nature is appreciated.

and the destruction of blood vessels interrupts the blood supply to overlying skin. This produces hemorrhagic blisters or necrosis with subsequent erosion and ulceration (see Figs. 6.6, 6.7, and 17.4).

Occasionally, leukocytoclastic vasculitis occurs in other areas and can be asymmetrical. Sometimes, lesions are barely palpable but, even if very subtle, any elevation or induration of purpuric lesions should raise the suspicion of leukocytoclastic vasculitis (Fig. 13.10).

Leukocytoclastic vasculitis of larger vessels can sometimes produce a livedo pattern of erythema, because of the alternating pattern of ischemia and normal blood flow from collateral vessels (see Figs. 6.4 and 6.5). This finding is suggestive of polyarteritis nodosa, lupus erythematosus, or rheumatoid arthritis as an underlying cause.

Often, leukocytoclastic vasculitis is limited to the skin. However, because vessels supply other epithelial surfaces and internal organs, leukocytoclastic vasculitis occurs systemically in about one-half of patients.[16] The sites most often affected are the joints, kidneys, lungs, gastrointestinal tract, heart, and peripheral nerves. This destruction of blood vessels can lead to distal ischemia and end-organ damage and dysfunction.

Differential Diagnosis

Leukocytoclastic vasculitis is sometimes clinically indistinguishable from lesions of sepsis, in which the organisms within vessels produce surrounding inflammation and vasculitis. Occasionally, the perivascular lymphocyctic inflammation associated with erythema multiforme is so intense as to produce some hemorrhage, particularly over the lower extremities, where hydrostatic pressure encourages extravasation of red blood cells.

Although punch biopsy of the skin is usually diagnostic, lesions older than 2 to 3 days may no longer reveal specific changes of leukocytoclastic vasculitis, but rather show primarily a lymphocytic infiltrate and reparative changes. Therefore, the patient should be advised, and the clinician should remember, that unless very early lesions are biopsied, a falsely reassuring biopsy may miss leukocyctoclastic vasculitis. In addition, leukocytoclastic

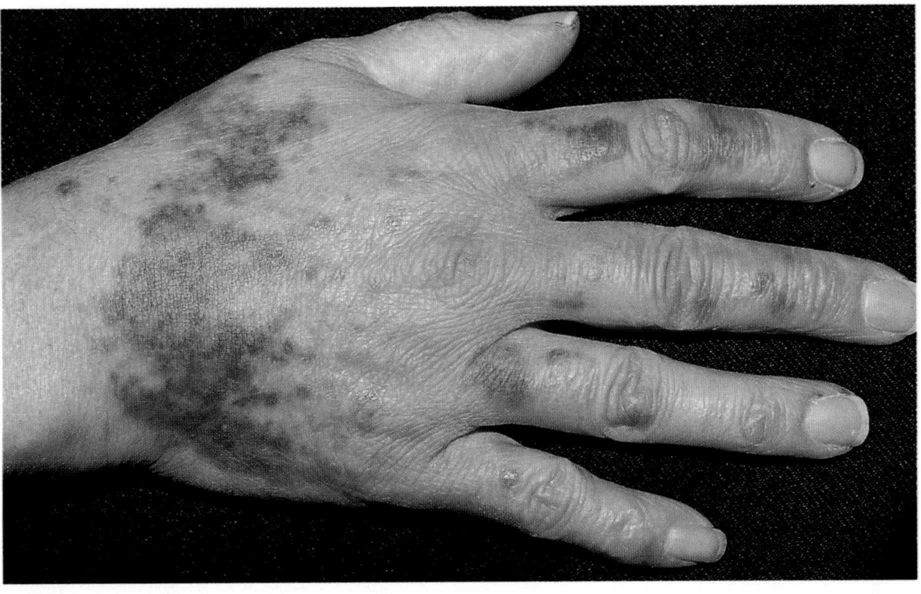

Figure 13.10 This nearly macular, purple plaque was very slightly indurated on palpation, and leukocytoclastic vasculitis was found on biopsy. The patient was also found to have significant kidney and joint involvement.

vasculitis of the larger vessels requires an incisional biopsy to fat for diagnosis.

Management

The treatment for leukocytoclastic vasculitis includes an investigation for, and the elimination of, a causative agent. The causes of leukocytoclastic vasculitis are the same as those of other vascular reactions. Medications, infections, and autoimmune diseases lead the list.

Second, a brief but immediate screen for systemic disease should be performed. This can be accomplished by a brief history and physical examination and limited laboratory testing. Clues to the diagnosis of systemic leukocytolastic vasculitis include joint pain, abdominal pain, melena, signs of kidney dysfunction, chest pain, shortness of breath, cough, arrhythmia, and neurologic symptoms. A directed physical examination should be performed, with particular attention to the identification of pulmonary infiltrates, which could be due to either infection or vasculitis, an abdominal examination for tenderness, inspection and palpation of joints for arthritis, and a brief neurologic screening. Palpation of lymph nodes, and liver and spleen can suggest the possibility of an associated lymphoreticular malignancy. Basic laboratory testing should include a stool guaiac done in the emergency department, a urine dipstick for blood and protein, and any testing indicated by positive findings in the history or physical examination. Patients not found to exhibit systemic involvement are unlikely to develop systemic leukocytoclastic vasculitis in the future.

Specific treatment for cutaneous leukocytoclastic vasculitis depends on the severity of the skin findings, as well as the presence of systemic vasculitis. If there is no sign of systemic vasculitis, and cutaneous vasculitic lesions are small, without significant necrosis, the patient can simply be reassured as the underlying infection resolves or the causative medication is withdrawn. If lesions are painful, large, or ulcerative, or if systemic vasculitis is present, oral prednisone is indicated. The usual dose is 40 to 60 mg each morning until healing begins, unless the patient is ill or aggressive systemic vasculitis is present. These patients should be evaluated for hospital admission and intravenous corticosteroid therapy, to include immediate consultation with a rheumatologist.

Patients with mild cutaneous vasculitis and a clear, self-limited, etiology should seek follow-up evaluation with a dermatologist in about 1 week, or sooner if lesions worsen. Those without a clear etiology should consult with a dermatologist or rheumatologist during the next few days for further evaluation. Patients with systemic vasculitis should be evaluated by a rheumatologist immediately if they are ill, and within 1 day if their systemic involvement appears mild.

Occasionally, chronic disease develops in patients with leukocytoclastic vasculitis as a result of an autoimmune disease, lymphoreticular malignancy, or unknown cause. These patients often benefit from the ongoing administration of colchicine or dapsone, medications that down-regulate the activation of neutrophils and that produce fewer morbid adverse reactions than occur with long-term administration of systemic corticosteroids.[17,18] Immunosuppressive agents such as azathioprine and cyclophosphamide can be used as well, but these drugs do have more troublesome possible side effects.

Course and Prognosis

Leukocytoclastic vasculitis produced by a medication or infection resolves after the elimination of the inciting agent. Because the hemosiderin deposition of purpura is relatively long lasting, especially on the lower extremities, complete clearing of the macular skin signs may require weeks. However, the appearance of new lesions ceases over several days, and the infiltrative inflammatory signs resolve rather quickly.

Those patients with leukocytoclastic vasculitis resulting from autoimmune disease or a lymphoreticular malignancy, or those with no identifiable etiology, are more likely to experience chronic or recurrent disease. Generally, control of the underlying disease minimizes the appearance of leukocytoclastic vasculitis.

LEUKOCYTOCLASTIC VASCULITIS

Clinical Manifestations

Pink to purple, nonblanching, palpable papules occurring most often over the lower extremities; occasionally associated with hemorrhagic blisters or erosions.

Management in the Emergency Department

1. *Identification and elimination of allergen when possible*
2. *Evaluation for systemic vasculitis by history and physical examination directed towards organ dysfunction, stool guaiac, urinalysis for red blood cells and protein, and other screening as dictated by abnormalities detected*
3. *Prednisone 40 to 60 mg/day for patients with more severe skin disease, and for patients who are not toxic but who show signs of systemic vasculitis*
4. *Hospital admission and intravenous corticosteroids for ill patients*
5. *Follow-up evaluation with regular health care provider or dermatologist in 1 week if disease is cutaneous only, and cause is evident and eliminated If cause is not evident, and the patient is not ill, follow-up evaluation with a dermatologist or rheumatologist should be sought within the next 1 or 2 days If the patient is ill, consultation with a rheumatologist in the emergency department is indicated*

RED, NONSCALING, FLAT-TOPPED DISEASES THAT ARE NOT HYPERSENSITIVITY REACTIONS

Several diseases exhibit red or pink, nonscaling, flat-topped lesions but do not represent hypersensitivity reactions. These diseases do not usually present a diagnostic dilemma because they are common and easily recognized.

Sunburn

Early or mild sunburn presents as painful, generalized pink or red skin in a sun-exposed distribution. Severe sunburn can produce blistering. The main diseases to be distinguished from sunburn are phototoxicity as a result of medications (especially tetracycline, doxycycline, NSAIDs, thiazides, griseofulvin, sulfonamides, and phenothiazines) or a hypersensitivity to sunlight with disease (e.g., lupus erythematosus or dermatomyositis). In addition, retinoids (Retin-A, Renova, Accutane, Tegison) increase the likelihood of a sunburn by producing desquamation of the stratum corneum, part of the natural ultraviolet (UV) protection.

The management of sunburn is primarily patient education regarding sun avoidance. Light-complexioned patients should become compulsive about the regular use of a sunscreen with a sun protection factor (SPF) of 15 or higher (Fig. 13.11). Blistering sunburns before the age of 14 years are associated with a significantly increased risk of cutaneous melanoma, an aggressive malignancy already occurring in about 1 per 100 white patients. In addition, excess sun exposure is well known to be associated with an increase in actinically induced squamous cell carcinomas and basal cell carcinomas. As important to some younger patients with confidence in their immortality is the unattractive dyspigmentation and wrinkling associated with chronic sun exposure.

Specific therapy in the emergency department is limited to the use of corticosteroids to decrease inflammation. Significant sunburn can be treated successfully with oral prednisone 40 to 60 mg each morning for a few days, if given early. This approach can abort blistering and, some theorize, decrease some of the later risk of cancer and sun damage. This may be because some DNA damage occurs from the inflammation of sunburn as well as the UV light. Patients who have a contraindication to prednisone can derive some improvement with triamcinolone (Kenalog) spray applied twice a day.

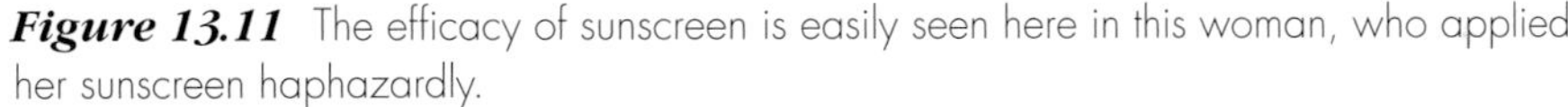

Figure 13.11 The efficacy of sunscreen is easily seen here in this woman, who applied her sunscreen haphazardly.

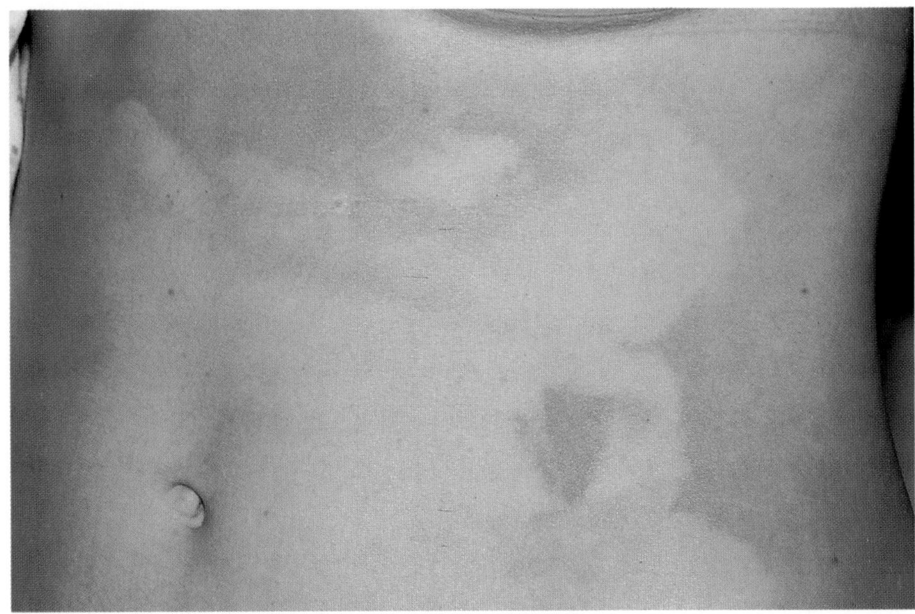

SUNBURN

Clinical Manifestations

Cutaneous erythema, ranging from tender, faint erythema to very painful, deep red color with blistering; seen in a sun-exposed distribution with sharp demarcation from skin shaded by clothing, hair, jewelry, etc. This usually begins about 6 hours after sun exposure and peaks about 24 hours after exposure.

Management in the Emergency Department

1. *Patient education (see the patient handout on* *p.364, Sunburn**)*
2. *If seen in the first 24 hours, consider prednisone 1 mg/kg/day (children) or 40 to 60 mg (adults) for 5 to 7 days*
3. *For less severe burn, consider Kenalog spray bid*
4. *NSAID for pain—narcotics if required*
5. *Over-the-counter diphenhydramine (Benadryl), or hydroxyzine HCl (Atarax) 25 to 75 mg at bedtime to induce sleep*

Cellulitis

Bacterial infection of the dermis and subcutaneous tissue produces cellulitis. This infection often begins following innoculation with bacteria through a break in the skin, such as lower-extremity cellulitis associated with foot eczema or fungal infection. This is especially likely to occur in an area of the body with poor lymphatic drainage and in patients who are debilitated or immunosuppressed. The responsible organism is usually streptococcal, with *Staphylococcus aureus* producing this disease as well. Children sometimes experience cellulitis on the basis of *Haemophilus influenza*, especially when occurring around the eyes.

Clinical Manifestations Cellulitis generally presents as localized erythematous, edematous skin over a painful area (Fig. 13.12). Cellulitis is often associated with fever, malaise, local lymphadenopathy, and a high WBC count. Periorbital cellulitis produced by *H. influenzae* in children classically

Figure 13.12 The relatively poor margination, associated edema, and toxicity of this patient suggest the correct diagnosis of cellulitis.

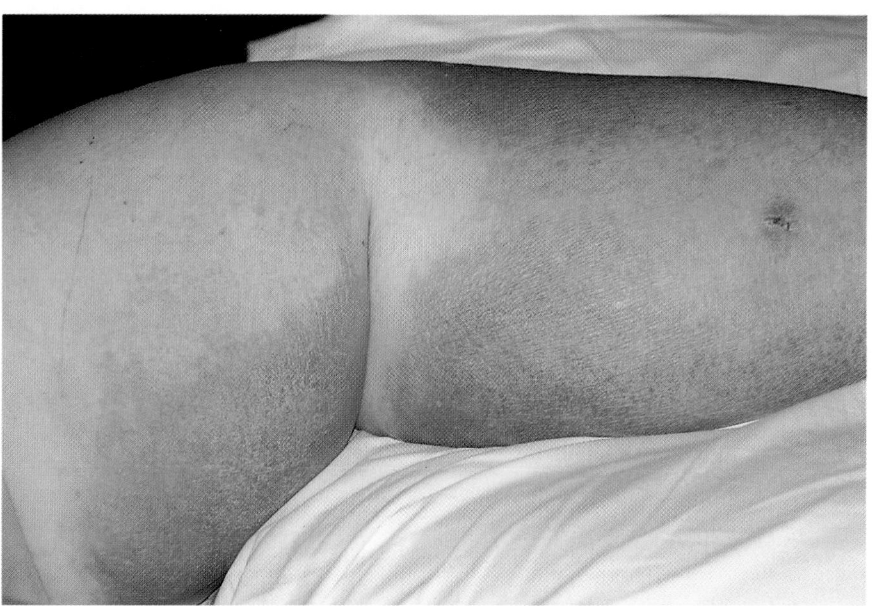

presents as edema and violaceous inflammation around an eye.

Differential Diagnosis Cellulitis can be confused with deep venous thrombosis, sometimes requiring special studies to rule this out. Severe cellulitis can produce blistering, occasionally with hemorrhage, that mimics necrotizing fasciitis. When these signs are present, a stab incision to rule out the presence of necrosis is mandatory (see Ch. 6, Hemorrhagic Bullous and Necrotic Diseases). Erysipelas is a dangerous bacterial infection of more superficial tissue that usually shows a deeper, red color with superficial edema and sharp demarcation. However, cellulitis and erysipelas exist along a spectrum, and differentiation is not always possible. Early acute allergic contact dermatitis can appear red and edematous before vesiculation occurs. This disease is usually extremely pruritic rather than painful, and the patient is not toxic.

Management Systemic antistaphylococcal antibiotics that also cover streptococcal infections constitute the primary therapy for cellulitis. For mild disease, cephalexin or dicloxacillin is reasonable therapy. Patients who are ill or who have more severe disease should be admitted to the hospital for intravenous therapy. Children should also receive an antibiotic that covers *H. influenzae*, such as ceftriaxone. Otherwise, elevation of the affected area helps decrease edema.

Course and Prognosis Rapid resolution after the institution of antibiotics is the usual course of cellulitis. Sometimes, cellulitis does not resolve as expected, with fever and other clinical signs relatively unchanged. This is sometimes due to the presence of very severe cellulitis or mild necrotizing fasciitis for which antibiotics are not reaching the affected area.

The inflammation of cellulitis, particularly over the lower extremity, sometimes produces scarring and lymphatic damage, resulting in permanent edema and an increased risk of additional episodes of cellulitis, which in turn cause further lymphatic damage. Patients with continuing edema should therefore wear elastic bandages or compression stockings to minimize edema and the future risk of cellulitis.

CELLULITIS

Clinical Manifestations

Localized erythema, pain, edema, heat; usually associated with fever, malaise, increased WBC count.

Management in the Emergency Department

1. *Antistaphylococcal antibiotics; oral cephalexin or dicloxacillin 500 mg qid if cellulitis is mild and patient compliant and not toxic; otherwise, hospital admission for intravenous administration until process begins to resolve*
2. *Elevation of affected area*
3. *Pain control*

Erysipelas

Erysipelas is an infection of the dermis usually caused by *Streptococcus pyogenes* or other streptococci.

Clinical Manifestation Most often, but not always occurring over the face, erysipelas presents as a relatively well-demarcated, edematous, deep red plaque that symmetrically affects the cheeks and bridge of the nose (Fig. 13.13). The onset is generally sudden, and patients are usually ill.

Differential Diagnosis Diseases confused with erysipelas include sunburn, photosensitivity, early acute allergic contact dermatitis, and cellulitis. The differentiation of these diseases is discussed above in the section on cellulitis.

Management Therapy for erysipelas is an intravenous antistreptococcal antibiotic, with penicillin as the first-line therapy. Some clinicians use an antistaphylococcal penicillin to cover any possibility of *S. aureas*, since this is such a common infecting agent in other settings.

Course and Prognosis Patients who receive appropriate antibiotics generally do very well without sequelae.

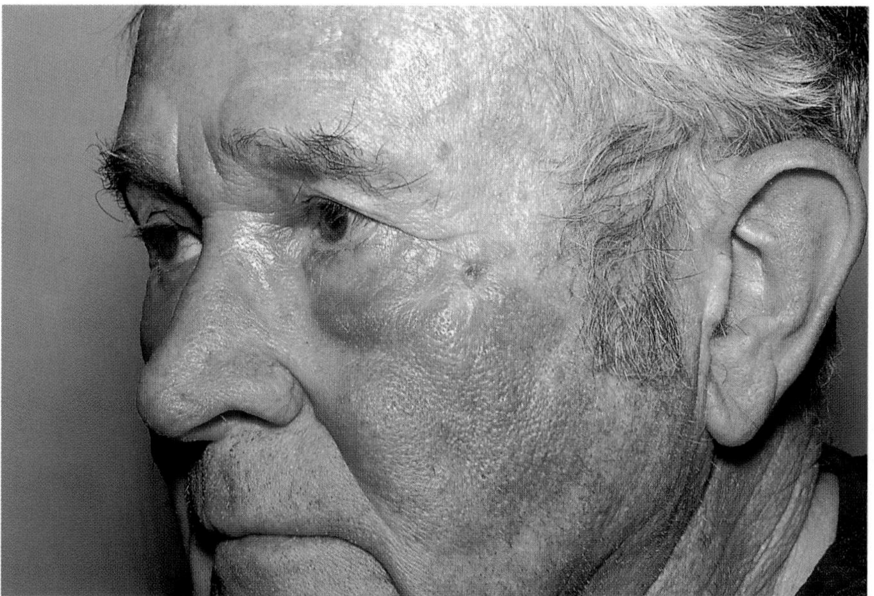

Figure 13.13 Erysipelas is more sharply demarcated than cellulitis and is more likely to occur on the face.

ERYSIPELAS

Clinical Manifestations

Well-demarcated, deeply erythematous, edematous plaque, most often over the face. Often occurs in an ill patient.

Management in the Emergency Department

1. *Hospital admission for intravenous penicillin therapy*
2. *Pain control*

TOXIC SHOCK SYNDROME

Classically occurring in menstruating women who wear tampons, toxic shock syndrome affects all ages and both genders, although childhood disease is unusual. This serious disease results from toxins produced by certain strains of *Staphylococcus aureus*. The infection itself can be mild or severe. Common sites of infection include skin, throat, vagina (in menstruating women), lung, joints, and sinuses.

Clinical manifestations include high fever, hypotension, diarrhea, malaise, and myalgias. Headache and confusion are common. The characteristic eruption is nonspecific and consists of generalized, blanchable erythema first occurring on the trunk, and later spreading to the extremities. The texture of the rash can become rough and sandpapery, similar to the rash of scarlet fever. Also, as occurs in scarlet fever, accentuation of the eruption over flexural skin folds is common and oral erythema with a strawberry tongue is usual. Conjunctivae are generally red as well. The diagnosis is made by application of specific criteria.

Therapy includes both antibiotic therapy with penicillinase-resistant antistaphylococcal antibiotics and aggressive supportive care for hypotension and the complications of renal and heart failure, and adult respiratory distress syndrome. The site of the infection should be identified so that foreign bodies can be removed and abscesses drained. Although the mortality rate was 10% when this disease was first recognized, this has decreased to about 3% with timely diagnosis and conscientious therapy.

CRITERIA FOR TOXIC SHOCK SYNDROME

1. *Fever >102°F, 39.9°C*
2. *Generalized erythematous rash*
3. *Hypotension, systolic <90 (adults), below tenth percentile for children under 16 years, or orthostatic*
4. *Three or more of the following:*
   - *vomiting or diarrhea at onset of the illness*
   - *severe myalgia or creatine phosphokinase level ≥ twice normal*
   - *vaginal, oropharyngeal, or conjunctival erythema*
   - *blood urea nitrogen or creatinine level ≥ twice normal, or >5 neutrophils high powered field in urine*
   - *total bilirubin, serum glutamic oxaloacetic transaminase, serum glutamic pyretic transaminase > twice normal*
   - *platelets <100,000/mm³*
   - *disorientation or altered consciousness with focal neurologic signs, when fever and hypotension are absent*
5. *Negative results of any bacterial cultures performed except for* Staphylococcus aureus, *and negative results of serologies for Rocky Mountain Spotted Fever, leptospirosis or measles, if obtained*

ERYTHEMA MIGRANS

Early Lyme borreliosis is a prominent cause of fever and an erythematous rash in Europe and in the northeastern United States, although cases also occur in the upper Midwest and West. This disease is produced by the spirochete *Borrelia burgdorferi*, and the vector is the tick. Both the specific tick and the strain of *Borrelia burgdorferi* vary with the locale, producing differences in disease manifestations. Prompt recognition and treatment are important to prevent long term morbidity in some patients.

Erythema migrans (erythema chronicum migrans, early Lyme borreliosis) begins as a red macule or papule that generally develops 8 or 9 days following the bite of an infected tick, although some lesions may follow as long as 4 weeks later. The lesion enlarges at a variable rate into a flat, nonscaling plaque that often exhibits central clearing. However, plaques are not always annular; many are solid (Fig. 13.7). Rarely, lesions may exhibit scale, hemorrhage, or vesicles. As many as half of patients develop disseminated infection manifested by multiple, usually smaller lesions that may exhibit variable morphology. Although these additional lesions are usually round or annular, some clinicians have reported even linear plaques suggestive of an allergic contact dermatitis such as poison ivy. Patients with Lyme borreliosis can also develop nonspecific cutaneous hypersensitivity vascular reactions such as urticaria, erythema nodosum, or atypical erythema multiforme.

Erythema migrans is often accompanied by constitutional symptoms that include malaise, myalgias, arthralgias, fever, headache, local lymphadenopathy, and gastrointestinal symptoms. Irritability and depression can also occur. These symptoms of early borrelia infection can occur unaccompanied by erythema migrans.

Acrodermatitis chronica atrophicans is a late cutaneous manifestation of Lyme borreliosis that occurs in Europe. These patients develop erythema and edema resembling cellulitis (when more inflammatory) or lymphedema (when inflammation is less marked). Fibrous dermal and subcutaneous nodules and bands can occur. Years later, affected areas develop atrophy manifested by crinkling of the skin, thinning, and laxity.

About a quarter of untreated patients with early Lyme borreliosis develop frank chronic or recurrent arthritis. Fewer patients experience lymphocytic meningitis, cranial neuritis manifested most often by a facial palsy, and peripheral neuropathy evidenced by radicular pain. Cardiac conduction abnormalities are an uncommon but dangerous complication, and still fewer patients develop carditis.

Other diseases to be differentiated from erythema migrans include granuloma annulare, which usually has a periphery composed of small coalescing papules, and annular subacute cutaneous lupus erythematosus, which generally shows multiple, coalescing, and scaling annular plaques.

The diagnosis of early Lyme borreliosis and erythema migrans can usually be made by the clinical presentation and morphology of the skin lesions. The histologic appearance of the lesion is nonspecific, but other diseases in the differential diagnosis can be ruled out on biopsy. When the diagnosis is unclear, absolute confirmation can be difficult. Seronegativity is common in patients with erythema migrans, and positive results are prevented by therapy. Lesional cultures are often negative as well. In addition, available serologic tests are poorly standardized and results are variable, with false positives occurring in both normal controls and in other disease settings such as lupus erythematosus.

The therapy of erythema migrans depends upon the age of the patient. Adults can be treated with doxycycline 100 mg two to three times a day or amoxicillin 500 mg four times a day for 10 to 28 days. Children and pregnant patients should receive amoxicillin or erythromycin. Amoxicillin is given at 20 to 40 mg/kg/day and erythromycin is given at 30 to 50 mg/kg/day, in divided doses, with the maximum dose being the same as the usual adult dose.

Following successful therapy, most patients with early Lyme borreliosis do well, although fatigue may continue for several months. The skin lesions generally resolve over days or weeks. Treatment failures occur, and therapy for later forms of Lyme borreliosis is less successful, sometimes with some sequelae persisting. Reinfection can occur.

ERYTHEMA MIGRANS (EARLY LYME BORRELIOSIS)

Clinical Manifestations

Red plaque or patch that usually develops central clearing as the lesion ages, often with a history of a tick bite 1 to 4 weeks prior to its appearance, seen in a patient who has recently been in an endemic area. Multiple lesions are common, and constitutional symptoms of malaise, headache, fever, myalgias, and gastrointestinal complaints are common.

Management in the Emergency Department

1. *When in doubt of the diagnosis, consider a skin punch biopsy of an area of active inflammation both for culture and to rule out other processes*
2. *Antibiotics for 10–28 days*
   - *Adults: doxycycline 100 mg two to three times a day, or amoxicillin 500 mg four times a day*

(Continues)

(Continued)

   - *Children ≤8 years and pregnant patients: amoxicillin at 20–40 mg/kg/day up to adult dose, or erythromycin at 30–50 mg/kg/day up to adult dose*
3. *Nonsteriodal anti-inflammatory medications or acetaminophen for constitutional symptoms*
4. *Call regular health care provider the next day to arrange follow up*

Nevus Flammeus

Nevus flammeus is a congenital patch of dilated blood vessels that produces an evenly pink, well-demarcated area of color change. Common over the eyelids and nape of the neck in newborns, larger and more permanent lesions can occur anywhere over the body, with the unilateral upper face (when it is sometimes a marker for tuberous sclerosus) and lower back common areas (for a detailed discussion of this entity, see Ch. 19, Pediatric Dermatology).

Actinic and Steroid Purpura

People who have experienced years of sun exposure or at least months of systemic corticosteroid excess, and especially those who have both risk factors, develop fragility of the skin. Even very mild trauma causes blood vessels to break, producing noninflammatory purpura. This usually occurs over the dorsal hands and arms, since minor trauma is more likely to occur here than over the equally sun-exposed face (Fig. 13.14).

This condition has no therapy except sun avoidance and patient education. Theoretically, topical tretinoin in conjunction with a sunscreen with a high SPF may help rejuvenate dermis and reverse some of the changes caused by sun exposure.

Acute Cutaneous Lupus Erythematosus

The acute cutaneous lesions of systemic lupus erythematosus are red patches and nearly flat plaques

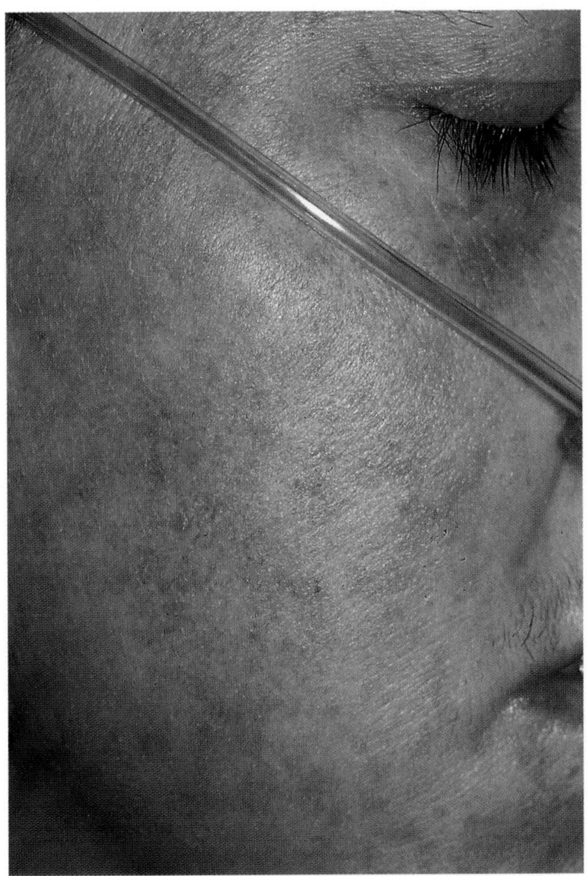

Figure 13.14 The acute cutaneous lesions of systemic lupus erythematosus often appear as a red, macular erythema and resolve without scarring.

over the face, and sometimes other sun-exposed skin, such as the dorsal hands and arms. Although the classic distribution is a malar butterfly eruption, often the only change seen is a pink flush (Fig. 13.14). Telangiectasias can be present, and erythema and telangiectasias over the upper eyelid margins and the posterior nail folds are frequently associated with systemic lupus erythematosus. Lesions resolve without scarring.

Diseases most often confused with acute cutaneous lupus erythematosus include sunburn, photosensitivity associated with medication, dermatomyositis, rosacea, chronic actinic damage with telangiectasias, and polymorphous light eruption, an uncommon disease of photosensitivity. The diagnosis is made by correlative signs and symptoms, positive serology for lupus erythematosus, or a skin biopsy (for a detailed discussion of cutaneous lupus erythematosus, see especially Ch. 14, Papulosquamous Diseases: Red, Scaling, Well-Demarcated Papules and Plaques).

Dermatomyositis

Dermatomyositis is an autoimmune disease of muscle and skin. Although the classic presentation includes both a rash and proximal muscle weakness, the latter finding can be subtle.

The eruption of dermatomyositis consists of a red, violaceous erythema of sun-exposed skin. The face, dorsal hands and arms, and V of the neck are usually involved (Fig. 13.15). Often, the eruption spares skin wrinkles and creases. The lesions over the dorsal hands and arms consist of coalescent, flat-topped papules (Gottron's papules) found preferentially over the joints. Violaceous erythema of the upper eyelids (a heliotrope rash) is associated with telangiectasias of the eyelid border; also seen are telangiectasias of the posterior nail folds, and unusually ragged cuticles are usual.

The skin findings associated with dermatomyositis are most easily confused both clinically and histologically with those of systemic lupus erythematosus. Eyelids affected by dermatomyositis are often more remarkably involved, and the rash is more pronounced over the finger joints rather than between the joints, as is often true of lupus erythematosus. The diagnosis is made by abnormal muscle enzymes and serologies.

Treatment of the skin disease of dermatomyositis is sun avoidance. The systemic corticosteroids used to treat muscle disease often secondarily treat the skin findings. Otherwise, antimalarial agents as used for cutaneous lupus erythematosus can be tried.

Dermatomyositis can be a chronic disease, or it can present explosively with rapid weakness that includes respiratory muscles. The mortality rate in adult dermatomyositis is up to 25%.[19] Dermatomyositis is associated with an internal malignancy in about 27% of patients.[20]

Please see patient information handouts for this chapter on pages 326, 335, 364, and 372.

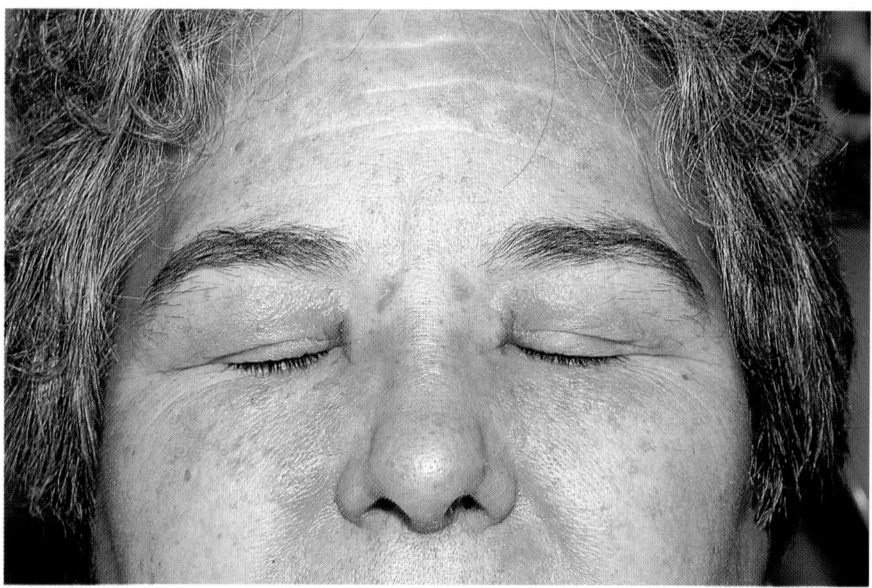

Figure 13.15 Violaceous erythema of the face is characteristic of dermatomyositis, especially when the upper eyelids are involved and there is sparing of the relatively sun-protected areas in the skin lines.

REFERENCES

1. Huff JC, Weston WL, Tonnesen MG: Erythema multiforme: a critical review of characteristics, diagnostic criteria, and causes. J Am Acad Dermatol 8:763, 1983
2. Bigby M, Jick S, Jeck H et al: Drug-induced cutaneous reactions: a report from the Boston Collaborative Drug Surveillance Program on 15,438 consecutive inpatients, 1975–1982. JAMA 256:3358, 1986
3. Correlia O, Chosidow O, Saiag P et al: Evolving pattern of drug-induced toxic epidermal necrolysis. Dermatology 186:32, 1993
4. Ekenstam E, Callen JP: Cutaneous leukocytoclastic vasculitis: clinical and laboratory features of 82 patients seen in private practice. Arch Dermatol 120:484, 1984
5. Soter NA, Wasserman SI: Clinical manifestations, pathogenesis, and therapeutic approaches in urticaria/angioedema. Dermatol Dig 18:17, 1979
6. Leigh IM, Mowbray JF, Levene GM et al: Recurrent and continuous erythema multiforme—a clinical and immunological study. Clin Exp Dermatol 10:58, 1985
7. Jacobson KW, Branch LB, Nelson JS: Laboratory tests in chronic urticaria. JAMA 243:1644, 1980
8. Monroe EW, Bernstein D, Bronsky E et al: A double-blind, randomized, placebo controlled, parallel study comparing the safety and efficacy of terfenadine 60 mg bid to hydroxyzine 25 mg qid administered for 6 to 12 weeks in the treatment of chronic idiopathic urticaria, abstracted. J Allergy Clin Immunol 89:248, 1992
9. Monroe EW, Fox R, Kalivas J et al: Comparative efficacy and safety of loratadine, hydroxyzine and placebo in chronic idiopathic urticaria, abstracted. J Allergy Clin Immunol 87:224, 1991
10. Kalivas J, Breneman D, Tharp J et al: Urticaria: clinical efficacy of cetirizine in comparison with hydroxyzine and placebo. J Allergy Clin Immunol 86:1014, 1990

11. Sullivan TJ: Pharmacologic modulation of the whealing response to histamine in human skin: identification of doxepin as a potent in vivo inhibitor. J Allergy Clin Immunol 69:260, 1982
12. Monroe EW: Chronic urticaria: Review of nonsedating H_1 antihistamines in treatment. J Am Acad Dermatol 19:842, 1988
13. Harvey RP, Wegs J, Schocket AL: A controlled trial of therapy in chronic urticaria. J Allergy Clin Immunol 68:262, 1981
14. Saihan EM: Ketotifen and terbutaline in urticaria. Br J Dermatol 104:205, 1981
15. Huff JC: Therapy and prevention of erythema multiforme with acyclovir. Semin Dermatol 7: 212, 1988
16. Sams WM Jr: Small vessel vasculitis. p. 543. In Sams WM Jr, Lynch PJ (eds): Principles and Practice of Dermatology. 2nd Ed. Churchill Livingstone, New York, 1996
17. Callen JP: Colchicine is effective in controlling chronic cutaneous leukocytoclastic vasculitis. J Am Acad Dermatol 13:193, 1985
18. Lang P: Sulfones and sulfonamides in dermatology today. J Am Acad Dermatol 1:479, 1979
19. Hockberg MC, Feldman D, Stevens MB: Adult onset polymyositis/dermatomyositis: an analysis of clinical and laboratory features and survival in 76 patients with a review of the literature. Semin Arthritis Rheum 15:168, 1986
20. Bernard P, Bonnetblanc J-M: Dermatomyositis and malignancy. J Invest Dermatol 100:128S, 1993

SUGGESTED READINGS

Urticaria

Juhlin L (ed): Urticaria. Semin Dermatol 6:271, 1987

Monroe EW: Chronic urticaria: review of nonsedating H_1 antihistamines in treatment. J Am Acad Dermatol 19:842, 1988

Urticarial Vasculitis

Soter NA: Urticarial vasculitis. p. 141. In Champion et al (eds): The Urticarias. Churchill Livingstone, Edinburgh, 1985

Erythema Multiforme

Ekenstam E, Callen JP: Cutaneous leukocytoclastic vasculitis: clinical and laboratory features of 82 patients seen in private practice. Arch Dermatol 120:484, 1984

Huff JC, Weston WL, Tonnesen MG: Erythema multiforme: a critical review of characteristics, diagnostic criteria, and causes. J Am Acad Dermatol 8:763, 1983

Vasculitis

Fauci AS, Haynes BF, Katz P: The spectrum of vasculitis. Ann Intern Med 89:660, 1978

CHAPTER 14

Papulosquamous Diseases: Red, Scaling, Well-Demarcated Papules and Plaques

The papulosquamous diseases are those skin diseases characterized by inflammatory, scaling, well-demarcated papules and plaques. Although usually red, these lesions often appear hyperpigmented in black patients. Papulosquamous diseases generally lack evidence of rubbing or scratching, such as excoriation or crusting, except in patients who are innately itchy and have secondarily scratched. The great majority of papulosquamous lesions are produced by five diseases, best remembered by the mnemonic, "3 L's, 2 P's, 1 F," representing the diseases *l*ichen planus, *l*upus erythematosus, and *l*ues (secondary syphilis); *p*soriasis, *p*ityriasis rosea; and *f*ungus. Morphologically, papulosquamous diseases can be divided into those conditions usually characterized by the presence of at least some larger plaques (psoriasis, lupus erythematosus, tinea) and those usually characterized by multiple, smaller papules (lichen planus, lues, and pityriasis rosea).

Scale is sometimes obvious and may be flaky, as is generally seen with psoriasis. Often, however, scale can be difficult to identify, as with the fine powdery "pityriasis" scale of pityriasis rosea or tinea versicolor (see Fig. 1.2), or the adherent, shiny "lichenoid" scale of lichen planus (see Fig. 1.6). Partial treatment and moisturization can also obscure scale. Even when scale is not visible, roughness of skin to the touch is a sign of scale.

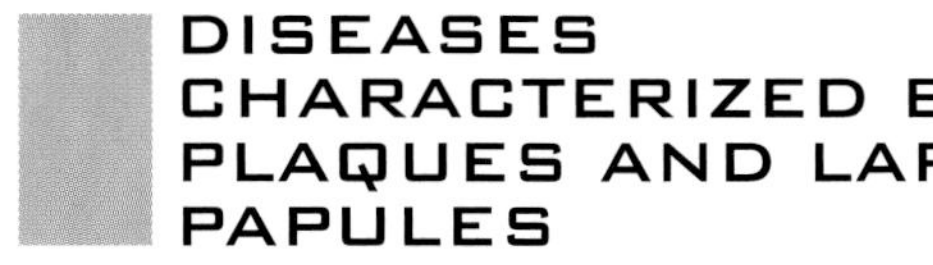

DISEASES CHARACTERIZED BY PLAQUES AND LARGE PAPULES

Some papulosquamous diseases typically present as large plaques. However, there is considerable overlap with those diseases that generally exhibit smaller plaques or papules. For example, psoriasis can be manifest only as 1 to 2 cm lesions (guttate psoriasis), and lichen planus can occasionally present with only large plaques. Therefore, the clinician should keep all these diseases in mind when generating a differential diagnosis for a papulosquamous disease.

Psoriasis

Psoriasis is the prototype for papulosquamous disease. It occurs in about 1 to 2% of the population, and there is a very strong familial predisposition for this disease. Although usually insidious in onset, psoriasis can present explosively after a severe sunburn, a streptococcal infection, or in patients with acquired immunodeficiency syndrome (AIDS).

Clinical Manifestations Psoriasis vulgaris (common psoriasis) is manifested by inflamed, thickened, sharply demarcated plaques with heavy, silvery scale (Fig. 14.1). Although papules and small plaques are often present, plaques of 10 cm or larger are common.

Common psoriasis has a very characteristic distribution. Essentially all patients have lesions in the scalp. In addition, elbows and knees are preferentially affected, as are the intergluteal cleft and the umbilicus. This distribution is at least partially explained by the Koebner phenomenon, in which the skin disease arises preferentially in an area of irritation, friction, or injury. The elbows and knees are likely common sites because these are frictional surfaces, and skin folds are often affected, as these

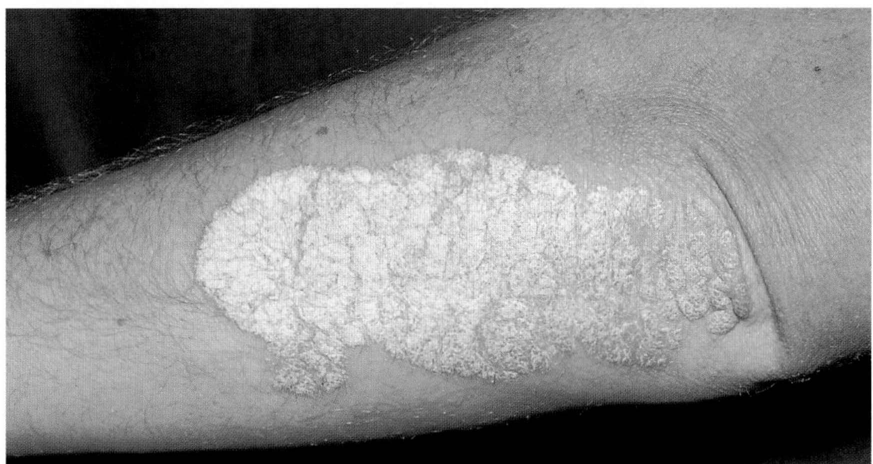

Figure 14.1 Untreated psoriasis is characterized by thick, inflamed plaques with heavy silvery scale, although even the use of emollients can minimize the silvery quality of the scale.

are areas of irritation and inflammation from both friction and retained heat and perspiration. Psoriasis also occurs in some patients within scars, sites of injury, and sunburns.

Some patients have limited disease, consisting of slight scalp scale and small papules on elbows and knees, but other patients can show rather extensive disease covering large portions of the body. When widespread, psoriasis and other causes of erythema and scale can confer considerable morbidity. The cutaneous inflammation results in increased cell turnover with loss of protein, iron, and folate, as well as obligatory vasodilation and increased cardiac output. Cutaneous infection becomes more likely and, with shunting of blood to the skin, there is sometimes significant shunting away from the intestines, resulting in malabsorption, and shunting away from the kidneys, resulting in a prerenal state. The patient's white blood cell (WBC) count may be elevated and, because of an inability to vasoconstrict and sometimes an inability to sweat, temperature stability may become a problem.

In addition to psoriasis vulgaris, psoriasis can occur in several other forms. *Guttate* (meaning "drop-like") psoriasis occurs as small, scattered papules, primarily over the trunk (Fig. 14.2). This is most common in children, classically occurring after a streptococcal infection or a sunburn. Often, those sites normally involved preferentially, such as the elbows and knees, are unaffected. *Inverse* psoriasis refers to disease occurring almost exclusively in skin folds, including the axillae, the crural creases, genital area, and intergluteal cleft. Because of the damp nature of skin folds, the scaly nature of psoriasis in these areas is much less well appreciated and lacks the silvery color (Fig. 14.3). *Erythrodermic* psoriasis occurs when most of the skin surface is involved. At this point, the scale becomes less characteristic, and the papulosquamous nature of the psoriasis is often obscured since the plaques become confluent, and the sharpness of the borders cannot be judged. Although Fig. 3.1 is actually a photograph of a patient with exfoliative erythroderma on the basis of atopic dermatitis, this clinical presentation is indistinguishable from generalized psoriasis. Finally, a life-threatening form of psoriasis, *pustular psoriasis*, occurs in some cases. This form of psoriasis is characterized by plaques studded with small, superficial pustules (see Fig. 7.6). As these break, the skin becomes exudative and crusted (see Fig. 7.7). Patients can appear toxic, febrile, and exhibit high WBC counts. Infection can become a significant concern, and these patients are sometimes medical emergencies.

Psoriasis, even when mild, can affect more than the skin. Most common are nail changes. Small, scattered pits are nearly pathognomonic of psoriasis (see Fig. 18.5). Other changes include "oil-drop"

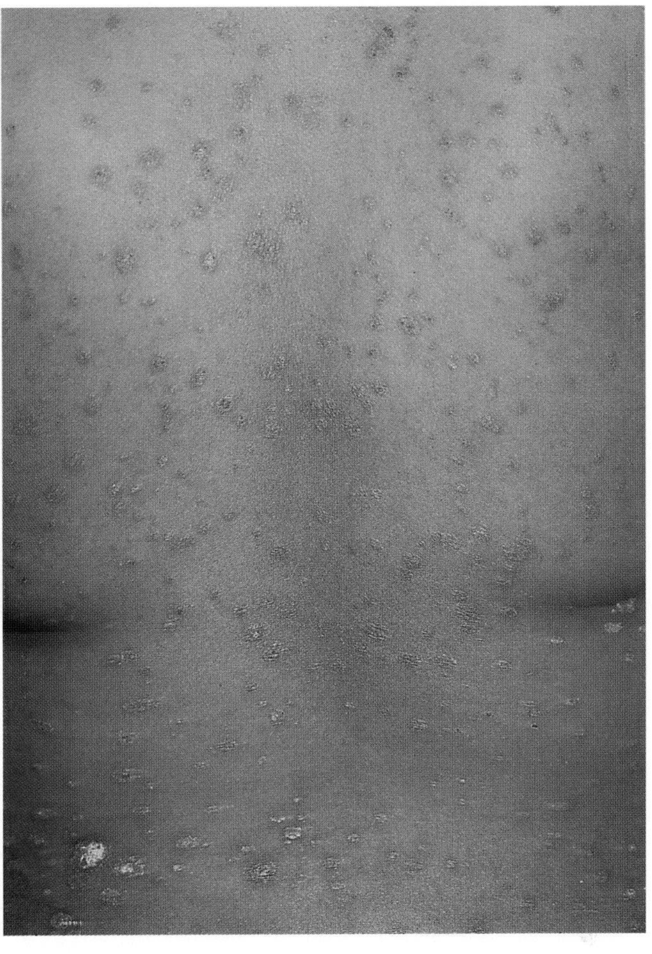

Figure 14.2 Scattered, small, well-demarcated papules are typical of guttate psoriasis, and these can mimic the eruptions of secondary syphilis, pityriasis rosea, or even eruptive lichen planus (cf. Figs. 14.12, 14.13, 14.14, 14.16, and 14.18). The few papules with typical silvery scale on the lower left back serve as a clue to the diagnosis.

spots, which signify psoriasis under the nail and appear as a brownish area (see Fig. 18.6). With more severe psoriasis under the nail, the nail plate may be lifted by underlying keratin debris. These latter changes can be indistinguishable from a fungal nail infection.

Psoriatic arthritis occurs in up to about 20% of patients with psoriasis.[1,2] Patients with nail involvement, those with severe disease, and those with pustular or erythrodermic disease have higher risks of associated arthritis. Patients with milder disease have a smaller, but difficult to measure, risk of arthritis. Most often, patients have non-debilitating joint aches that could also represent common osteoarthritis. However, some patients develop a severe and deforming arthritis with bone resorption. Psoriasis, especially pustular psoriasis, exists on a spectrum with other seronegative spondyloarthropathies, including Reiter's disease and ankylosing spondylitis (see Ch. 7, Pustular Diseases).

Differential Diagnosis When psoriasis has been untreated, including no lubrication, the thick, silvery scale and distribution usually make this diagnosis easy. However, most patients will have applied some medications or emollients to their skin, changing the character of the scale. In addition, psoriasis on the face, in skin folds, and over the genitalia characteristically shows much less scale (Fig. 14.3).

The differential diagnosis of psoriasis includes other papulosquamous diseases. Common psoriasis, with its larger scaling plaques, is most often confused with a superficial dermatophyte infection (tinea), particularly when the scalp, groin, and nails are involved. Tinea usually produces far

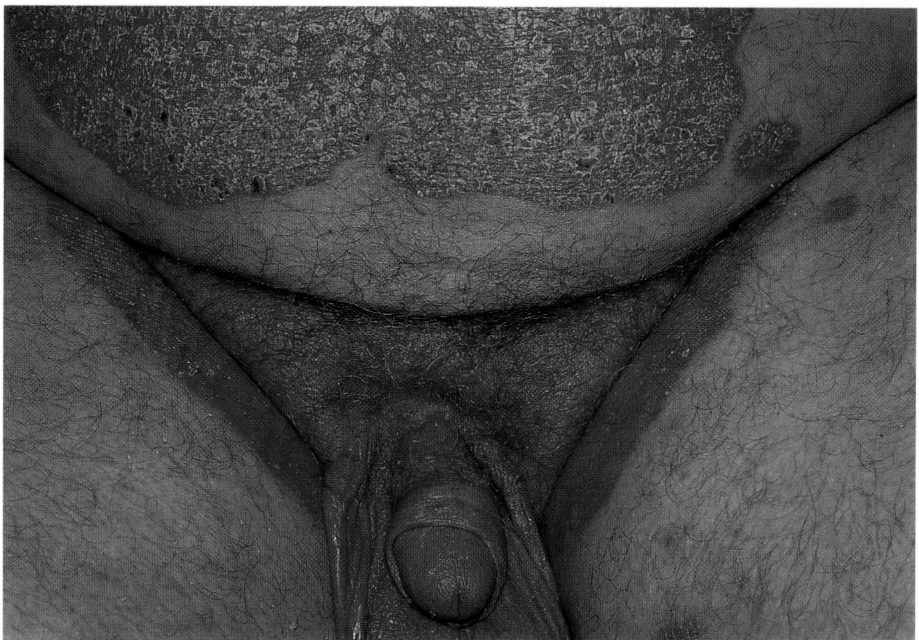

Figure 14.3 Inverse psoriasis preferentially affects skin folds, where the natural dampness obscures scale. More typical psoriasis over the abdomen is also present in this patient.

fewer and thinner plaques, does not preferentially affect elbows and knees, and is more likely to be annular in immunocompetent patients, although psoriasis is occasionally annular also. In experienced hands, a potassium hydroxide preparation can reveal fungi in the case of tinea. Subacute and chronic (discoid) cutaneous lupus erythematosus sometimes mimic psoriasis without showing other cutaneous or extracutaneous signs of lupus erythematosus. Chronic (discoid) cutaneous lupus erythematous is usually confined to the face and scalp; well-developed lesions show central scarring with surrounding hyperpigmentation (Fig. 14.4). Subacute cutaneous lupus erythematosus is usually restricted to the dorsal arms and upper trunk and is manifested by thinner plaques with less scale (Figs. 14.5 and 14.6). All these diseases except fungal infection lack nail changes and the characteristic distribution of psoriasis.

Guttate psoriasis is most easily confused with papulosquamous diseases that usually exhibit papules and small plaques, such as lichen planus, pityriasis rosea, and secondary syphilis. The scale of lichen planus is usually adherent and shiny, and the color of the papules is usually a deeper, more violaceous red. Sometimes there are characteristic oral mucous membrane changes of lichen planus. Pityriasis rosea usually has very thin, extremely lightly scaling papules, generally limited to the trunk and proximal extremities. Secondary syphilis usually shows discrete palmar lesions, finer scale, and generalized lymphadenopathy. Syphilis serology is a dependable test for this disease and should be performed when any doubt exists.

Inverse psoriasis is most often confused with a fungal infection, either candidiasis or dermatophytosis. This is further complicated by the fact that skin fold areas of psoriasis are sometimes secondarily infected with a fungus. A potassium hydroxide preparation, fungal culture, or response to empirical therapy is useful in making the correct diagnosis.

The differential diagnosis of erythrodermic psoriasis can be much broader. A generalized exfoliative erythroderma can occur with any inflammatory skin disease that becomes widespread and chronic, most often eczema or psoriasis, and with medication reactions (see Ch. 15, Eczematous Diseases).

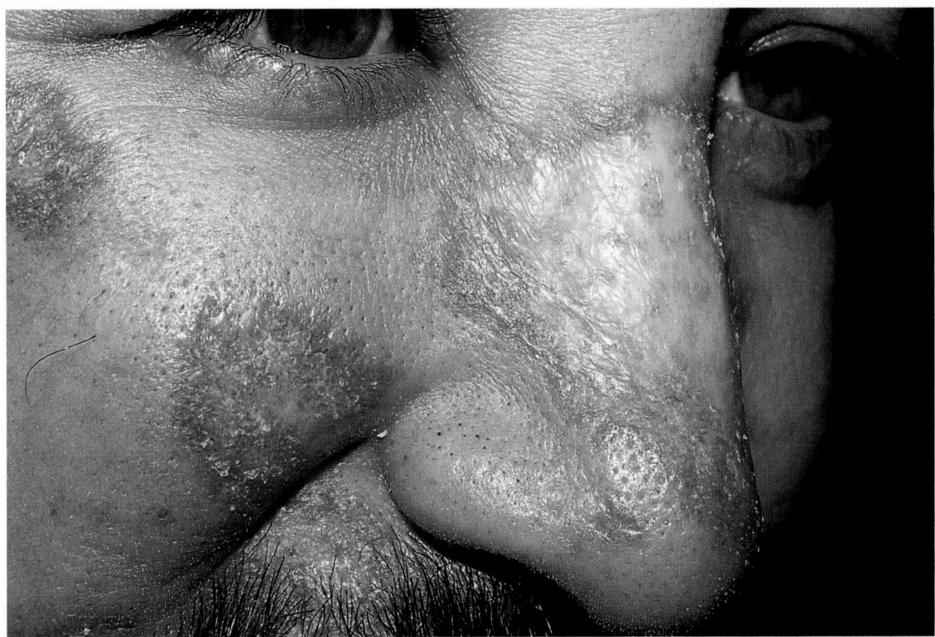

Figure 14.4 Early chronic cutaneous lupus erythematosus, such as that seen on the medial cheeks, shows solid, red plaques with scale/crust. Depigmentation and central scarring occur later, producing the annular appearance of the lesions on this patient's nose. Peripheral hyperpigmentation is common.

The correct diagnosis can be impossible in the absence of a previous history of psoriasis, pathognomonic nail changes, or a diagnostic skin biopsy.

Pustular psoriasis is most easily confused with infection, particularly in the presence of fever and a high WBC count. Patients in whom pustular psoriasis is a diagnostic possibility should be evaluated promptly by a dermatologist.

Management First-line therapy for most patients with psoriasis, and the only treatment appropriate for the emergency department, is *topical therapy*. Psoriasis is moderately steroid responsive. A midpotency corticosteroid such as triamcinolone (Kenalog) 0.1% cream or ointment is a reasonable initial choice, with progression to a high-potency corticosteroid such as fluocinonide (Lidex) 0.05% preparation for more resistant lesions and palms and soles. Although creams and ointments are useful for keratinized skin in most areas of the body, a gel, lotion, or solution is best for hairy areas such as the scalp. Betamethasone valerate (Valisone) 0.1% lotion is an inexpensive, effective, and cosmetically acceptable topical preparation for the scalp that is a midpotency strength. Skin fold and facial lesions are best treated initially with lower strength hydrocortisone cream 1% or 2.5% twice daily. The patient should be warned that, although dramatic improvement is common initially, topical corticosteroids often become less effective over time. Still, for the average patient with mild to moderate psoriasis, this "band-aid" therapy is perfectly appropriate for the urgent care setting, with follow-up evaluation in a dermatologist's office planned two to four weeks later.

Other topical therapies include tar (Estar gel, T-Derm), which improves some cases when applied once or twice daily, particularly when applied 1 to 2 hours before exposure to sunlight. Shampoos with keratolytic agents or antiproliferative medications such as salicylic acid, pyrithione zinc, or tar are beneficial for scalp disease. Effective and widely available choices include T-Gel, Ionil T Plus, T-Sal, and Zincon.

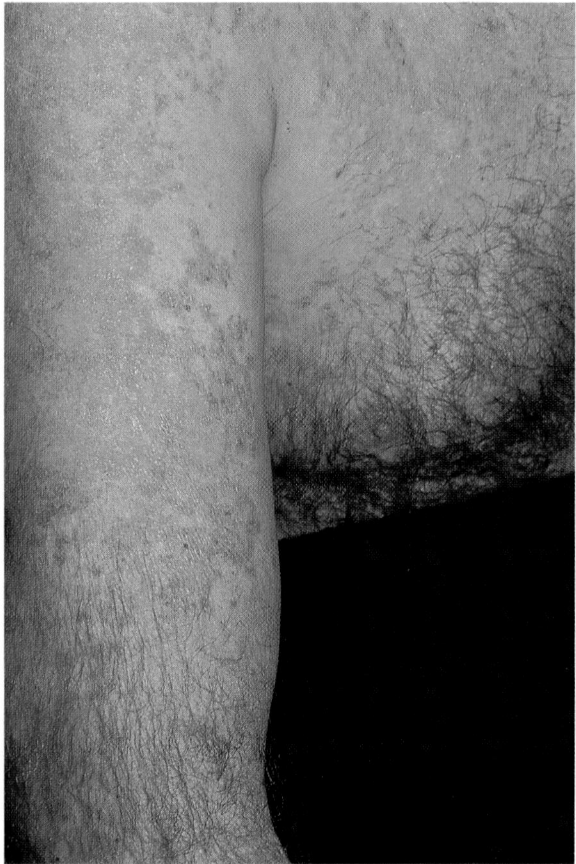

Figure 14.5 Red, often violaceous, sharply demarcated, scaling, coalescing papules and plaques located predominantly over the upper trunk, shoulders, and dorsal arms are most typical of papulosquamous subacute cutaneous lupus erythematosus.

Calcipotriene (Dovonex) ointment is a new topical antipsoriatic agent. This vitamin D analog is as effective as midpotency corticosteroids in some patients.[3] It has the advantage of retaining its activity over time rather than becoming less effective, as corticosteroids tend to do. Also, the adverse reactions associated with topical corticosteroids, such as cutaneous atrophy, striae, and systemic absorption of steroid do not occur. However, calcipotriene can be absorbed when applied over large areas of skin, and hypercalcemia has been reported. Improvement from calcipotriene is slower than that achieved with corticosteroids, and this is an expensive (about $1/g) therapy for psoriasis.

Anthralin (Dithrocream) is an antimetabolite that is often beneficial for more hyperkeratotic, thickened plaques of psoriasis. It has the significant disadvantages of permanently staining clothes, surrounding skin, and even bathtubs, as well as producing local irritation. Because it is irritating, anthralin is applied for short periods of time that are gradually increased. This is not an appropriate medication for the usual emergency department setting because it requires very careful patient education and patients frequently call back with questions or complications.

Ultraviolet light therapy is more effective than topical therapy and is relatively safe, but it is very time consuming and expensive. Treatments usually begin at frequencies of three to five times each week, sometimes ultimately requiring only one treatment per week to retain the beneficial effect. Ultraviolet B (UVB) therapy employs the same wavelength that normally causes sunburn, tanning, and skin cancers. The effects of UVB therapy can be enhanced by the application of a topical tar preparation. The second type of light therapy is psoralens and ultraviolet A (PUVA) light therapy. Ultraviolet A light is very low energy so that the patients must use medication (psoralens) to make DNA more vulnerable to damage by UV light, resulting in an antiproliferative effect. Psoralens are most often administered orally, but topical use is also possible. Because psoralens taken orally are deposited in the eye, patients should wear UVA-protective goggles for 1 day after ingesting psoralens.

The third general type of antipsoriatic therapy is *oral medication*. The vitamin A analog, etretinate (Tegison), methotrexate, cyclosporine (Sandimmune), and sulfasalazine (Azulfidine) are all beneficial therapies for psoriasis which also carry significant risks.[4,5] These are inappropriate therapies in the emergency department setting because of the extremely careful and frequent mandatory follow-up requiring laboratory testing and examinations.

Many psoriasis specialists feel that corticosteroids, especially when administered systemically, should be avoided in the treatment of psoriasis. Corticosteroid therapy can sometimes make psoriasis more resistant to therapy in general. Also, although many patients are nursed through a flare of their psoriasis by an injection of triamcinolone acetonide (Kenalog), an occasional patient experi-

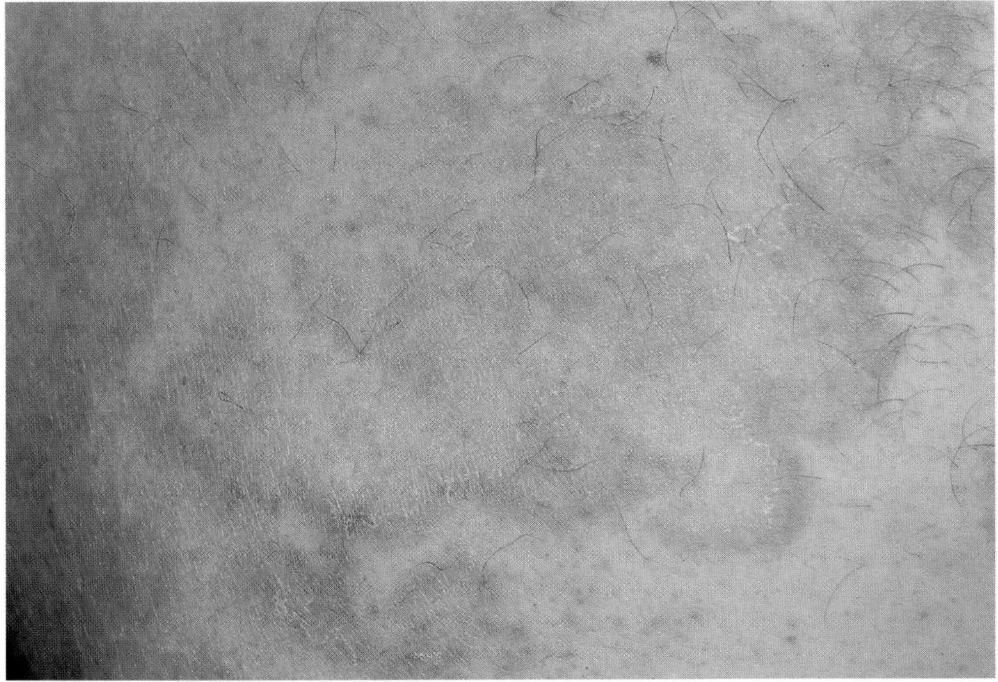

Figure 14.6 Subacute cutaneous lupus erythematosus can appear annular, with coalescing plaques producing an arcuate morphology.

ences a pustular flare as the effect of the medication wears off, and the prescribing clinician is credited. A corticosteroid applied over extensive areas of inflamed skin also results in systemic absorption.

Many patients with erythrodermic psoriasis and pustular psoriasis should be admitted to the hospital and their skin care supervised by a dermatologist. In general, oral retinoids or methotrexate are most effective for these patients, but care should be taken to identify and treat infections and fluid or electrolyte abnormalities.

Course and Prognosis Psoriasis is not a curable disease. Although some patients may be lucky enough to experience a remission of their disease, most patients continue to have visible lesions that improve in the summer and worsen every winter and with stress.

Some patients experience significant and disabling pruritus. Other patients have painful lesions. Crusting and inflammatory plaques over palms and soles are especially crippling and can prevent some from performing normal daily functions.

For many people, psoriasis is psychologically debilitating. The striking appearance of the lesions and the quantity of scale left on clothing and furniture by the patient can be humiliating. Even patients with limited or mild disease are often extremely upset by the appearance of their psoriasis.

Also, some patients have severe and extensive disease with crippling arthritis. Fortunately, psoriasis in most patients can be controlled, but the toll in time, expense, and adverse reactions to therapies is high.

PSORIASIS

Clinical Manifestations

Classic, untreated psoriasis vulgaris exhibits well-demarcated, inflamed plaques with dense silvery scale, located preferentially over the scalp, elbows, and knees. Nail pitting is pathognomonic, and other nail dystrophies are common.

(Continues)

(Continued)

Management in the Emergency Department
Patients with pustular psoriasis or erythrodermic psoriasis who are ill should be evaluated immediately by a dermatologist, and hospital admission is usual

1. *Topical corticosteroids:*
   - *Triamcinolone ointment 0.1% (most body areas) bid*
   - *Hydrocortisone cream 1% or 2.5% (face, skin folds) bid*
   - *Betamethasone valerate lotion 0.1% (scalp) bid*
2. *Nighttime sedation with diphenhydramine, hydroxyzine, or amitriptyline 25 to 75 mg at bedtime if itchy*
3. *Follow up with regular health care provider in one month (if mild), or dermatologist at earliest convenience (if severe).*
4. *Patient education (see patient handouts on p. 358, Psoriasis, and on p. 368, Topical Cortisone Creams, Ointments, and Solutions.)*

Cutaneous Lupus Erythematosus

Cutaneous lupus erythematosus is an autoimmune disease that can present in any of several characteristic fashions. The clinical morphology of lesions correlates roughly with the presence of systemic disease. Cutaneous lupus erythematosus is relatively common, and the skin lesions are often a presenting feature of this disease.

Clinical Manifestations *Chronic cutaneous lupus erythematosus* (CCLE, discoid LE) is generally associated with minimal or no systemic disease. Most often, erythematous, scaling, crusted papules and plaques occur predominantly over the lateral face (Fig. 14.4). As the disease progresses, central scarring and hypopigmentation are usual and may give lesions an annular appearance. The erythema of these lesions is dusky or slightly violaceous, and often hyperpigmentation is present at the periphery. The scalp is sometimes affected, and a scarring, permanent hair loss ensues. In rare cases, chronic cutaneous lupus erythematosus can affect other parts of the body, especially the dorsal arms and shoulders.

Most patients with only a few lesions report no symptoms of systemic lupus erythematosus and there is generally no evidence of significant systemic disease on laboratory testing. Many even lack antinuclear antibodies (ANA). However, patients with many lesions and those with extrafacial involvement are much more likely to exhibit at least some evidence of systemic disease.

Subacute cutaneous lupus erythematosus (SCLE) is a less common and more recently recognized variant of this disease. Although usually associated with at least some laboratory evidence of lupus erythematosus, these lesions are usually not associated with significant kidney or central nervous system involvement.

Subacute cutaneous lupus erythematosus occurs in two main morphologic varieties. The first is *papulosquamous SCLE*, which presents as coalescing, erythematous, scaling plaques most often distributed over the upper trunk and dorsal arms (Fig. 14.5). *Annular SCLE* consists of red, scaling, annular, and arcuate plaques in this same distribution (Fig. 14.6). Neither the annular nor the papulosquamous form of subacute cutaneous lupus erythematosus exhibits the extreme inflammation, crusting, or scarring of chronic cutaneous lupus erythematosus.

The lesions of *acute systemic lupus erythematosus* are often the most subtle, most evanescent, and least scaling of the forms of cutaneous lupus erythematosus. This eruption forms the classic "butterfly" rash consisting of dusky red erythema over the central face and malar areas (see Fig. 13.14). Although the distribution is characteristic, the eruption itself is not specific. Like subacute cutaneous lupus erythematosus, it is a nonscarring eruption.

Both SCLE and lesions of acute systemic lupus erythematosus are often associated with other skin findings of systemic lupus erythematosus. These include erythema over the posterior nail folds of the fingernail (the skin surrounding the cuticles) as well as erythema or telangiectasis at the lid margin of the upper eyelids. Some patients also show evidence of vasculitis in the form of palpable purpura or small cutaneous infarctions primarily over the fingers and toes. Another nonspecific finding in some patients with systemic lupus erythematosus is livedo reticularis, a dusky red mottling of the skin that represents a deep vasculitis (see Fig. 6.5).

Differential Diagnosis Early lesions of chronic cutaneous lupus erythematosus that simply show scaling papules over the lateral aspects of the face can be confused with actinic keratoses, seborrheic dermatitis, and tinea infection. More developed, indurated lesions are sometimes confused with sarcoidosis. Subacute cutaneous lupus erythematosus can be confused with partially treated psoriasis or very extensive tinea corporis.

The erythema of the acute lesions of systemic lupus erythematosus is sometimes indistinguishable from rosacea, chronic sun damage, seborrheic dermatitis, or a photosensitive eruption associated with some medications such as tetracycline or hydrochlorothiazide.

In the absence of diagnostic laboratory tests or a previous, known diagnosis of lupus erythematosus, a skin biopsy should be performed. Fortunately, a punch biopsy of involved skin is nearly always specific for cutaneous lupus erythematosus.

Management Appropriate therapy for the lesions of chronic cutaneous lupus erythematosus and subacute cutaneous lupus erythematosus in the emergency department is topical corticosteroids. A midpotency preparation such as triamcinolone (Kenalog) cream 0.1% can be used on involved skin of any area, taking care to avoid surrounding, normal skin. Some patients with cutaneous lupus erythematosus require ultrahigh-potency topical corticosteroids, but this should be done with careful follow-up evaluation by a dermatologist. Some patients derive adequate benefit from these measures alone, but most require additional therapy that should be initiated in a physician's office, for ongoing follow-up evaluation.

If a patient with acute cutaneous lesions of systemic lupus erythematosus has significant signs of systemic disease, the patient will receive systemic corticosteroids, which provide secondary treatment of the skin.

Other medications which are useful for cutaneous lupus erythematosus include oral antimalarial medications, particularly hydroxychloroquine (Plaquenil) and oral retinoids (e.g., isotretinoin and etretinate).[6]

Course and Prognosis The usual course for lesions of chronic cutaneous lupus erythematosus is stabilization or slow progression with increasing numbers of lesions, larger lesions, and progressive hypopigmentation and scarring. These lesions can be extremely disfiguring, particularly in black patients. In general, patients with CCLE who develop significant signs of systemic lupus erythematosus do so within the first year.

Patients with subacute cutaneous lupus erythematosus experience waxing and waning of their skin lesions but generally do not experience significant improvement without therapy. Although people with subacute cutaneous lupus erythematosus generally exhibit systemic disease also, severe systemic lupus erythematosus with serious kidney or central nervous system disease is unusual.

Patients with acute lesions of systemic lupus erythematosus usually exhibit significant systemic disease. Their skin lesions are usually a minor part of the overall process, and the prognosis depends on the progress of the systemic disease and on the patient's response to therapy.

CHRONIC CUTANEOUS (DISCOID) LUPUS ERYTHEMATOSUS

Clinical Manifestations

Inflamed, scaling papules and plaques with central scarring and hypopigmentation, located preferentially over the lateral face and often on the scalp, but can occur anywhere.

Management in the Emergency Department

1. *Triamcinolone cream 0.1% bid*
2. *Sun avoidance*
3. *Punch skin biopsy to confirm diagnosis, or refer for this*
4. *Referral to dermatologist at earliest convenience for additional therapy*
5. *Patient education (see the patient handouts on p. 337, Cutaneous Lupus Erythematosus, and on p. 368, Topical Cortisone Creams, Ointments, and Solutions)*

SUBACUTE CUTANEOUS LUPUS ERYTHEMATOSUS

Clinical Manifestations

Solid or annular, coalescing, inflamed, lightly scaling, nonscarring plaques located primarily over the upper shoulders, trunk, and dorsal arms.

Management in the Emergency Department

1. *Confirmation of diagnosis with skin biopsy, antinuclear antibodies (ANA), or refer for this*
2. *If ill, immediate screen for significant systemic disease*
3. *Triamcinolone cream 0.1% bid*
4. *Sun avoidance*
5. *Follow up with a dermatologist or rheumatologist at earliest convenience*
6. *Patient education (see the patient handouts on* *p. 337, Cutaneous Lupus Erythematosus, and on p. 368, Topical Cortisone Creams, Ointments, and Solutions**)*

ACUTE CUTANEOUS LUPUS ERYTHEMATOSUS

Clinical Manifestations

Inflamed, violaceous, nonscaling plaques and patches over the face, associated with posterior nail fold erythema and other signs of systemic lupus erythematosus.

Management in the Emergency Department

1. *Confirmation of the diagnosis*
2. *Therapy and follow-up evaluation for systemic disease*

Fungal Infection

Fungal infection comprises both dermatophyte (often called "ringworm") and yeast infections. Tinea properly refers to dermatophyte infections of the scalp (tinea capitis), feet (tinea pedis), hands (tinea manum), face (tinea faciei), inner thighs (tinea cruris), and keratinized body skin (tinea corporis). However, pityriasis "tinea" versicolor is a misnomer, referring not to a dermatophyte infection, but rather to a yeast infection caused by *Pityrosporum ovale* (also called *Malassezia furfur*). This becomes important during therapy, since not all antifungal medications effectively treat both dermatophytes and yeast.

Most tinea infections exhibit papulosquamous morphology. However, fungal infections involving follicular epithelium can be pustular (see Fig. 7.2), and very inflammatory infections exhibiting crusting and exudation can be classified in the eczematous group. Pityriasis "tinea" versicolor often appears hypopigmented or hyperpigmented, thus appearing in the white or brown lesion groups, but it is frequently pink as well, placing it in the papulosquamous group. Therefore, fungal diseases, like many skin diseases, can exhibit variable morphologies that allow them to fit into any of several groups.

Clinical Manifestations Classic tinea infection is an annular, inflamed, scaling plaque that is single or few in number. Scale is most prominent at the periphery (Fig. 14.7). However, when occurring over the feet, hands, groin, and scalp, the annular nature is often more subtle, and annularity is not always present in any area. Pustules and crusted papules within plaques represent follicular involvement; this occurs most often in hairy areas (see Fig. 7.2).

When occurring over the genital area, plaques are generally solid rather than annular, but scale is nonetheless more prominent at the periphery (Fig. 14.8). Much more common in men than women, and essentially confined to postpubertal patients, tinea cruris does not extend to the scrotum or penis unless the patient is immunosuppressed or the eruption has been treated with a topical corticosteroid.

Tinea pedis is often, but not always, less well demarcated. Usually associated with fungal nail disease, erythema and scale over a moccasin distribution and between toes is usual (Fig. 14.9). Tinea manum generally occurs only on one hand, and always with tinea pedis, producing *two-foot, one-hand disease.* Again, nails may be affected.

Tinea faciei in children usually presents with typical annular morphology, but in adults (especially within the beard area of men), follicular involvement often produces infiltrated, inflamed plaques with minimal scale and annularity.

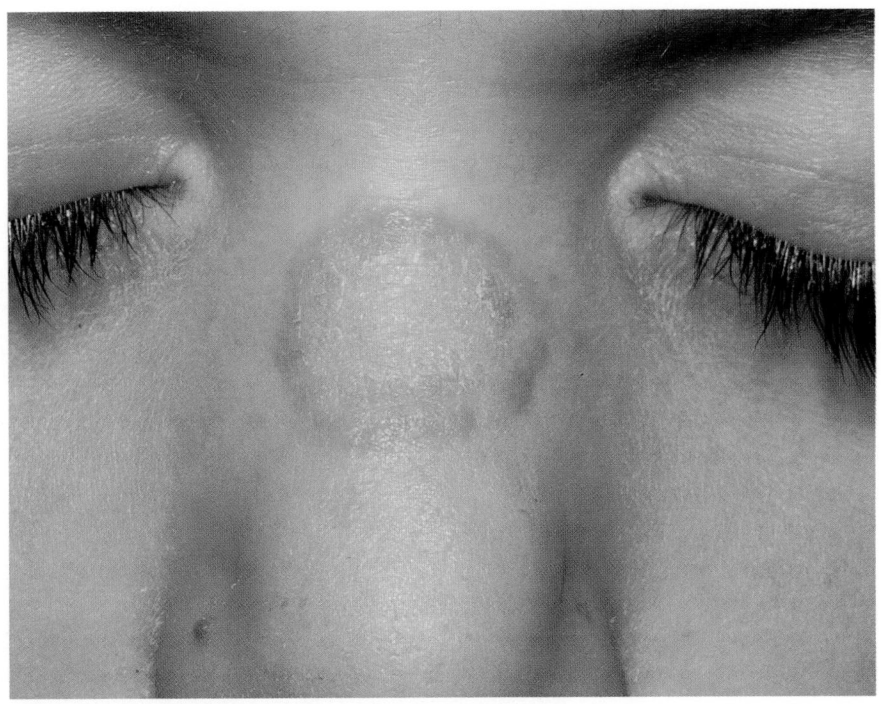

Figure 14.7 Tinea corporis consists of red, well-demarcated scaling plaques with central clearing, producing the annular appearance that confers the name "ringworm."

Figure 14.8 Tinea cruris, seen primarily in men, often exhibits less annularity but scale is nonetheless accentuated at the borders (arrow). Unlike neurodermatitis, the borders are sharply demarcated, and the scrotum and penis are largely spared.

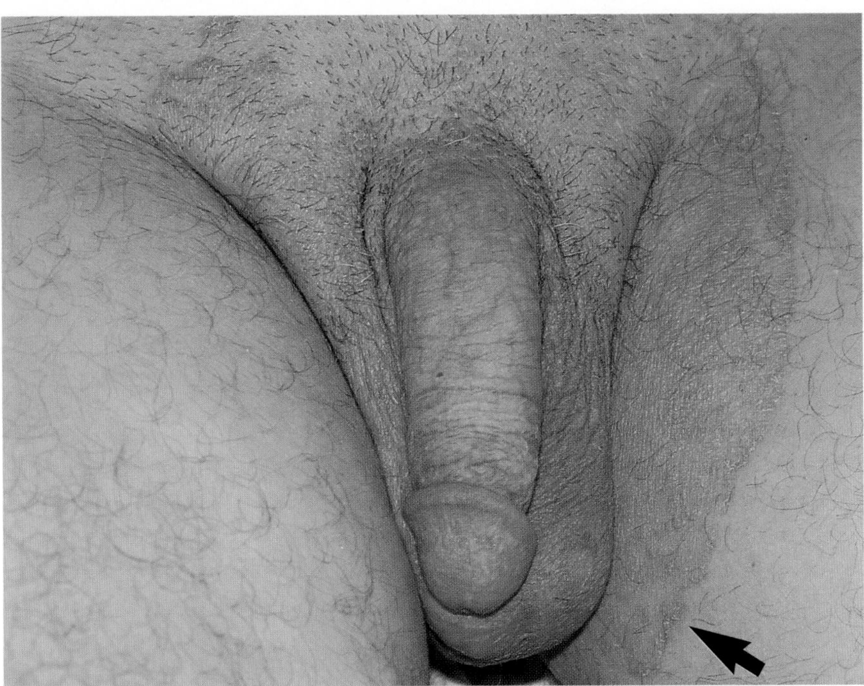

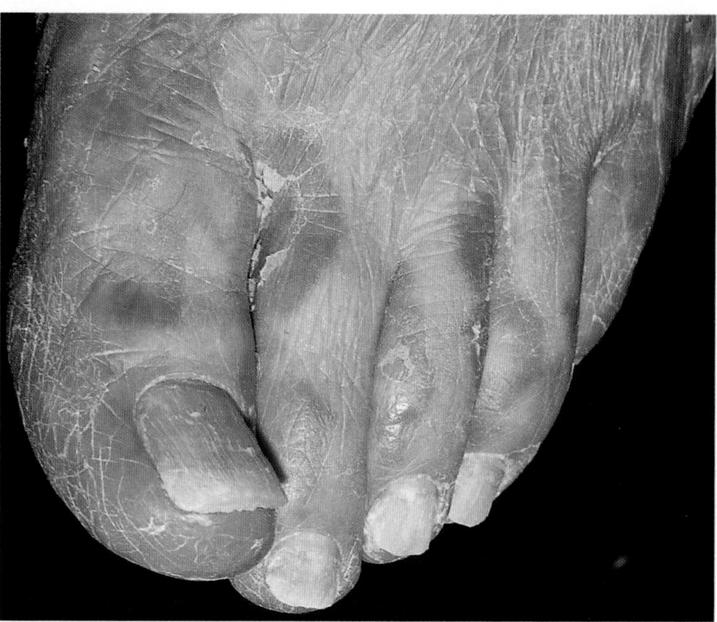

Figure 14.9 Tinea pedis shows red, scaling plaques often associated with onychomycosis. Fine white scale often collects in skin lines.

Tinea capitis is confined almost entirely to children, and it is much more common in black children. Usually associated with hair loss, scalp dermatophyte infection exists on a spectrum from nearly normal-appearing skin with minor scale or "black dots" produced by hair broken off at the skin surface, to scaling and crusted, boggy plaques (*kerion*) (Figs. 14.10 and 14.11).

Pityriasis "tinea" versicolor occurs primarily over the central trunk as small, round, subtly scaling papules coalescing into larger plaques. These can be light tan-pink, hypopigmented (see Fig. 9.6), or hyperpigmented (see Fig. 11.3). There is no annularity (for a detailed discussion, see Ch. 9, White Lesions, and Ch. 11, Brown Lesions).

Differential Diagnosis Obviously, a positive potassium hydroxide (KOH) preparation of scale or a fungal culture is the definitive test to differentiate fungal disease from other morphologically similar skin conditions. However, few nondermatologists can interpret a fungal smear, and the results of a fungal culture are far too delayed for decisions made in the emergency department. Therefore, the following discussion concentrates on the morphologic differences among similar diseases.

Classic tinea corporis (ringworm) can be confused with many annular, inflamed diseases. Psoriasis, chronic (discoid) and annular subacute cutaneous lupus erythematosus, and even lichen planus can be annular (see Figs. 14.4 and 14.6). Like tinea corporis, all of these diseases exhibit scale, but unlike tinea corporis, these diseases usually have many more lesions and other signs of the specific diseases, such as the nail changes of psoriasis, or mucous membrane lesions of lichen planus.

Granuloma annulare and sarcoidosis are inflammatory diseases that are often annular, but these are more infiltrated and lack scale (see Fig. 12.2).

Tinea cruris can be difficult to distinguish from neurodermatitis/eczema, another inflamed, scaling disease with a predisposition for this area. However, neurodermatitis is poorly demarcated, lichenified or excoriated, and preferentially affects the scrotum and vulva, whereas tinea cruris generally spares these areas. Another disease easily confused with tinea cruris is erythrasma. This superficial bacterial infection is a tan-pink, lightly scaling, sharply demarcated plaque that covers the upper, inner thighs. There is coral pink fluorescence under a Wood's lamp.

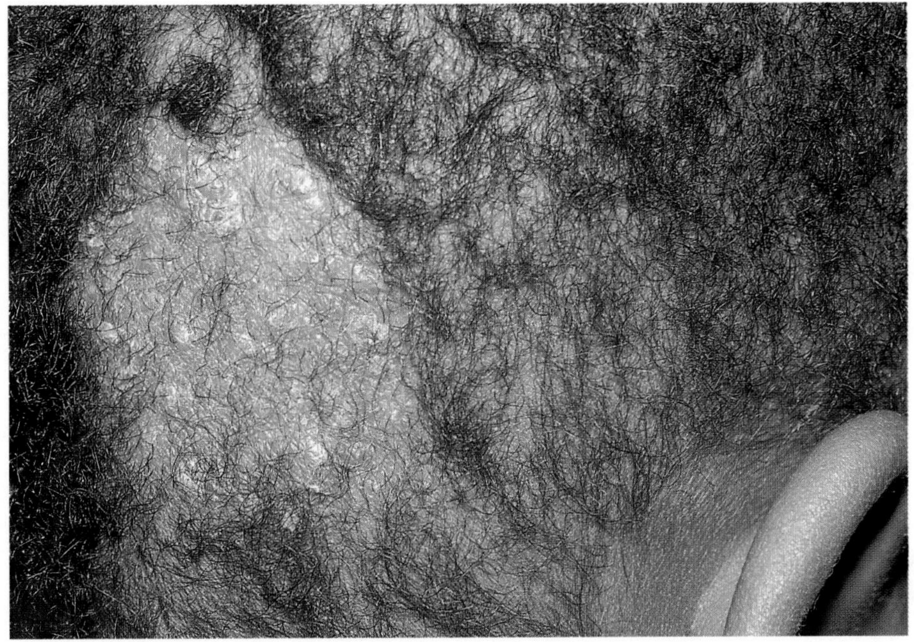

Figure 14.10 Tinea capitis is almost the only cause of scale and hair loss in children; borders are usually well defined.

Figure 14.11 Some dermatophytes create remarkable inflammation, resulting in a kerion. This crusted plaque can easily scar and produce permanent hair loss unless the child receives prednisone as well as an oral antifungal medication initially. (Photograph courtesy of Ronald C. Hansen, MD, Tucson, Arizona)

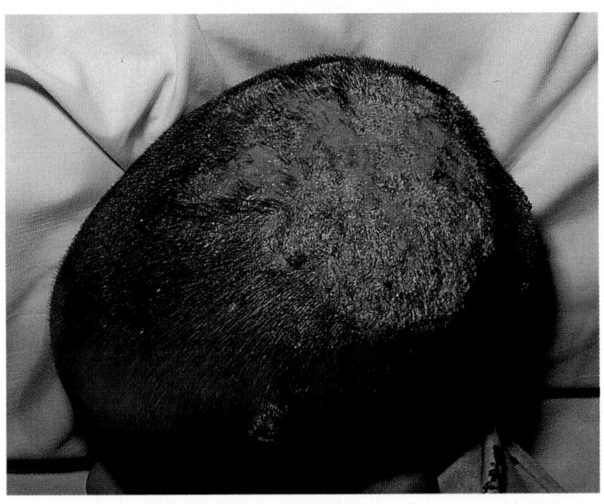

Tinea pedis and manum are most often confused with, and often coexist with, neurodermatitis/eczema. Typically, the borders of tinea are well demarcated, whereas those of dermatitis are poorly demarcated. Often, however, this distinction cannot be made without positive fungal smears or cultures.

Tinea faciei can resemble chronic cutaneous (discoid) lupus erythematosus, but the latter disease usually has several associated lesions. Sarcoidosis, seborrheic dermatitis, and actinic keratoses can also appear similar to tinea faciei.

Tinea capitis is by far the most common cause of well-demarcated plaques of scale and hair loss in children. Seborrhea produces poorly demarcated areas of scale without hair loss, and psoriasis, although associated with well-demarcated scaling plaques, does not produce hair loss. The very confusing morphologic picture of local eczema with broken hairs from rubbing results in the name *tinea amiantacea.* Differentiation from true tinea infection requires a history, other areas of eczema, and, often, a fungal culture or poor response to fungal therapy.

Management Limited areas of superficial tinea infection that lack deeper hair follicle involvement can usually be treated topically. Many good antifungal therapies are available (see Ch. 3, Medical Therapy).

Clotrimazole and miconazole creams are available over the counter, and these azoles treat both dermatophyte and yeast fungi (and are therefore useful for pityriasis "tinea" versicolor as well) when applied twice a day. Other prescription azoles such as econazole and oxiconazole have the advantage of once-daily dosing for dermatophyte infections. Nystatin is not effective for tinea infections.

For widespread disease, dermatophyte infections in hairy areas, exudative disease, or plaques of tinea with papules, nodules, or pustules indicative of deeper involvement, systemic therapy is required. Even when follicular involvement is not appreciated clinically, tinea in areas of coarse hairs such as the scalp, beard area of an adult, and, sometimes, the genital area often have inapparent disease in areas not reached by topical medication. Therefore, these patients should be treated orally until the skin appears normal and without scale. Griseofulvin 500 mg PO bid for adults or 20 mg/kg/day for children, with meals, is usually effective and very safe. Although laboratory testing is not needed for patients receiving this medication, side effects of nausea, headache, or hives prevent many patients from taking griseofulvin. Second-line therapies are fluconazole (Diflucan) and itraconazole (Sporanox) at 200 mg/day for adults and 3 to 5 mg/day for children.[7]

Children with very inflammatory tinea capitis (a kerion) should receive prednisone 1 to 2 mg/kg up to 40 mg each morning for 7 to 10 days, in addition to an oral antifungal to prevent permanent scarring and alopecia. Often, the intense inflammation causes concern for bacterial superinfection as well. When in doubt, initial therapy can include cephalexin or another antistaphylococcal antibiotic. These children should be seen by a dermatologist in one week to assess the need to continue or adjust the dose of prednisone.

Course and Prognosis Very inflammatory tinea generally resolves without recurrence, as do most tinea corporis and tinea capitis. However, patients should be advised that tinea cruris and tinea pedis are likely to recur, and they should use a topical antifungal medication as needed. Those patients with tinea pedis and onychomycosis should be advised to use a topical antifungal daily, as recurrence is very likely.

TINEA CORPORIS, TINEA CRURIS, TINEA PEDIS, TINEA MANUM, TINEA CAPITIS

Clinical Manifestations

Well-demarcated, scaling plaques with peripheral scale and, often, central clearing; associated with a positive fungal smear or culture.

Management in the Emergency Department

Localized, without involvement of follicles or areas of terminal hair, without pustules or blistering

1. *Topical antifungal therapy such as clotrimazole cream (OTC) twice a day or econazole cream (prescription) once a day until clear*
2. *Patient education regarding chronicity and recurrence in the case of tinea pedis and tinea cruris (see the patient handout on p. 367, Tinea Capitis)*
3. *Follow up in one month if not clear, or in 1 to 2 weeks if worsening or not improving*

Widespread, involvement of follicles, located in areas of terminal hair, or presence of pustules or blistering

1. *Oral antifungal until clear:*
   - *Griseofulvin 500 mg bid (adults); 20 mg/kg/day (children) with meals*

   OR

   - *Fluconazole 200 mg/day (adults); 3 to 5 mg/kg/day (children)*
2. *If intensely inflamed (crusted, pustular, vesicular), add prednisone 40 mg/day (adults) or 1 mg/kg/day (children) for 1 week*
3. *Follow up with personal health care provider or dermatologist in 3 to 4 weeks if not on prednisone, or in 1 week if on prednisone*

DISEASES CHARACTERIZED BY PAPULES OR SMALL PLAQUES

Some papulosquamous diseases are characterized by smaller plaques and papules. However, most diseases can present atypically, and these diseases sometimes overlap with papulosquamous diseases that usually present with larger plaques. For example, syphilis can exhibit larger plaques, especially in patients with AIDS, and lichen planus sometimes occurs as large plaques rather than papules.

Pityriasis Rosea

Pityriasis rosea is a common disease of unknown (but perhaps viral) cause that is easily recognized when it presents in its classic form. However, pityriasis rosea can present a diagnostic dilemma when occurring in an atypical form, as it often does. The primary importance of this disease derives from its similarity to secondary syphilis.

Clinical Presentation Occurring most often in children and young adults, pityriasis rosea is asymptomatic except for itching that occurs in some people. Typical pityriasis rosea involves the trunk primarily, with extension to the proximal extremities only. The generalized eruption is often preceded by a larger (about 3- to 7-cm), often annular, scaling plaque, referred to as a *herald patch*. Even when there is no particular lesion that is identified by the patient as being first, there is often one plaque which is larger and fits this description.

The majority of the eruption consists of small (1- to 3-cm) pink, very lightly scaling, oval papules and plaques (Fig. 14.12). The long axis of the oval lies in skin lines so that lesions lie roughly parallel to each other, forming a "fir tree" or "Christmas tree" pattern. At times, the scale is nearly inapparent and can be demonstrated only by scraping the surface with a fingernail. Sometimes, lesions exhibit a peripheral rim of scale that is very typical of pityriasis rosea. Although the individual lesions are typically well demarcated, some patients (particularly those who are itchy and are scratching) exhibit papules with poorly demarcated borders.

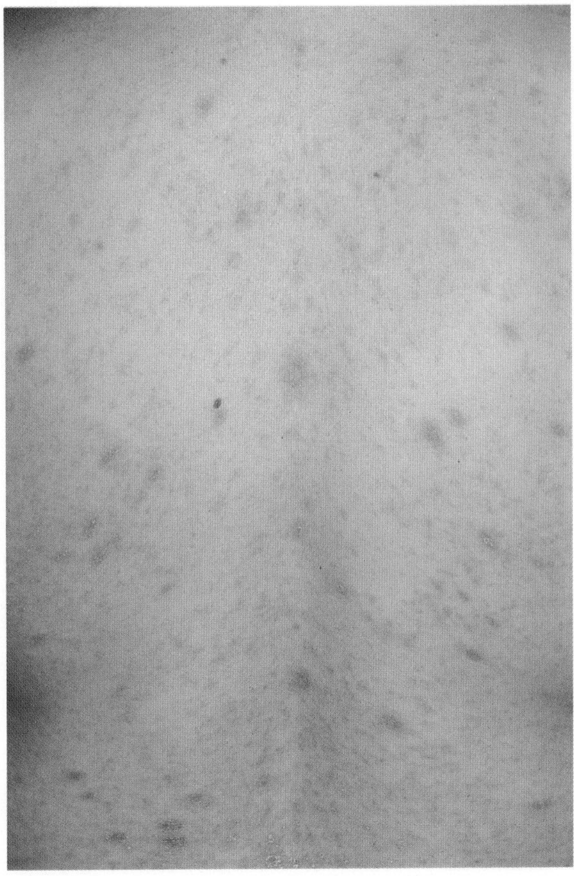

Figure 14.12 Small, oval, relatively well-demarcated papules with very subtle scale over the trunk are typical for pityriasis rosea. The long axis of the oval generally lies in natural skin lines, producing a "fir tree" pattern.

There are several well-recognized, atypical presentations of pityriasis rosea. The first is *inverse* pityriasis rosea, where distal extremities are preferentially affected with relative sparing of the trunk. A second form of pityriasis rosea is *purpuric*. This purpura does not represent serious underlying disease, but at times it must be differentiated from important causes of purpura including leukocytoclastic vasculitis. A relatively common form of pityriasis rosea, most often seen in black patients, is pityriasis rosea occurring as very small (1- to 2-mm) papules over the trunk in a distribution that appears *follicular* (Fig. 14.13). The most common typical presentation of pityriasis rosea is disease

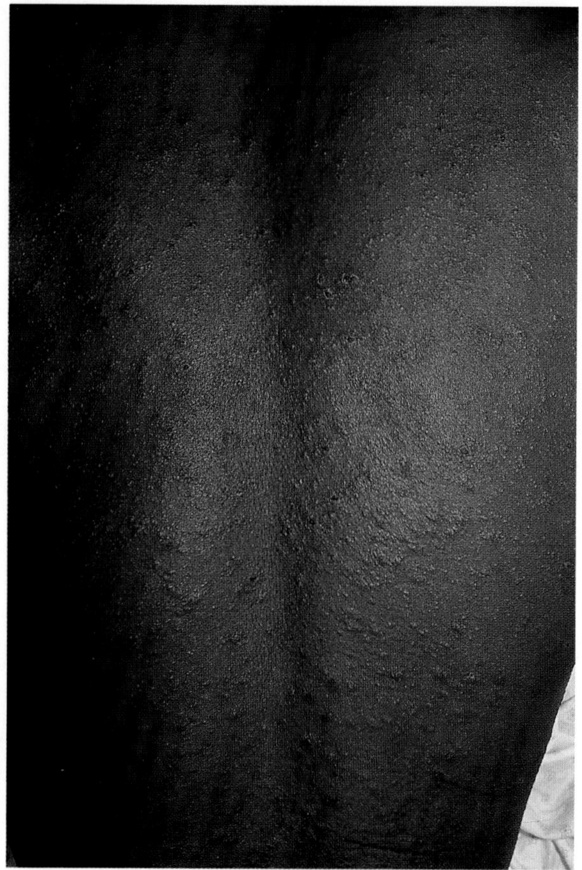

Figure 14.13 When occurring in a follicular pattern or secondarily eczematized, pityriasis rosea can be difficult to diagnose.

that has been changed by rubbing and scratching so that *secondary eczematization* coexists. As a result of scratching, borders are often poorly demarcated, scale may be more apparent, and excoriations or lichenification may be present.

Differential Diagnosis The differential diagnosis of pityriasis rosea includes other papulosquamous diseases, papular and common atopic dermatitis, and nummular eczema. Pityriasis rosea is most often confused with those papulosquamous diseases that can occur as papules or small plaques; namely, secondary syphilis, guttate psoriasis, pityriasis "tinea" versicolor, and eruptive lichen planus (Figs. 14.2, 14.12, 14.14, 14.16, and 14.18). Usually, secondary syphilis shows rounder rather than oval lesions, palmar and plantar scaling papules, and associated lymphadenopathy. However, the absence of these findings does not rule out the possibility of secondary syphilis, and most patients with pityriasis rosea should undergo syphilis serology. All patients with a rash due to secondary syphilis have positive serologies except for those occasional patients who are seronegative as a result of acquired immunodeficiency syndrome (AIDS).

Patients with generalized lichen planus are rare and usually have lesions that are darker or more violaceous in color, as well as mucous membrane disease. Those with guttate psoriasis usually exhibit silvery-white scale and nearly always show scalp disease or signs of fingernail psoriasis.

Pityriasis rosea can be indistinguishable from small plaque (digitate) parapsoriasis, a very uncommon and medically benign disease of unknown cause. Although a skin biopsy can differentiate these diseases, this is generally unnecessary initially, since a diagnosis of parapsoriasisis is only entertained when the eruption fails to remit as expected.

There are reports of pityriasis rosea-like eruptions occurring with some medications, especially those also reported to cause lichenoid (lichen planus-like) eruptions. These include captopril, gold, D-penicillamine, barbiturates, and metronidazole.[8–10]

In predisposed patients, pityriasis rosea produces itching and precipitates an itch–scratch cycle that results in secondary eczematization. If a typical lesion of pityriasis rosea cannot be found after a careful search, patients can be treated with a topical corticosteroid and reevaluated several days later when the eczematous component has improved.

Management There is no effective treatment for pityriasis rosea, but patients with pruritus benefit from symptomatic therapy. A midpotency topical corticosteroid such as triamcinolone 0.1% (for adults) or hydrocortisone 1% (for children) in conjunction with moisturization often decreases itching substantially. Nighttime sedation also can help itching and permit patients to sleep. Exposure to natural sunlight or ultraviolet B wavelength light hastens resolution.[11]

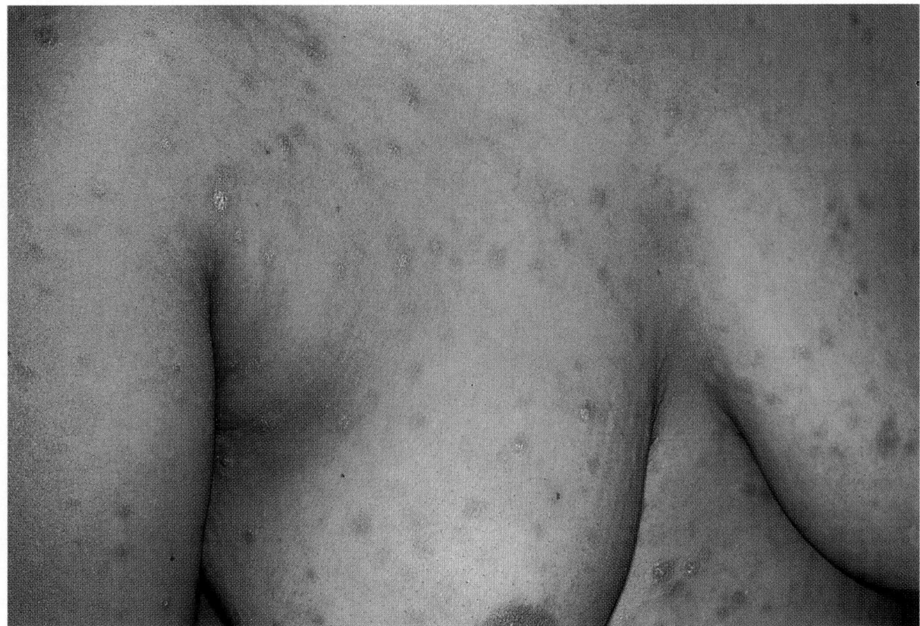

Figure 14.14 Secondary syphilis, as in this patient, can appear identical to pityriasis rosea. Nearly every patient with pityriasis rosea should undergo syphilis serology testing.

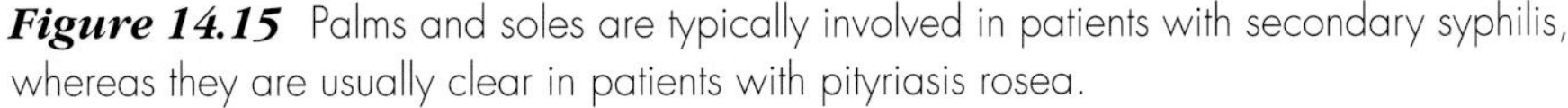

Figure 14.15 Palms and soles are typically involved in patients with secondary syphilis, whereas they are usually clear in patients with pityriasis rosea.

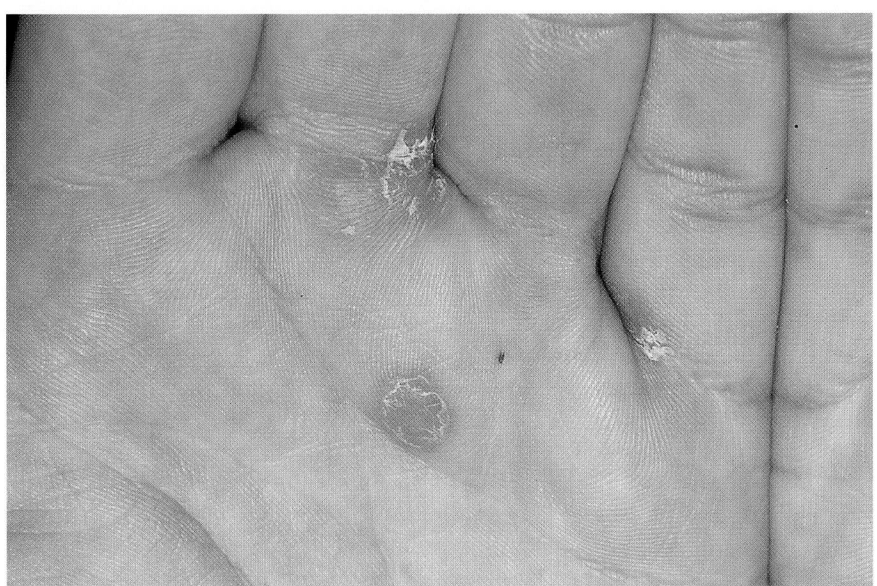

Course and Prognosis Pityriasis rosea generally resolves spontaneously in 1 to 2 months. Those patients with apparent pityriasis rosea continuing longer than 3 or 4 months nearly always have small plaque (digitate) parapsoriasis.

APITYRIASIS ROSEA

Clinical Manifestations

Pink, lightly scaling, oval papules with long axis in skin lines of the trunk; often accompanied by a larger, sometimes annular "herald patch." Palm and sole lesions, but lymphadenopathy usually absent. Negative syphilis serology.

Management in the Emergency Department

1. *Venereal Disease Research Laboratories (VDRL) or rapid plasma reagin (RPR)*
2. *Reassurance and patient education (see the patient handout on p. 354, Pityriasis Rosea)*
3. *If itchy, triamcinolone ointment 0.1% (adults) or hydrocortisone 1% or 2.5% (children), and nighttime diphenhydramine, hydroxyzine HCl, or amitriptyline at sedating doses of 25 to 75 mg*
4. *Exposure to natural sunlight may hasten resolution*
5. *No follow-up visits necessary unless eruption fails to resolve in 2 to 3 months*

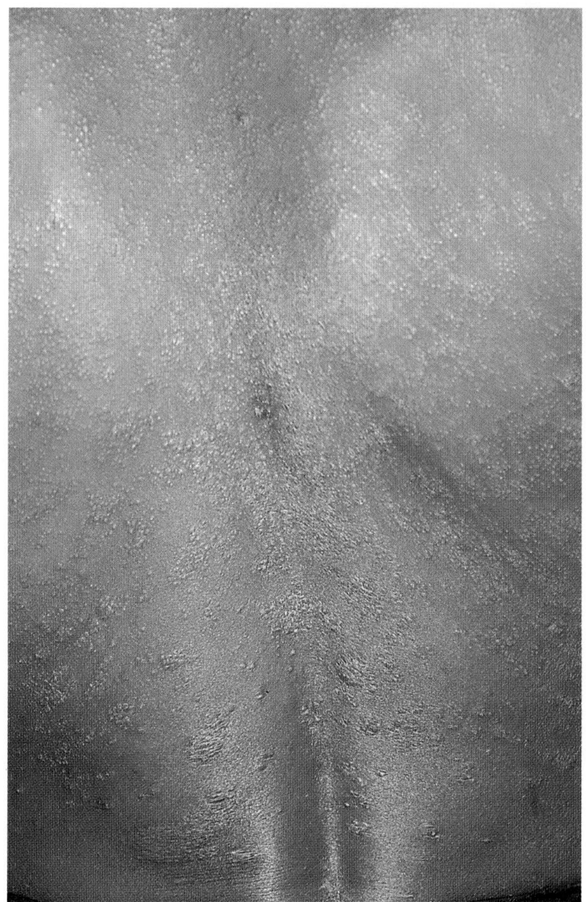

Figure 14.16 Rubbing and scratching can produce lesions of secondary syphilis that are less well demarcated than usual. Some patients, particularly black patients, exhibit tiny scattered papules that appear follicular. Typical lesions over the lower back of this patient suggest a (correct) diagnosis of secondary syphilis, or perhaps pityriasis rosea.

Secondary Syphilis (Lues)

Although often unimpressive clinically, the lesions of secondary syphilis are the most important to differentiate from other papulosquamous diseases in the emergency department. Even without treatment, these lesions disappear, but the infection may remain in a latent form and produce late, life-threatening disease.

Clinical Manifestations Although secondary syphilis can present with any of several different types of lesions, the most common are small, pink, relatively well-demarcated scaling papules. These are scattered over the skin surface, including the palms, soles, and face (Figs. 14.14 and 14.15). When prompted, many patients remember, the genital ulcer of a chancre in the recent past. Others have no such recollection, particularly women who may have had vaginal or cervical lesions.

Sometimes, the papules of secondary syphilis are infiltrated and display only minimal scale, mimicking sarcoidosis. Secondary syphilis can also present as annular papules and plaques, particularly around the mouth. Not infrequently, individual lesions in black skin may be very small and appear follicular (Fig. 14.16). Patients with AIDS may exhibit larger, infiltrated, crusted plaques similar to psoriasis.

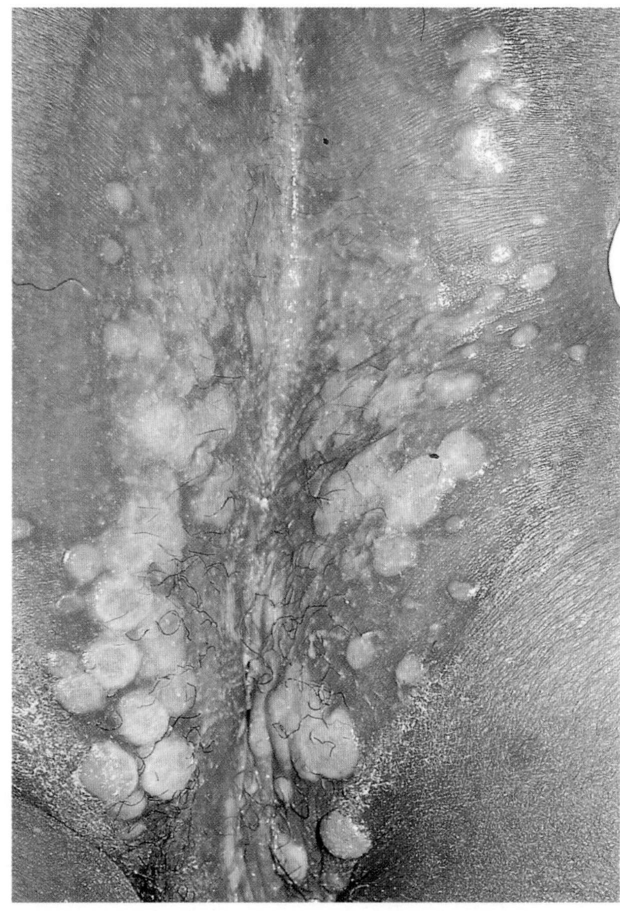

Figure 14.17 These white and skin-colored, flat-topped, moist papules over the vulva and perianal region are typical of condylomata lata, lesions specific for secondary syphilis.

In addition to the generalized rash, some patients with secondary syphilis have patchy hair loss, white papules over the oral mucosa, and the skin-colored or white, infiltrated, flat-topped papules of condylomata lata (Fig. 14.17). Most patients with secondary syphilis exhibit generalized lymphadenopathy.

Differential Diagnosis The most common disease that resembles secondary syphilis is pityriasis rosea (see Figs. 14.12 and 14.13). These diseases can be nearly identical in presentation. However, patients with pityriasis rosea generally do not have lesions on face, palms, or soles, and they usually lack lymphadenopathy. In addition, the lesions of secondary syphilis are not oval but rather round and more haphazardly distributed and oriented, lacking the distinctive "fir tree" pattern of pityriasis rosea. Sometimes, guttate psoriasis and eruptive lichen planus can also be indistinguishable from secondary syphilis (Figs. 14.2 and 14.18).

The more infiltrative and less scaling papules of secondary syphilis can be indistinguishable from sarcoidosis, and even a biopsy can show a similar granulomatous picture. The fine papular pattern of secondary syphilis can be indistinguishable from a follicular pattern of pityriasis rosea, and it can be very similar to that of papular atopic dermatitis. The annular form of secondary syphilis can usually be distinguished from other common, annular diseases such as tinea corporis and annular subacute cutaneous lupus erythematosus by the very indurated nature of the lesions and scattered distribution.

Fortunately, syphilis serology is uniformly positive in patients with a skin lesion with the rare exception of some patients with AIDS.

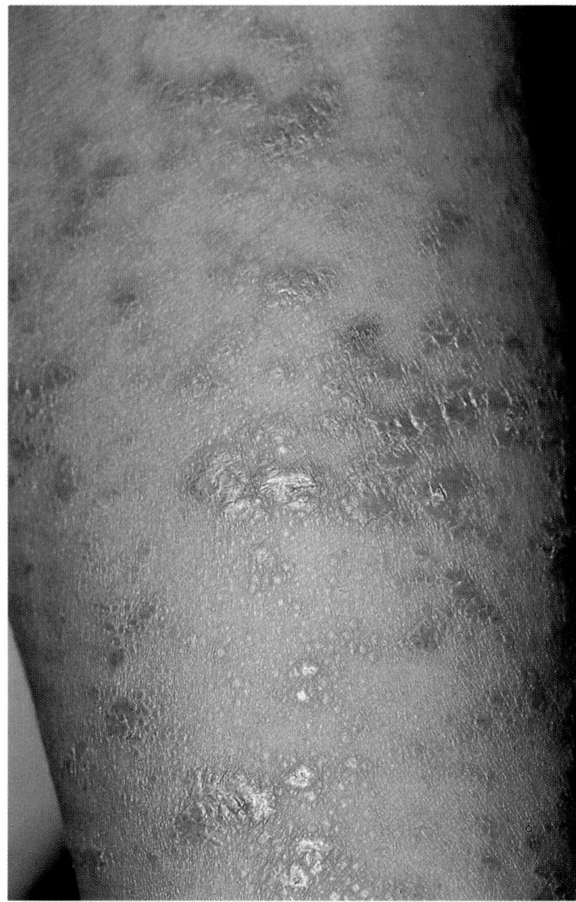

Figure 14.18 Eruptive lichen planus is unusual, but it can also mimic guttate psoriasis, secondary syphilis and pityriasis rosea (cf. Figs. 14.2, 14.12, and 14.14).

Management The treatment of choice for secondary syphilis is penicillin. Benzathine penicillin G (L-A Bicillin) 2.4 million units is administered intramuscularly once. Some patients experience a Jarisch-Herxheimer reaction with fever and chills soon after treatment, with resolution within 1 or 2 days. Those patients allergic to penicillin can be treated with tetracycline or erythromycin at 500 mg qid, or doxycycline 100 mg bid for 2 weeks.

Patients with the acquired immunodeficiency syndrome are less likely than immunocompetent patients to have a fourfold decrease in RPR titer to show an adequate response to therapy after four months.[12] Therefore, some clinicians treat patients with secondary syphilis and HIV disease with benzathine penicillin G 2.4 MU IM weekly for 3 weeks; careful follow-up management is especially important.

Patients with secondary syphilis who have been treated should be followed up in about three months either with their primary care physician, their dermatologist, or at the health department. Many patients with this diagnosis are reluctant to follow up with their personal physician. Serology should be repeated at that time to ensure a loss of positivity or at least a sustained fourfold drop in titer.

Course and Prognosis The lesions of secondary syphilis resolve whether or not the patient is treated. Without therapy, the rash disappears in one to three months. About 25% of untreated patients experience at least one recurrence of secondary syphilis. When the signs of secondary syphilis abate, untreated patients enter a latent phase, and 15 to 40% develop tertiary syphilis.[13]

With proper therapy, the eruption resolves quickly. Infection is not protective against subsequent syphilis infection.

SECONDARY SYPHILIS

Clinical Manifestations

Scattered, lightly scaling, round and oval papules that affect trunk, extremities, palms and soles, as well as the face. Usually associated with lymphadenopathy, and sometimes associated with white mucous patches and condylomata lata. Annular, scaling papules may occur, and infiltrated papulonodules may also occur. Positive VDRL or RPR.

Management in the Emergency Department

1. *Benzathine penicillin 2.4 MU IM (if allergic to penicillin, tetracycline or erythromycin 500 mg qid or doxycycline 100 mg bid for 2 weeks)*
2. *Serology for human immunodeficiency virus, and screen for other sexually transmitted diseases*
3. *Patient education (see the patient handout on p. 365, Syphilis)*
4. *Follow up in 3 months with health department or personal physician for repeat serology to confirm adequate treatment*
5. *Report occurrence to Health Department*

Lichen Planus

Lichen planus is a disease of probable autoimmune origin that exhibits widely variable symptoms and appearance.

Clinical Manifestations The lesions of lichen planus vary widely, depending partly upon location. In its classic form, lichen planus presents as small, flat-topped, shiny papules, most often over the inner wrists. The shiny color is indicative of adherent, lichenoid scale, although occasionally the scale may be flaky. The lesions are generally well-demarcated and pink or red with lavender or purple hues (Fig. 14.18 and 14.19). However, lichen planus in black patients often shows primarily deep brown-black hyperpigmentation. Because lichen planus exhibits the Koebner phenomenon (the tendency of a skin disease to occur or worsen in areas of injury), a careful search occasionally reveals irregular or linear lesions produced by trauma as minor as a scratch. Individual lesions that have resolved often leave striking hyperpigmentation in all skin types.

Lichen planus can appear anywhere and everywhere. When occurring over the shins, it is especially likely to be itchy. Scratching worsens the disease and extends the area of involvement into larger plaques, again due to the Koebner phenomenon. Scratching also produces excoriations, more obvious scale, and poorly demarcated borders, so that underlying lichen planus is obscured by changes which are more characteristic of eczema. In these cases, a high index of suspicion, the purplish color, and a poor response to therapy for eczema can suggest to the careful examiner that a biopsy is indicated. Less frequent morphologic variations of lichen planus may occur, the most common being *hypertrophic* lichen planus. In this case, lesions are unusually thick and sometimes nodular, occasionally with hyperkeratosis. Occasionally, *eruptive* lichen planus occurs, with uncountable, widespread lesions (see Fig. 14.18). Lichen planus occasionally affects the scalp and presents with erythema and scale/crust around

Figure 14.19 Classic lichen planus is manifested by purplish, shiny, flat-topped, well-demarcated papules. The surface sometimes shows overlying white discoloration or striae.

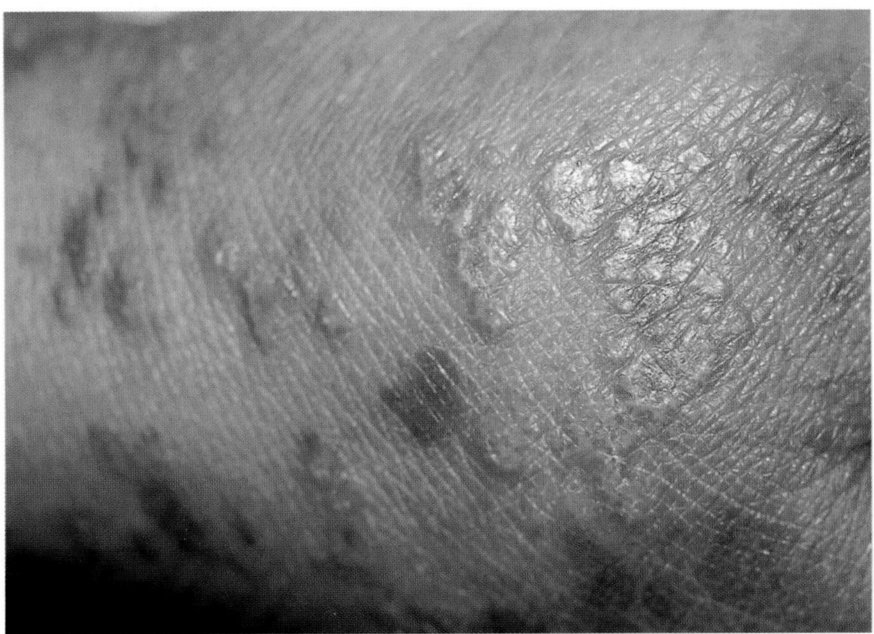

each follicle (*lichen planopilaris*). Gradually, scarring and permanent hair loss occur. Other, rarer forms of lichen planus include *atrophic* (thinned) and *bullous* disease.

Even mucous membranes can be affected. The appearance of lichen planus when it occurs on mucous membranes is quite different, and consists of white lesions and/or erosions (see Chapters 9 and 17). The white lesions of papular lichen planus generally occur in a reticulate, lacy, or fern-like pattern (see Fig. 9.8). Erosive mucosal lichen planus sometimes presents as nonspecific, superficial erosions. Often, however, surrounding white, frequently streaky, epithelium typical of papular lichen planus enables the clinician to make the correct diagnosis. The posterior buccal mucosa is the most commonly affected mucous membrane surface. However, lichen planus (particularly erosive disease) can also affect the gingiva, and both papular and erosive lichen planus are sometimes found on the tongue and on both the keratinized and unkeratinized aspects of the lips (see Fig. 17.9).

Both the keratinized skin and the mucous membrane portion of the genitalia are sometimes affected with lichen planus also. The glans penis is a common site, usually showing pink, well-demarcated, flat-topped papules and plaques, although erosive lesions with scarring can occur. Both white lesions and erosions similar to those found in the mouth occur over the vulva and vagina. Patients with erosive vulvovaginal disease usually have oral involvement as well, but they lack lichen planus of the keratinized epithelium.

Differential Diagnosis Other papulosquamous diseases are in the differential diagnosis of lichen planus. Psoriasis can usually be distinguished by its silvery scale but, especially when partially treated or moisturized, the appearance may be very similar. Lichen planus is far less likely to exhibit scalp disease and nail changes, and the occasional presence of pathognomonic mucous membrane lesions is usually helpful in distinguishing this disease from psoriasis. Chronic cutaneous (discoid) lupus erythematosus and fungal infections can occasionally be confused with lichen planus. Pityriasis rosea, secondary syphilis, and guttate psoriasis can resemble eruptive lichen planus.

A lichenoid medication reaction can be indistinguishable from lichen planus, with differentiation made by a history of medication ingestion. Any patient with lichen planus should be questioned for exposure to gold, antimalarial medications including hydroxychloroquine, thiazide diuretics, tetracycline, phenothiazines, chlorpropamide, penicillamine, propranolol, captopril, levamisole, or furosemide.[14]

When scale is subtle, lichen planus can be confused with granuloma annulare and sarcoidosis.

Therapy First-line therapy for lichen planus is topical corticosteroids. Usually, a midpotency or high-potency topical corticosteroid such as triamcinolone 0.1% (Kenalog, Aristocort) or fluocinonide 0.05% (Lidex) cream or ointment on keratinized skin is indicated. Although topical steroids often improve itching and flatten individual lesions somewhat, they do not produce resolution of the underlying disease process.

Mucosal lesions are more difficult to treat topically. Although creams are sometimes used in the mouth, gels, solutions (sometimes under damp cotton ball occlusion), or Kenalog in Orabase are preferred in this area. The genital mucosa is generally intolerant of gels, solutions, and Orabase so that ointments or creams should be used for vulvovaginal and penile lichen planus. Patients with significant and painful mucosal ulcerations benefit from oral prednisone at 40 to 60 mg each morning to induce healing. Systemic medication is discontinued as soon as possible and the patient maintained on topical therapy.

For limited areas of significant erosion, intralesional corticosteroids can be useful. Triamcinolone acetonide 3 to 3.3 mg/ml (TAC-3, or Kenalog 10, 1 ml, mixed with injectable saline, 2 ml) is injected around and underneath the ulcer using a 30-gauge needle. Normally only 0.1 to 1.0 ml of the mixture is required.

Oral prednisone (40 to 60 mg each morning) is sometimes useful also for eruptive lichen planus. This condition is generally self-limited, but resolution can be very slow. A short course of oral prednisone can sometimes induce faster resolution.

Options for patients who are not controlled with topical corticosteroids are limited. There are conflicting reports that suggest oral griseofulvin at 500 mg bid may be useful.[15] Topical tretinoin (Retin-A) 0.05% cream or gel is sometimes used on oral lichen planus.[16] There have also been reports of patients improving while on oral retinoids such as isotretinoin (Accutane) or etretinate (Tegison).[17] Cyclosporine (Sandimmune) applied topically to oral disease has been shown to be useful although extremely expensive.[18] The patient swishes 100 mg cyclosporine 4 times a day, holds the medicine as long as 15 minutes in the mouth, then spits, tapering the frequency as lesions improve. Other medications reported to be useful include cyclophosphamide (Cytoxan), azathioprine (Imuran), and hydroxychloroquine (Plaquenil).[19,20]

Course and Prognosis Papular lichen planus is generally self-limited, with remissions occurring in most patients in about 1 to 2 years. Those with significant itching and scratching are more likely to experience persistent disease, and erosive mucosal disease is chronic and unremitting. In rare cases, squamous cell carcinomas can arise in chronic, erosive mucosal lichen planus, so patients should be advised to keep routine follow-up appointments with their dermatologists for ongoing surveillance. In addition, severe scarring can occur over the genitalia in the presence of erosive disease, more often in women than in men. Loss of the labia minora and covering of the clitoris under scar are common consequences of erosive lichen planus. Chronic vaginal erosions may eventuate in scarring of the vaginal walls with obliteration of the vaginal space.

LICHEN PLANUS

Clinical Manifestations

Violaceous, well-demarcated, flat-topped, shiny papules with white film or striae over the surface. When appearing on mucous membranes, linear, lacy, or reticulate white striae are typical and sometimes associated with erosions or ulcerations.

Management in the Emergency Department

NONMUCOUS MEMBRANE LICHEN PLANUS

1. *Triamcinolone cream 0.1% bid*
2. *Follow up with a dermatologist in 1 month*
3. *Patient education (see the patient handouts on p. 352, Lichen Planus, and on p. 368, Topical Cortisone Creams, Ointments, and Solutions)*

(Continues)

(Continued)

ORAL MUCOSAL LESIONS: WHITE PAPULES OR MILD EROSIONS

1. *Fluocinonide 0.05% gel qid*
2. *Follow up with a dermatologist in 1 month*
3. *Patient education (see the patient handout on p. 352, Lichen Planus)*

ORAL MUCOSAL LESIONS: SEVERE EROSIONS

1. *Prednisone 40 to 60 mg each morning for 1 week*
2. *Pain control:*
   - *Oral analgesics*
   - *Topical diphenhydramine elixir or topical lidocaine jelly 2% prn*
3. *Follow-up with dermatologist in 1 week*
4. *Patient education (see the patient handout on p. 352, Lichen Planus)*

Guttate Psoriasis

Psoriasis sometimes presents with widely scattered, scaling, sharply demarcated papules, often without the typical distribution that includes the knees and elbows, and often without the typical, heavy, silvery scale (see Fig. 14.2). A discussion of this pattern, called guttate psoriasis, is included in the first section of this chapter on psoriasis.

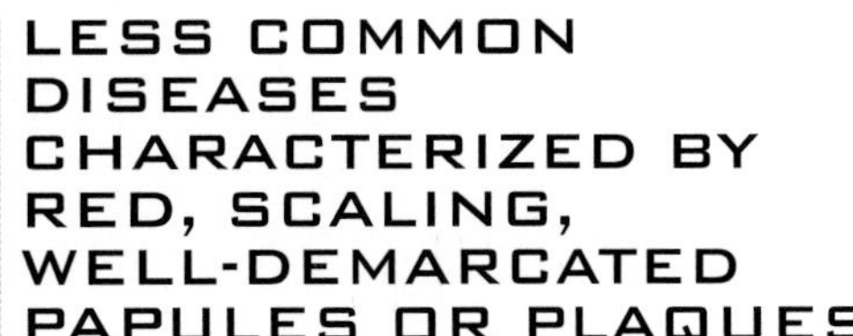

LESS COMMON DISEASES CHARACTERIZED BY RED, SCALING, WELL-DEMARCATED PAPULES OR PLAQUES

Pityriasis Rubra Pilaris

Pityriasis rubra pilaris is an uncommon disease that begins as follicular, red, scaling papules that coalesce into plaques that cover most of the body. Classic morphologic features include well-demarcated islands of normal skin within plaques of pityriasis rubra pilaris, and an orange hue to the inflammation of lesions. Remarkable scalp involvement is usual, and hyperkeratosis of the palms and soles are regular features. Topical corticosteroids, oral methotrexate, and oral retinoids such as isotretinoin (Accutane) and etretinate (Tegison) are the most common therapies. Generally, pityriasis rubra pilaris remits spontaneously within about 3 years.

Parapsoriasis

Parapsoriasis is an uncommon group of diseases of unknown cause. There are two main forms. The first is small-plaque (digitate) parapsoriasis, morphologically consisting of pink, oval, lightly scaling papules over the trunk, often indistinguishable from pityriasis rosea except for its chronic course. For those wishing therapy, topical corticosteroids can improve itching, and PUVA (oral psoralens followed by UVA light) can improve the eruption. Methotrexate can also be used, but this is not appropriate in the emergency department.

The second form of parapsoriasis consists of larger plaques, and presages the development of cutaneous T-cell lymphoma (mycosis fungoides). This is a disease of older patients that, because of its gradual onset and minimal symptoms, does not usually present to an emergency department. Skin lesions are primarily truncal and consist of thin, finely scaling, dusky pink, and often overlapping plaques. These plaques gradually become either more infiltrative, or exhibit the finding of poikiloderma (thinning, mottled hyperpigmentation, telangiectasias) heralding transformation into mycosis fungoides (Fig. 14.20). The therapy of large plaque parapsoriasis consists of topical corticosteroids for itching and PUVA, or oral psoralens and UVA light therapy (see above, under Management of Psoriasis). PUVA is also beneficial for mycosis fungoides, as are topical nitrogen mustard, electron beam therapy, and oral retinoids such as isotretinoin.[21]

Figure 14.20 These large, overlapping, thin, brown-pink plaques of cutaneous T-cell lymphoma (mycosis fungoides) in this patient began as pink, lightly scaling plaques.

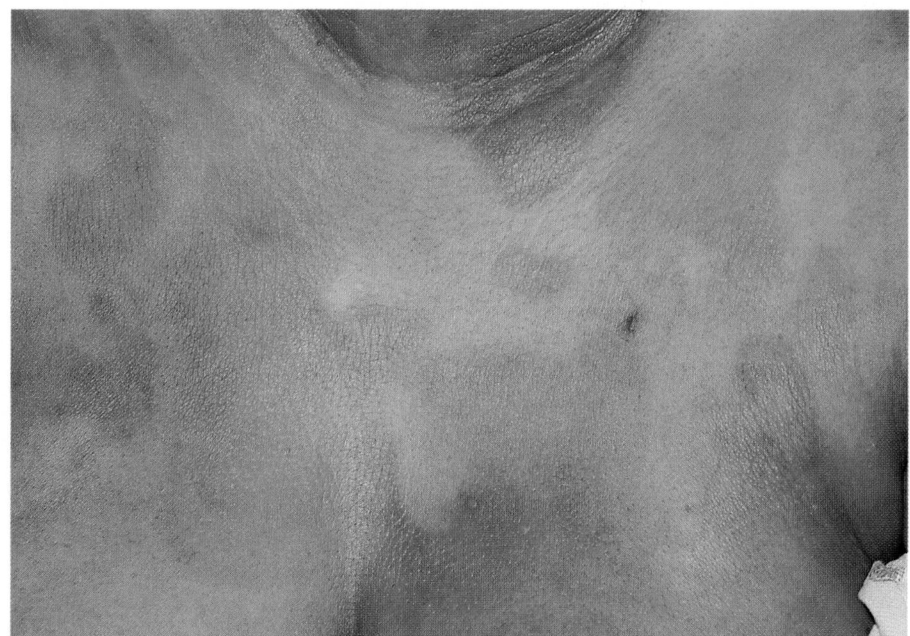

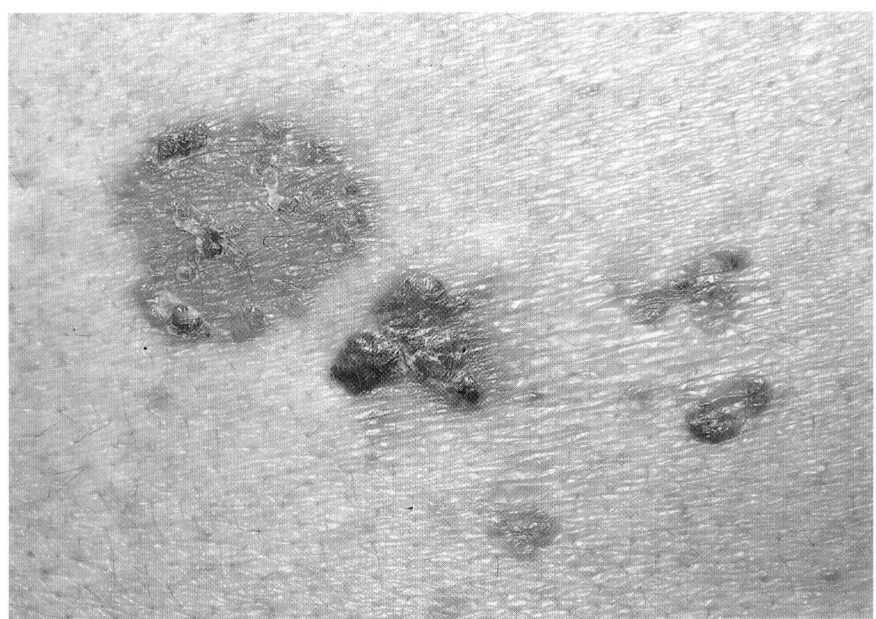

Figure 14.21 Superficial basal cell carcinomas present as scaling, well-demarcated papules or plaques. Shown here also are pigmented basal cell carcinomas, which can mimic melanoma.

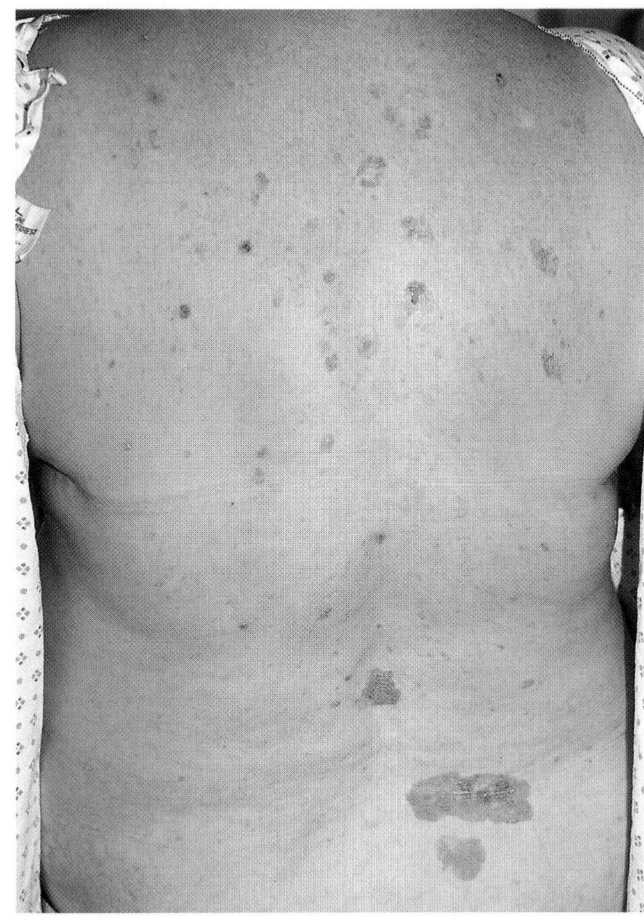

Figure 14.22 Bowen's disease, or squamous cell carcinoma in situ, is manifested as red, sharply demarcated, scaling, and sometimes hyperkeratotic papules or plaques.

Other Skin Malignancies

Several other skin malignancies also can mimic inflammatory papulosquamous disease. *Superficial basal cell carcinomas* are sharply demarcated, lightly scaling, rough, or thinned papules (Fig. 14.21). *Bowen's disease* (squamous cell carcinoma in situ) is also a scaling, well-marginated, red lesion (Fig. 14.22). These malignancies are usually single or few in number and do not have associated features suggestive of other common papulosquamous diseases. They may even improve slightly with a topical corticosteroid, but significant and long-lasting improvement does not occur. The diagnoses are by skin biopsy since these skin cancers are most often flesh colored (for detailed discussion of these lesions, see Ch. 8, Skin-Colored Lesions).

Paget's disease, a low-grade malignancy of probable apocrine gland origin, is manifested by an inflammatory, scaling or glistening, well-demarcated plaque or plaques over the breast or perineum/genitalia. When present over the breast, it is a sensitive and predictable sign of underlying breast cancer. When occurring in the genital area, an underlying genitourinary malignancy is sometimes, but not always, present. The diagnosis is by skin biopsy.

Please see patient information handouts for this chapter on pages 337, 352, 354, 358, 365, and 367.

REFERENCES

1. Stern RS: The epidemiology of joint complaints in patients with psoriasis. J Rheumatol 12:315, 1985
2. Zanolli MD: Joint complaints in psoriasis patients. Int J Dermatol 31:488,1992
3. Kragballe K: Treatment of psoriasis with calcipotriol and other vitamin D analogues. J Am Acad Dermatol 27:1001, 1992
4. Mrowietz U, Farger L, Henneicke-von Zepelin H-H et al: Long-term maintenance therapy with cyclosporine and posttreatment survey in severe psoriasis: results of a multicenter study. J Am Acad Dermatol 33:470, 1995
5. Skinner RB Jr, Rosenberg EW, Noah PW: Antimicrobial treatment of psoriasis. Dermatol Clin 13:909, 1995
6. Newton RC, Jorizzo JL, Solomon AJ et al: Mechanism-oriented assessment of isotretinoin in chronic or subacute cutaneous lupus erythematosus. Arch Dermatol 122:170, 1986
7. Elewski BE, Weil ML: Dermatophytes and superficial fungi. p. 155. In Sams WM Jr, Lynch PJ (eds): Principles and Practice of Dermatology. 2nd Ed. Churchill Livingstone, New York, 1996
8. Wilkin JK, Kirkendall WM: Pityriasis rosea-like eruption from captopril. Arch Dermatol 118: 186, 1982
9. Corke CF, Meyrick TR, Huskisson EC et al: Pityriasis rosea-like rashes complicating drug therapy for rheumatoid arthritis. Br J Rheumatol 22:187, 1983
10. Milikan LE: Drug eruptions (dermatitis medicamentosa). p. 432. In Moschella SL, Hurley HJ (eds): Dermatology. 2nd Ed. WB Saunders, Philadelphia, 1985
11. Fitzpatrick TG, Johnson RA, Polano MK et al: Pityriasis rosea. p. 58. In Color Atlas and Synopsis of Clinical Dermatology: Common and Serious Diseases. 2nd Ed. McGraw-Hill, New York, 1992
12. Yinnon AM et al: Serologic response to treatment of syphilis in patients with HIV infection. Arch Intern Med 156:321, 1996
13. Sanchez M, Luger AFH: Syphilis. p. 2703. In Fitzpatrick TB, Eisen AZ, Wolff K, Freedberg IM, Austen KF (eds): Dermatology in General Medicine. 4th Ed. McGraw-Hill, New York, 1993
14. Blacker KL, Stern RS, Wintroub BU: Cutaneous reactions to drugs. p. 1783. In Fitzpatrick TB, Eisen AZ, Wolff K, Freedberg IM, Austen KF (eds): Dermatology in General Medicine. 4th Ed. McGraw-Hill, New York, 1993
15. Massa MC, Rogers RS III: Griseofulvin therapy in lichen planus. Acta Derm Venereol (Stockh) 61:547, 1981
16. Giustina TA, Stewart JCB, Ellis CN et al: Topical application of isotretinoin gel improves oral lichen planus. Arch Dermatol 122:534, 1986

17. Laurberg, G, Geiger JM, Hjorth N et al: Treatment of lichen planus with acitretin: a double-blind, placebo-controlled study in 65 patients. J Am Acad Dermatol 24:434, 1991
18. Eisen D, Ellis CN, Duell EA et al: Effect of topical cyclosporine rinse on oral lichen planus. N Engl J Med 323:290, 1990
19. Paslin DA: Sustained remission of generalized lichen planus induced by cyclophosphamide. Arch Dermatol 121:236, 1985
20. Eisen D: Hydroxychloroquine sulfate (Plaquenil) improves oral lichen planus: an open trial. J Am Acad Dermatol 28:609, 1993
21. Holloway DB, Flowers FP, Ramos-Caro FA: Therapeutic alternatives in cutaneous T-cell lymphoma. J Am Acad Dermatol 27:367, 1992

SUGGESTED READINGS

Psoriasis

Boyd AS, Menter A: Erythrodermic psoriasis. Precipitating factors, course, and prognosis in 50 patients. J Am Acad Dermatol 21:985, 1989

Lebwohl M, Zanolli M (eds): Psoriasis. Dermatol Clin 13:717, 1995

Zelickson BD, Muller SA: Generalized pustular psoriasis. A review of 63 cases. Arch Dermatol 127:1339, 1991

Cutaneous Lupus Erythematosus

Callen JP: Treatment of cutaneous lesions in patients with lupus erythematosus. Dermatol Clin 8:355, 1990

Lee LA: Lupus erythematosus. p. 581. In Sams WM Jr, Lynch PJ (eds): Principles and Practice of Dermatology. 2nd Ed. Churchill Livingstone, New York, 1996

Sontheimer RD, Euwer RL, Geppert TD, Cohen SB: Connective tissue disease. p. 1217. In Moschella SL, Hurley HJ (eds): Dermatology. 3rd Ed. WB Saunders, Philadelphia, 1992

Fungal Infections

Faergemann J, Gothenburg S: *Pityrosporum* infections. J Am Acad Dermatol 31:S18, 1991

Hay RJ: Treatment of dermatomycoses and onychomycoses—state of the art. Clin Exp Dermatol, suppl. 17:2, 1992

Honig PJ, Caputo GL, Leyden JJ et al: Treatment of kerions. Pediatr Dermatol 11:69, 1994

Rippon JW: Forty four years of dermatophytes in a Chicago clinic (1944–1980). Mycopathologia 119:25, 1992

Smith EB: Topical antifungal drugs in the treatment of tinea pedis, tinea cruris, and tinea corporis. J Am Acad Dermatol 28:S24, 1993

Pityriasis Rosea

Allen RA, Janniger CK, Schwartz RA: Pityriasis rosea. Cutis 56:198, 1995

Parsons JM: Pityriasis rosea update: 1986. J Am Acad Dermatol 15:159, 1986

Secondary Syphilis

Hira SK, Patel JS, Bhat SG et al: Clinical manifestations of syphilis. Int J Dermatol 26:103, 1987

Hook EW III, Marra CM: Acquired syphilis in adults. N Engl J Med 326:1060, 1992

Lichen Planus

Boyd AS, Neldner KH: Lichen planus. J Am Acad Dermatol 25:593, 1991

Irvine C, Irvine F, Champion RH: Long-term follow-up of lichen planus. Acta Derm Venereol (Stockh) 71:242, 1991

Parapsoriasis/Mycosis Fungoides

Lorincz AL: Cutaneous T-cell lymphoma (mycosis fungoides). Lancet. 1:871, 1996

CHAPTER 15

Eczematous Diseases

Eczema and dermatitis are interchangeable terms that are defined on the basis of their morphology. Eczema consists of poorly demarcated inflamed plaques that exhibit evidence of scratching in the form of excoriations or lichenification (i.e., thickening of the epithelium in response to rubbing). Most of the diseases in this group are forms of atopic dermatitis, including neurodermatitis, lichen simplex chronicus, neurotic excoriations, and prurigo nodules. However, this group comprises several other unrelated diseases, including seborrheic dermatitis, allergic contact dermatitis, and nummular eczema.

ATOPIC DERMATITIS

Pruritus is the hallmark of atopic eczema. Therefore, the rash of eczema is characterized by evidence of scratching and rubbing. Sometimes, eczema is called "the itch that rashes" because itching precipitates the scratching that produces the rash. Although atopic dermatitis does not result from an allergy to a specific antigen, it generally does occur in atopic patients; that is, in patients with an allergic diathesis. These patients usually have a personal or family history of allergic rhinitis, asthma, or food, or drug allergies.[1] For these patients, irritation is often perceived as an itch, rather than as pain or soreness.[2] In addition, scratching is exquisitely pleasurable to atopic people, so that the combination of itching and pleasure upon scratching produces an itch-scratch cycle that perpetuates the disease.

Clinical Manifestations

The skin lesions of eczema are produced by rubbing and scratching, and the appearance may differ from one patient to the next. Patients who predominantly scratch exhibit poorly demarcated, red, scaling plaques with excoriations (Figs. 15.1 and 15.2). Patients who predominantly rub their itchy skin develop thickened skin with accentuation of normal skin markings, producing a texture that resembles elephant hide. This change is called lichenification (Fig. 15.3). Although lichenified skin sometimes appears to lack scale, scale is present but subtle. Lichenoid scale is closely adherent to underlying epithelium, and the absence of air between the scale and skin confers a shiny, rather than scaling, appearance.

A variant that is common in black skin, particularly the skin of small children, is papular atopic dermatitis. Papular eczema is composed of tiny, monomorphous, follicular, shiny (with lichenoid scale) papules that may represent lichenification of the follicles (Fig. 15.4). In black skin, eczema often produces apparent hyperpigmentation, rather than the erythema that occurs in lighter skin. In reality, inflammation is often marked, only appearing as hyperpigmentation because of the natural brown color of the skin (Figs. 15.3 and 15.4).

Eczema exists on a wide spectrum of severity. When disease is widespread, it is generally referred to as *atopic dermatitis*. When plaques are localized and scratching is influenced by stress and habit, as well as response to inflammation, the lesions are termed *neurodermatitis* (Fig. 15.5). Some patients, especially those with stronger components of stress and habit, not only scratch, but also pick. These *neurotic excoriations* are manifested by linear erosions with minimal surrounding inflammation and scale (see Fig. 17.12). No "primary" lesions are present, meaning that all lesions are picked. When one or a few lichenified, rather than excoriated, plaques are present, the process is referred to as *lichen simplex chronicus* (Fig. 15.6). Some patients rub and pick small areas, producing a lichenified

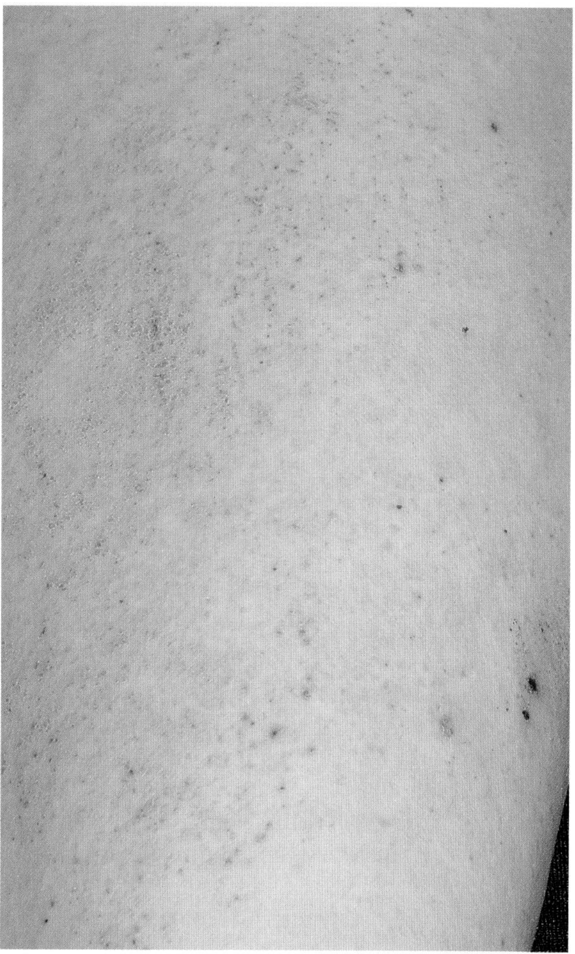

Figure 15.1 Poorly demarcated, inflamed, scaling plaques with evidence of excoriation or crusting are typical of atopic dermatitis, because the eruption is produced by rubbing or scratching.

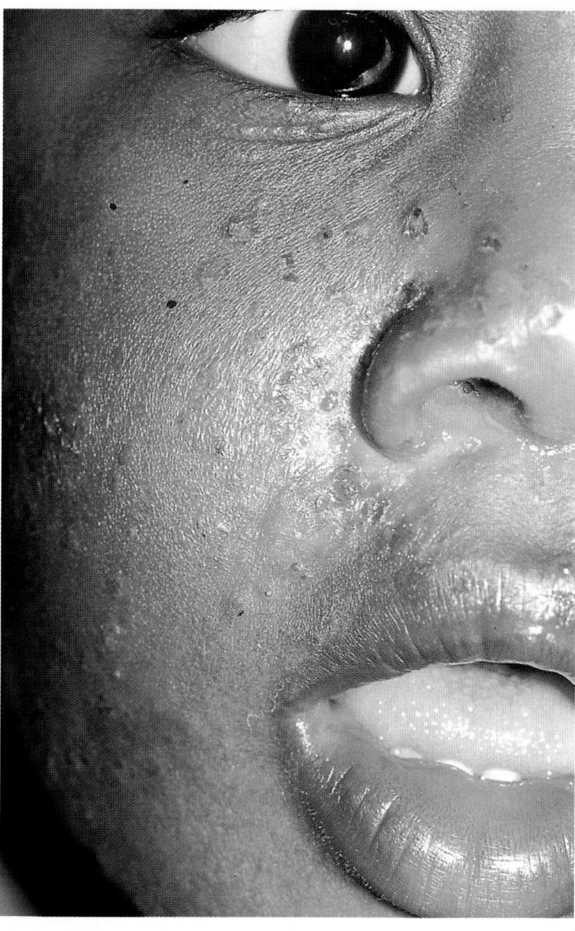

Figure 15.2 The cheeks are a common site of atopic dermatitis in babies, at least in part because the cheeks are irritated by contact with sheets. Yellow crusting is a sign of secondary staphylococcal infection.

nodule, rather than a plaque. These *prurigo nodules* are analogous to neurotic excoriations, signifying a strong component of habit and stress. Like neurotic excoriations, these lesions are found only in areas the patient can reach and they are not accompanied by primary lesions (see Fig. 8.5). Excoriated folliculitis can mimic neurotic excoriations and prurigo nodules, but a careful examination usually reveals a pustule, a red papule, or a collarette.

Although eczema can occur anywhere on the body, there is a characteristic distribution, depending on the patient's age and habits. Although newborns rarely experience atopic dermatitis, older infants develop lesions over the cheeks and extensor surfaces of the extremities first. These areas are more likely to be irritated by contact with bed clothes and are the most easily scratched by rubbing against sheets. Older children and adolescents are especially likely to have plaques of eczema over the antecubital fossae and popliteal fossae. In this age group and in adults, the most affected areas are those most easily irritated, depending on a person's activities and habits.

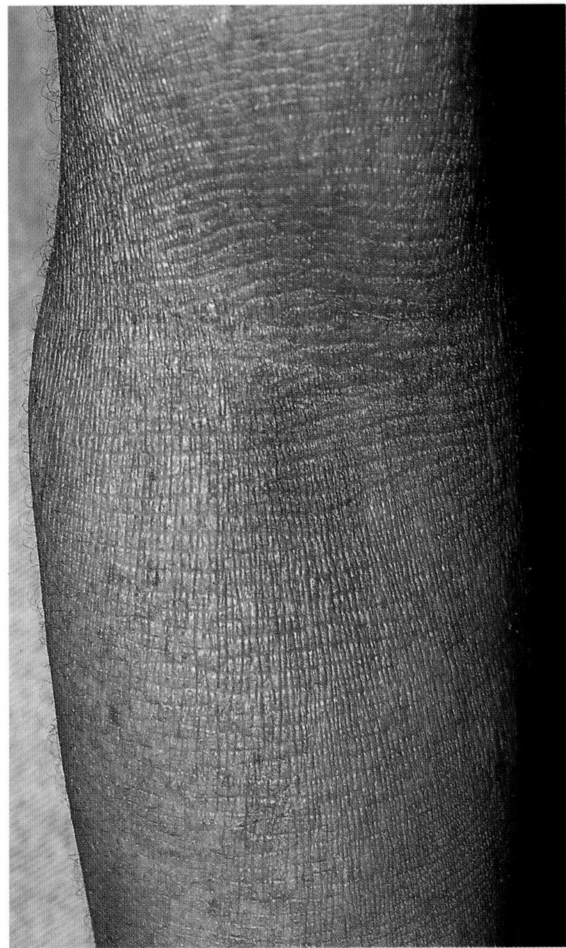

Figure 15.3 Lichenification is thickened eczema produced by rubbing. Lichenoid scale on this skin is discernible by the shiny appearance of the adherent scale. Although the skin is inflamed, it appears only hyperpigmented because the natural dark color of the skin disguises inflammation.

Differential Diagnosis

Because eczema is a red, scaling disease produced by rubbing or scratching, other red scaling diseases should be considered in the differential diagnosis. This can be especially confusing in atopic patients who may experience itching with any inflammation. Therefore, these patients sometimes scratch skin irritated by the presence of another dermatosis and produce superimposed eczema. In this event, the more symptomatic component is usually eczema, and often the eczema must be treated before the primary underlying skin disease is apparent.

The primary diseases to be differentiated from eczema are psoriasis, tinea infection, and lichen planus. When typical, these papulosquamous diseases are sharply demarcated without evidence of rubbing or scratching. When secondarily rubbed or scratched, the distinguishing characteristics may be lost. In these patients, efforts to make the diagnosis on the basis of distribution, history, character of the scale, and examination of the scalp, nails, and mouth are often extremely helpful.

Fingernail pitting, silvery scale, and elbow, knee, or scalp involvement suggest psoriasis. Violaceous color, typical oral lesions, and areas of lichenoid scale suggest lichen planus and lupus erythematosus. Pityriasis rosea is often secondarily eczematized, so that the primary papules and plaques of pityriasis rosea may be quite subtle and obscured by secondary changes. This can also be true of secondary syphilis but, because of the widespread nature of the papules and plaques of these diseases, there are usually some areas typical of the underlying disease. In addition, typical, noneczematized palm and sole lesions are often present in patients with secondary syphilis.

An extremely common problem is the differentiation of eczematized tinea (fungal eczema) from atopic eczema, particularly when the hands, feet, or genitalia are affected. Because of a minor alteration in the immunity of atopic patients, these people are more susceptible to cutaneous infections, including superficial fungal, viral, and bacterial infections.[3] Therefore, atopic patients are more likely to contract superficial fungal infections and subsequently to rub, scratch, and eczematize the area. Even for an experienced microscopist, a microscopic fungal preparation of a very inflammatory, eczematized fungal infection may produce a false-negative result simply because of the degree of inflammation. Therefore, foot eczema in association with obvious fungal nails should be treated for both eczema and fungus. In the genital area, eczema occurs primarily on the scrotum and vulva, while tinea cruris is nearly always confined to the proximal inner thighs and crural crease.

Other skin diseases that typically produce itching may precipitate eczema even in a nonatopic

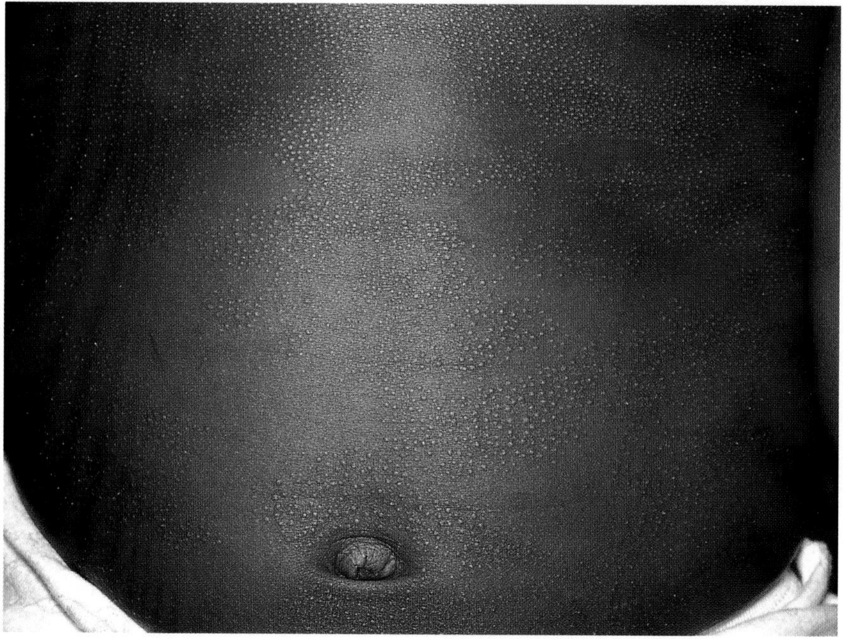

Figure 15.4 Papular atopic dermatitis is a variant particularly common in black children. Rubbing the skin preferentially lichenifies hair follicles, producing plaques of shiny, monomorphous papules.

patient. For example, the intense itching associated with scabies often produces nearby eczema. In fact, nearly all of the rash seen in patients with scabies is a result of scratching, rather than of the mite itself, since most patients with scabies have only about 10 mites over their entire skin surface. This diagnosis is suggested by the distribution, which is unusual for most other forms of eczema. Scabies preferentially affects the web spaces between fingers and the skin folds of the axilla, as well as the groin and under the breasts. The face and scalp are spared, except in infants and bedridden patients. Allergic contact dermatitis, such as that caused by poison ivy, is often prolonged by itching and scratching long after the original vesicles have disappeared. Again, history, distribution, and pattern are often useful in diagnosing these patients.

Although other, exotic diseases can sometimes mimic eczema, these are uncommon and beyond the scope of this book. None of these diseases constitutes an acute emergency and, because atopic dermatitis is a chronic disease and patients require follow-up evaluation, these diagnoses can be left to the dermatologist who evaluates recalcitrant cases.

Management

Treatment of mild and moderate eczema is fun and rewarding, particularly to the clinician, who is able to see the happy, grateful patient in follow-up. Treatment for severe eczema is an art that requires not only appropriate and sometimes aggressive medical therapy, but patience, understanding, and careful follow-up management.

The eczematous diseases are the only truly steroid-responsive skin conditions. However, a common mistake in the treatment of eczema is the dependence on corticosteroids, to the exclusion of other very important factors. For rapid and maximal benefit, topical corticosteroids must be used in

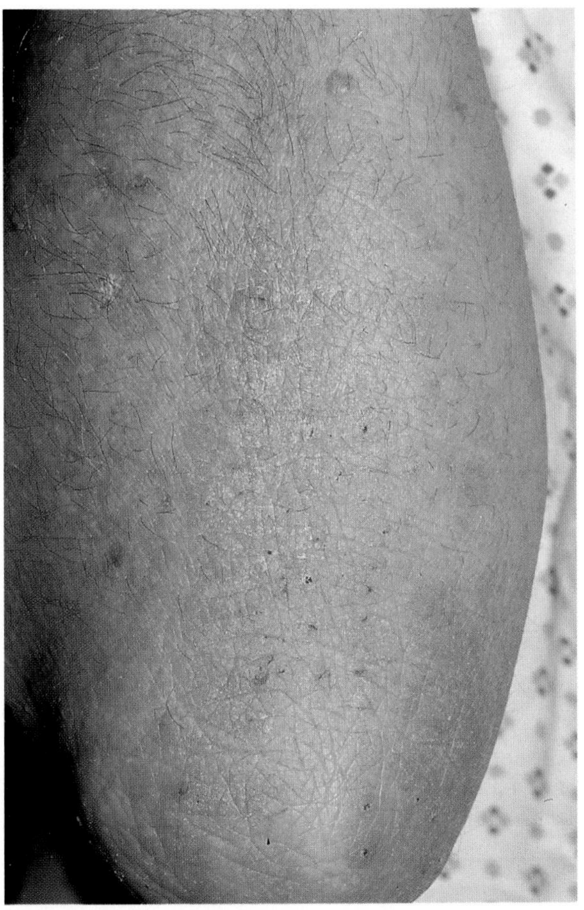

Figure 15.5 Neurodermatitis refers to localized eczema and, like atopic dermatitis, consists of poorly demarcated, inflamed, scaling plaques with evidence of scratching or rubbing. Although this plaque resembles psoriasis in its location and scale, the poorly demarcated borders and excoriations exhibit the eczematous nature.

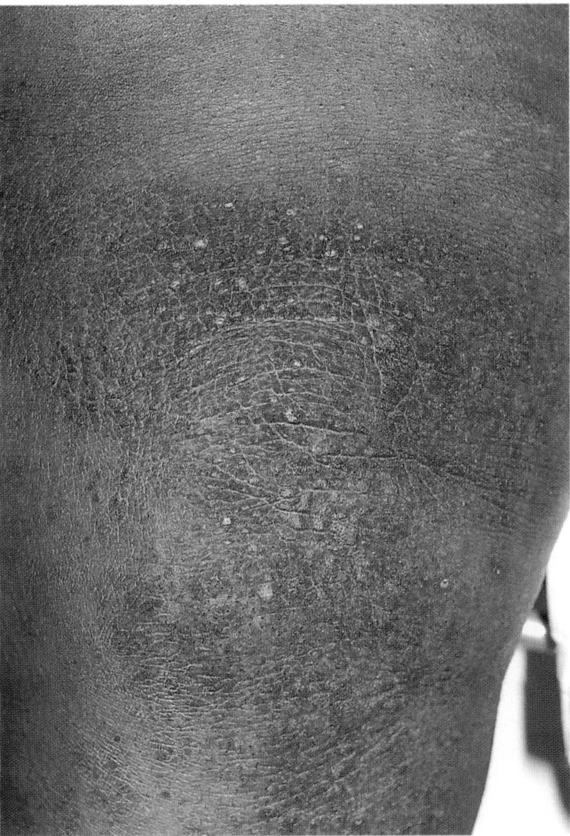

Figure 15.6 This lichenified, localized eczema is called lichen simplex chronicus.

conjunction with supportive measures, including moisturization, avoidance of irritants, nighttime sedation, and infection control.

Most childhood eczema improves nicely with a low-potency corticosteroid preparation. This is true also of eczema on thin skin in adults, including the face, axilla, and groin. The most commonly used and inexpensive low-potency corticosteroid is hydrocortisone 1%, which is available over the counter, and hydrocortisone 2.5%, which is available only by prescription. Despite the differing percentages, these corticosteroids are approximately equal in biologic potency, so that the choice is one of convenience and finances. A midpotency corticosteroid such as triamcinolone (Kenalog, Aristocort) 0.1% is generally used for mild or moderate skin disease on adult nonfacial, non-skin-fold areas of the body. A medium-potency corticosteroid is also appropriate for short-term use in more severe disease in childhood or on adult faces and skin fold areas. Palms and soles as well as extremely lichenified skin generally require the use of a high-potency corticosteroid such as fluocinonide 0.05% (Lidex). When a midpotency corticosteroid is used on small children or on normally thin adult skin, and when a high-potency steroid is used on areas other than palms and soles, follow-up evaluation with a dermatologist should be planned within 2 or

3 weeks because of the risk of local, and occasionally systemic, side effects.

An ointment vehicle is most soothing to very inflamed and excoriated skin, while also providing more lubrication than a cream. Creams generally contain alcohols, and can therefore produce burning on inflamed or broken skin. However, unless very inflamed, the face and skin fold areas are best treated with a cream vehicle. In addition, many patients prefer a cosmetically appealing cream vehicle as their eczema improves and moisturization is less crucial.

In a patient with exudative disease or widespread, extremely pruritic disease, a course of systemic corticosteroids can be more quickly and efficiently effective than topical therapy. When systemic steroids are used for widespread disease, topical steroids should be prescribed as well, both to hasten improvement and to avoid the psychological pitfall of patients always wanting "those pills, because they are what really work and they are so much easier." The usual dose of prednisone in children is 1 to 2 mg/kg up to 40 mg. The dose for adults is 40 to 60 mg each morning, depending on whether the patient is a small or large individual. The prednisone can be abruptly discontinued in 7 to 10 days. Prednisone is usually preferred over dose packs by dermatologists because dose packs deliver an insufficient starting dose of corticosteroid and a too-rapid taper. Generally, oral prednisone also is preferred over intramuscular injections of triamcinolone acetonide (Kenalog). Relatively slow absorption from intramuscular administration results in a delay in the clinical response as compared to oral prednisone. Also, the initial dose delivered intramuscularly is lower than the dose generally prescribed for oral prednisone. Thus, improvement over the first few days is often more rapid with oral prednisone. Many patients require systemic therapy only for 7 to 10 days, whereas the corticosteroid effect of intramuscular triamcinolone lasts about 1 month. Finally, the natural tapering that occurs with intramuscular medication is generally not needed with eczema, since use of the topical medication provides a tapering effect, with little or no adrenal suppression. In addition to the usual side effects of corticosteroids, patients who receive intramuscular medication should be advised of the uncommon adverse experience of an abscess or late atrophy at the injection site. Patients who develop adverse reactions with intramuscular corticosteroid should also understand that the medication gradually dissipates over a 1-month period. Despite these limitations, intramuscular triamcinolone is preferred over prednisone in patients who are likely to be noncompliant and in those whose personal experience has led them to know that this method is beneficial for them. The normal adult dose of intramuscular triamcinolone acetonide is 40 to 80 mg.

Most clinicians are aware that corticosteroids are the first-line therapy for eczema. Most therapeutic failures occur when patients are given simply a corticosteroid without adequate education and adjunctive measures. These measures are extremely important not only in making a flare more bearable during its acute phase, but also in the long-term control of the disease, as well as for the physical and emotional comfort for the patient.

Lubrication is extremely important and is often forgotten.[4] Fissures and excoriations expose unprotected dermis to the air, increasing inflammation. Covering dry, cracked skin and open erosions with a soothing layer of lubrication minimizes itching and soreness. In addition, when the lubricant is applied over the medication, it can enhance penetration of the topical steroid. One simple way of enhancing lubrication is by dispensing the corticosteroid in an ointment vehicle. However, additional lubrication is required for significant eczema. The most effective lubricants are thick creams or ointments, rather than lotions that are thinned by the addition of water and alcohol. In fact, patients with extremely inflamed and eroded skin may experience stinging with application of the thinner lotions. As the eczema improves, these lotions may be substituted for the less cosmetically acceptable and greasy creams and ointments. Examples of effective, thick moisturizers include petrolatum (Vaseline Petroleum Jelly), Eucerin cream (not lotion), Aquaphor, and even vegetable shortening from the grocery store.

Also important for patients with eczema is evening sedation to prevent nighttime scratching and to ensure adequate sleep.[5] This can usually be achieved with sedating doses of diphenhydramine (Benadryl), hydroxyzine HCl (Atarax), doxepin (Sinequan), or amitriptyline (Elavil) at doses of 25 to 75 mg. These tricyclic medications produce the benefits of deeper sleeping as compared to other antihistamines. Patients require sufficient medication to sleep soundly. Although antihistamines are commonly known as anti-itch medications, their anti-itch properties are achieved primarily by sedation, so they have limited benefit during the day. However, some patients report slight relief with low-dose, daytime diphenhydramine or hydroxyzine.

Antibiotics are the third important adjunctive treatment for patients with secondary infection. Any significant crusting or exudation suggests a secondary staphylococcal infection (Fig. 15.2). These infections generally resolve as skin improves with eczema therapy, whether treated with antibiotics or not, but the use of antibiotics can hasten healing significantly. The usual medications are cephalexin (Keflex), dicloxacillin, and, depending on the patterns of bacterial resistance in the area, erythromycin. Because any superinfection is generally minor, the medication can be given in two divided doses rather than four, resulting in increased compliance in most patients. Less common but important causes of failed therapy for eczema are superinfections with *Candida*, tinea, or herpes simplex virus (HSV) (Fig. 4.6).

Finally, patient education is crucial. The patient must understand that eczema is a chronic disease and that, although there is no cure, careful skin care and avoidance of irritation can minimize disease activity. The most common irritant is washing with soap and water. Although itching may be lessened initially, water exposure, even with little or mild soap, removes natural oils from the skin and worsens roughness and fissuring, increasing irritation and pruritus as an end result. Patients should be advised to bathe no more often than two to three times a week, using tepid rather than hot water and a mild soap such as Dove. Stiff fabrics and wool worn against the skin can cause irritation and increase itching. Heat and perspiration can increase both itching and irritation, causing a flare in some patients during the summer months. Parents should be cautioned not to overdress, and thereby overheat, their children. In winter, central heating decreases the amount of moisture in the air, tending to dry the skin, making increased use of lubrication important. Atopic patients with eczema also have an increased susceptibility to the development of allergic contact dermatitis, and unnecessary topical agents should be avoided. Fragrances, medications, and preservatives in skin care products can sometimes be responsible for flares in disease activity.

Patients with mild atopic dermatitis who are given a low-potency topical corticosteroid can be reassured that follow-up management is unnecessary if they respond comfortably to therapy and are able to control their disease with measures suggested in the patient handout on p. 331. Those requiring a mid- or high-potency topical corticosteroid should be instructed to seek follow-up evaluation in 1 to 4 weeks, depending on the severity of their disease and their response to therapy. Even those who respond well to therapy should see a health care provider for reinforcement of patient education and for tapering of the potency of the topical corticosteroid to the safest, lowest effective strength.

Several aggressive therapies are not appropriate for the emergency department. Cyclosporin A, antimetabolites such as azathioprine, ultraviolet light therapy, and interferon-γ (IFN-γ), have all been reported to be useful in the treatment of severe atopic dermatitis.[6–8]

Patients requiring systemic corticosteroid therapy and small children requiring high potency topical corticosteroids should be re-evaluated in 1 week by a dermatologist, both to ensure adequate response to therapy to monitor systemic effects and to ascertain the necessity of ongoing aggressive therapy.

Course and Prognosis

Atopic dermatitis is a chronic disease. Because these patients have sensitive, easily itchy skin, anything that irritates the skin may precipitate and perpetuate eczema. Fortunately, the course of eczema in babies and small children is usually one of gradual improvement. Some patients completely "outgrow" eczema, but they remain at risk of future eczema under the right circumstances. Some children with severe disease experience lifelong disfiguring, and miserably pruritic eczema.

Those with mild disease often maintain clear skin simply by moisturization and avoidance of irritants. Occasional flares are easily controlled with intermittent use of low- or midpotency topical corticosteroids and lubrication.

Severe eczema can be recalcitrant and debilitating, with widespread inflamed or lichenified areas that periodically flare, become superinfected, and may be excruciatingly pruritic. The consequences are not only the physical disability from the disease but also complications from medical therapy, including systemic steroids and sometimes cytotoxic agents. In addition, the psychological effects of disfigurement, the depression from ongoing itchiness and sleeplessness, and the constant inconvenience of frequent application of unpleasant, greasy topical medications can exact a tremendous toll from the patient.

ATOPIC DERMATITIS, ECZEMA, AND NEURODERMATITIS

Clinical Manifestations

Poorly demarcated, inflamed, scaling plaques with evidence of rubbing or scratching in the form of excoriations or lichenification.

Management in the Emergency Department

CHILDREN

1. *Corticosteroids*
   - *Mild to moderate eczema: hydrocortisone ointment 1% or 2.5% ointment applied sparingly twice daily*
   - *Moderate to severe or recalcitrant eczema: triamcinolone 0.1% ointment applied sparingly twice daily*
   - *Severe eczema: add prednisone 1 mg/kg/day for 1 week to a triamcinolone 0.1% ointment applied twice daily*
2. *Moisturization with Vaseline Petroleum Jelly or Eucerin cream (not lotion) over corticosteroid and any time the skin dries*
3. *Nighttime diphenhydramine at sedating doses, starting at twice the usual antihistamine dose for the child's age, increasing dose until the child sleeps well*
4. *Treat superinfections with cephalexin or dicloxacillin*
5. *Decrease irritants, such as frequent bathing, scratchy fabrics, and heat*

(Continues)

(Continued)

6. *Patient education (see the patient handouts on p. 331, Atopic Dermatitis, Eczema, and Neurodermatitis, on p. 357, Prednisone (Cortisone Pills), and on p. 368, Topical Cortisone Creams, Ointments, and Solutions)*
7. *Follow up in 1 month with regular health care provider for mild or moderate eczema, or in 1 week with a dermatologist for severe eczema treated with oral corticosteroids*

ADULTS

1. *Corticosteroids*
   - *Moderate eczema: triamcinolone 0.1% ointment applied sparingly twice daily, except hydrocortisone cream 1% or 2.5% for skin folds and face*
   - *Severe eczema: prednisone 40 mg/day (small adult), or 60 mg/day (large adult) for 1 week in addition to topical corticosteroid ointment*
2. *Moisturization with Vaseline petroleum jelly or Eucerin cream (not lotion) over corticosteroid and any time the skin dries*
3. *Nighttime diphenhydramine, hydroxyzine HCl, doxepin, or amitriptyline 25 to 75 mg at bedtime to sleep without scratching*
4. *Treat superinfections with cephalexin or dicloxacillin 500 mg bid*
5. *Decrease irritants, such as frequent bathing, scratchy fabrics, and heat*
6. *Patient education (see the patient handouts on p. 331, Atopic Dermatitis, Eczema, and Neurodermatitis, on p. 357, Prednisone (Cortisone Pills), and on p. 368, Topical Cortisone Creams, Ointments, and Solutions)*
7. *Follow-up evaluation in 1 month with regular health care provider for mild or moderate eczema, or in 1 week with a dermatologist for severe eczema treated with oral corticosteroids*

ECZEMATOUS PATTERNS

In predisposed people, eczema, or atopic dermatitis, is especially likely to occur in predictable settings that regularly produce irritation and precipitate itching. These can be considered simply as recognizable patterns of atopic dermatitis, responsive to the same therapy discussed above for eczema/neurodermatitis. However, those factors that precipitated that particular pattern must be discovered and addressed.

Stasis Dermatitis

Stasis dermatitis refers to eczema that occurs in a setting of edema. Although the classic cause of lower leg edema is venous stasis, swelling also often occurs as a result of injury, scarring of lymphatics from recurrent cellulitis, and other causes. Stasis dermatitis is precipitated by inflammation that occurs when edema stretches the skin, producing small fissures. An atopic person perceives this inflammation as pruritus, and the resulting scratching initiates an itch-scratch cycle. Because edema is most common and the skin is least elastic over the lower leg, this is the most common location for stasis dermatitis (Fig. 15.7). Healing is delayed in areas of edema, as fissures and erosions are stretched wider by the swelling. This is one reason that patients with stasis dermatitis are at risk of stasis ulcers.

Figure 15.7 Stasis dermatitis is eczema of the lower leg precipitated by edema that produces fissuring and inflammation that initiates itching.

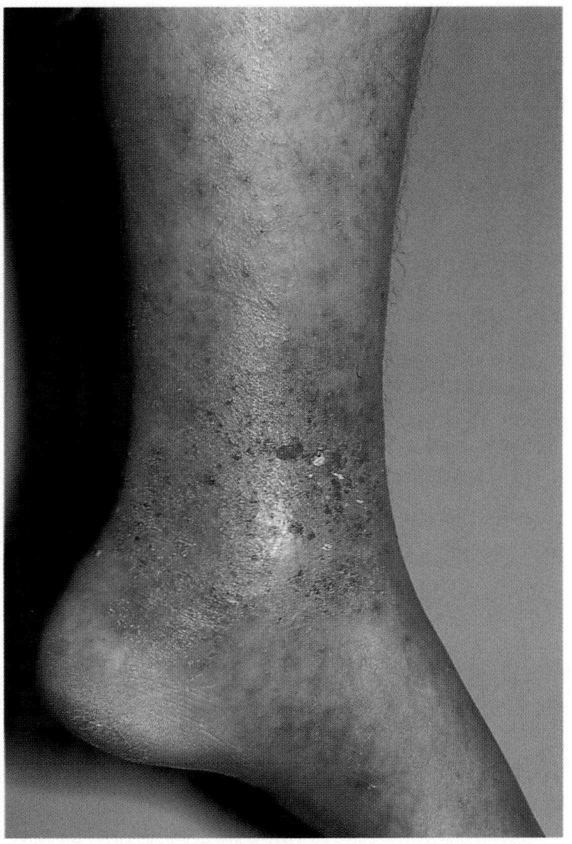

By definition, patients with stasis dermatitis have evidence of present or recent edema. Sometimes this can be ascertained from a history, although physical findings usually yield this information as well. Most patients show frank edema on the physical examination. Others may show patchy hyperpigmentation due to hemosiderin remaining from leakage of blood into the dermis, as a result of hydrostatic pressure and edema.

Otherwise, stasis dermatitis is characterized by the same poorly demarcated, red, scaling plaques, with evidence of rubbing or scratching in the form of excoriations or lichenification. As is true of other inflammatory diseases, black patients often appear to have hyperpigmented plaques rather than red plaques.

The management of stasis dermatitis begins with control of local edema. When possible, the cause of the edema should be corrected. Meantime, mechanical measures should be introduced in the form of compression stockings, elastic wraps, or Unna's boots. Otherwise, therapy for stasis dermatitis follows that for atopic dermatitis, including a topical corticosteroid, lubrication, infection control, and nighttime sedation. As stasis dermatitis usually occurs on the lower legs, a midpotency corticosteroid such as triamcinolone 0.1% ointment applied sparingly twice a day is usually sufficient. The ointment base is more soothing to cracked and broken skin than alcohol-containing creams; it also helps provide the essential extra lubrication that can lead to rapid improvement. Most patients require additional moisturization in the form of a thick emollient such as Vaseline or Eucerin cream applied over the corticosteroid and at any other time that the skin becomes rough, scaling, and dry in appearance.

As in the case of atopic dermatitis, control of secondary infection and the institution of bedtime sedation with high doses of antihistamines in patients who itch at night are important in the total care of a patient with stasis dermatitis.

When effective edema control with compression is combined with topical corticosteroids and emollients, patients generally improve dramatically and quickly. However, because dependent edema is generally chronic, stasis dermatitis is also a chronic condition unless the edema can be controlled.

Patients with stasis dermatitis relatively often develop a superimposed allergic or irritant contact dermatitis. This may occur because of overwashing or when patients unintentionally expose their skin to many allergens by applying multiple medications to the areas. These factors should be considered when patients have an unexplained flare or do not respond to what should be appropriate therapy.

Hand or Foot Dermatitis

Sometimes, eczema affects the hands and/or feet preferentially, producing hand or foot dermatitis (dyshidrosis, pomphylox). Hand and foot eczema often represents atopic dermatitis, probably because these areas are subject to trauma and other irritants. However, allergic and irritant contact dermatitis can produce the same clinical picture, making the term hand or foot eczema imprecise. Eczema of the hands and feet, in addition to erythema, scale, and erosions, often exhibits small vesicles. These typically occur in the normally thickened palmar and plantar epithelium as a result of the intense loculated edema fluid due to the inflammation of eczema (see Figs. 4.18 and 4.19).

First-line therapy in the emergency department for eczema of the hands and feet is the same as for eczema in other areas of the body. A high-potency topical corticosteroid is useful for those with mild to moderate disease, but patients with significant pain or itching on the basis of very inflammatory disease or exudation should receive a burst of prednisone at 40 to 60 mg/day for about 1 week, with follow-up evaluation by a dermatologist at that time. The diagnosis of allergic contact dermatitis should be seriously considered in patients who do not respond well to basic therapy.

Scabies

Scabies is an extraordinarily pruritic mite infestation. The resulting scratching produces eczema that often obscures the characteristic burrows of the mite. Most patients have only 8 to 10 mites on their body, despite often widespread excoriations, erythema, and scale produced by scratching. Otherwise healthy patients have a characteristic pattern of involvement, with no disease above the neck, and marked disease in skin folds such as the digit web spaces, the axillae, groin, penis, and (in women) inframammary skin. Often, a few oval, edematous 1- to 3-mm papules that represent burrows that have not yet been removed by fingernails can be found on a careful examination (Fig. 15.8). A scraping of the burrow with a No. 15 scalpel blade sometimes yields the mite, ova, or mite feces, confirming the diagnosis (see Fig. 2.5). A negative scraping should not dissuade the clinician.

The treatment of scabies consists of 5% permethrin cream (Elimite) applied overnight to the patient and to all members of the household.[9] Lindane (Kwell) lotion is rarely indicated now because of neurotoxic side effects in babies and debilitated patients, and crotamiton cream is seldom used because it is not very effective.[10,11] One dose of oral ivermectin has been reported to be a very effective therapy that may become available in the United States in the future.[12] In addition to elimination of the mite in the skin, clothes worn by each family member during the previous 24 hours, as well as all towels and bed linens, should be washed in hot water. Because pruritus results from an immunologic response to the mite, and the dead mite remains embedded in the skin until the skin is shed, itching often persists for a week or two. Secondary eczematization should be treated as discussed above for atopic dermatitis, with a topical corticosteroid, lubrication, and nighttime sedation with an antihistamine.

Xerotic Eczema

Xerotic eczema occurs when the irritation from cracking and fissuring of extremely dry skin precipitates eczema in the predisposed person. In addition to the usual erythema, scale, and excoriation, there are often characteristic, adherent flakes of skin with lifted edges that give the skin the appearance of a dried river bed. Xerotic eczema is most common over the lower legs and over any area, such as the hands, that may receive sufficient exposure to water

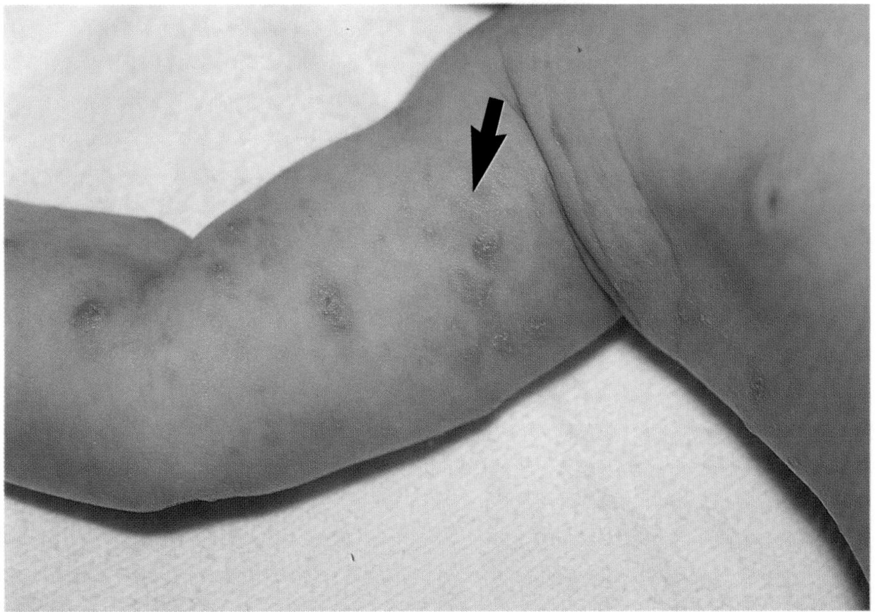

Figure 15.8 This poorly demarcated, scaling eruption is suggestive of scabies as an underlying condition because of the distribution and the oval edematous papules (burrows; see arrow).

or overwashing to defat the skin. The treatment is the same as for eczema in other circumstances: avoidance of water and soap, aggressive lubrication, and a topical corticosteroid ointment.

Nummular Eczema

Nummular eczema is a pattern of eczema that occurs as one to several fairly sharply demarcated, round plaques. These are sometimes very inflammatory and may appear vesicular and crusted. Nummular dermatitis can sometimes resemble inflammatory tinea corporis; occasionally, it is confused with guttate psoriasis. Because nummular eczema can sometimes be precipitated by xerosis, frequent lubrication is extremely important for successful therapy.

Infectious Eczematoid Dermatitis

Infectious eczematoid dermatitis is eczema produced by irritation from draining body fluids. Often, there is no direct infectious component to the skin findings, but the drainage (as occurs with an external otitis) produces maceration and irritation (Fig. 15.9). At other times, such as with chronic drainage from an ostomy, no infection is present. The diagnosis is by the setting and morphology, and the management includes protection of the skin and control of drainage.

Fungal Eczema

Fungal eczema is an extremely common condition, occurring when an atopic patient scratches his tinea. This situation is most common on the feet and in the groin. Atopy is associated with a minor T-cell abnormality that predisposes to superficial fungal and viral skin infections. In addition, atopic people perceive any inflammation as an itch, so that the inflammation of a tinea infection precipitates scratching. Since eczema is produced by scratching, superimposed eczema is common in these patients. A high index of suspicion is required to make the diagnosis of fungal eczema, since a fungal preparation can be difficult to perform and interpret. When in doubt, the patient

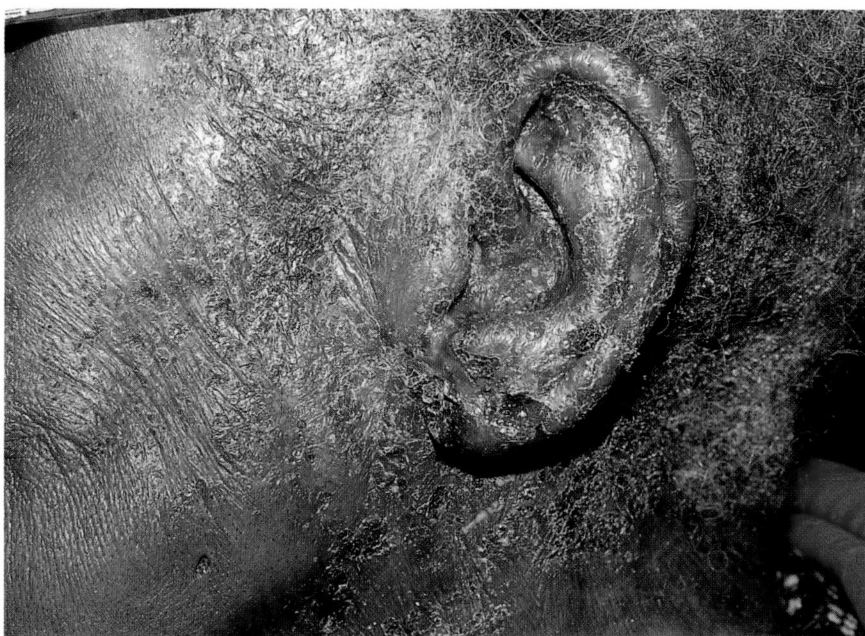

Figure 15.9 This patient developed surrounding eczematous changes because of drainage from otitis externa.

should receive both an antifungal medication and, initially, a topical corticosteroid. Generally, the corticosteroid can be discontinued after the patient improves substantially, so that it does not interfere with elimination of the fungus.

Miscellaneous Dermatoses

Any dermatosis can precipitate itching in an atopic patient, producing secondary eczematization. Psoriasis, pityriasis rosea, and lichen planus are especially common diseases to cause itching in predisposed patients. Because these papulosquamous diseases are only moderately steroid responsive, the underlying disease becomes apparent as the eczema clears with topical steroid therapy.

STASIS DERMATITIS

Clinical Manifestations

Poorly demarcated erythema, scale, and lichenification or excoriations over the lower legs, in association with edema or evidence of past edema.

(Continues)

(Continued)

Management in the Emergency Department

1. *Elimination of edema with elastic wraps, support stockings, or Unna's boots*
2. *Triamcinolone ointment 0.1% applied sparingly twice daily and covered with moisturizer such as Vaseline petroleum jelly or Eucerin cream (not lotion)*
3. *Nighttime sedation with diphenhydramine, hydroxyzine HCl, amitriptyline, or doxepin 25 to 75 mg*
4. *If infection is suspected, treat with oral cephalexin or dicloxacillin 500 mg bid*
5. *Patient education regarding eczema and importance of edema control (see the patient handout on p. 331, Atopic Dermatitis, Eczema, and Neurodermatitis and on p. 369, Topical Cortisone Creams, Ointments, and Solutions)*
6. *Follow-up evaluation with primary care provider for medical control of edema at earliest convenience*

(Continues)

(Continued)

SCABIES

Clinical Manifestations

Excruciatingly itchy disease characterized by scattered excoriations and papulovesicular lesions distributed especially in skin folds, genital area, finger web spaces, and wrists.

Management in the Emergency Department

1. *Permethrin cream 5% (Elimite) to patient and all household members overnight*
2. *Wash all bedclothes, linens, clothes, and so forth, that came in contact with the patient or family members in the previous 24 hours*
3. *Patient education (see the patient handout on p. 361, Scabies)*
4. *Triamcinolone 0.1% (adults) or hydrocortisone 1% or 2.5% (children) cream twice daily for scaling, inflamed, and itchy areas*
5. *Nighttime sedation with diphenhydramine, hydroxyzine HCl, doxepin, or amitriptyline 25 to 75 mg for sleeping if needed*

SEBORRHEIC DERMATITIS

Seborrheic dermatitis, or "inflammatory dandruff," is an extraordinarily common skin condition that is unrelated to atopic dermatitis. Generally not particularly pruritic, seborrheic dermatitis is found primarily in neonates and in postpubertal patients. The etiology is believed by some to be secondary inflammation resulting from the buildup of scale trapped by hair or within skin folds. Others believe that this is an infection caused by *Malassezia furfur* (also called *Pitysporum ovale*), the causative organism of pityriasis "tinea" versicolor.[13]

Very severe seborrhea is found in debilitated patients and other conditions (e.g., homelessness, institutionalization, neurologic diseases) that discourage regular effective shampooing. In addition, patients with acquired immunodeficiency syndrome (AIDS) can develop unusually severe seborrheic dermatitis with exudative crusting.

Clinical Manifestations

Because seborrheic dermatitis is not usually pruritic, signs of rubbing and scratching are absent, except in atopic patients who perceive any inflammation as pruritic. Seborrheic dermatitis presents as poorly demarcated, red, scaling plaques in the scalp, especially at the hairline around the face. The scale usually has a subtle yellow color and a slightly greasy texture (Fig. 15.10). The scale is also often prominent in the skin folds behind the ear, and often in the ear itself. In more severe seborrheic dermatitis, the lesions can extend to the skin of the face around the scalp, in the eyebrows, and over the central face, including the nasolabial folds. Occasionally, especially in men, the red, scaling plaques also involve the central chest, but only very rarely and in extremely severe disease does seborrheic dermatitis involve other skin folds, such as the axilla and genital area. There are rare reports of generalized erythroderma and scaling from seborrheic dermatitis. Sometimes, when seborrheic dermatitis involves areas other than the scalp, the individual lesions can be sharply demarcated and appear to be a papulosquamous condition rather than eczematous. Occasionally, black patients exhibit sharply demarcated, hypopigmented, scaling papules or plaques (Fig. 15.11).

When seborrheic dermatitis occurs in infants, the appearance can vary slightly. The earliest scalp scale is often more generalized, rather than confined to the hairline, and the retained scale is often more thickened into what is commonly called "cradle cap." In more severe disease, the face becomes involved but the distribution is less remarkably central facial (see Fig. 20.7). Other intertriginous areas of the body are often involved, and generalized seborrheic dermatitis is far more common in infants than in adults.

Differential Diagnosis

The disease most often confused with seborrheic dermatitis in adults is psoriasis, because psoriasis almost always affects the scalp. However, psoriasis usually manifests as sharply demarcated, scattered plaques with dense silvery scale. Other red, scaling diseases that can occur in the scalp include atopic dermatitis and its variants, such as neurodermatitis

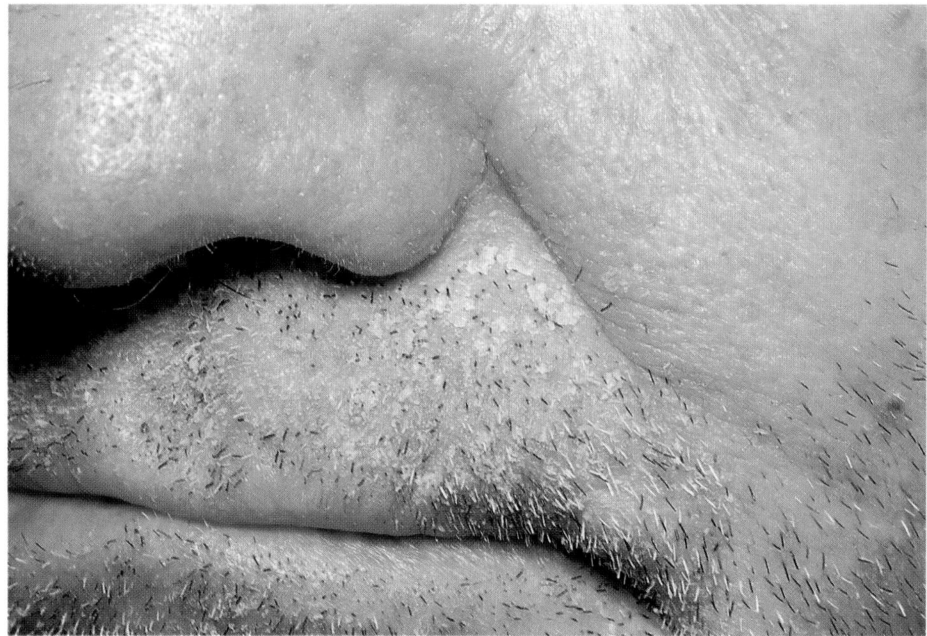

Figure 15.10 Seborrheic dermatitis presents with yellowish scaling at the hairline, followed in more severe disease by scaling in the eyebrows, in and behind the ears, and in the nasolabial folds.

Figure 15.11 Black patients often exhibit well-demarcated, central facial, finely scaling papules and plaques of seborrheic dermatitis that may mimic secondary syphilis.

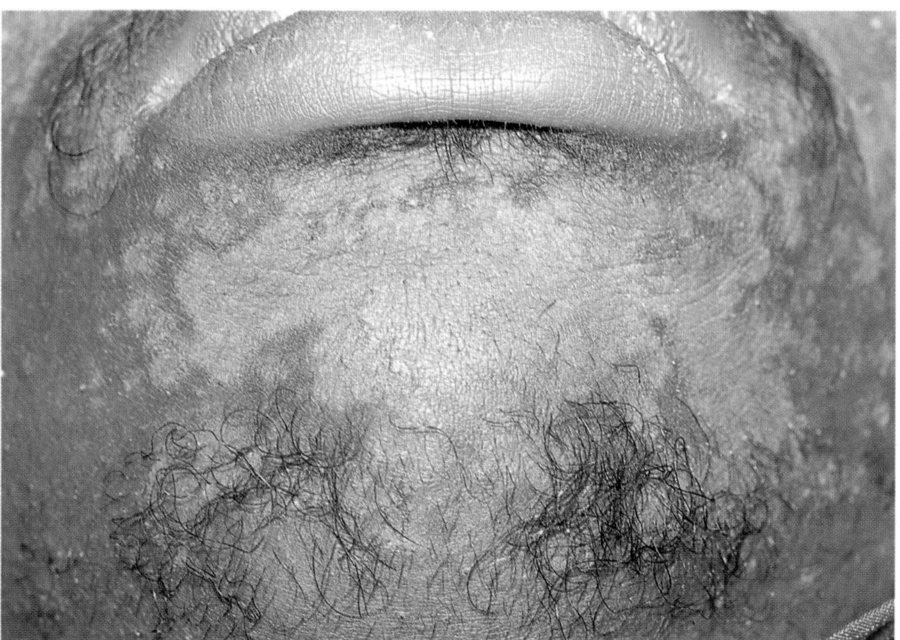

and lichen simplex chronicus. Tinea capitis, discoid lupus erythematosus, and rarely lichen planus can produce scaling scalp disease. These diseases can usually be distinguished by their distribution and setting and, in children (who are most susceptible to tinea capitis but rarely have seborrheic dermatitis), by fungal culture.

Seborrheic dermatitis in infants is most often confused with atopic dermatitis. When seborrheic dermatitis is severe in infants, the appearance is sometimes indistinguishable from atopic dermatitis. The diagnosis is made on the basis of the age of the infant, response to therapy, and lack of recurrence as the child ages. Most dermatitic eruptions during the first 2 months of life are seborrheic dermatitis; most eruptions after 5 months of age are atopic dermatitis.

Management

First-line therapy for seborrheic dermatitis in both adults and infants is daily or alternate-day mechanical removal of scalp scale. In adults, this is best accomplished by frequent, vigorous shampooing, preferably with an antiseborrheic shampoo. Antiseborrheic shampoos contain antiproliferative agents, such as coal tar or pyrithione zinc, to reduce the production of scale, or keratolytic agents, such as salicylic acid, to dissolve scale. Common antiseborrheic shampoos include T-Gel, T-Sal, Ionil T Plus, and Zincon (all over the counter), and Selsun (for those who are financially better served by a prescription medication). These shampoos are scrubbed into the scalp and allowed to remain for about 5 minutes; scalp scales are then mechanically removed with the fingernails. In infants, these harsher agents are generally not used; instead, baby shampoo or mineral oil is applied to the scalp to soften the scale. The scale is then removed with a soft brush or gentle rubbing with the fingernails. Because inflamed skin is associated with an increased rate of cellular turnover and increased scale, this process must be repeated frequently. Unfortunately, black patients develop unacceptable dryness and brittleness of the hair when shampooing frequently, so that shampooing should be limited to twice a week for these patients until they improve. They can be counseled that moisturizing their hair is acceptable but that they should avoid the use of heavy grease on the skin of the scalp itself.

Patients with significant seborrheic dermatitis also require the use of a topical corticosteroid. Hydrocortisone cream 1% or 2.5% is usually sufficient for the face of adults and for all involved areas in infants. For severe recalcitrant facial seborrheic dermatitis, short-term use of a midpotency topical corticosteroid such as triamcinolone 0.1% is sometimes indicated, but a follow-up visit for re-evaluation should be prompt. A very common corticosteroid preparation for the scalp is betamethasone valerate (Valisone) lotion 0.1%, a cosmetically elegant midpotency topical corticosteroid that is inexpensive and widely available in a generic form. Corticosteroids are applied twice each day.

An alternative therapy for seborrheic dermatitis is ketoconazole (Nizoral) shampoo. This medicated shampoo is used twice a week for 4 weeks and then as needed. The mechanism of action is believed to be as a fungicide, eliminating the *Pityrosporum* organisms that may be involved in the pathogenesis of seborrheic dermatitis. In addition, ketoconazole has anti-inflammatory effects.

Mild or moderate seborrhea can usually be controlled with over-the-counter hydrocortisone and shampoo; follow-up is unnecessary. Those treated with midpotency corticosteroids or those who are not controlled with over-the-counter medications should seek follow-up evaluation with their usual health care provider or with a dermatologist for re-evaluation and therapy. Patients with extremely severe or recalcitrant seborrhea should be considered for testing for the human immunodeficiency virus (HIV).

Course and Prognosis

Seborrheic dermatitis is a chronic disease in adults. It tends to wax and wane, requiring intermittent therapy. Seborrheic dermatitis in infants is less likely to recur, as long as the scalp is kept free of scale. The tendency for the accumulation of scalp scale and the development of seborrheic dermatitis declines sharply as circulating levels of maternal sex hormones disappear.

SEBORRHEIC DERMATITIS

Clinical Manifestations

Yellow scaling, often over mildly inflamed papules and plaques located predominantly at the hairline, behind and in the ears, and over the central face. Black patients often exhibit well-demarcated, finely scaling, hypopigmented, coalescing papules. Infants manifest cradle cap and red papules and plaques with yellowish scale.

Management in the Emergency Department

ADULTS (FOR CHILDREN, SEE CH. 19)

1. *Antiseborrheic shampoo daily (twice weekly for black patients), scrubbed into scalp, left 5 minutes, then rinsed out, while mechanically removing scale with fingernails*
2. *Topical corticosteroids*
   - *Betamethasone valerate 0.1% to scalp qid-bid*
   - *Hydrocortisone cream 1% or 2.5% to affected nonhairy skin twice daily*
3. *Patient education (see the patient handout on p. 327, Adult Seborrheic Dermatitis)*

CONTACT DERMATITIS

Eczema precipitated or caused by direct contact of the skin to an external substance is called contact dermatitis. Contact dermatitis occurs in two forms. The first is irritant contact dermatitis, in which exposure to irritating substances produces inflammation and itching, particularly in patients with atopic dermatitis or an atopic diathesis. The subsequent scratching initiates a superimposed itch–scratch cycle and the development of eczema.

The second form of contact dermatitis is allergic contact dermatitis, in which a patient with prior hypersensitivity to a specific allergen experiences inflammation and edema in response to direct contact with the skin. Usually, the resulting pruritus initiates an itch–scratch cycle that eventuates in the skin changes of eczema. However, in very acute disease with a potent allergen, the edema can actually produce clinical vesicles or bullae (see Ch. 4, Vesicular Diseases).

Irritant Contact Dermatitis

Irritant contact dermatitis occurs in areas that have been exposed to an irritating substance or event. Sometimes, the distinction between atopic dermatitis/neurodermatitis initiated or perpetuated by an irritant such as dryness or overwashing and that due to mild irritant contact dermatitis is a fine one that is unimportant. However, even patients who are not atopic develop changes of eczema with severe irritants. An irritant contact dermatitis in a patient who is not atopic generally produces more irritation and burning than itching, whereas an allergic contact dermatitis is pruritic in everyone.

A mild irritant, such as soap and water, produces dermatitis after repeated exposure, so that the etiology may not be obvious to the patient. A very caustic irritant produces immediate symptoms and the equivalent of a chemical burn.

Clinical Manifestations Lesions of an irritant contact dermatitis are poorly demarcated scaling, inflammatory papules and plaques. In atopic patients, this "chapping" is accompanied by pruritus, as evidenced by excoriation or lichenification. The hands are an extremely common location for irritant contact dermatitis since the hands are at great risk of exposure to irritants. Frequent hand washing or exposure to harsh chemicals can produce erythema, cracking, and scale. Similar changes may appear around insect bites or minor abrasions that have been treated by the patient with repeated applications of alcohol or other irritating substances. Even mechanical irritation from pressure or friction can produce an irritant contact dermatitis, such as the changes of eczema over the stump of an amputee under a prosthetic device. One of the most well-recognized examples of an irritant contact dermatitis is diaper dermatitis, in which irritation and maceration from feces, perspiration, and urine held against the skin produce poorly demarcated erythema and scale. Although this is most common in babies, it occurs in incontinent adults as well.

Differential Diagnosis The diagnosis of irritant contact dermatitis is made when changes of eczema are identified in an area that comes into contact with an irritant. The diseases most commonly confused with an irritant contact dermatitis are atopic dermatitis and allergic contact dermatitis. Patients with atopic dermatitis and atopic patients with irritant contact dermatitis describe greater itching and exhibit more marked physical findings due to rubbing and scratching, such as excoriation and lichenification, than do nonatopic patients with an irritant contact dermatitis. Patients with an irritant contact dermatitis often can identify the offending agent because immediate burning, stinging, or pain frequently occur with exposure. Allergic contact dermatitis differs from irritant contact dermatitis in that symptoms are delayed hours to days after exposure to the contactant.

Management Nonatopic patients who have not initiated an itch–scratch cycle usually experience resolution with removal of the irritant. However, in addition to eliminating the offending irritant, a topical corticosteroid ointment applied twice a day and covered with a moisturizer (except in skin folds, where maceration is a concern) can reduce pruritus and hasten improvement. Hydrocortisone 1% or 2.5% is appropriate for children, skin fold areas, or the face. A midpotency corticosteroid such as triamcinolone 0.1% (Kenalog, Aristocort) ointment for other areas is best for most areas of skin in adults. A cream vehicle can be used in naturally moist areas that are not eroded.

As is true of other skin conditions, sedating doses of antihistamines for those with nighttime pain and itching are an important adjunct. Good choices include diphenhydramine (Benadryl), hydroxyzine HCl (Atarax), doxepin (Sinequan), or amitriptyline (Elavil) 25 to 75 mg at bedtime. Any patient with crusting or exudation suggestive of a superinfection should receive an oral antistaphylococcal medication such as cephalexin or dicloxacillin 500 mg bid. In some areas, such as the genitalia and feet, fungal superinfection is common and should be treated.

Follow-up management is unnecessary if the condition clears on the above therapy. However, patients should be instructed that if there is no improvement after 1 week, or if the skin is not clear after 3 weeks, follow-up evaluation with a primary care physician or a dermatologist is warranted.

Course and Prognosis Once the disease has cleared, irritant contact dermatitis usually does not recur if the offending irritant and similar substances can be avoided. However, irritant dermatitis on the hands and in the genital area of incontinent patients is often recurrent or chronic, as the precipitating irritants cannot always be completely eliminated.

Allergic Contact Dermatitis

Although acute allergic contact dermatitis, such as that caused by poison ivy or poison oak, is usually easy to diagnose by the presence of small blisters in characteristic patterns, the more common chronic allergic contact dermatitis causes a much less specific clinical picture that resembles atopic dermatitis.

Clinical Manifestations Patients experience inflammation and pruritus without vesiculation in areas of contact with a less potent allergen than poison ivy or poison oak. The resulting poorly demarcated, scaling papules and plaques are usually associated with excoriation or lichenification. These plaques occur roughly in the area of contact, but rubbing and scratching often extend the boundaries to other areas.

The location of the allergic contact dermatitis depends on the offending substance. For example, eczematous changes around previous skin trauma may be due to an allergy to adhesive from a dressing, to sensitivity to a topical antibiotic, or to a reaction to a preservative in a medication that has been applied. Even corticosteroids are well documented to produce allergic contact dermatitis in some people.[14] Inflammation and scaling on the back of the wrist, over the earlobes, and over the central abdomen are frequently caused by contact with nickel in watches, earrings, and belt buckles[15] (Fig. 15.12). Eczema and edema of the eyelids are classically associated with an allergy to fingernail polish. Even minute amounts of weak allergens inadvertently transferred to very thin, fragile skin of the eyelids can create a reaction in the absence of eczema around the fingers, where larger amounts were applied. Often, plaques of allergic contact dermatitis are randomly scattered where substances

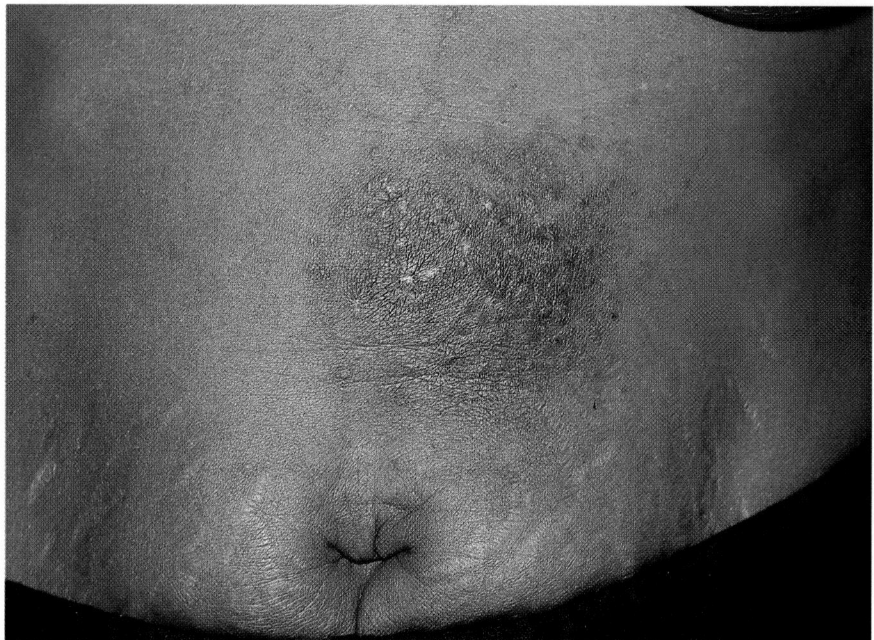

Figure 15.12 This poorly demarcated lichenified plaque occurred from a contact allergy to nickel in the patient's belt buckle.

have brushed against the skin or have been inadvertently carried to the skin by the patient's fingers and hands. Contact dermatitis is a common cause of hand eczema as well. Classically, allergic contact dermatitis begins on the dorsum of the hands, because the skin of the palms is thicker and penetration of an allergen is more difficult (Fig. 15.13).

Differential Diagnosis The differential diagnosis of an allergic contact dermatitis includes an irritant contact dermatitis, which can be very difficult to distinguish. This differentiation is generally made by history, location, and allergy patch testing when needed. Atopic dermatitis can also be extremely difficult to differentiate and, because patients with allergic contact dermatitis are by definition atopic, these diseases often exist together, with one complicating the other. Patients with apparent atopic dermatitis may worsen as they develop an allergy to a corticosteroid, preservative, or fragrance in medications. Once again, distribution, history, and patch testing may be required to sort out this question. Other scaling diseases, such as tinea infection and psoriasis, can sometimes be confused with, or complicated by, allergic contact dermatitis. Appropriate testing and further clinical evaluation of other skin surfaces can usually differentiate these diseases when location or appearance is confusing.

Management The identification and elimination of the allergen(s) in allergic contact dermatitis is essential and often difficult, especially when there is more than one allergen and the disease is chronic. Unless there is one obvious offender, such as poison ivy, nickel, or leather, patients require more definitive evaluation by a dermatologist.

A topical corticosteroid ointment will hasten improvement. Although hydrocortisone 1% or 2.5% is the preferred potency for the face, skin folds, and children, a midpotency corticosteroid such as triamcinolone ointment 0.1% is reasonable for other areas. In addition to the usual advantages of an ointment, such as increased moisturizing effect and less irritation due to the lack of alcohol as compared to creams, ointments also contain fewer preservatives and other possible exacerbating allergenic substances.

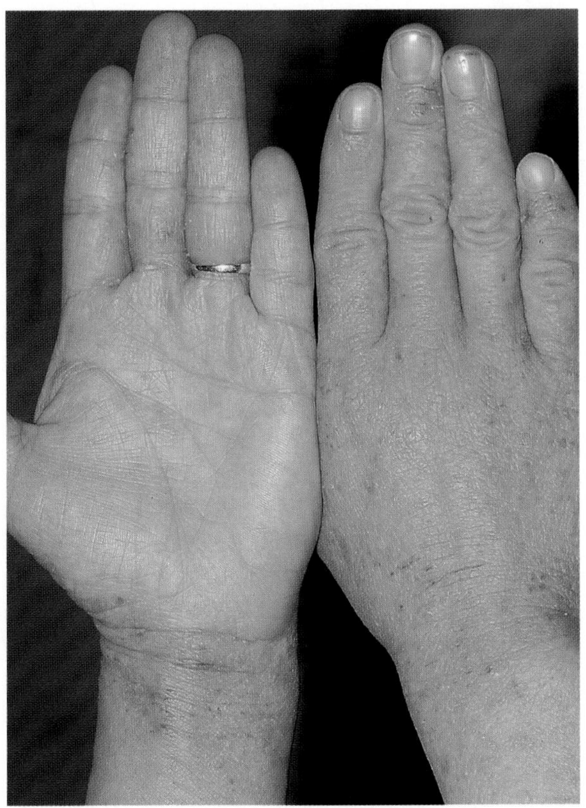

Figure 15.13 This patient experienced an allergic contact dermatitis of the hands, with sparing of the palms, where the thicker skin was relatively protective.

As is usual for other forms of eczema, areas other than the face and intertriginous zones should also receive moisturization, possible superinfection should be treated, and patients with nighttime itching or pain should receive evening sedation with an antihistamine, such as diphenhydramine, hydroxyzine HCl, amitriptyline, or doxepin 25 to 75 mg.

Course and Prognosis When an allergic contact dermatitis results from exposure to one identifiable, specific allergen, avoidance of that allergen usually produces significant improvement or clearing of the disease. However, all too often, allergic contact dermatitis is due to more than one allergen, and cross-reactions with other substances occur. These patients tend to have recurring or chronic problems. In addition, some allergens are ubiquitous and unavoidable, resulting in recurrent or chronic disease. Finally, when allergic contact dermatitis is very chronic, even total avoidance of the irritant may not result in complete clearing or even dramatic improvement. This disease can sometimes become self-perpetuating.

ALLERGIC CONTACT DERMATITIS

Management in the Emergency Department

1. *Stop any identified allergen*
2. *Application of a topical corticosteroid: hydrocortisone 1% or 2.5% for children, or to adult face and skin folds; or triamcinolone 0.1% for other areas in adults*
3. *Lubrication of scaling skin with Vaseline petroleum jelly or Eucerin cream*
4. *Nighttime sedation with diphenhydramine, hydroxyzine HCl, doxepin, or amitriptyline at 25 to 75 mg*
5. *If the allergen is not easily identified, or if the patient does not respond well to therapy, follow-up evaluation with a dermatologist should be sought, with the timing depending on the severity of the disease*
6. *Patient education (see the handout on p.336, Contact Dermatitis)*

Please see patient information handouts for this chapter on pages 327, 331, 336, and 361.

REFERENCES

1. Lammintausta K, Kalimo K, Raitala R, Forsten Y: Prognosis of atopic dermatitis. A prospective study in early adulthood. Int J Dermatol 30:563, 1991
2. Rajka G: Atopic dermatitis. An evaluation of clinical and laboratory findings. Int J Dermatol 26:27, 1986
3. Hanifin JM: Immunological aspects of atopic dermatitis. Dermatol Clin 8:747,1990
4. Lazar AP, Lazar P: Dry skin, water, and lubrication. Dermatol Clin 9:45, 1991

5. Healsmith M, Berth-Jones J, Graham-Brown RAC: Histamine, antihistamines and atopic dermatitis. J Dermatol Treat 1:325, 1991

6. Taylor RS, Cooper KD, Headington JT et al: Cyclosporin therapy for severe atopic dermatitis. J Am Acad Dermatol 21:580, 1989

7. Jekler J, Larko O: Combined UVA-UVB versus UVB phototherapy for atopic dermatitis. J Am Acad Dermatol 22:49, 1990

8. Hanifin JM, Schneider LC, Leung DYM et al: Recombinant interferon gamma therapy for atopic dermatitis. J Am Acad Dermatol 28:189, 1993

9. Schultz MW, Gomez M, Hansen RC et al: Comparative study of 5% permethrin and 1% lindane lotion for the treatment of scabies. Arch Dermatol 126:167, 1990

10. Taplin D, Meinking T: Infestations. p. 1347. In Schachner LA, Hansen RC (eds): Pediatric Dermatology. 2nd Ed. Churchill Livingstone, New York, 1996

11. Taplin D, Meinking TL, Chen JA, Sanchez R: Comparison of crotamiton 10% cream (Eurax) and permethrin 5% cream (Elimite) for the treatment of scabies in children. Pediatr Dermatol 7:67, 1990

12. Meinking TL, Taplin D, Hermida JL et al: The treatment of scabies with ivermectin. N Engl J Med 333:26, 1995

13. Heng MCY, Henderson CL, Barker DC et al: Correlation of *Pityrosporum ovale* density with clinical severity of seborrheic dermatitis as assessed by a simplified technique. J Am Acad Dermatol 23:82, 1990

14. Dooms-Groossens AC, Degreef HJ, Marien KJC, Coopman SA: Contact allergy to corticosteroids: a frequently missed diagnosis? J Am Accad Dermatol 21:538, 1989

15. McDonagh AJG, Wright AL, Cork MJ: Nickel sensitivity: the influence of ear piercing and atopy. Br J Dermatol 126:16, 1992

SUGGESTED READINGS

Atopic Dermatitis/Neurodermatitis

Cooper KD: Atopic dermatitis: recent trends in pathogenesis and therapy. J Invest Dermatol 102: 128, 1994

Frank LA: Atopic dermatitis. Clin Dermatol 12:565, 1994

Rothe MJ, Grant-Kels JM: Atopic dermatitis: an update. J Am Acad Dermatol 35:1, 1996

Williams RE, MacKie RM: The staphylococci. Importance of their control in the management of skin disease. Dermatol Clin 11:201, 1993

Scabies

Elgart M: Scabies. Dermatol Clin 8:253, 1990

Orkin M, Maibach HI: Cutaneous Infestations and Insect Bites. Marcel Dekker, New York, 1985

Seborrheic Dermatitis

Rebora A, Rongioletti F: The red face: seborrheic dermatitis. Clin Dermatol 11:243, 1993

Webster G: Seborrheic dermatitis. Int J Dermatol 30:843, 1991

Contact Dermatitis

Adams RM (ed): Occupational Skin Disease. WB Saunders, Philadelphia, 1990

Adams RM, Nethercott JR: Contact dermatitis. Dermatol Clin 8:1, 1990

Marks JG, DeLeo VA: Contact and Occupational Dermatology. Mosby-Year Book, St. Louis, 1992

CHAPTER 16

Purpura

Purpura, or bleeding into the skin, is a finding that sometimes heralds serious or even life-threatening disease. At other times, it has no medical significance. Therefore, the differentiation among causes of purpura is very important. Generally, very small flecks of purpura are termed *petechiae.* Larger areas of superficial purpura are called *ecchymoses.* A *contusion* (bruise) is a purpuric area that is deep, less well demarcated, and blue-purple initially, later showing shades of green and yellow. Superficial purpura is bright red or purple initially, with the color gradually becoming yellow or brown before clearing.

Purpura results from any of three circumstances, each producing a characteristic morphology. First, the fracture of blood vessels allows extravasation of blood. This may be due to significant crush trauma to normal vessels, creating contusions. However, several specific diseases produce fragility of the supporting tissue around vessels, allowing even minor trauma to rupture superficial vessels. This produces well-demarcated flat and nonpalpable ecchymoses. Second, abnormalities of clotting can produce exaggerated bruising as well as oozing from mucous membrane sites, such as the gingivae and nasal mucosae. Finally, destruction of vessel walls by inflammation or ischemia produces extravasation of blood cells. Purpura produced by destruction of small, superficial vessels is manifested by small, well-demarcated papules and plaques. Deeper vessel involvement is often manifested by a reticulate pattern of purpura, often with areas of necrosis.

Most of the diseases highlighted in this chapter are presented in greater detail in the chapters referred to. This chapter is designed primarily to help the physician sort through the differential diagnosis of purpura, rather than discuss specific diseases.

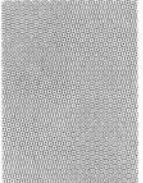

PURPURA DUE TO FRAGILITY OF BLOOD VESSEL-SUPPORTING TISSUES

Bruising develops predictably when trauma sufficient to disrupt blood vessels occurs. More remarkable is purpura resulting from minor trauma to vessels surrounded by fragile tissue. These lesions are characterized by superficial, well-demarcated, nontender patches of purple ecchymoses.

Steroid and Actinic Purpura

Steroid and actinic purpura are the best known examples of purpura caused by fragile supporting tissue of vessels. In these conditions, normally elastic supporting and protective dermis is replaced by fragile, inelastic surrounding tissue. Trivial injury, especially over the sun-exposed dorsal arms and hands, produces well-demarcated purple ecchymoses (Fig. 16.1). This type of purpura is superficial and macular, rather than palpable. The skin appears very thin, and fragility is often obvious from tears in the skin and multiple old scars. Actinic purpura is limited to the dorsal, sun-exposed surface of the hands and arms and, much less often the face, because of the infrequency of trauma. Steroid purpura is usually remarkably

PURPURA DUE TO FRAGILITY OF BLOOD VESSEL SUPPORTING TISSUE

Steroid purpura
Actinic purpura
Immunocyte derived amyloidosis
Lichen sclerosus et atrophicus

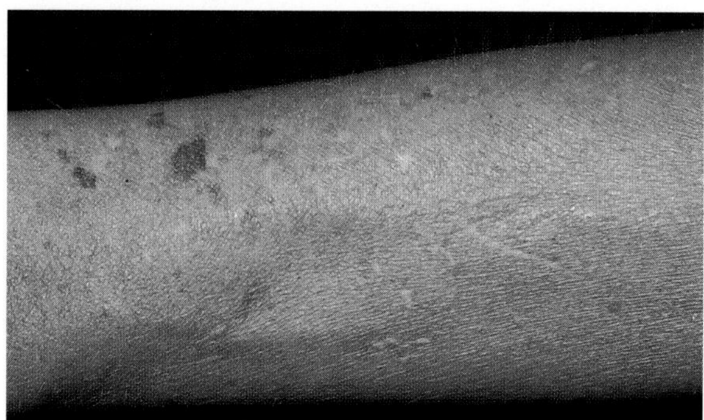

Figure 16.1 Actinic and steroid purpura present as flat, purple, well-demarcated patches that are most marked over the dorsal forearms and hands. Old scars and fragility are often obvious. Those with actinic purpura also exhibit mixed hyperpigmentation and hypopigmentation from sun damage, and actinic keratoses are common.

potentiated by sun damage, so that these changes are accentuated over these areas in the case of steroid purpura as well as actinic purpura.

There is no effective therapy for actinic and steroid purpura. Careful avoidance of sun minimizes further thinning; discontinuation of corticosteroids, when possible, results in eventual improvement. Theoretically, nightly application of topical tretinoin (Retin-A, Renova) may improve these conditions. Histologically, thickening of the epidermis and ultrastructural improvement in dermal collagen in sun-damaged skin has been shown to occur in response to tretinoin, but clinical improvement is arguable.[1,2] If this is used, conscientious use of a sunscreen each morning is important, since tretinoin desquamates the stratum corneum, part of the skin's natural sunscreen.

ACTINIC PURPURA

Clinical Manifestations
Well-demarcated, purple or red macular, noninflammatory ecchymoses over the dorsal hands and forearms, often with associated scarring from tears due to fragile skin.

Management in the Emergency Department
1. *Reassurance*

(Continues)

(Continued)

2. *Sun avoidance using a daily sunscreen with a sun protection factor (SPF) of 15 or higher, and long-sleeved clothing*

STEROID PURPURA

Clinical Manifestations
Well-demarcated patches of purple or red macular purpura, especially marked over extensor surfaces of sun-exposed skin, where mild trauma is most likely and where actinic damage accentuates fragility.

Management in the Emergency Department
1. *Reassurance*
2. *Avoidance of topical and systemic corticosteroids, when possible*
3. *Sun protection, including daily use of a sunscreen with SPF 15 or higher, and long-sleeved clothing*

Immunocyte-Derived Amyloidosis

Idiopathic or multiple myeloma-associated systemic *amyloidosis* can produce deposits of amyloid around blood vessels. Amyloid is fragile, fractures easily, and cannot provide the spongy protective cushion of normal dermis. Therefore, a classic presentation for these forms of amyloidosis is noninflammatory ecchymoses. Postproctoscopic palpebral purpura is a classic sign of amyloidosis. Before the advent of flexible sigmoidoscopy, patients who were positioned for proctoscopic examination with their heads down and their buttocks raised developed periorbital purpura from the increased intravascular pressure of the position and increased intra-abdominal pressure. Occasionally, with late disease, the skin has a yellowish, infiltrated texture that represents amyloid deposition (see Fig. 10.3). The diagnosis is made by a biopsy of purpuric skin (see also Chapter 10, Yellow Lesions).

Lichen Sclerosus (et Atrophicus)

Lichen sclerosus (et atrophicus) is a skin disease found primarily over the vulva. This condition is characterized by hypopigmentation and remarkable thinning of the epidermis that produces shiny skin or fine crinkling (see Ch. 9, White Lesions). Edema and mucin deposition in the dermis provides poor support for dermal blood vessels, so that minor trauma fractures blood vessels and produces superficial, well-demarcated purpura. Because the skin is fragile and often pruritic, erosions and excoriations are common. When lichen sclerosus is left untreated, scarring occurs, with resorption of the labia minora and narrowing of the introitus. The diagnosis is made by a skin biopsy, unless the skin findings are very characteristic. Therapy consists of a limited course of a topical superpotent corticosteroid such as clobetasol propionate (Temovate) cream under close supervision by a clinician who is experienced with this disease.[3]

PURPURA DUE TO COAGULOPATHIES

The second general cause of purpura is a coagulopathy. Thrombocytopenia, hemophilia, consumption coagulopathy, and anticoagulant usage are states that produce purpura. These patients are especially likely to experience oozing from mucous membranes, such as gingival bleeding after brushing the teeth. Patients with clotting abnormalities also develop exaggerated purpura following minor injury and needle sticks. Easy bruisability is typical.

These diseases are classified as hematologic abnormalities, rather than as dermatologic abnormalities, so that the correct laboratory evaluation should be sought from a hematology source. Screening laboratory work initially includes a complete blood count, prothrombin time, and partial thromboplastin time.

PURPURA DUE TO COAGULOPATHIES

Thrombocytopenia

Genetic deficiencies of clotting factors (hemophilia)

Anticoagulant medications

Consumptive coagulopathy

PURPURA CAUSED BY A COAGULOPATHY

Clinical Manifestations

Bleeding from gums, conjunctivae; exaggerated bruising from mild trauma and needle sticks.

Management in the Emergency Department

1. *Evaluation of the severity and cause of coagulopathy*
2. *Specific therapy directed toward the cause and correction of coagulopathy*

PURPURA DUE TO DESTRUCTION OF BLOOD VESSELS

The third general cause of purpura is destruction of blood vessels by inflammation or ischemia. Skin lesions produced by destruction of blood vessels result from extravasation of blood from the destroyed vessel. If many vessels or large vessels are destroyed, necrosis due to interrupted blood flow produces blistering, black eschars, or ulcers (see Ch. 6, Hemorrhagic Bullous and Necrotic Diseases; and Ch. 17, Ulcers).

Inflammatory Destruction

Vasculitis Vasculitis, an intense immune-mediated inflammation of a vessel, produces purpura when vessel walls are disrupted and red blood cells extravasate (see box on p. 239). Acute, noninfectious, necrotizing forms of vasculitis, including

PURPURA FROM DESTRUCTION OF VESSELS

Inflammation

- *Hypersensitivity vasculitis*
- *Septic vasculitis*
- *Necrotizing soft tissue infection*

Vaso-occlusive disease

- *Thrombi*
- *Emboli—cholesterol, septic*

leukocytoclastic vasculitis and polyarteritis nodosa, are examples (see Ch. 6, Hemorrhagic Bullous and Necrotic Diseases; Ch. 13, Vascular Reactions and Other Flat-Topped, Nonscaling Patches and Plaques; and Ch. 17, Ulcers). The edema and inflammatory cellular infiltrate of vasculitis provide a palpable component. (For a discussion of the most common form of vasculitis, small vessel leukocytoclastic vasculitis, see Ch. 13, Vascular Reactions and Other Flat-Topped, Nonscaling Patches and Plaques.) This is manifested as small palpable purpuric papules or plaques that usually occur first and are most noticeable over the lower extremities (see Figs. 13.9 and 13.10). The destruction of larger vessels produces ischemia of the overlying skin because of the disruption of blood flow. Pale or mottled ischemic skin later develops ecchymoses, often followed by hemorrhagic blistering or necrosis in a setting of surrounding purpura (see Figs. 6.6, 6.7, and 17.4). When only a few vessels are affected, and healthy, intact vessels contribute collateral blood flow, an irregular, livedo pattern can occur (see Figs. 6.4 and 6.5). These diseases are discussed in greater detail in Chapters 6 and 13. Much less often, other types of vascular inflammation, including granulomatous inflammation such as Churg-Strauss disease and Wegener's granulomatosis, can produce hemorrhagic papules and nodules as well (see Ch. 17, Ulcers).

Septic Vasculitis Septic vasculitis is produced by direct infection of the vessel, rather than by an immune-mediated hypersensitivity response. This can begin either with direct seeding of bacteria or fungus in a septic patient, or when septic vegetations embolize and lodge in vessels. First, these events produce scattered, nonspecific red papules that often resemble insect bites. These papules become purpuric as infection and inflammation destroy the vessel and extravasation occurs (Fig. 16.2). These are the earliest skin lesions of Rocky Mountain spotted fever and acute meningococcemia. The primary, characteristic lesions of Rocky Mountain spotted fever are pink, blanching, tiny macules that appear acrally. These macules then become petechial and palpable (Fig. 16.3). The initial lesions of meningococcemia are also scattered pink papules. These papules may become petechial or pustular. Because these lesions of Rocky Mountain spotted fever and acute meningo-

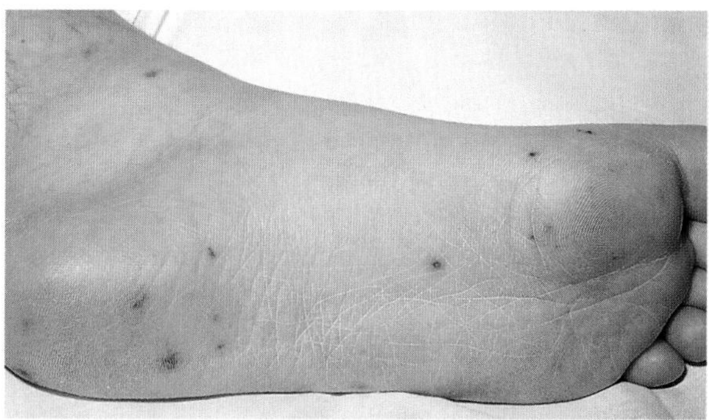

Figure 16.2 Septic emboli, like hypersensitivity leukocytoclastic vasculitis, present as palpable purpura. When small vessels and small emboli are involved, purpuric macules occur, becoming papular as inflammatory cells are recruited locally, producing septic vasculitis.

Figure 16.3 Unfortunately, the lesions of Rocky Mountain spotted fever are characteristic but not diagnostic. Tiny, pink macules over the hands and feet evolve into petechiae that also exhibit characteristic, but not diagnostic, biopsy findings. (From Sams and Lynch,[7] with permission.)

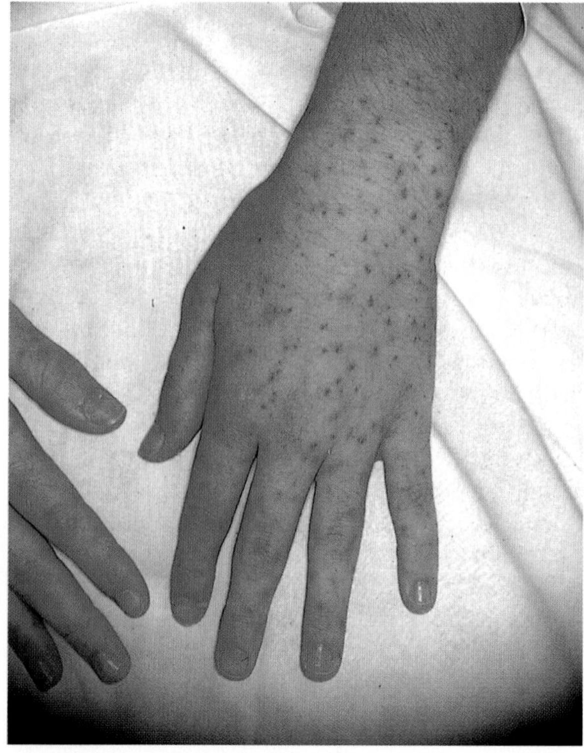

coccemia are not diagnostic, but only characteristic, the diagnosis rests on the presentation of the illness and the history, in association with confirmatory tests (Fig. 16.4). These diseases, especially meningococcemia, can eventuate in purpura fulminans (see below).

Vaso-occlusive Disease

Large thrombi and *emboli* interrupt blood flow and produce ischemia of the vessel and of overlying skin. Thrombi can occur from hypercoagulable states such as cryoglobulinemia, disseminated intravascular coagulation (DIC), and protein C or S deficiency. These emboli most often result from dislodged clots, septic vegetations, or cholesterol. The skin lesions of these conditions that produce vascular occlusion begin as irregular, often stellate or reticulate purpuric patches (Fig. 16.5). These progress to ecchymoses with central necrosis, followed by erosion and, sometimes, ulceration. Biopsies of early lesions reveal noninflammatory thrombi, but the cause of the thrombi requires further evaluation. Management consists of identification and elimination of the underlying cause of the thrombi.

Blood flow can also be interrupted by *extravascular infection*. A necrotizing soft tissue infection disrupts blood vessels, producing ischemia and worsening infection (see Figs. 6.1 to 6.3).

Figure 16.4 Bland, pink, nonspecific papules are the earliest skin findings in meningococcemia. These become purpuric and may evolve into pustules. Patients with severe disease can develop purpura fulminans (see Fig. 16.6).

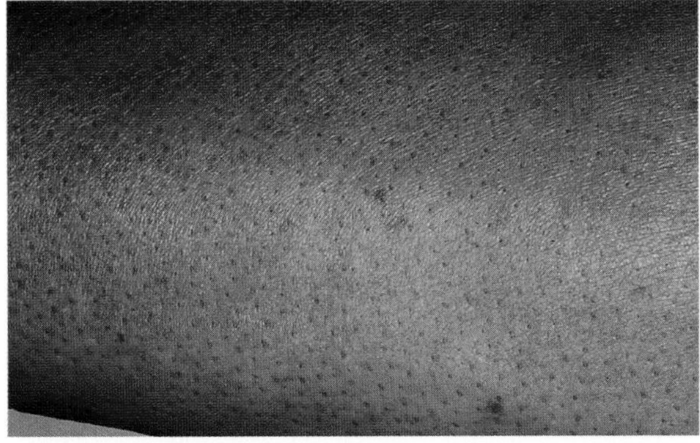

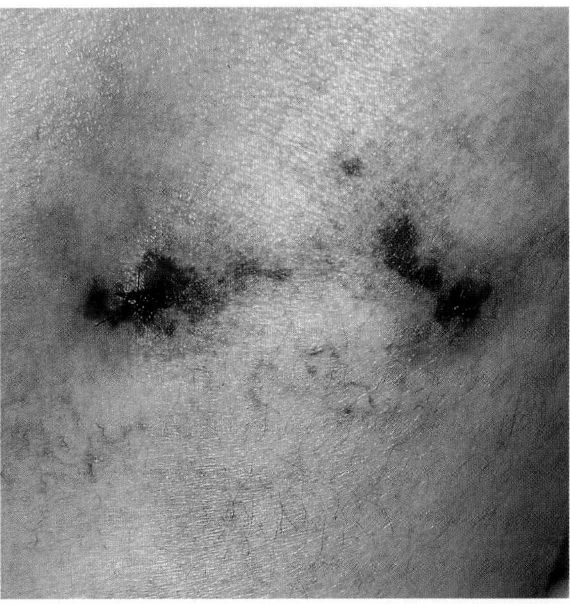

Figure 16.5 This patient with cholesterol emboli following a cardiac catheterization shows irregular purpura in a livedo pattern that developed central necrosis.

Streptococcal infection is a common initiating organism, but secondary bacteria including anaerobes invade, and infections generally become polymicrobial.[4] Antibiotics are not delivered appropriately to the infection because blood flow is interrupted as vessels are destroyed. Ischemia from the lack of blood flow to overlying skin first produces pale, painful skin, followed by anesthetic, purpuric skin that develops purpuric bullae and necrosis. The diagnosis is made by a surgical incision that reveals necrosis, rather than inflammation. Therapy requires immediate surgical debridement, intravenous antibiotics, and aggressive supportive care.[5]

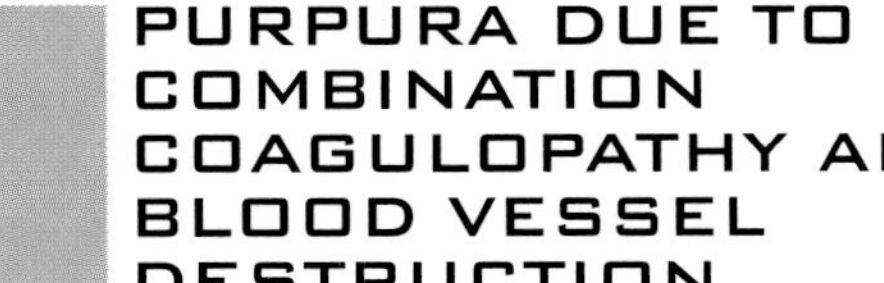

PURPURA DUE TO COMBINATION COAGULOPATHY AND BLOOD VESSEL DESTRUCTION

Purpura fulminans is a nonspecific, dramatic sign of sepsis that usually portends a grave prognosis. Closely related or identical to peripheral symmetric

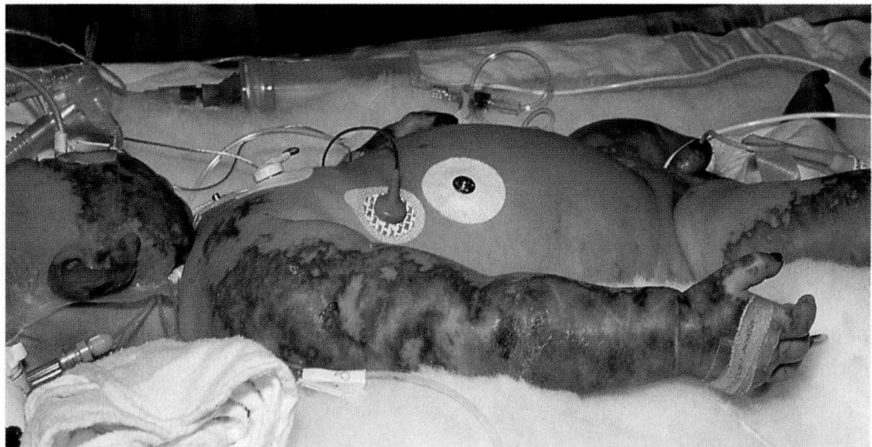

Figure 16.6 This infant with acute meningococcemia developed classic purpura fulminans, showing well-demarcated plaques of purple, stellate purpura and necrosis.

gangrene or peripheral symmetric purpura, this can occur with any of several infections, including group A streptococcal, staphylococcal, and pneumococcal infections, Rocky Mountain spotted fever, acute meningococcemia, and following a varicella infection, although this may be related to a secondary streptococcal infection.[6,7] Other causes of DIC can rarely cause purpura fulminans also, including spider and scorpion venoms, and some neoplasms.[8] Purpura fulminans results from destruction of a vessel by a thrombus from the first, hypercoagulable phase of disseminated intravascular coagulation. The extravasation of red blood cells from the damaged vessel is exaggerated by the coagulopathy that occurs as clotting factors and platelets are consumed. Ischemia and necrosis of lesions occurs because the blood supply is interrupted as vessels are destroyed. Morphologically, purpura fulminans consists of irregular, stellate patches of purpura surrounding central necrosis (Fig. 16.6). Initially, this necrosis appears as dusky purple, or gray discoloration that then evolves into a black eschar, hemorrhagic blistering, epithelial sloughing, or ulceration.

Any patient with purpura fulminans should be evaluated for sepsis and should receive broad-spectrum antibiotic coverage, with particular attention paid to diseases with stronger associations with purpura fulminans. Those patients who are likely to have Rocky Mountain spotted fever should receive doxycycline or tetracycline, unless pregnant or younger than 9 years of age. Those patients should receive chloramphenicol. Some, however, believe that the danger of chloramphenicol and the rarity of adverse effects of short courses of tetracycline on children justifies the use of a tetracycline even in children for this disease. Very ill patients should receive intravenous chloramphenicol, 100 mg/kg/day up to 3 g/day, decreasing the dose to 50 mg/kg/day after improvement is evident. Patients with possible meningococcemia should receive initial broad-spectrum antibiotics that cover other likely organisms. Infants should receive ampicillin and an aminoglycoside, or ampicillin and ceftriaxone, cefuroxime, or cefotaxime. Older patients should receive ampicillin and cephalosporin or a third-generation antibiotic. Intravenous penicillin G should be substituted when the diagnosis is firm. In addition, aggressive general medical supportive care is essential.

PURPURA FULMINANS

Clinical Manifestations

Irregular, stellate, well-demarcated plaques of purple purpura, with central gray, dusky, deep purple, or black necrosis; associated with serious sepsis, and DIC in a gravely ill patient

(Continues)

(Continued)

Management in the Emergency Department

1. *Evaluation of, and therapy for, cause of sepsis*
2. *Aggressive supportive care*

ROCKY MOUNTAIN SPOTTED FEVER

Clinical Manifestations

Patient, usually young, with fever, chills, malaise, severe headache, myalgia, and arthralgia, usually in association with tiny pink or petechial papules concentrated over the wrists and ankles, progressing to involve hands and feet, then centripetally toward trunk. Occurring most often in the spring or summer, sometimes with a history of tick exposure.

Management in the Emergency Department

1. *Confirmation of diagnosis if possible; for rapid results, skin biopsy for frozen-section routine histology (characteristic but not diagnostic) and direct immunofluorescence (30% false-negative immunofluorescence, 100% specific); acute serology*
2. *Chloramphenicol 100 mg/kg/day up to 3 g IV for ill patients. For others, tetracycline 10 to 20 mg/kg/day q6h or oral chloramphenicol (50 mg/kg/day) for children and pregnant patients, continuing therapy for 4 days after afebrile*
3. *General medical supportive care if needed*

ACUTE MENINGOCOCCEMIA

Clinical Manifestations

Abrupt onset of malaise, fever, headache, myalgia, arthralgia, nausea and vomiting, associated with scattered pink or purpuric papules that may become vesicular or pustular. Rapid progression to obtundation and signs of meningitis. About one-half of patients are small children. Followed sometimes by purpura fulminans.

Management in the Emergency Department

1. *Initial choice depends on age: aminoglycoside and ampicillin, or third-generation cephalosporin and ampicillin (infants), chloramphenicol and ampicillin (older patients); after initial broad-spectrum coverage before the diagnosis is*

(Continues)

(Continued)

indisputable, intravenous penicillin G 300,000 U/kg/day divided q4h, up to 2 million units/day.

2. *Latex agglutination for soluble antigens in the cerebrospinal fluid can provide rapid diagnosis. Also, a smear of a petechial lesion for organisms, or skin biopsy for frozen-section analysis for characteristic histology, and Gram stain can be helpful.*
3. *Blood cultures*
4. *Vigorous general medical supportive care*

REFERENCES

1. Ellis CN, Weiss JN, Hamilton TA et al: Sustained improvement with prolonged topical tretinoin (retinoic acid) for photoaged skin. J Am Acad Dermatol 23:629, 1990
2. Weinstein GD, Nigra TP, Pochi PE et al: Topical tretinoin for treatment of photodamaged skin. Arch Dermatol 127:659, 1991
3. Bracco GL, Carli P, Sonni L et al: Clinical and histologic effects of topical treatments of vulval lichen sclerosus. A critical evaluation. J Reprod Med 38:37, 1993
4. Kaldjian LC, Andriole VT: Necrotizing fasciitis: use of computed tomography for noninvasive diagnosis. Infect Dis Clin Pract 2:325, 1993
5. Sudardky LA, Laschinger JC, Coppa GF, Spencer FC: Improved results from a standardized approach in treating patients with necrotizing fasciitis. Ann Surg 206:661, 1987
6. Adcock DM, Hicks MJ: Dermatopathology of skin necrosis associated with purpura fulminans. Semin Thromb Hemost 1990;16:283
7. Hirschmann JV: Cutaneous signs of systemic bacterial infection. p. 91. In Sams WM Jr, Lynch PJ (eds): Principles and Practice of Dermatology. 2nd Ed. Churchill Livingstone, New York, 1996
8. Faria DT, Fivenson DP, Green H: Peripheral vascular diseases. p. 1145. In Moschella SL, Hurley HJ (eds): Dermatology. 3rd Ed. WB Saunders, Philadelphia, 1992

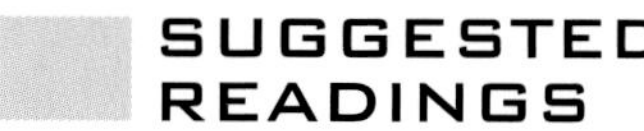

SUGGESTED READINGS

General

Lotti T: The purpuras. Int J Dermatol 33:1, 1994

Piette WW: The differential diagnosis of purpura from a morphologic perspective. Adv Dermatol 9:3, 1994

Schreiner DT: Purpura. Dermatol Clin 7:481, 1989

Purpura from Destruction of Vessels

Cohen RD Conn DL, Ilstrup DM: Clinical Features, prognosis and response to treatment in polyarteritis. Mayo Clin Porc 55:146, 1980

Fauci AS, Haynes BF, Katz P: The spectrum of vasculitis. Ann Intern Med 89:660,1978

Galen WK, Cohen I, Rogers M, Smith MHD: Bacterial infections. p. 1169. In Schachner LA, Hansen RC (eds): Pediatric Dermatology. 2nd Ed. Churchill Livingstone, New York, 1996

Hunder GG, Arend WP, Bloch DA, et al: The American College of Rheumatology 1990 criteria for the classification of vasculitis. Arthritis Rheum 33:1065, 1990

Kirk JL, Fine DP, Sexton DJ et al: Rocky Mountain spotted fever. A clinical review based on 48 confirmed cases, 1943–1986. Medicine (Baltimore) 69:35, 1990

Pottola H: Meningococcal disease: still with us. Rev Infect Dis 5:71, 1983

Prose NS, Resnick SD: Cutaneous manifestations of systemic infection in children. Curr Prob Dermatol 5:81, 1993

Weber DDJ, Walker DHD: Rocky mountain spotted fever. Infect Dis Clin North Am 5:19, 1991

CHAPTER 17

Ulcers and Erosions

An ulcer is a loss of surface tissue that extends into, or even through, the dermis. Generally, the differential diagnosis for ulcers differs from that for erosions, which involve a loss of epithelium only. Erosions most often result from blisters (for a more detailed discussion of diseases, see Ch. 4, Vesicular Diseases; and Ch. 5, Bullous Diseases).

Ulcers can be caused by many different processes, including infections, trauma, sterile inflammatory diseases, and ischemia. The diagnosis of the cause of an ulcer is difficult, since morphologically the clinician sees a lack of tissue, rather than a change in tissue. However, the location, adjacent skin abnormalities, and setting provide important clues. A biopsy is often indicated to rule out some diseases, but biopsy results are often nonspecific, with the inciting cause no longer visible.

No matter what the cause, there are several complications of ulcers that the clinician should know and consider, especially when an ulcer does not respond well to therapy. Ulcers, especially leg ulcers, are at high risk of a superimposed irritant or allergic *contact dermatitis*. One reason for this is that patients typically have used numerous soaps, antiseptics, and medications. Another reason is the frequent accompanying stasis dermatitis and fissures that allow for greater permeability of the skin. *Secondary infection* sometimes complicates ulcers. Bacterial infection is most common in leg ulcers, although tinea infections may occur when topical corticosteroids are used and the patient has tinea pedis. *Candida* is most common in oral or genital ulcers, especially when the patient is being treated with a topical corticosteroid. A third, much less common but more dangerous, complication is the development of a *secondary squamous cell carcinoma*. This occurs only after years of chronic ulceration, but it should always be considered in a nonhealing ulcer.

The differential diagnosis of ulcers can be grouped by location. Although most diseases that cause ulcers can produce them anywhere on the body, there is usually a predilection of specific diseases for different places.

LEG AND FOOT ULCERS

Although all causes of leg ulcers can produce ulcers in other areas of the body, some ulcers nearly always occur on the leg.

Stasis Ulcers

Stasis ulcers occur in an area of chronic swelling. Occurring most often around the ankle, stasis ulcers appear within skin that exhibits signs of stasis dermatitis and past or present edema (see also the section on stasis dermatitis, Ch. 15, Eczematous Diseases). The surrounding skin usually shows mottled dyspigmentation from hemosiderin deposition and postinflammatory changes (Fig. 17.1). Active stasis dermatitis may be present, manifested as erythema and scale. The ulcer itself generally exhibits irregular borders. When an ulcer occurs in a setting of edema with signs of present or past stasis dermatitis in an otherwise healthy patient, the diagnosis is presumptive and response to therapy confirms that diagnosis (Fig. 17.1).

Management requires the elimination of edema. This is generally best accomplished by the application of an Unna's boot for immediate edema control, while allowing the patient to remain mobile. A topical corticosteroid ointment such as triamcinolone 0.1% applied to surrounding, dermatitic skin decreases inflammation and improves the

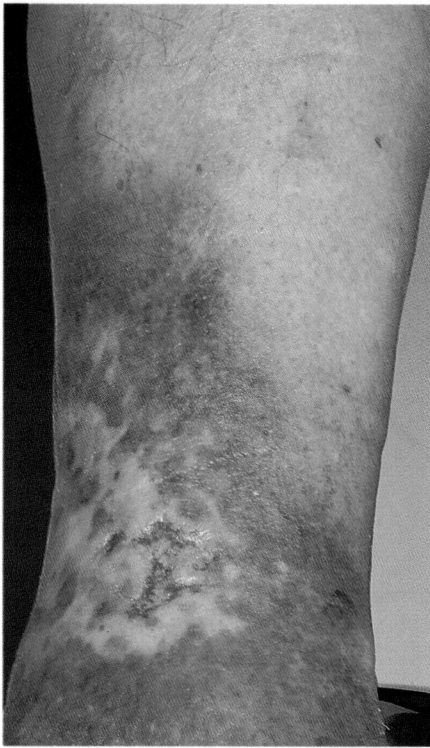

Figure 17.1 The remarkable skin changes of mottled hyperpigmentation, edema, erythema, and scale in asssociation with an irregular ankle ulcer indicate the diagnosis of a stasis ulcer.

environment to maximize healing. An occlusive dressing, such as the hydrocolloid Duoderm or the hydrogel Vigilon applied to the ulcer maintains moisture, decreases exudate production, and enhances healing.[1] However, if maceration of surrounding skin occurs, zinc oxide paste applied to the skin can protect from the moisture.

If the ulcer appears to be secondarily infected, the patient should be seen in 2 or 3 days. Otherwise, patients should follow up with their usual health care provider in 1 week for replacement of the Unna's boot and evaluation of healing. Also at that time, medical therapy can be initiated to improve underlying causes of edema when possible. The boot normally is changed weekly, and most patients experience steady healing of their venous stasis ulcer.

STASIS ULCERS

Clinical Manifestations

Irregular ulcerations of the lower leg in association with signs of current or past edema of any cause; also usual are the erythema and scale of stasis dermatitis, generally accompanied by dyspigmentation from chronic dermatitis.

Management in the Emergency Department

1. *Control of edema with Unna's boot; second choice is an elastic wrap*
2. *If active dermatitis is present, apply triamcinolone ointment 0.1% sparingly on dermatitic skin, avoiding the ulcer, before application of the Unna's boot*
3. *Hydrocolloid dressing (e.g., Duoderm) to ulcer to maintain moist environment*
4. *If superinfected: antistaphylococcal antibiotic such as cephalexin or dicloxacillin 500 mg bid or, for more significant infection, qid for 10 to 14 days*
5. *Patient education regarding necessity of long-term edema control*
6. *Follow-up evaluation with primary health care provider in 1 week to change Unna's boot, institute other medical management of edema, and monitor progress; if significantly infected, follow-up in 2 to 3 days*

Vascular Occlusion

Arterial Insufficiency Occlusion of blood vessels produces ischemia that may result in ulcers. Ulcerations that occur from the arterial insufficiency of atherosclerotic disease are painful and occur in a setting of poor or absent peripheral pulses. Possible physical findings include thinning of the skin, hair loss, and thick toenails. When the feet are elevated, the skin becomes quite pale, but the feet are suffused when they are lowered. The diagnosis is made on the basis of the clinical setting and by the demonstration of an inadequate arterial blood supply. Therapy consists of medical or surgical management of the arterial insufficiency and local supportive care.

Thrombi and Emboli Other causes of vaso-occlusive disease include cryofibrinogenemia, cholesterol emboli, and hypercoagulable states, such as sickle cell disease, cryoglobulinemia, polycythemia vera, protein C deficiency, and antiphospholipid antibody syndrome. These ulcers are not inflammatory. Purpura and livedo reticularis may be present as a result of ischemia and necrosis, but surrounding skin changes of remarkable erythema and induration are absent (Fig. 17.2; see also Fig. 16.5). An incisional skin biopsy to fat that includes the edge of the ulcer in early disease shows bland vascular occlusion. The diagnosis of cholesterol emboli is made by a history of recent vascular instrumentation and a biopsy submitted with a specific request to evaluate for cholesterol emboli. The biopsy specimen should not be placed in formalin; rather, it should be transported immediately to a laboratory, on damp gauze or in transport medium. Otherwise, the specific cause is generally discovered as a result of laboratory testing to investigate for the presence of cryofibrinogenemia or the above causes of a hypercoagulable state. Therapy depends on the cause of the disease.

Figure 17.2 Stellate purpura with central necrosis is typical of ulcerations resulting from vascular occlusion by thrombi or cholesterol emboli.

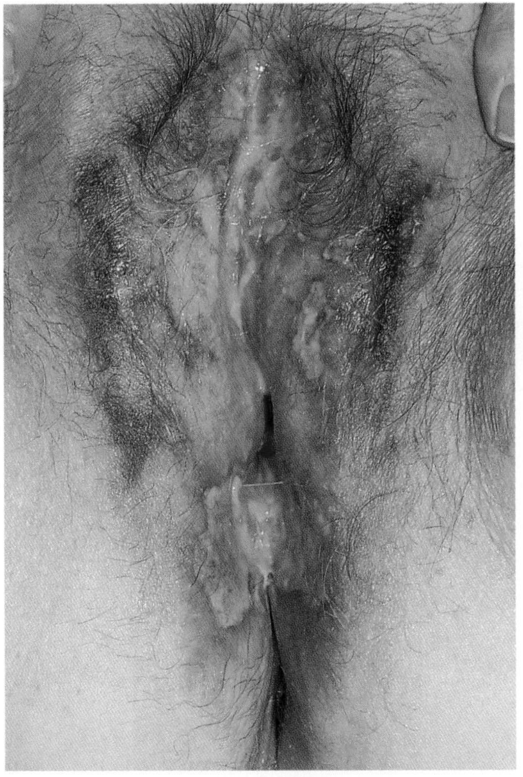

Atrophie Blanche Atrophie blanche, also called livedoid vasculitis or segmental hyalinizing vasculitis, produces characteristic irregular, stellate ulcers over the ankle or lower leg. These ulcers heal with irregular white, depressed scars surrounded by small spots of bright red telangiectasias. The underlying cause is debated. Despite the designation of vasculitis, vessels are not destroyed by inflammation. However, vessel occlusion by fibrinoid material and microthrombi are usual on biopsy. There is no uniformly effective therapy, but management commonly consists of careful local skin care as well as trials of oral dipyridamole and aspirin.[2] Other medications that have been tried include combination treatment with phenformin and ethylestrenol and low-dose intravenous recombinant tissue plasminogen activator.[3,4]

ULCERS CAUSED BY ARTERIAL INSUFFICIENCY

Clinical Manifestations

Ankle and foot ulcers caused by arterial insufficiency usually occur in the setting of poor peripheral pulses and a cool foot that becomes pale when elevated and suffused when the leg is lowered; associated claudication is common, and toenails are often thickened. The diagnosis is confirmed by the demonstration of arterial disease.

Management in the Emergency Department

1. *Timely referral for workup and correction of arterial disease*
2. *Supportive care including treatment of any secondary infection and avoidance of compression dressings and constricting shoes*

ULCERS CAUSED BY VESSEL OCCLUSION

Clinical Manifestations

Noninflammatory, irregular, often stellate purpura with central ulceration.

Management in the Emergency Department

1. *Immediate referral for evaluation of cause of occlusion, to include deep incisional biopsy to evaluate for the presence of occlusion, and laboratory testing for protein C or S deficiency, cryoglobulins, etc.*
2. *Supportive care, including treatment of any secondary infection*

Ulcers Due to Sensory Neuropathy

Patients with a sensory neuropathy are at risk of the development of ulcers that result from unappreciated trauma, especially pressure. When neurotropic ulcers occur in skin overlying the metatarsal heads, these lesions are called mal perforans ulcers. Neurotropic ulcers are especially common on the feet of diabetic patients, although any cause of decreased sensation is likely to lead to erosions and ulcerations. The diagnosis is made by the demonstration of decreased sensation in the area and by the recognition of a site prone to trauma or pressure, such as skin overlying bony prominences (Fig. 17.3) or areas that rub against a shoe . Therapy consists of alleviation of pressure with special shoes or padding devices.

NEUROPATHIC ULCERS

Clinical Manifestations

Ulcers over pressure points such as the metatarsal heads, in a setting of sensory neuropathy.

Management in the Emergency Department

1. *Alleviation of pressure with padding, shoe inserts, etc.*
2. *Supportive local therapy such as treatment of secondary infection*

Inflammatory Ulcers

Intense inflammation can produce necrosis and ulceration, even when the inflammation is not

Figure 17.3 Deep ulcers over the ischial tuberosities are present in this quadriplegic patient who sat for long periods because of lack of pain from pressure.

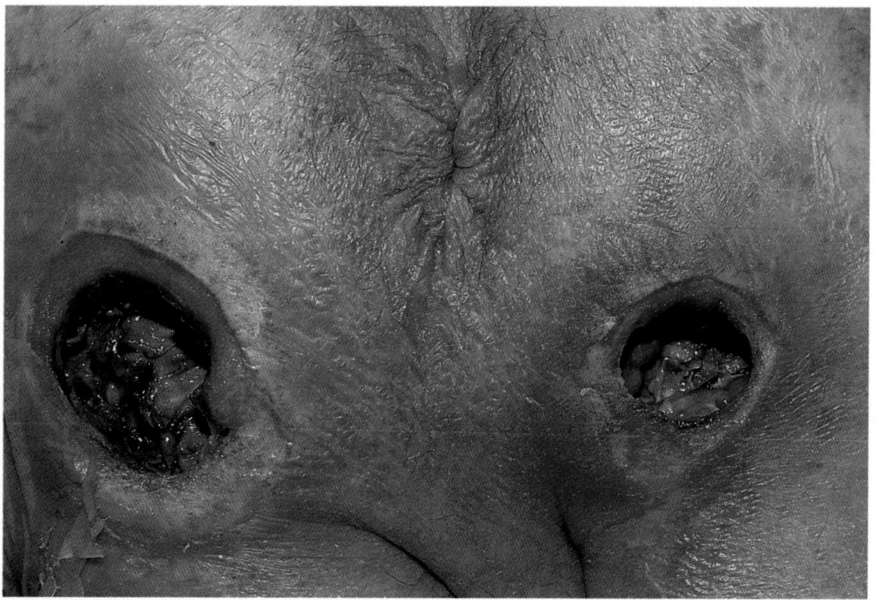

associated with infection. Several sterile, inflammatory processes that regularly create ulcers are most common on the lower extremities.

Vasculitic Ulcers Vasculitic ulcers occur as a result of immune-mediated destruction of blood vessels and tissue (see also the sections on vasculitis in Ch. 6, Hemorrhagic Bullous and Necrotic Diseases and Ch. 13, Vascular Reactions and Other Flat-Topped, Nonscaling Patches and Plaques). This inflammation most often results from a hypersensitivity reaction to a medication or infection, or it can be an autoimmune phenomenon. Vasculitic ulcers occurring most often on the legs usually result from small vessel leukocytoclastic vasculitis or, less often, polyarteritis nodosa. However, granulomatous vasculitides (e.g., Wegener's granulomatosis, granulomatosis of Churg-Strauss) are also rare causes of ulcers, but these are less specifically found on the lower extremities.

Ulcers of leukocytoclastic vasculitis generally begin as palpable purpura or hemorrhagic blisters (see Figs. 6.6, 6.7, 13.9, and 13.10). These necrose and ulcerate, typically producing lesions with punched out, violaceous borders (Fig. 17.4). Although a recently initiated medication, an infection, or an autoimmune disease such as lupus erythematosus or rheumatoid arthritis can often be identified, an obvious underlying etiology is often absent.

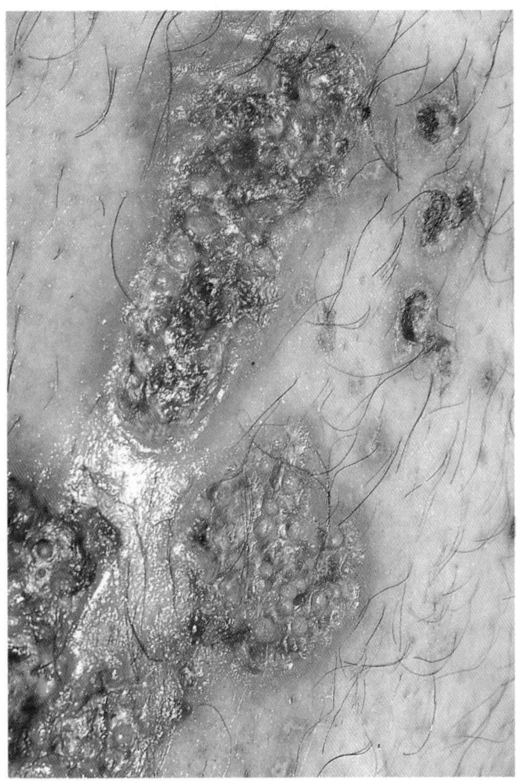

Figure 17.4 Punched-out ulcers with violaceous borders are characteristic of lesions occurring on the basis of inflammation, such as these vasculitic ulcers.

The diagnosis can be made easily when surrounding, typical leukocytoclastic vasculitis is evident, but histologic confirmation is usually sought because chronic corticosteroids are generally needed for healing. A biopsy performed from any typical surrounding palpable purpura is most useful. Otherwise, the edge of an ulcer should be sampled. The clinician should not be surprised if a nonspecific result is returned, since the original vasculitis may no longer be evident.

The management of ulcers due to leukocytoclastic vasculitis consists of a screen for systemic vasculitis as well as systemic corticosteroids. Patients should be referred to a dermatologist or a rheumatologist for this workup and therapy.

Polyarteritis Nodosa Polyarteritis nodosa, an autoimmune disease that manifests as leukocytoclastic vasculitis of larger vessels, can produce deeper purpuric nodules that can occasionally necrose, blister, and form ulcers (see Fig. 6.4). Surrounding livedo reticularis is sometimes a morphologic clue to this condition (see Fig. 6.5) (for further discussion of this disease, see Ch. 6, Hemorrhagic Bullous and Necrotic Diseases).

Granulomatous Vasculitis Ulcers resulting from granulomatous destruction of blood vessels can have variable morphology, including palpable purpura, ulcerated nodules, or ulcers with violaceous, undermined borders. Systemic disease is regularly present in Churg-Strauss syndrome, consisting of asthma, recurrent pneumonia, and peripheral eosinophilia, although other organs can be affected. Wegener's granulomatosis is a systemic disease also, with hallmarks of respiratory tract involvement and renal disease. These diagnoses are made on the basis of biopsy and correlation with systemic disease.

Pyoderma Gangrenosum Pyoderma gangrenosum is also an ulcer produced by a sterile, neutrophilic infiltrate, but inflammation is not angiocentric as it is in vasculitis (see also Ch. 6). The name is a misnomer, since the disease is neither pyogenic nor gangrene.

The most common underlying causes of common pyoderma gangrenosum are inflammatory bowel disease, rheumatoid arthritis, and chronic active hepatitis, although about one-half of patients have no underlying associated disease.[5] Classic pyoderma gangrenosum begins as a pustule that proceeds to ulcerate, forming a well-demarcated ulcer with violaceous, slightly underlined borders, and a clean base (Fig. 17.5). This disease can mimic a pyogenic, deep fungal, or mycobacterial infection. Therefore, in the absence of previous pyoderma gangrenosum, patients require a tissue biopsy for routine histology and for cultures. Myeloproliferative diseases and malignancies are associated with an atypical form of pyoderma gangrenosum that overlaps with an atypical form of Sweet syndrome (see Ch. 6). Pyoderma gangrenosum on the basis of myeloproliferative diseases often begins as a hemorrhagic blistering process (see Fig. 6.8). This form of pyoderma gangrenosum often becomes an ulcerated, boggy plaque with some areas healing, while other areas progress.

Management of pyoderma gangrenosum consists of an evaluation for an underlying, associated medical disease, if this is not already known. Screening includes a careful history and physical examination, as well as a complete blood count, screening blood chemistries, antinuclear antibodies, rheumatoid factor, hepatitis profile, a serum protein electrophoresis, and a urinalysis. The most predictably effective therapy is systemic corticosteroids, although some patients respond to oral dapsone.[6] Less often used therapies that are useful in some patients include cyclophosphamide, cyclosporine, and pulsed doses of intravenous corticosteroids.[7–9] Skin grafts are generally rejected.

Figure 17.5 The well-demarcated, purple, undermined borders of this ulcer are classic for pyoderma gangrenosum, but infectious causes must be ruled out.

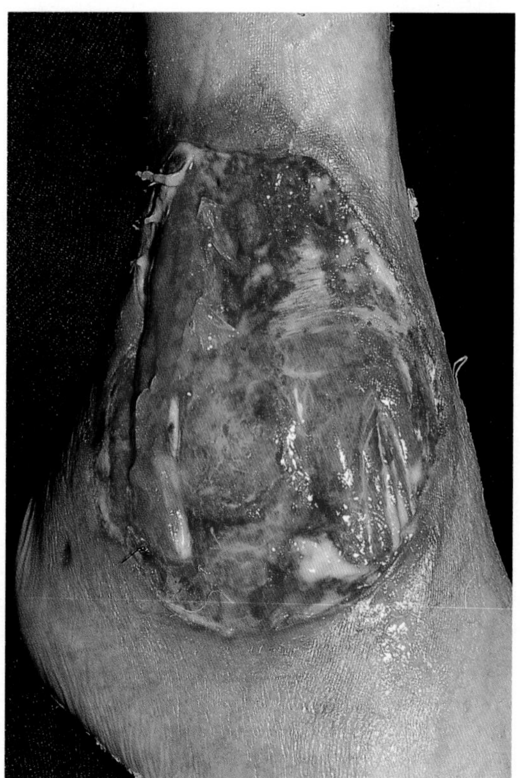

ULCERS DUE TO LEUKOCYTOCLASTIC VASCULITIS

Clinical Manifestations

Palpable purpura, most often but not always on the lower extremities, with central necrosis and ulceration.

Management in the Emergency Department

1. *Establish diagnosis either by referral or in the emergency department by setting, morphology, and biopsy*
2. *Screen for systemic vasculitis (urinalysis, stool guaiac, review of systems, physical examination)*
3. *Treat any underlying autoimmune disease, or remove causative antigen (e.g., a medication; see Ch. 13, Vascular Reactions and Other Flat-Topped, Nonscaling Patches and Plaques)*
4. *Prednisone 40 mg (small adults) or 60 mg (large adults) each morning*
5. *Treat any secondary infection with an antistaphylococcal antibiotic such as cephalexin or dicloxacillin 500 mg bid or qid, depending on severity*

(Continues)

(Continued)

6. *Immediate follow-up evaluation with usual primary care provider (if patient not ill, and cause is obvious and corrected); rheumatologist (if patient is ill), rheumatologist or dermatologist (if patient is not ill, but cause is obscure)*

PYODERMA GANGRENOSUM

Clinical Manifestations

Pustule that enlarges to form an ulcer with violaceous, undermined borders; often associated with inflammatory bowel disease or rheumatoid arthritis; sometimes associated with underlying hematologic malignancies or dyscrasias, especially when borders are infiltrated and purpuric.

Management in the Emergency Department

1. *Confirm diagnosis by morphology, biopsy, cultures*
2. *Prednisone 40 mg (small adult), 60 mg (large adult)*
3. *Follow up immediately with dermatologist or primary care provider*

ORAL AND GENITAL ULCERS AND EROSIONS

Although the first diseases to be considered when ulcerations occur on the genitalia are sexually transmitted diseases (STDs) other, noninfectious diseases should be considered as well. Ulcerations of the oral mucosa are not generally infectious. In fact, although oral erosions (shallow loss of epithelium only) are characteristic of many diseases, oral ulcerations (deeper tissue loss) are uncommon, except for aphthae.

Oral and Genital Ulcers

Aphthous Ulcers Aphthous ulcers are an extremely common cause of oral ulcerations, occurring in about one-half of people at some time. They are an occasional cause of genital ulcers. When occurring in the mouth, these are usually small, 2 to 5 mm round, regular, well-demarcated erosions over the inner lips, tongue, or buccal mucosa. There is a rim of erythema and a

Figure 17.6 Aphthae are usually small erosions with a peripheral red flare and a white fibrin base.

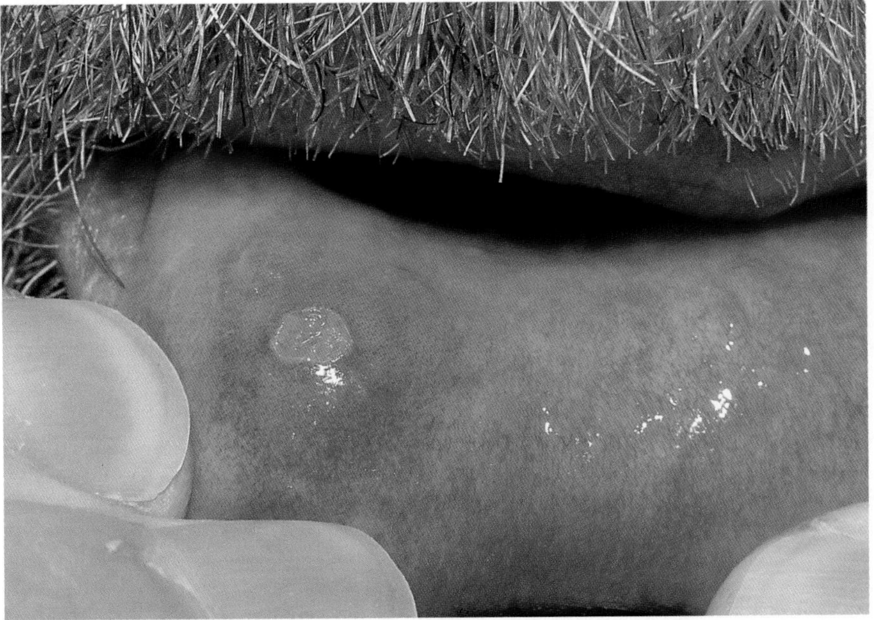

white (less often, red) fibrin base (Fig. 17.6). Aphthae are often exquisitely painful, even when small. These occur only within the mouth, sparing the external surface of the lips. Aphthae also spare mucous membranes over bone, such as the gingiva and hard palate. Occasionally, ulcers can be large (aphthae major), causing considerable pain and scarring.

Genital aphthae are usually larger than oral aphthae, and the base of these larger ulcerations can be red or covered with white fibrin. Genital lesions are usually well demarcated, but the borders may be more irregular than those of smaller, oral aphthae (Fig. 17.7). Genital aphthae occur most often over the modified mucous membranes of the vulva, but they also affect the scrotum and labia majora. Most patients with genital aphthae have experienced oral aphthae at some point, either concomitantly or in the past. This combination is called complex aphthosis.

Figure 17.7 Aphthae major are larger and more irregular, and very large aphthae may have a red rather than white base. Sexually transmitted causes of ulcers must be ruled out in patients with recent onset of large genital aphthae.

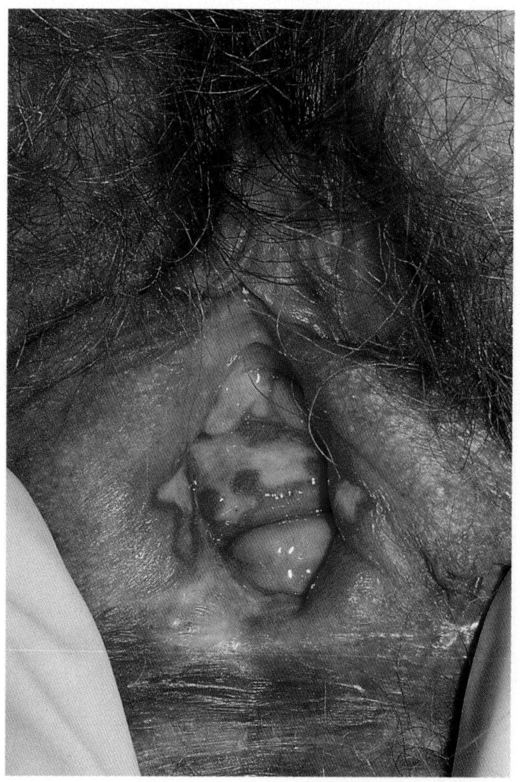

The diagnosis of oral aphthae is generally made on the clinical morphology, since no other diseases mimic this condition routinely. A diagnosis of Behçet disease should be considered when aphthae are unusually large or recalcitrant. A diagnosis of Behçet disease requires at least three of the following criteria: oral aphthae, genital aphthae, uveitis, cutaneous pustular vasculitis, synovitis, and meningoencephalitis. Patients with two of these criteria should be followed for the development of others. Behçet disease in Western countries is generally a much less severe condition than described in Japan and the eastern Mediterranean areas. Herpes simplex gingivostomatitis produces intraoral erosions, but this occurs only with the primary infection, and herpes simplex virus (HSV) infection affects both the external surface of the lips and the normal, keratinized skin surrounding the mouth. Unlike aphthae, herpes stomatitis affects mucous membranes over bone. Hand, foot, and mouth disease causes oral vesicles and erosions, but these are generally associated with a mild viral illness, and blisters on the hands and feet are regularly present.

The differential diagnosis for genital aphthae is broader and includes the sexually transmitted causes of ulcerations discussed above. Patients who present for the first time with genital aphthae require evaluation for these STDs.

The initial treatment of small, minor oral aphthae includes the application of a superpotent topical corticosteroid such as clobetasol propionate (Temovate) gel or cream qid. Covering the applied medication with a damp cotton ball enhances the effect. Kenalog in Orabase is often used for oral lesions as well. Stinging or pain often occurs with the application of these medications on the genitalia unless the ointment forms are used. Corticosteroid side effects are not a problem on the oral mucosa, but the long-term use of potent formulations on the genitalia should be avoided. Patients with large, multiple, or very painful disease benefit from prednisone at 40 to 60 mg each morning with abrupt discontinuation when pain is controlled and healing is well under way. This is efficient, effective, and safe in those patients who have occasional outbreaks. However, some patients experience frequently recurrent aphthae, and frequent courses of oral prednisone are inadvisable. Chronic therapy with oral dapsone or colchicine administered by a clinician who can follow the patient sometimes prevents the appearance of new aphthae.[10,11] Oral thalidomide has also been reported to be beneficial.[12]

> **APHTHOUS ULCERS**
>
> ***Clinical Manifestations***
>
> *Two- to 5-mm round, well-demarcated erosions with a white fibrin base and a red rim located over the mucous membranes of the mouth, but sparing skin fixed to bone. When occurring on the genitalia, aphthae are often larger, with irregular borders, and associated with either concomitant or discordant oral aphthae.*
>
> ***Management in the Emergency Department***
>
> 1. *Mild to moderate oral disease: clobetasol propionate gel or cream topically, covered with a damp cotton ball for 15 min qid; mild to moderate genital disease: clobetasol propionate ointment four times a day (prescribe one small tube without refills)*
> 2. *Severe, widespread, or very painful disease: prednisone 40 mg (small adult) to 60 mg (large adult) each morning for 3 to 7 days, until pain is controlled and healing has begun*
> 3. *Follow-up evaluation with a dermatologist if episodes are frequent or severe disease does not respond promptly*
> 4. *Patient education (see the patient handout on p. 330, Apthous Ulcers)*

Herpes Simplex Virus in an Immunosuppressed Patient Although less classic than syphilis, a much more common cause of genital ulceration is an HSV infection occurring in an immunosuppressed patient (see Ch. 20, Cutaneous Signs of Immunosuppression and AIDS). This infection produces chronic, large, often deep, well-demarcated ulcerations with irregular, arcuate borders that suggest coalescence of the original blisters (see Fig. 20.1). The diagnosis is presumptive in a patient with morphologically consistent genital ulcers who is known to be immunosuppressed. Otherwise, a culture or a biopsy from the edge of a blister confirms the diagnosis.

Chancres Chancres, produced by infection with *Treponema pallidum* (see Ch. 14, Papulosquamous Diseases: Red, Scaling, Well-Demarcated Papules and Plaques), occur most often on the genitalia, but these can occur at any site of inoculation, including the mouth. The chancre of primary syphilis classically presents as an indurated ulcer that is usually nontender. The borders are sharply marginated, raised, and regular. The base can be smooth or covered with necrotic gray material or a hemorrhagic crust (Fig. 17.8). Painless local lymphadenopathy is usual. Although usually single, several ulcers may be present. Other diseases to be considered in the differential diagnosis of primary syphilis include chancroid, aphthae, ulcerative HSV infection in an immunosuppressed host, and granuloma inguinale. The diagnosis is made by the characteristic appearance and a positive darkfield examination, because syphilis serologies become positive only about 2 weeks after the appearance of the ulcer. The chancre heals without therapy in about 3 weeks, but this does not signify elimination of the spirochete.

Treatment consists of benzathine penicillin 2.4 million units IM. For patients who are allergic to penicillin, tetracycline, or erythromycin 500 mg qid or doxycycline 100 mg bid for 2 weeks are alternatives. The clinician should also consider testing for the human immunodeficiency virus (HIV) because of shared risk factors.

> **CHANCRE**
>
> ***Clinical Manifestations***
>
> *Firm, painless, well-demarcated ulcer with regular, elevated borders; usually associated with painless local lymphadenopathy.*
>
> ***Management in the Emergency Department***
>
> 1. *Confirm diagnosis with a darkfield examination if possible, or a biopsy with special stains to identify the organism*
>
> *(Continues)*

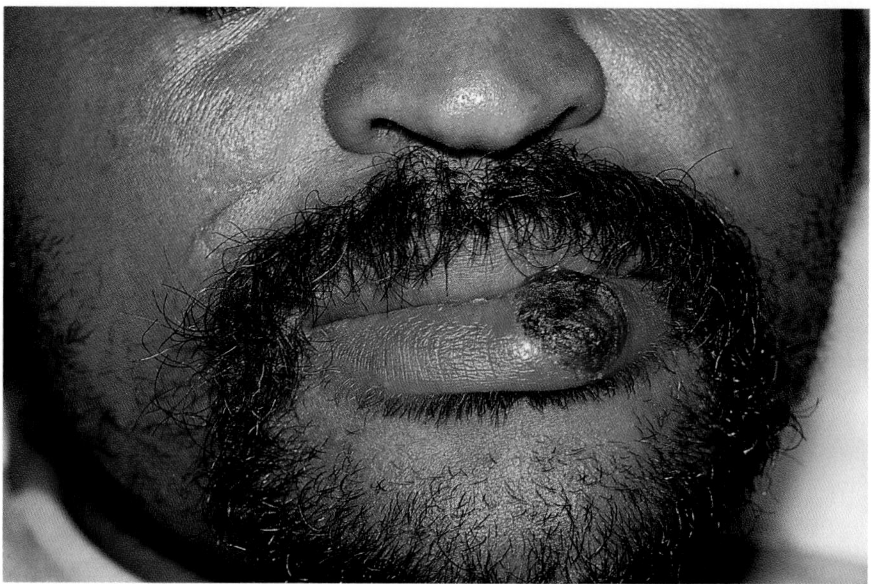

Figure 17.8 Although in an atypical location, the nontender, indurated sharply demarcated and regular borders of this ulcer are typical for a chancre.

(Continued)

2. *Benzathine penicillin 2.4 million units IM, or, for patients allergic to penicillin, tetracycline or erythromycin 500 mg qid or doxycycline 100 mg bid for 2 weeks*
3. *Report to Health Department*
4. *Consider testing for HIV and other STDs*
5. *Patient education*
6. *Follow-up evaluation with Health Department or personal health care provider in 1 month*

Chancroid Less common is chancroid, an ulcer produced by infection with *Haemophilus ducreyi*. These ulcers are seen more often in men than women, and the most common locations are the coronal sulcus and frenulum. Frequently, several ulcers begin as pustules that erode into sharply demarcated, very painful ulcers. Undermining of the borders occurs, producing ragged edges. Remarkable, painful, and sometimes suppurative local lymphadenopathy can occur. The diagnosis of chancroid is made by the exclusion of syphilis and by either a positive culture or smear of a lymph node aspirate. Management consists of laboratory screening for other STDs, since one chancroid patient in seven has concomitant syphilis. Specific antibiotic therapies include a 2-week course of tetracycline 500 mg qid or trimethoprim/sulfamethoxazole double strength bid, or ceftriaxone 250 mg IM once.

Granuloma Inguinale Granuloma inguinale, or donovanosis, is another infectious cause of genital ulcers. This STD is produced by *Calymmatobacterium granulomatis*. A small inflamed papule appears 2 to 4 weeks after exposure and develops into one of several morphologic variants. Most common are ulcerovegetative lesions that are well-demarcated lesions that resemble nodules of eroded, exophytic granulation tissue. Lesions occur most often on the shaft of the penis or the labia majora. Firm subcutaneous granulomas that mimic lymphadenopathy may occur, although true lymph node enlargement is uncommon. Chronic ulceration and edema may result. The diagnosis is made on the basis of the morphologic characteristics and by the identification of organisms on biopsy or a touch preparation. Therapy consists of tetracycline

500 mg qid, doxycycline 100 mg bid, or trimethoprim/sulfamethoxazole bid for 2 weeks.

Oral and Genital Erosions

Herpes Simplex Virus Infection An HSV infection is a frequent cause of genital erosions (see Ch. 4, Vesicular Diseases). Herpes labialis is also a very common cause of perioral erosion or crusting. Typically, HSV infection on mucous membranes or modified mucous membranes begins as scattered (in the case of a primary HSV infection) or grouped (in recurrent disease) vesicles. These immediately slough to form erosions with an arcuate border that reveal the coalescing nature of smaller lesions (see Fig. 4.2). The erosions remain superficial in most patients with healing occurring over several days for those with recurrent disease (for a discussion of this therapy, see Ch. 4).

HERPES SIMPLEX VIRUS INFECTION

Clinical Manifestations

Small, round, discrete, and coalescing erosions; sometimes associated with vesicles on surrounding keratinized skin. Intraoral HSV occurs only in children and exhibits lip and facial involvement.

Management in the Emergency Department

Primary herpes simplex virus infection (mouth: intraoral erosions; genital: scattered vesicles, erosions)

1. *Pain control, with narcotic analgesia often required*
2. *Local, supportive care*
   - *cold, bland liquids and ice for the mouth*
   - *cool tap water soaks for the genitalia*
3. *Acyclovir 5 mg/kg up to 200 mg five times a day (or famciclovir, valacyclovir) for 10 days*
4. *Patient education (see patient handout on p. 345, Genital Herpes Simplex Virus Infection)*

Recurrent herpes simplex virus infection (mouth: lip erosion, crust; genitalia: grouped vesicles or erosions)

1. *Pain control; cool soaks and acetaminophen or nonsteroidal anti-inflammatory medications usually adequate*

(Continues)

(Continued)

2. *Early, significant disease (first 48 hours): acyclovir 200 mg five times per day for 5 days*
3. *Frequently recurent or severe recurrences: acyclovir 400 mg bid chronically*
4. *Patient education (see patient handout on p. 345, Genital Herpes Simplex Virus Infection)*

Erosive Lichen Planus Several less common diseases can cause nonspecific, superficial erosions, rather than well-demarcated discrete ulcers or erosions. These are most often seen in the mouth, but the genitalia can be affected. Erosive lichen planus is a common cause of nondescript, irregular mucous membrane erosions and ulcerations. Usually, there is surrounding white epithelium that provides a clue to the diagnosis, particularly when white, reticulate, or fern-like papules and plaques occur (Fig. 17.9). However, when this white epithelial change is absent, the morphology is nonspecific. When erosive lichen planus occurs on the genitalia, scarring is common, producing resorption of the labia minora, narrowing of the introitus, and covering the clitoris under a resorbed clitoral hood. Because the vagina can be affected as well, erosions and scarring of the vaginal walls can occur with synechiae formation and even eventual obliteration of the vaginal space. In men, the glans penis can scar to the prepuce. However, scarring from oral lichen planus is generally minor. The diagnosis of erosive lichen planus can be made with relative certainty when there are typical, white, reticulate striae of lichen planus associated with the erosions. Without these typical white lesions, a biopsy is required for diagnosis. The biopsy should sample the edge of an erosion, including some intact epithelium, since the presence of epithelium is required for a histologic diagnosis of lichen planus. Unfortunately, sometimes several biopsies are required for diagnosis (for a discussion of this disease, including therapy, see Ch. 14, Papulosquamous Diseases: Red, Scaling, Well-Demarcated Papules and Plaques).

Cicatricial Pemphigoid Cicatricial pemphigoid (see Ch. 5, Bullous Diseases) can produce nondescript erosions unaccompanied by white reticulate papules or plaques. These can be identical to the

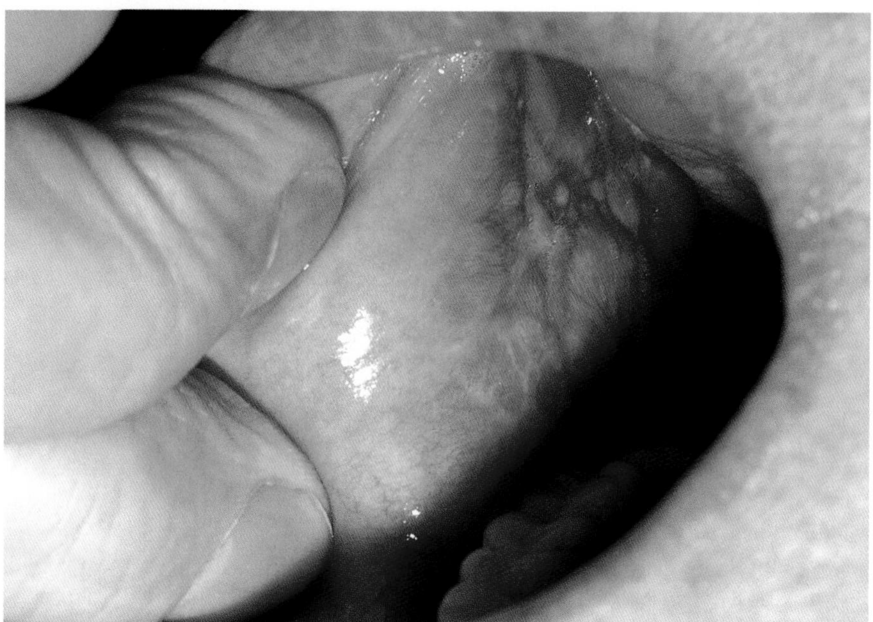

Figure 17.9 Mucosal lichen planus is more often erosive than ulcerative, but severe disease may ulcerate. When present, the surrounding white, streaky epithelium is pathognomonic for lichen planus.

more nonspecific lesions of erosive lichen planus. This disease also causes scarring and, unlike lichen planus, shows a distinct predilection for the eye, sometimes causing blindness. The diagnosis is made by a biopsy from the edge of an erosion.

EROSIVE MUCOUS MEMBRANE LICHEN PLANUS

Clinical Manifestations

Erosions, usually with associated white streaky, lacey, or reticulate epithelium.

Management in the Emergency Department

1. *Mild to moderate oral disease: fluocinonide gel or cream topically, covered with a damp cotton ball for 15 minutes qid; mild to moderate genital disease: fluocinonide ointment qid (prescribe one small tube without refills)*
2. *Severe, widespread, or very painful disease: prednisone 40 mg (small adult) to 60 mg (large adult) each morning for 7 days*

(Continues)

(Continued)

3. *Follow-up evaluation with a dermatologist in 1 week if treated with prednisone or if not improving*
4. *Patient education regarding the chronic nature of the problem*

Pemphigus Vulgaris Pemphigus vulgaris (see Ch. 5, Bullous Diseases) produces nonspecific oral, gingival, and genital erosions. These can be indistinguishable from those of lichen planus and cicatricial pemphigoid, but pemphigus vulgaris is usually associated with flaccid, cutaneous bullae and erosions. However, these nonmucous membrane lesions may not be present at presentation. Generally these erosions do not produce scarring. The diagnosis is made by a biopsy from the edge of an erosion.

Erythema Multiforme Blistering forms of erythema multiforme (see Ch. 5; and Ch. 13, Vascular Reactions and Other Flat-Topped, Nonscaling

Patches and Plaques) regularly affect the mouth and genitalia, and sometimes the mucous membranes of the eyes. Although the oral and genital erosions are often indistinguishable from those of pemphigus vulgaris, cicatricial pemphigoid, and erosive lichen planus, the explosive onset and usual presence of other cutaneous blisters, especially over the palms and soles, suggest this diagnosis. Sometimes, however, a biopsy is required for differentiation.

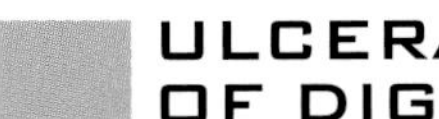

ULCERATIONS OF DIGIT TIPS

Vasculitis

Vasculitis (see Ch. 13) can preferentially affect the tips of fingers and toes, especially when leukocytoclastic vasculitis is associated with systemic lupus erythematosus. On fingers, vasculitis lesions begin as purpuric papules or macules that may necrose, become crusted, and ulcerate. These fingertip ulcers heal with scarring. The diagnosis may require a biopsy, unless characteristic lesions of palpable purpura occur in the setting of systemic lupus erythematosus. Therapy consists of treatment for, or removal of, underlying causes of hypersensitivity, and systemic corticosteroids. Sometimes, oral dapsone or colchicine can control chronic vasculitis.

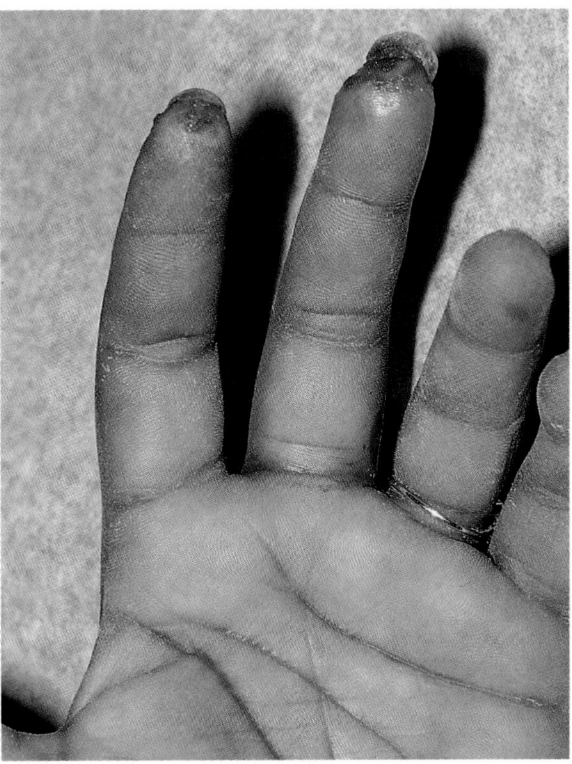

Figure 17.10 Ragged digit tip ulcerations and irregular scars are typical for lesions of Raynaud's phenomenon and disease, and lesions are generally accompanied by a history of color changes on the fingers in response to cold.

Emboli

Small emboli, including thromboemboli, cholesterol emboli, and septic emboli sometimes produce distal, digital infarcts that can erode or ulcerate. The diagnosis is generally made by the setting. Although a biopsy is sometimes required, histology is often nondiagnostic. Therapy is directed at eliminating underlying causes of emboli and local care.

Vasospasm

Vasospasm is a well-known cause of infarcts and fingertip ulceration. Raynaud's phenomenon (e.g., associated with lupus erythematosus, scleroderma) and Raynaud disease (idiopathic) can produce either short-lived color and temperature changes of the digits in response to cold, or ischemia sufficient to cause necrosis and ulceration (Fig. 17.10). Therapy includes the treatment of secondary infection and control of any associated disease. Cold avoidance and the elimination of tobacco use are important. Calcium channel blockers such as nifedipine (Procardia) up to 20 mg tid can be beneficial, and there are reports of benefit from oral diltiazem.[13,14] Topical nitroglycerin is used by some, and the vasodilators reserpine and prazosin are sometimes tried. Sympathectomies are used as a last resort, but benefits are usually short lived.

Trauma Due to Neuropathy or Fragility

Another cause of digital ulceration is trauma, either over joints of patients with fibrotic, fragile, bound down skin (as occurs over the interphalangeal joints of patients with scleroderma) or in the setting of poor sensation (Fig. 17.11). In the United States, diabetes melitis is a prime cause of peripheral neuropathy, but Hansen's disease (leprosy) is a major cause worldwide. Cigarette burns on fingertips and ulcerations from pinches and cuts are very common. Ulcers on the toes and feet are generally pressure ulcers that occur because the normal painful warnings of ischemia and trauma are absent. The diagnosis is made by the demonstration of the peripheral neuropathy, the setting, the morphologic appearance of the ulceration, and the frequent presence of scarring from old injuries. Therapy consists of the recognition of the cause of the lesions and of patient education to enhance protection from further injury.

ULCERS WITHOUT CHARACTERISTIC LOCALIZED DISTRIBUTIONS

Some ulcers have no particular distribution, and diseases that produce ulcers in characteristic locations generally can produce ulcers in other locations at times. Erosions and ulcers with either no particular site predilection or a tendency to become generalized include infectious ulcers and factitial disease. In addition, ulcerated skin cancers are distributed primarily over the sun-exposed skin.

Neurotic Excoriations

Neurotic excoriations are erosions and ulcerations produced by fingernails. Most often, there is a minor pre-existing skin irregularity, and the patient picks at it, producing the excoriation. When the inevitable crust forms, the patient again efficiently removes it with fingernail surgery. Often, the inciting skin lesions cannot be identified, although acne is a common association. Occasionally, underlying folliculitis can be itchy and precipitate picking and scratching. Most often, however, neurotic excoriations are a manifestation of stress. Excoriations are characteristically irregular, and with some linear or triangular lesions (Fig. 17.12). There is minimal surrounding inflammation, and accompanying scars are common. Neurotic excoriations are most often located over the upper shoul-

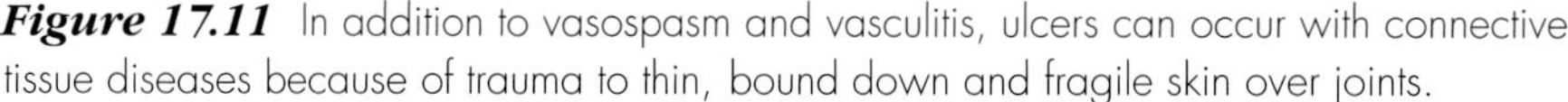
Figure 17.11 In addition to vasospasm and vasculitis, ulcers can occur with connective tissue diseases because of trauma to thin, bound down and fragile skin over joints.

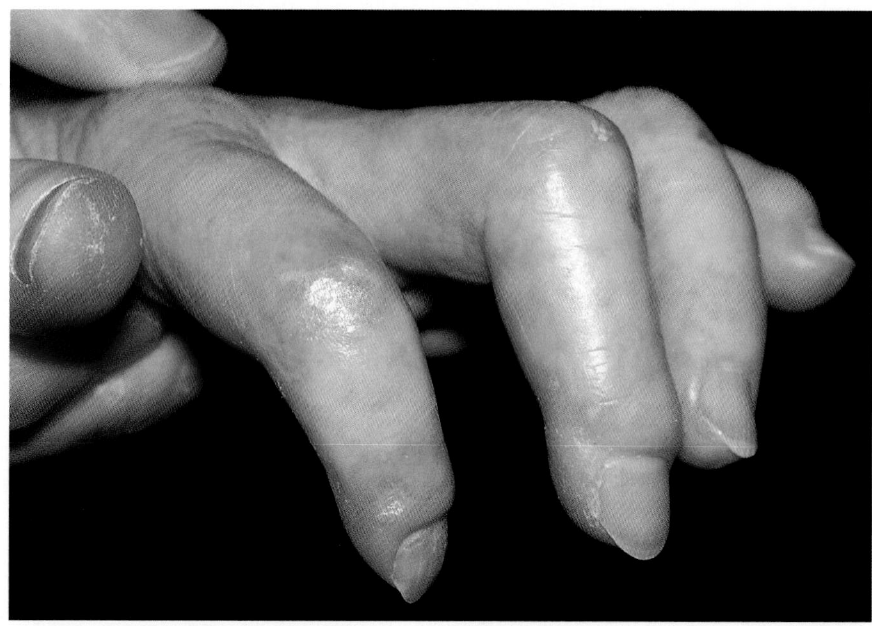

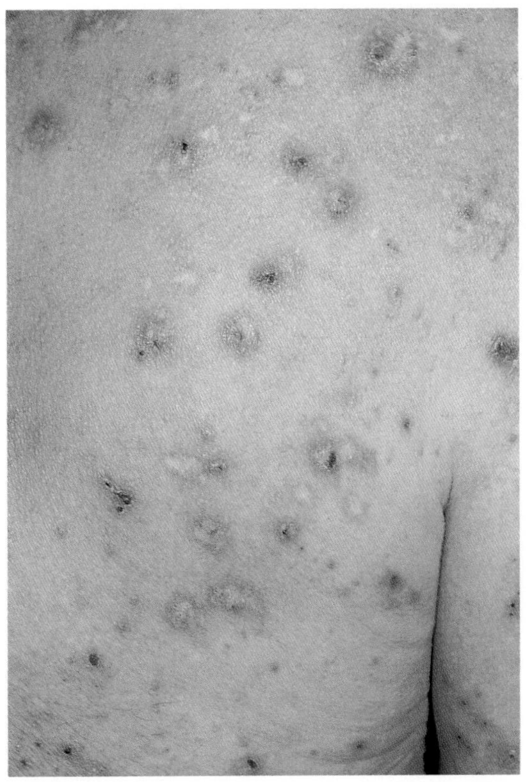

Figure 17.12 Neurotic excoriations are characterized by erosions that show linear or angular edges, no primary (unscratched) lesions, little surrounding inflammation, and a distribution in areas the patient can reach. White scars also attest to the ongoing and chronic nature of this entity.

ders, upper back, and upper arms, sparing the scapulae where fingernails do not easily reach.

The diagnosis is made by the clinical morphology. A history of picking may or may not be elicited because of the patient's embarrassment or denial. Management differs according to the individual patient or the severity of the condition. Any underlying skin disease such as acne or folliculitis should be treated. Sometimes, simply eliminating the acne breaks the picking cycle. Otherwise, for those patients with only a few excoriations, patient education sometimes suffices. Often, however, denial is such that the patient must be gradually led into the diagnosis. The application of a nonremovable dressing, such as an Unna's boot, prevents picking. This can be applied and changed in 1 week, and the absence of new lesions plus substantial healing of old ones often arouse the patient's suspicion of the diagnosis of picking. In addition, occlusion allows any underlying primary lesions such as folliculitis to remain intact long enough to be appreciated and recognized.

NEUROTIC EXCORIATIONS

Clinical Manifestations

Irregular erosions or ulcerations with minimal surrounding inflammation and no primary papules, pustules, or vesicles. Some lesions with a linear or triangular border, often associated with one or more prurigo nodules.

Management in the Emergency Department

1. *Reassurance and, if appropriate, tactful patient education*
2. *Referral to a dermatologist for significant disease (by your or the patient's estimation)*

Skin Malignancies

Skin malignancies can outgrow their blood supply; the resulting necrosis sometimes produces ulceration. Usually, the borders of the tumor are intact so that the presence of an underlying tumor is appreciated. Basal cell carcinomas classically ulcerate when they enlarge, becoming "rodent ulcers" because of the gnawed appearance (Fig. 17.13). Squamous cell carcinomas often ulcerate also, but a more common concern is the development of a squamous cell carcinoma as a result of the chronic irritation of a pre-existing ulcer. Ulceration only occurs very late in melanomas. Benign tumors can necrose also, but ulcer formation is unusual. More often, a skin tag twists and infarcts, or trauma to a lesion results in erosion. The diagnosis of a skin cancer producing an ulcer is made by a biopsy from the edge of the ulcer where the tumor is intact. Therapy consists of removal of the tumor.

Skin Infections

Skin infections can sometimes produce ulceration. Ecthyma, chronic deep fungal infections, mycobacterial infections, and sometimes parasitic infections are most likely to develop ulcers. Ulcerated infec-

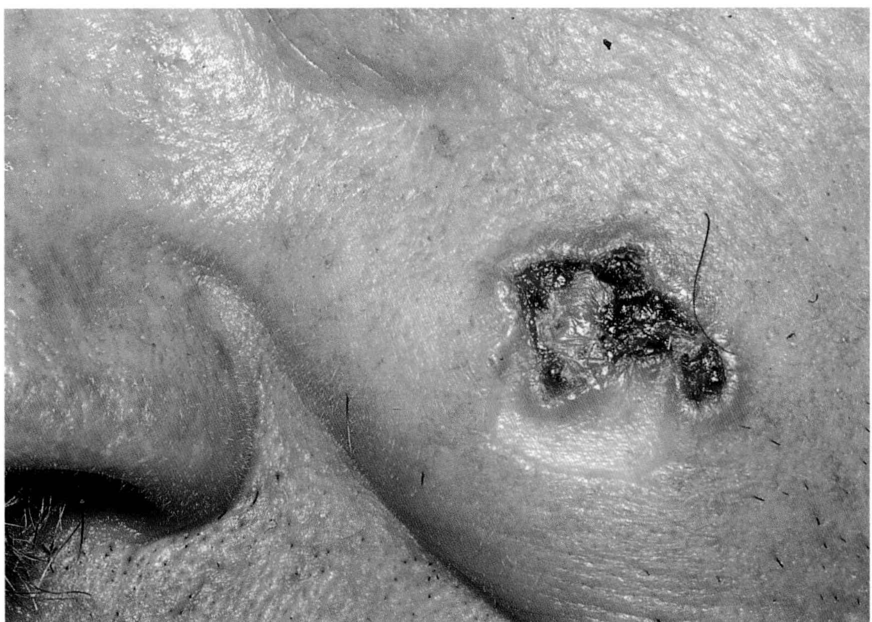

Figure 17.13 Skin cancers can ulcerate when they outgrow their blood supply or are traumatized. In spite of the ulceration, the shiny, rolled borders of this ulcer reveal the diagnosis of a basal cell carcinoma.

tions are generally infiltrated and indurated, and often there are few specific morphologic features that indicate the etiologic agent (see Fig. 12.8). When an infection is suspected, a punch biopsy for routine histology and special smears for organisms should be performed, with the specimen transported to the laboratory in a jar containing formalin. In addition, another punch biopsy should be obtained and transported in a bottle with nonbacteriostatic saline for culture for bacteria, mycobacteria, and deep fungi. The therapy depends on the cause of the infection.

Decubitus Ulcers

Decubitus ulcers are ulcers that occur as a result of chronic pressure in patients unable to protect their skin by shifting the pressure occasionally, either because of a debilitated state or poor sensation. These ulcers occur most often over the sacral area or heels, where bony prominences put overlying skin at risk (Fig. 17.3). However, decubitus ulcers are simply a variant of those ulcers discussed under the above headings of neuropathic and traumatic ulcers. The diagnosis is made by the location and setting, and therapy consists of the alleviation of pressure and local care.

Please see patient information handout for this chapter on pages 330 and 345.

REFERENCES

1. Thomas S, Fear M, Humphreys J et al: The effect of dressings on the production of exudate from venous leg ulcers. Wounds 8:145, 1996
2. Yamamoto M, Danno K, Shio H et al: Antithrombotic treatment in livedo vasculitis. J Am Acad Dermatol 18:57, 1988
3. Shornick JK, Nicholes BK, Bergstresser P et al: Idiopathic atrophie blanche. J Am Acad Dermatol 8:792, 1983
4. Klein KL, Pittelkow MR: Tissue plasminogen activator for treatment of livedoid vasculitis. Mayo Clin Proc 67:923, 1992

5. Sams WM Jr: Inflammatory ulcers. p. 917. In Sams WM Jr, Lynch PJ (eds): Principles and Practice of Dermatology. 2nd Ed. Churchill Livingstone, New York, 1996
6. Powell F, Perry H: Pyoderma gangrenosum in childhood. Arch Dermatol 120:959, 1984
7. Ko CB, Walton S, Wyatt EH: Pyoderma gangrenosum: associations revisited. Int J Dermatol 31:574, 1992
8. Goldberg NS, Ottuso P, Petro J: Cyclosporine for pyoderma gangrenosum. Plast Reconstr Surg 91:91, 1993
9. Johnson R, Lazarus G: Pulse therapy. Therapeutic efficacy in the treatment of pyoderma gangrenosum. Arch Dermatol 118:76, 1982
10. Mangelsdorf HC, White WL, Jorizzo JL: Behçet's disease. Report of twenty-five patients from the United States with prominent mucocutaneous involvement. J Am Acad Dermatol 34:745, 1996
11. Ruah CB, Stram JR, Chasin WD: Treatment of severe recurrent aphthous stomatitis with colchicine. Arch Otolaryngol Head Neck Surg 114:671, 1988
12. Revuz J, Guillaume JC, Janier M et al: Crossover study of thalidomide vs placebo in severe recurrent aphthous stomatitis. Arch Dermatol 126:923, 1990
13. Rodeheffer RJ, Rommer JA, Wigler F et al: Controlled, double-blind trial of inifedepine in the treatment of Raynaud's phenomenon. N. Engl J Med 308:880, 1983
14. Kahan A, Amor B, Menkes CJ: A randomized double-blind trial of diltiazem in the treatment of Raynaud's phenomenon. Ann Rheum Dis 44:30, 1085

SUGGESTED READINGS

Leg Ulcers

Chow RK, Ho VC: Treatment of pyoderma gangrenosum. J Acad Dermatol 36:1047, 1996

Cohen RD, Conn DL, Ilstrup DM: Clinical features, prognosis, and response to treatment in polyarteritis. Mayo Clin Proc 55:146, 1980

Fauci AS, Haynes BF, Katz P: The spectrum of vasculitis. Ann Intern Med 89:660, 1978

Hunder GG, Arend WP, Bloch DS, et al: The American College of Rheumatology 1990 criteria for the classification of vasculitis. Arthritis Rheum 33:1065, 1990

Milstone LM, Braverman IM, Lucky P, Fleckman P: Classification and therapy of atrophie blanche. J Am Acad Dermatol 119:963, 1983

Ouahes N, Phillips TJ: Leg ulcers. Curr Probl Dermatol 7:114, 1995

Phillips TJ, Dover JS: Leg ulcers. J Am Acad Dermatol 25:965, 1991

Oral and Genital Ulcers

Buntin DM, Rosen T, Lesher JL et al: Sexually transmitted diseases: bacterial infections. J Am Acad Dermatol 25:287, 1991

Camisa C, Rindler JM: Diseases of the oral mucous membranes. Curr Probl Dermatol 8:41, 1996

Hook EW, Marra CM: Acquired syphilis in adults. N Engl J Med 326:1060, 1992

Johnson RA, White M: Syphilis in the 1990s: cutaneous and neurologic manifestations. Semin Neurol 12:287, 1992

Jones C, Rosen T, Clarridge J, Collins S: Chancroid: results from an outbreak in Houston, Texas. South Med J 83:1384, 1990

Miles DA, Rogers RS III: Disorders affecting the oral cavity. Dermatol Clin 14:205, 1996

Porter SR, Scully C: Aphthous stomatitis—an overview of aetiopathogenesis. Clin Exp Dermatol 16:235, 1991

Sehgal VN, Sharma HK: Donovanosis. J Dermatol 19:932, 1992

Oral and Genital Erosions

Bricker SL: Oral lichen planus: a review. Semin Dermatol 13:87, 1994

Mangelsdorf HC, White WL, Jorizzo JL: Behçet's disease. Report of twenty-five patients from the United States with prominent mucocutaneous involvement. J Am Acad Dermatol 34:745, 1996

Pelisse M: The vulvo-vaginal-gingival syndrome: a new form of erosive lichen planus. Int J Dermatol 28:381, 1989

Other

Koblenzer CS: Neurotic excoriations and dermatitis artefacta. Dermatol Clin 14:447, 1996

CHAPTER 18

Diseases of the Hair and Nails

Hair loss and nail disease are unlikely to be common presenting complaints for patients in the emergency department. However, these abnormalities are common, and striking scalp disease, hair loss, or nail abnormalities can confound the diagnosis of other diseases. Hair and nail diseases cannot be categorized by the presence of redness, scale, blisters, and the other morphologic characteristics that provide diagnostic clues to skin diseases. Therefore, these diseases are discussed together in this chapter. However, more complete discussions of some of these entities can be found in other chapters.

ALOPECIA

The myriad of different causes of hair loss can be narrowed down by dividing diseases into four subgroups; patchy or diffuse hair loss with normal skin over the scalp, and patchy or diffuse hair loss with skin disease.

Several specific elements should be addressed in the evaluation of alopecia. First, is the scalp normal? Is there any erythema or scale? Is scarring present? Although late scarring is often obvious, scarring can be subtle. Very early scarring is characterized by more than one hair in some follicles. Also, follicles can become atretic and disappear simply from disuse, as occurs in some men with shiny scalps from male-pattern alopecia.

Second, is hair loose? Patients may describe increased hair loss because now that their hair is thin, they become more aware of hair loss. Average hair loss is about 100 hairs each day. A firm tug of a lock of hair normally releases about one club hair (a hair with an intact root) for each five pulls. This test is less helpful in black patients, whose hair is likely to be more fragile due to its structure and the use of hair-straightening permanents.

The character of the hairs should be evaluated. Are the tips broken, suggesting trichotillomania (compulsive pulling of hair), or are the short hairs fine and tapered, suggesting alopecia areata and pattern baldness?

Patchy Hair Loss Without Scalp Disease

Alopecia Areata Alopecia areata is a relatively common, probably autoimmune, disease that produces well-demarcated patches of hair loss[1] (Fig. 18.1). Children occasionally exhibit patches of hair loss that are somewhat less well demarcated, with a more moth-eaten appearance. When alopecia areata is active, hair with intact roots (club hairs) can be very easily detached with a very slight tug. Regrowing hair is fine and tapered and often shows a lighter color initially. The severity of disease ranges from a small patch that regrows promptly to eventual total and permanent hair loss of the scalp (alopecia totalis) or loss of all body hair (alopecia universalis). Extensive and disfiguring hair loss is rare.

The natural history of the disease in most patients is one of waxing and waning. Old areas regrow, while new areas may or may not appear, with ultimate regrowth over the next year usual but certainly not guaranteed. Patients with many or large patches have a poor prognosis, and alopecia totalis and universalis rarely improve significantly. Therapy may not affect the eventual outcome of the disease, but several available treatments induce at least temporary hair growth. Many physicians believe that induction of hair growth sometimes prompts resolution of the disease. The most common therapies include topical corticosteroids[2] and intralesional triamcinolone acetonide (Kenalog) injections at a dose of 3 to 5 mg/ml. This regularly

HAIR LOSS WITHOUT SCALP DISEASE

Patchy

- *Alopecia areata: well-demarcated patches of total hair loss, regrowing hair is fine, with tapered tips*
- *Trichotillomania: patches of hair uniformly broken off close to the scalp, with broken tips visible microscopically*
- *Secondary syphilis: moth-eaten, incomplete patches of hair loss of recent onset, associated with other stigmata of secondary syphilis and positive serology*
- *Traction alopecia: patches of hair loss around hairline in black girls and women with a history of braiding*
- *Male pattern alopecia: bitemporal and vertex thinning of gradual onset*

Generalized

- *Telogen effluvium: sudden, recent, generalized increase in hair loss following a significant physical insult*
- *Medications: dramatic and complete hair loss (chemotherapies) or more gradual and incomplete but often severe alopecia with other medications*
- *Hypothyroidism: gradual onset of generalized thinning of the hair, associated with other physicial and laboratory signs of hypothyroidism*
- *Female-pattern hair loss: generalized thinning beginning at the vertex in women with family history of pattern hair loss, most marked after menopause or in women with diseases of androgen excess*
- *Breakage: fragile hair that breaks easily when pulled; often with a history of coloring, straightening, permanents; common in black women*

HAIR LOSS WITH SCALP DISEASE

Patchy

- *Tinea capitis: well-demarcated scaling or crusted plaques in children*
- *Discoid lupus erythematosus: well-demarcated scaling or crusted plaques in an adult, with peripheral hyperpigmentation and central, depigmented scarring*

Diffuse

- *Follicular degeneration syndrome: red papules, pustules, crusts over vertex with scarring, in a black patient*
- *Lichen planopilaris: red scale and crust around follicles with scarring and hair loss, often associated with other signs of lichen planus such as buccal mucosa lesions*
- *Dissecting cellulitis of the scalp: inflamed, draining nodules over the scalp with associated scarring alopecia, in black men*

Figure 18.1 Well-demarcated patches of hair loss without associated visible scalp skin disease are characteristic of alopecia areata.

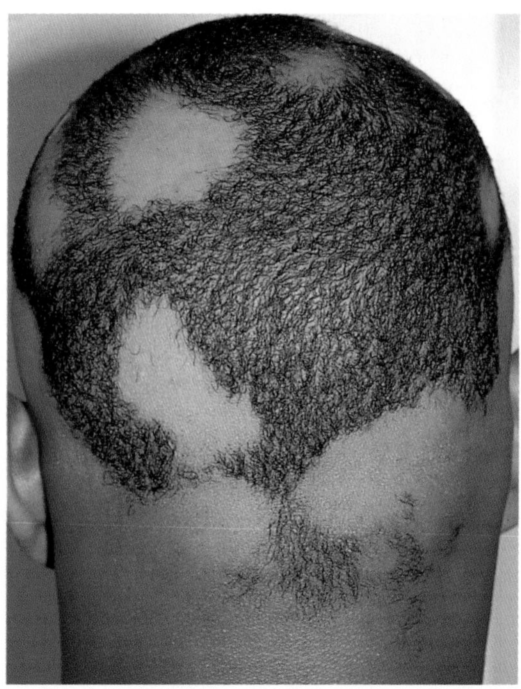

induces regrowth that is visible at a 1-month check, but this new hair is generally lost without either follow up injections every 4 to 6 weeks or spontaneous remission. This is a very practical and effective therapy for small areas, but it is neither reasonable nor safe for large areas. Oral prednisone induces hair growth, but chronic administration is required and the benefit generally does not justify the risk of adverse reactions. The application of very irritating substances, such as anthralin, to produce a chronic irritant contact dermatitis can be beneficial although uncomfortable.[3] Sensitizing chemicals applied to produce an ongoing allergic contact dermatitis can also induce hair growth.[4] Topical minoxidil is sometimes beneficial.[5] The topical or oral administration of psoralens, a photosensitizing chemical, followed by irradiation with ultraviolet A light (PUVA) has been reported to improve some patients,[6] although a recent survey of 102 patients suggests that this therapy is not particularly helpful.[7]

Alopecia areata is occasionally associated with other autoimmune diseases, but the only association strong enough to warrant laboratory testing is thyroid disease.

Significant hair loss is emotionally traumatic for some, and sensitive patient education is important. The National Alopecia Areata Foundation is a nationwide network of support groups for these patients (see the patient handout on p. 329, Alopecia Areata).

ALOPECIA AREATA

Clinical Manfestations

Well-demarcated patches of hair loss without scale or visible scalp disease.

Management in the Emergency Department

1. *Triamcinolone cream 0.1% to the affected area bid*
2. *Patient education (see the patient handout on p. 329, Alopecia Areata)*
3. *Referral to a dermatologist, with follow-up evaluation in 1 month*

Trichotillomania Trichotillomania causes patchy hair loss without significant scalp disease as patients twist or pull hair, breaking it off close to the skin surface. This habit can be as psychologically insignificant as nail biting or a compulsion deserving of medication and professional psychiatric care. Patches of trichotillomania are chronic and fairly stable. Although the patient or family members are often aware of the habit of pulling or twisting, occasionally this history is absent. Nevertheless, the diagnosis can be made by the presence of hairs broken off at about the same length, since the patient breaks the hair as soon as it is long enough to grasp. Tugging on hair does not reveal easily detached strands as occurs with alopecia areata. In addition, a microscopic examination of the tips of hairs shows broken ends, rather than the slender, tapered hairs regrowing within patches of alopecia areata. Therapy consists of tactful and nonjudgmental patient education and of follow-up management with a dermatologist, if the patient does not exhibit signs of significant psychological dysfunction. Follow-up management can be arranged with the patient's personal physician or a therapist for those who require psychotropic medication or counseling.

Secondary Syphilis Secondary syphilis occasionally produces "moth-eaten alopecia" (see Ch. 14, Papulosquamous Diseases: Red, Scaling, Well-Demarcated Papules and Plaques). Small, irregular patches of incomplete hair loss occur in a generalized pattern, with no areas of complete hair loss as occurs in patients with alopecia areata. Patients normally exhibit other signs of secondary syphilis, such as a papulosquamous eruption over the skin surface, or white mucous membrane patches. Lymphadenopathy is usual, and syphilis serologies are routinely positive except for a very rare patient with the acquired immunodeficiency syndrome (AIDS). Treatment consists of benzathine penicillin 2.4 million units IM. For those patients allergic to penicillin, tetracycline, or erythromycin 500 mg qid or doxycycline 100 mg bid for 2 weeks are alternative therapies. Repeat serologies to ensure response to therapy should be performed about 3 months later.

Traction Alopecia Traction alopecia is hair loss caused by chronic tension on hair that is left braided for long periods. Limited almost entirely to black girls and women, this hair loss is manifested primarily by a receding hairline around the face (Fig. 18.2). Generally, a fringe of short hair at the

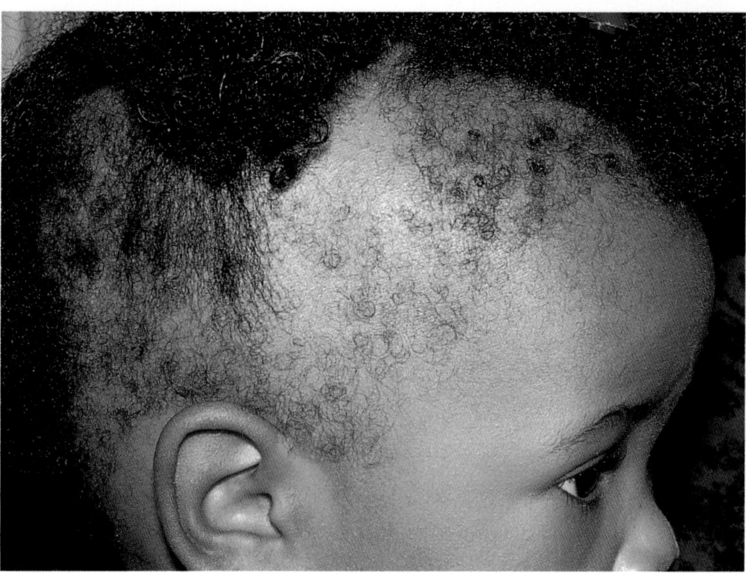

Figure 18.2 Traction alopecia presents as incomplete hair loss around the edges of the scalp of black girls whose hair is pulled tightly or braided for prolonged periods.

very edge is unaffected, since these hairs are too short to remain in braids. A zone of hair loss that ranges from slight thinning to wide complete alopecia is present. The parietal area bilaterally is especially affected. The treatment in children consists of braiding the hair more loosely or eliminating this hair style. Hair follicles can ultimately be destroyed by constant tension, so there is no good nonsurgical therapy for adult women with hair loss resulting from traction during childhood. This condition is most easily confused with alopecia areata, particularly the ophiasis pattern of alopecia areata that occurs over the parietal area bilaterally.

Male Pattern Alopecia Male-pattern alopecia (androgenic alopecia) is the most common and most easily recognized form of patchy alopecia, although late disease becomes more generalized. Beginning bitemporally and on the vertex, areas expand and coalesce to a variable degree. Although male pattern alopecia is thought to be a deficiency of regrowth of hair, rather than of increased loss, many patients report increased hair loss as well. This type of alopecia occurs as a result of familial predisposition and androgenic effects. Treatments consist of hair transplants, especially single-hair transplants) from the always-unaffected lower posterior scalp and sides, excision of bald skin so that hairbearing skin is stretched over a wider area (scalp reduction), or topical minoxidil 2% (Rogaine) applied twice daily on a chronic basis.[8] Minoxidil, now available over the counter, produces regrowth in about one-third of men with intact follicles, prevents further loss in about one-third, and has no significant effect on the remaining one-third. Discontinuation of minoxidil results in loss of new growth. Systemic antiandrogen therapies also show promise.[8,9]

Generalized Hair Loss Without Scalp Disease

Telogen Effluvium Telogen effluvium is a form of generalized thinning of scalp hair that results from a major systemic trauma. A significant insult such as a myocardial infarction, a high fever, a severe injury, delivery of a baby, and sometimes even a psychological blow can induce the body to cycle hair follicles into a resting phase as though to reserve all possible energies for healing. At 1 to 3 months after this resting phase, hair follicles release hair so that a sudden, dramatic increase in hair loss occurs. Patients do not become bald, but they may lose a great deal of their hair. Most often, casual observers do not notice a difference, but the patient is extremely aware of the dramatic decrease in scalp hair. Hair loss continues for several months until hair again recycles into growing phases. Because this is a gradual process, patients often do not recognize new growth and a return of hair for more than a year. Treatment consists of reassurance that hair will return and that they will not lose all scalp hair.

MEDICATIONS CAUSING HAIR LOSS

Anticoagulants[a]
Anticonvulsants: phenytoin, valproic acid
b-Blockers
Bromocriptine in women
Chemotherapy[a]*: doxorubicin, vincristine; cyclophosphamide less likely*
Lithium
Nonsteroidal anti-inflammatory drugs
Retinoids: isotretinoin, etretinate
Sex/steroid hormones
[a] *High likelihood of hair loss*

Alopecia Due to Medications Specific medications sometimes cause hair loss. Some medications, such as certain chemotherapies, cause this change abruptly, dramatically, and completely in most or all patients. Other medications, such as sex hormones, anticoagulants, and nonsteroidal anti-inflammatory drugs (NSAIDs), cause hair thinning of slower onset, only in selected patients, and rarely resulting in total baldness. Therapy consists of identification and elimination of the causative medication.

Hypothyroidism Hypothyroidism sometimes causes generalized thinning of scalp hair. This is insidious in onset and rarely produces complete baldness, although thinning may be noticeable by casual observers. Therapy consists of thyroid hormone replacement.

Female-Pattern Alopecia Although less obvious and usually later in onset than male-pattern baldness, female-pattern baldness (androgenic alopecia) is nevertheless a frequent condition. Most often seen in postmenopausal women who have unopposed androgen effects, patients experience generalized thinning over the top half of the scalp (Fig. 18.3). Women with a strong family history or a disorder of androgen excess may develop female-pattern alopecia much earlier and more severely. The diagnosis is made by the setting and the pattern of hair loss. Therapy consists of twice-daily topical minoxidil 2% solution, which is more effective for women with androgenic alopecia than for men.[8] If the medication is discontinued, hair loss recurs.

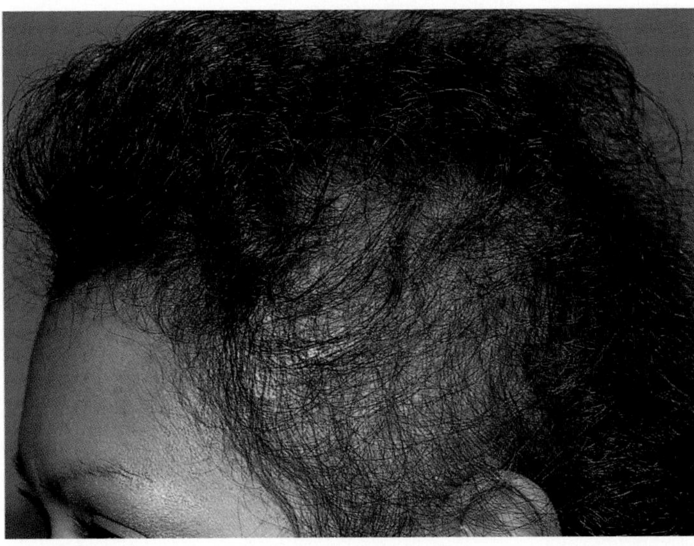

Figure 18.3 Androgenic alopecia in women consists of generalized thinning of the hair, beginning over the crown, without associated skin disease.

Breakage Generalized hair loss can also occur as a result of breakage of the hair. This is especially associated with damage to the hair caused by aggressive coloring, straightening, and the use of permanents. This is especially common in the hair of blacks, which, because of its tight curl, is more likely to knot and break, and simple combing causes more pulling and friction. Diagnosis is by the setting and by observation of fragile hair that often breaks in response to tugging.

Patchy Hair Loss Associated With Scalp Disease

Most skin diseases of the scalp do not produce hair loss. Seborrheic dermatitis and psoriasis, which have well-known predilections for the scalp, almost never produce hair loss, even when severe. Eczema is occasionally associated with hair loss that occurs from breakage of hair due to rubbing and scratching. The treatment is a topical corticosteroid such as betamethasone valerate 0.1% lotion, a very cosmetically acceptable preparation for hairy areas, in conjunction with an antihistamine, such as diphenhydramine (Benadryl), hydroxyzine HCl (Atarax), doxepin (Sinequan), or amitriptyline (Elavil) 25 to 75 mg for nighttime sedation to prevent rubbing and scratching during sleep. However, five skin diseases regularly and directly produce hair loss: tinea capitis, discoid (chronic) lupus erythematosus, follicular degeneration syndrome, lichen planopilaris, and dissecting cellulitis of the scalp.

Tinea Capitis Tinea capitis is the most common cause of hair loss in children (see also Ch. 14, Papulosquamous Diseases). Most often presenting as a round plaque, this scalp disease ranges from very subtle scale or texture change to extremely inflammatory crusting lesions with associated induration, bogginess, and drainage (see Figs. 14.10 and 14.11). Tinea capitis with subtle scale can sometimes mimic alopecia areata, so the examiner must be careful to ascertain the presence of any skin change and to obtain a fungal culture when the diagnosis is unclear. The elimination of tinea capitis requires oral therapy since fungus within hair follicles is not treated adequately by topical agents (see also Ch. 3, Medical Therapy). First-line therapy is oral griseofulvin at 20 mg/kg/day until the scalp appears normal (usually 2 to 3 months). No laboratory monitoring is necessary, but the parents should be warned about possible nausea, headache, photosensitivity, or urticaria.[10] For resistant disease, and for patients intolerant of griseofulvin, oral fluconazole (Diflucan) or itraconazole (Sporanox) at 3 to 5 mg/kg/day for one month is usually effective.[11] Because itraconazole is only available as 100-mg capsules that cannot be divided, children may require alternate-day dosing. Nausea and rash are the more common side effects, and laboratory monitoring is not required in otherwise healthy people. A 1-month course of terbinafine (Lamisil) has recently been reported to be effective at a dose of 62.5 mg/day (if 10 to 20 kg) 125 mg/day (if 20 to 40 kg), or 250 mg/day (for patients weighing more than 40 kg).[12]

Some children develop crusted, exudative tinea capitis (a kerion) in response to very inflamogenic dermatophyte organisms. These patients are at high risk of the development of scarring and permanent alopecia. Those children with a kerion should receive prednisone 1 to 2 mg/kg each morning for the first week, in addition to the oral antifungal therapy to quickly blunt this inflammatory response. Often, the inflamed, boggy plaque may present concerns of a secondary bacterial infection as well. Oral cephalexin or dicloxacillin can be added to the regimen for the first week for these children. The patient should be re-evaluated in a week to determine the need of further anti-inflammatory therapy.

TINEA CAPITIS

Clinical Manifestations

Well-demarcated plaques of hair loss with scale, and sometimes crust, occurring in children and confirmed by a fungal culture.

Management in the Emergency Department

1. *Griseofulvin 20 mg/kg/day up to 500 mg bid for 2 to 3 months*
2. *For kerions (very inflammatory, crusting disease), add prednisone 1 to 2 mg/kg/day up to 40 mg for the first week to decrease inflammation*

(Continues)

> *(Continued)*
>
> *and decrease the risk of permanent alopecia due to scarring*
>
> 3. *Follow-up evaluation with personal health care provider or a dermatologist in 1 week if on prednisone, or otherwise in 1 month*
> 4. *Patient education (see the patient handout on p. 366, Tinea Capitis)*

Chronic Cutaneous (Discoid) Lupus Erythematosus Discoid lupus erythematosus often occurs in the scalp and heals with scarring that is hairless (see also Ch. 14). Lesions are intensely inflammatory with peripheral erythema or hyperpigmentation and central crust that eventually produces white, atrophic scars. Scalp disease is usually associated with lesions over the lateral face. Therapy consists of high-potency topical corticosteroids such as fluocinonide (Lidex) 0.05% cream or solution bid. Most patients require the addition of oral hydroxychloroquine (Plaquenil) administered by a dermatologist or a personal physician.

> **DISCOID LUPUS ERYTHEMATOSUS**
>
> ***Clinical Manifestations***
>
> *Well-demarcated red, scarring, and crusted plaques with complete hair loss, often with central depigmentation and peripheral hyperpigmentation, confirmed by biopsy.*
>
> ***Management in the Emergency Department***
>
> 1. *Triamcinolone cream 0.1% to the scalp bid*
> 2. *Screening for the presence of systemic lupus erythematosus, or follow-up evaluation with a dermatologist at earliest convenience*
> 3. *Patient education (see the patient handout Cutaneous Lupus Erythematosus, on p. 337)*

Follicular Degeneration Syndrome Follicular degeneration syndrome is a relatively common condition of black women (and, rarely, men) that results in scarring alopecia. Patients exhibit follicular pustules or crusts as a result of sterile inflammation, rather than infection. The process begins at the top of the head and gradually progresses peripherally until generalized hair loss is present. The cause is not understood, but many clinicians believe that this entity represents a condition previously called hot comb alopecia. Theoretically, heat and occlusion from hot oils dripped on the scalp produced follicular damage and scarring alopecia. However, this pattern of alopecia persists despite the fact that hot combs are no longer in widespread use. The treatment includes a biopsy to rule out other diseases, such as lichen planus, and chronic administration of an anti-inflammatory antibiotic, as is used for acne.[13] These antibiotics include twice daily tetracycline or erythromycin 500 mg, doxycycline 100 mg, minocycline 100 mg, clindamycin 150 mg, or double-strength trimethoprim/sulfamethoxazole. In addition, a topical corticosteroid such as betamethasone valerate (Valisone) lotion 0.1% can be beneficial in halting progression of the skin lesions and hair loss.

> **FOLLICULAR DEGENERATION SYNDROME**
>
> ***Clinical Manifestations***
>
> *Occasional red papules, pustules, or crusts over the vertex of the scalp of black patients, producing hair loss with scarring that eventually becomes generalized.*
>
> ***Management in the Emergency Department***
>
> 1. *Tetracycline or erythromycin 500 mg bid, chronically*
> 2. *Betamethasone valerate (Valisone) 0.1% lotion bid to scalp*
> 3. *Referral to a dermatologist, with follow-up evaluation in 1 month*

Diffuse Alopecia With Scalp Disease

The skin diseases in this section often begin in one area as a patchy alopecia. However, these diseases progress to affect much or all of the scalp, rather than producing well-made plaques.

Follicular Degeneration Syndrome Follicular degeneration syndrome is discussed primarily in the preceding section, because it affects the vertex first and only becomes more generalized later. This disease of follicular inflammation and scarring occurs in black patients.

Lichen Planopilaris Lichen planopilaris, or lichen planus of hair follicles, is a rare disease that occurs most often in older women. Clinically, this disease is manifested by perifollicular erythema and scale or crust. Gradually, individual follicles scar and the potential for hair growth in these follicles is lost. The diagnosis is made by skin biopsy. Initial therapy in the emergency department consists only of topical corticosteroids such as betamethasone valerate 0.1% lotion. However, topical corticosteroids rarely produce satisfactory improvement. Aggressive systemic therapies that are sometimes beneficial, but that require careful monitoring, include oral retinoids, hydroxychloroquine, and antimetabolites.

Dissecting Cellulitis of the Scalp By far most common in black men, dissecting cellulitus of the scalp (perifolliculitis capitis abscedens et suffodiens) is not, despite its name, a bacterial cellulitis (see also Ch. 12, Red Papules and Nodules). Rather, this sterile, inflammatory process represents cystic acne of the scalp. Hair follicles are distended with keratin, producing epidermal cysts (see Fig. 12.7). When these cysts rupture, an inflammatory response ensues. Inflammatory and fluctuant cysts coalesce and create chronic draining sinus tracts. This intense inflammation results in scarring alopecia. The treatment of dissecting cellulitus of the scalp includes ongoing twice-daily oral administration of antibiotics with those medications known to benefit acne: tetracycline or erythromycin 500 mg, doxycycline or minocycline 100 mg, or clindamycin 150 mg. In addition, incision and drainage of fluctuant nodules followed by an injection of triamcinolone acetonide (Kenalog) 3.3 to 5.0 mg/ml into the cyst wall can temporarily improve disease. This corticosteroid solution is prepared by mixing 0.2 to 0.4 ml of Kenalog 10 with 0.4 ml of normal saline. Alternatively, TAC-3 is a different brand name of triamcinolone that is available in this strength. The amount injected depends on the size and number of cysts, with 0.2 to 0.3 ml injected into each inflamed cyst. Isotretinoin (Accutane) can produce beneficial effects in this disease.[14] However, most clinicians find that these effects are short lived, therefore, for ongoing benefit, this teratogenic medication must be given chronically, usually in lower doses. This is not an appropriate therapy to begin in the emergency department. Frequent and careful follow-up monitoring is required because of the many adverse reactions that can occur, including increased triglyceride levels and bony exostoses.

DISSECTING CELLULITIS OF THE SCALP

Clinical Manifestations

Chronic, inflamed, fluctuant nodules (perifolliculitis capitis abscedens et suffodiens) with draining sinus tracts over the scalp of black men, eventuating into boggy plaques with multiple sinus tracts and overlying hair loss.

Management in the Emergency Department

1. *Tetracycline or erythromycin 500 mg bid ongoing*
2. *Conservatively incise and drain fluctuant cysts*
3. *Triamcinolone acetonide 3.3 to 5 mg/ml injected into cyst walls (see text for instructions)*
4. *Patient education (see the patient handout on p. 339, Dissecting Cellulitis of the Scalp)*
5. *Follow-up evaluation with a dermatologist in 2 months*

SKIN DISEASES OF THE SCALP

Several skin diseases preferentially affect the scalp but generally do not cause hair loss unless they are extraordinarily severe or superinfected.

Seborrhea

Seborrheic dermatitis is an extraordinarily common cause of scaling of the scalp (see Ch. 15, Eczematous Diseases). This disease is manifested by yellowish scale that sometimes exhibits a slightly greasy texture, hence the term "seborrheic" (see Fig. 15.10). Scale is most prominent around the hairline, particularly anteriorly, and scale is generally associated with mild erythema. Erythema and scale behind and in the ears and on the central face occur with more severe disease.

Psoriasis

Nearly every patient with psoriasis has prominent scalp involvement. Psoriasis of the scalp is characterized by sharply demarcated, heavily scaling or hyperkeratotic, red plaques. Seborrhea and psoriasis often occur together, and a definitive diagnosis can be difficult. Such terms as *sebopsoriasis* and *seborriasis* are often used to denote disease with features of both. Often, an examination of other areas of the body for psoriasis yields a definitive diagnosis (for a discussion of the treatment of psoriasis, see Ch. 14).

Acne Keloidalis

Acne keloidalis is a skin disease found almost exclusively in black men. Representing neither acne nor keloid scarring, small, skin-colored or hyperpigmented, nonscaling, shiny, dome-shaped follicular papules occur over the occiput (Fig. 18.4). These increase in number, and scarring occurs, producing secondary alopecia. This condition remains localized to the occiput. Although topical corticosteroids, intralesional steroids, and oral anti-inflammatory antibiotics such as tetracycline or erythromycin 500 mg bid or doxycycline or minocycline 100 mg bid can retard the appearance of new lesions, definitive therapy requires excisional surgery to fat with healing by secondary intention. Laser therapy can be helpful as well.[15]

Several other diseases classically affect the scalp in addition to other areas. These include mycosis fungoides (cutaneous T-cell lymphoma) and pityriasis rubra pilaris, a self-limited, often miserably pruritic disorder, vaguely related to psoriasis. However, these diseases are very uncommon and do not fall within the scope of this book.

SCALP PRURITUS

Itching of the scalp without obvious scalp disease is an occasional symptom that is poorly tolerated by patients. Sometimes, very subtle seborrhea or eczema can produce itching, and a presumptive therapeutic trial with a topical corticosteroid such as betamethasone valerate (Valisone) lotion 0.1% bid is reasonable.

Head Lice

Head lice are an infestation that generally do not cause obvious scalp disease but sometimes produce itching with evidence of scratching. Those patients who are sensitive to the bite of the louse

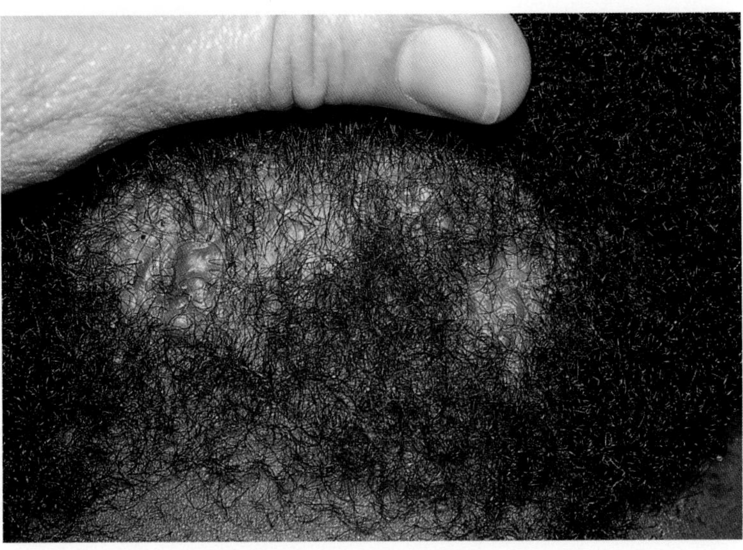

Figure 18.4 Acne keloidalis is manifested as occipital, dome-shaped papules and nodules with hair loss and scarring, seen primarily in black men or in men with dark natural complexions.

develop a small red papule at the site. The small, 2- to 3-mm lice are present only in small numbers, and they often are not observed. However, the nits (eggs) are usually easily seen cemented to hair follicles, appearing as gray-white nodules. These nits are close to the scalp in recent infections but, as hair grows, they appear farther from the skin. Therapy for head lice consists of a 10-minute application of permethrin 1% (Nix), which is available over the counter. Nits remain on the hair, although they are killed.

Psychogenic Pruritus

Scalp pruritus or burning is sometimes psychogenic. Itching in the absence of physical findings is known to be associated in some patients with depression or anxiety, but a careful examination for erythema, scale, and lice should be performed. Whereas a trial of a topical corticosteroid to treat any subclinical disease is reasonable, attention must also be directed toward the patient's psychological symptoms. A tricyclic antidepressant, such as amitriptyline (Elavil), doxepin (Sinequan), or despiramine (Norpramine), is effective for several reasons. First, these are very potent antihistamines and they produce nighttime sedation, so that the patient can sleep rather than scratch. The obvious antidepressant and anxiolytic properties are very useful in some patients. Finally, in the event that scalp pruritus could sometimes be due to a neuropathy, tricyclic antidepressants are known to be effective for neuropathic symptoms.

DISEASES OF THE NAILS

Nails are structures that are produced by skin. Thus, abnormalities of the nails may occur with some skin diseases or some systemic diseases or may be due to local infections or trauma.

Psoriasis

Psoriasis often causes classic nail findings. Nail pits (small, well-demarcated, 1-mm pits) are nearly pathognomonic of psoriasis (Fig. 18.5). Psoriasis under the nail produces "oil drop spots," yellow brown discoloration under the nails (Fig. 18.6). As disease worsens, the nail loses its attachment to the underlying nail bed and becomes lifted by scale collecting under the nail. This nail deformity can be indistinguishable from a tinea (dermatophyte) nail infection, or onychomycosis. The differentiation is made by a nail culture positive for a dermatophyte or the presence of other signs of psoriasis, although a nail bed biopsy is sometimes required. Not all patients with psoriatic nail disease exhibit skin findings of psoriasis.

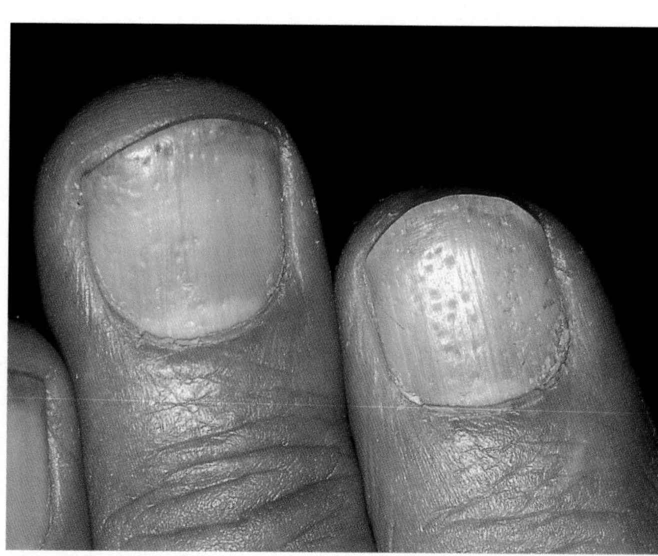

Figure 18.5 Discrete, tiny pits are characteristic of psoriasis.

There is no safe, effective, reasonably priced therapy for psoriasis of the nails. Topical medications and ultraviolet light are ineffective. Oral methotrexate, cyclosporine, or etretinate are often useful, but these medications are too toxic to use for nail disease alone and should not be used in the emergency department setting.

Lichen Planus

Lichen planus occasionally causes very characteristic nail disease. The cuticle remains attached to the nail plate, so that as the nail grows, a wing of skin from the posterior nail fold is pulled distally, covering part of the nail. The diagnosis is made by the identification of associated oral or cutaneous lichen planus, or by a nail biopsy. There is no reasonable, effective therapy.

Onychomycosis

Onychomycosis (dermatophyte fungal infection of the nail) is a very common cause of nail thickening and detachment (see Fig. 14.9). Occurring almost exclusively in toenails, classic onychomycosis begins with detachment of the distal nail plate, and subsequent buildup of scale and keratin debris under the nail. There may or may not be associated tinea pedis. Fingernail involvement occurs only in the presence of fungal infection of the feet or toenails. In the absence of cutaneous psoriasis, nail pits, and oildrop spots, the diagnosis of onychomycosis can be made with relative certainty. However, a diagnosis of psoriasis should be considered in those patients not responding to appropriate oral antifungal therapy.

The treatment of onychomycosis requires oral therapy. Griseofulvin, 500 mg bid is a safe and effective therapy for this disease. Although there is no need for laboratory testing in healthy patients receiving griseofulvin, nausea, headaches, hives, or photosensitivity can make this medication poorly tolerated in many adults. Therapy must be continued until nails appear normal; about 3 months for fingernails and 1 year for toenails. About 80% of nails clear with this regimen, but about 80% of those patients whose condition clears will experience recurrence of onychomycosis. Newer and better tolerated therapies that require only four months of therapy are itraconazole (Sporanox) and terbinafine (Lamisil). Itraconazole is given either as 200 mg/day for 4 months, or 200 mg bid for the first week of each month for four courses.[16] Although there are few day-to-day side effects,

Figure 18.6 Psoriasis also produces onycholysis (lifting of the nail plate from underlying skin) resembling a fungal infection, and yellowish color change of the nail adjacent to detachment. These yellowish "oil drop spots" are seen only with psoriasis, and help to differentiate psoriasis of the nails from onychomycosis.

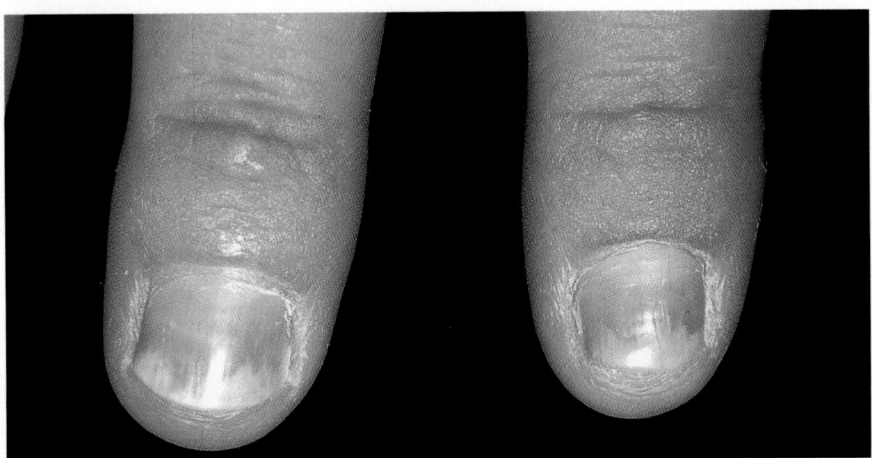

there are several drug interactions that can be dangerous. Itraconazole raises levels of terfenadine, cisapride, and, possibly, astemazole, all of which prolong Q-T levels and at high levels can produce cardiac arrhythmias.[17] Oral terbinafine has recently become available in the United States. A dose of 250 mg each day for 12 weeks clears more than 80% of nails.[18] Like itraconazole, its great advantage over griseofulvin is the shorter total dosing schedule. The drug interactions of itraconazole are not a problem with terbinafine. More recently, the older medication, fluconazole, has been reported to clear fungal nails at a dose of 300 mg/week or 100 mg every other day. The medication is continued until the nails are clear.[19]

ONYCHOMYCOSIS (TOENAIL FUNGUS)

Clinical Manifestations

Thickened nail plate that is lifted from the surface of the skin, with subungual debris, in the absence of cutaneous or nail changes of psoriasis.

Management in the Emergency Department

1. *Reassurance if only cosmetic, without pain or surrounding inflammation*
2. *For those who want treatment:*
   Griseofulvin 500 mg bid until clear (about 1 year)
   OR
   Itraconazole 200 mg bid for the first week of each month for 4 months
   OR
   Terbinafine 250 mg qd for 12 weeks
3. *Patient education, including the likelihood of recurrence and adverse reactions to medication*
4. *Follow-up evaluation with personal health care provider or dermatologist in 1 to 2 months*

Beau's Lines

Several nail deformities may produce concern in some patients. Patients who experience a severe physical trauma, such as life-threatening disease or chemotherapy, sometimes develop Beau's lines, in which growth of the nail plate was interrupted during the stressed period. This sometimes consists of a horizontal, depressed ridge, or more remarkable changes are characterized by a disruption of the nail plate (Fig. 18.7). Therapy is neither required nor effective, but the abnormal nail eventually grows out leaving a normal nail plate.

Linear Leukonychia

Linear leukonychia consists of irregular, white, well-demarcated color change on the nails. This

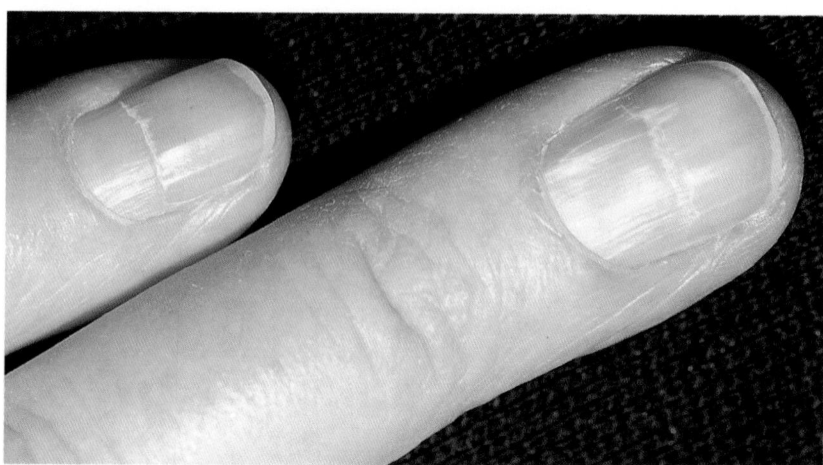

Figure 18.7 Beau's lines demonstrate an interruption in the growth of the nail during times of significant physical stress.

change is produced by trauma to the proximal nail fold, such as over grooming of cuticles, during production of the nail. The white color grows out with the nail.

Habit Tic

A habit tic is a wide, depressed, irregular vertical ridge composed of short, closely set horizontal ridges (Fig. 18.8). Most common on the thumbnail, this defomity is produced by chronic trauma at the posterior nail fold. The therapy consists of patient education and avoidance of trauma.

Median Canal Dystrophy

Median canal dystrophy is a raised, vertical ridge that tents up the thumbnail (Fig. 18.9). The cause is unknown and there is no effective therapy.

Brittle Nails

Brittle nails, characterized by splitting of the tips, are a common complaint, especially of older women. Therapy consists of using nail hardeners (a fingernail polish designed to add strength), soaking fingernails before trimming, and shortening nails by filing rather than cutting. Oral supplements, such as calcium, iron, and gelatin, are not useful.

NAIL FOLD ABNORMALITIES

The skin around nails can sometimes provide information regarding systemic diseases. Also, this skin can become inflamed due to disease or infection.

Collagen Vascular Diseases

Collagen vascular diseases often produce proximal nail fold changes. *Systemic lupus erythematosus* is often associated with telangiectasias that make this skin at the base of the nail appear red (Fig. 18.10). By contrast, the proximal nail fold telangiectasias associated with *dermatomyositis* are often more discrete and prominent, so that individual vessels are very easily appreciated.

Paronychia

A paronychia is an infection of the nail fold itself. The moisture trapped between the nail and surrounding skin provides a favorable environment for the growth of yeast and bacteria, especially *Pseudomonas aeruginosa.* Edematous, red skin surrounding the nail is characteristic of a *Candida* infection, unlike the normal skin surrounding nails infected with a dermatophyte (onychomycosis). A chronic paronychia of any kind produces an irregular nail from nonspecific inflammation. When

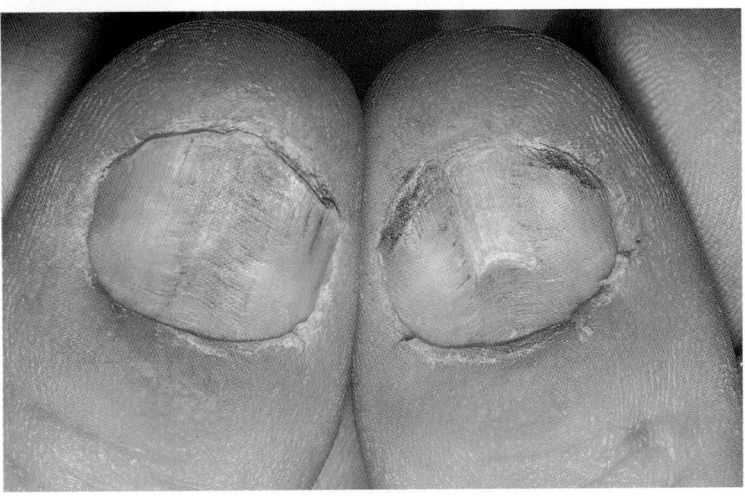

Figure 18.8 A habit tic exhibits a central longitudinal depression in the nail, produced by multiple small horizontal lines from repetitive manipulation of the cuticle.

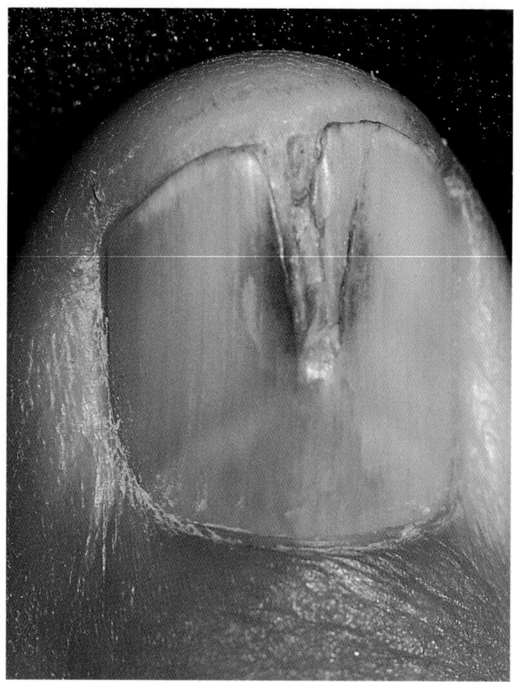

Figure 18.9 Median canal dystrophy is characterized by a nail that tents up in a central longitudinal ridge, often producing a central crack.

Pseudomonas complicates this infection, the nail often takes on a green hue. The treatment of a *Candida* paronychia includes keeping the area dry, topical anticandidal agents such as miconazole or clotrimazole, and the application of a desiccant such as thymol 4% in chloroform. Resistant cases may require fluconazole 100 mg/day. Griseofulvin, however, does not eliminate yeast. When *Pseudomonas* is present, oral ciprofloxacin can be added initially, although the infection clears without this antibiotic.

Herpetic Whitlow

A herpetic whitlow, a herpes simplex virus infection of this area, is characterized by deep-seated vesicles or pustules with surrounding erythema and edema (see Fig. 4.5). A paronychia with vesicles or pustules should be assumed to be viral rather than bacterial or candidal. Typically, a HSV infection of the fingertip or nail fold, is recurrent. Therapy requires an oral antiviral medication such as acyclovir 200 mg 5 times a day, or famciclovir 125 mg 3 times a day.

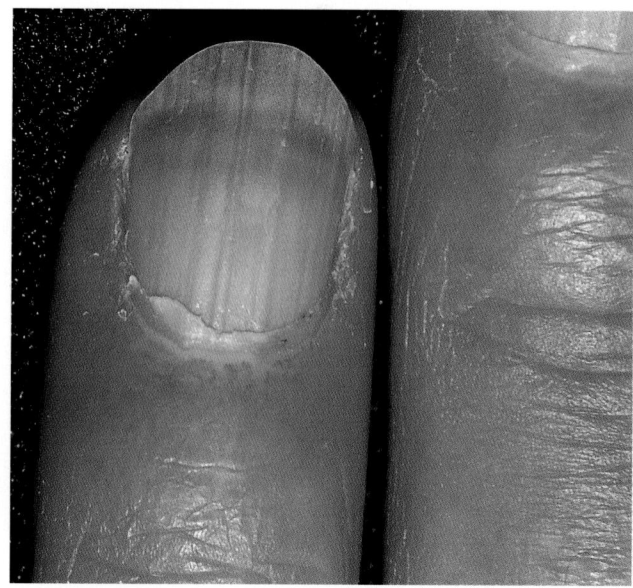

Figure 18.10 Collagen vascular diseases often show erythema of the posterior nail folds and edges of the eyelids. This erythema is produced by small telangiectasias, which are sometimes visible.

Myxoid Cysts

Myxoid cysts (mucous cysts) are small, pink or skin-colored, dome-shaped nodules at the proximal nail fold or over the distal interphalangeal joint. These cysts are sometimes produced by herniations of synovium, requiring surgery that involves the joint. At other times, there is no connection and the cyst can be removed by simpler maneuvers. These include cryosurgery, repeated draining by a needle puncture, curettage, and electrodesiccation, or intralesional corticosteroid. There are no tests that can predict whether a connection will be found during surgery.[20]

Please see patient information handouts for this chapter on pages 329, 337, 339, and 366.

REFERENCES

1. Tobin DJ, Orentreich N, Fenton DA, Bystryn J-C: Antibodies to hair follicles in alopecia areata. J Invest Dermatol 102:721, 1994
2. Fiedler VC: Alopecia areata. A review of therapy, efficacy, safety, and mechanism. Arch Dermatol 128:1519, 1992
3. Price VH, Khoury EL: Alopecia areata. Prog Dermatol 25:1, 1991
4. Van der Steen PHM, Van Baar HMJ, Perret CM, Happle R: Treatment of alopecia areata with diphenylcyclopropenone. J Am Acad Dermatol 24:253, 1991
5. Fiedler-Weiss VC: Topical minoxidil solution (1% and 5%) in the treatment of alopecia areata. J Am Acad Dermatol 16:745, 1987
6. Orecchia G, Douville H, Marelli MA: PUVA treatment in extensive alopecia areata. Ann Ital Derm Clin Sper 42:66, 1987
7. Healy E, Rogers S: PUVA treatment for alopecia areata—does it work? A retrospective review of 102 cases. Br J Dermatol 129:42, 1993
8. Shupack JL, Stiller MJ: Status of medical treatment for androgenetic alopecia. Int J Dermatol 32:701, 1993
9. Sawaya M, Hordinsky M: The antiandrogens. Dermatol Clin 11:65, 1993
10. Sherertz EF: Are laboratory studies necessary for griseofulvin therapy? J Am Acad Dermatol 22:1103, 1990
11. Elewski BE, Weil ML: Dermatophytes and superficial fungi. p. 155. In Sams WM Jr, Lynch PJ (eds): Principles and Practice of Dermatology. 2nd Ed. Churchill Livingstone, New York, 1996
12. Haroon TS, Hussain I, Mahmood A et al: An open clinical pilot study of the efficacy and safety of oral terbinafine in dry non-inflammatory tinea capitis. Br J Dermatol, suppl 39. 126:47, 1992
13. Sperling LC, Sau P: The follicular degeneration syndrome in black patients: "hot comb alopecia" revisited and revised. Arch Dermatol 128:68, 1992
14. Bjellerup M, Wallengren J: Familial perifolliculitis capitis abscedens et suffodien in two brothers successfully treated with isotretinoin. J Am Acad Dermatol 23:752, 1990
15. Kelly AP: Acne and related disorders. p. 801. In Sams WM Jr, Lynch PJ (eds): Principles and Practice of Dermatology. 2nd Ed. Churchill Livingstone, New York, 1996
16. De Doncker P, Decroix J, Pierard GE et al: Antifungal pulse therapy for onychomycosis: a pharmacokinetic and pharmacodynamic investigation of monthly cycles of 1 week pulse therapy with itraconazole. Arch Dermatol 132:34, 1996
17. von Moltke LL, Greenblatt DJ, Duan SX et al: Inhibition of terfenadine metabolism in vitro by azole antifungal agents and by selective serotonin reuptake inhibitor antidepressants: relation to pharmacokinetic interactions in vivo. J Clin Psychopharmacol 16:104, 1996
18. Schroeff JG, Cirkel PKS, Crijns MB et al: A randomised treatment duration-finding study of terbinafine in onychomycosis. Br J Dermatol, suppl 39. 126:36, 1992
19. Assaf RR, Elewski BE: Intermittent fluconazole dosing in patients with onychomycosis: results of a pilot study. J Am Acad Dermatol 35:216, 1996

20. Norton LA: Tumors. p. 202. In Scher RK, Daniel CR III (eds): Nails: Therapy, Diagnosis, Surgery. WB Saunders, Philadelphia, 1990

SUGGESTED READINGS

Alopecia

Fiedler VC: Alopecia areata. A review of therapy, efficacy, safety, and mechanism. Arch Dermatol 128:1519, 1992

Honig PJ, Caputo GL, Leyden JJ et al: Treatment of kerions. Pediatr Dermatol 11:69, 1994

Shupack JL, Stiller MJ: Status of medical treatment for androgenetic alopecia. Int J Dermatol 32:701, 1993

Sperling LC: Evaluation of hair loss. Curr Probl Dermatol 8:101, 1996

Sperling LC, Sau P: The follicular degeneration syndrome in black patients: "hot comb alopecia" revisited and revised. Arch Dermatol 128:68, 1992

Nails

Daniel CR III: Diagnosis of Onychomycosis and Other Nail Disorders: A Pictorial Atlas. Springer, New York, 1996

Hay RJ: Onychomycosis: agents of choice. Dermatol Clin 11:65, 1993

Scher RK, Daniel CR III: Nails: Therapy, Diagnosis, Surgery. WB Saunders, Philadelphia, 1990

Nail Fold Disease

Daniel CR III: Paronychia. p. 249. In Greer K (ed): Common Problems in Dermatology. Year Book Medical Publishers, Chicago, 1988

CHAPTER 19

Pediatric Dermatology

Although most skin diseases that occur in children also occur in adults, some diseases are either more common in children or require special consideration in children. Many of these diseases have been discussed in greater detail in the appropriate morphologic chapter, but some are so specific to childhood that they have been grouped here together.

SKIN DISEASES IN INFANCY

Discrete Inflammatory Papules/Vesicles/Pustules

With the trend to early discharge of newborns from the hospital, families are likely to present more often to an emergency department for common and trivial neonatal skin findings.

Erythema Toxicum Neonatorum Erythema toxicum neonatorum is a very common rash characterized by red papules and pustules scattered over the skin surface, particularly the trunk. Lesions are generally 1 to 3 mm, with a surrounding red flare. The eruption generally appears during the first week of life and resolves within 2 or 3 days. The etiology is unknown, and the only importance of this disease is that it should be differentiated from the uncommon but dangerous neonatal herpes simplex virus (HSV) infection. Staphylococcal folliculitis, miliaria, and transient neonatal pustular melanosis can also resemble erythema toxicum. Fortunately, the diagnosis can be made easily by scraping a pustule with a #15 scalpel blade, removing the pustule roof with some contents. A smear of the pus reveals sheets of eosinophils, rather than organisms or giant cells, when examined microscopically.

The eruption resolves spontaneously over the first few days of life. Therapy consists of reassurance.

Miliaria Miliaria (prickly heat) is a common condition produced by heat. It is most common in infancy, when small children who cannot communicate their discomfort or who have no choice are dressed too warmly, or when they are febrile. As children perspire and the skin is occluded by clothing or bedsheets, eccrine sweat glands can become inflamed by retained perspiration. This inflammation produces scattered, tiny, red papules located primarily on the trunk and in areas of greatest warmth.

Miliaria can be confused with erythema toxicum and transient neonatal pustular melanosis in the first few days of life and with folliculitis, insect bites, and early varicella in older children. However, the very small size of individual lesions and the large number of lesions occurring in an otherwise healthy (but recently warm) infant are usually diagnostic.

Therapy consists of reassurance and of keeping the infant cool.

Transient Neonatal Pustular Melanosis Transient neonatal pustular melanosis is characterized by small, scattered, relatively noninflammatory vesicles, pustules, and/or collarettes similar to those of erythema toxicum neonatorum. This disease of unknown etiology is most often recognized in infants with a darker natural skin color. Most prominent on the palms, soles, lower back, and face, these superficial lesions are short-lived, leaving hyperpigmented macules. Sometimes, intact lesions have disappeared by the time a baby is born, with the only findings the brown, scattered macules of postinflammatory hyperpigmentation.

This trivial disease also resembles folliculitis, miliaria, and neonatal HSV infection. Generally, the presence of typical lesions with accompanying brown macules in a healthy infant make the diagnosis straightforward. The diagnosis is confirmed by the presence of multiple neutrophils without organisms on a microscopic examination of a smear of the contents of a pustule.

Therapy consists of reassurance, with the caution that brown macules may take several weeks to months to fade completely.

Neonatal Herpes Simplex Virus Infection Neonatal HSV infection, an often devastating disease, is generally acquired during delivery through a birth canal affected with a primary HSV type II infection, although congenital cases have been reported. A neonatal HSV infection can be strictly cutaneous, but a large proportion of infants experience systemic disease, with death or permanent, severe neurologic sequelae occurring in most babies. Therefore, even apparently healthy infants with lesions suggestive of HSV infection should be evaluated and treated aggressively and immediately. About one-half of patients with neonatal HSV infection exhibit skin lesions.

Skin lesions usually occur at 5 to 12 days after delivery. Patients exhibit small, pink, edematous papules, vesicles, and crusts that can be scattered widely without grouping of individual lesions, or lesions can be zosteriform or grouped. Mucous membranes are often involved. Although skin disease can occur without systemic involvement, infants are often ill. Multiorgan dysfunction is common, especially lungs, liver, and coagulation abnormalities. Central nervous system involvement, a frequent complication, carries the highest risk of permanent morbidity.

The diagnosis is made by the clinical presentation and the presence of a positive culture of a skin lesion for HSV. Unfortunately, a culture takes several days to yield a final result; some hospitals report significant numbers of false-negative cultures. A reliable method of making a presumptive diagnosis of a herpesvirus infection in the emergency department is by a skin biopsy submitted for frozen sections. A biopsy is very specific for a herpesvirus, although it does not differentiate between HSV infection and varicella zoster virus (VZV) infection. However, other diseases in the differential diagnosis can be ruled out. A Tzanck preparation is also a viable but less dependable test for clinicians or laboratories comfortable in the interpretation of these smears. A microscopic smear obtained by scraping the base of the lesions with a #15 scalpel blade and stained with Giemsa shows multinucleated epithelial cells in a herpesvirus infection. This examination also detects herpesvirus without distinguishing between HSV and VZV. Finally, the identification of HSV by the polymerase chain reaction (PCR) technique is exquisitely sensitive and specific for HSV, and this test can be performed within several hours at some hospitals. However, it is not yet widely available and most hospitals are not prepared to perform this in an urgent situation, particularly at nights or on weekends. Fortunately, a skin biopsy or a Tzanck preparation generally yields test results that narrow diagnostic possibilities to HSV infection or varicella. Usually, differentiation can be made on the basis of clinical setting and a history of chickenpox or active HSV in the mother.

Infants with neonatal HSV infection require hospital admission for therapy with intravenous acyclovir and general supportive care. The prognosis associated with this disease is grave; most affected infants either die or experience severe, permanent neurologic sequelae.

Birthmarks

Several different kinds of pigmented or red lesions are present at birth or shortly thereafter in a small but significant percentage of newborns. Although these lesions are often innocuous, they are sometimes of great concern to parents, and some are actually associated with serious diseases or complications. Any congenital lesion overlying the spinal cord, and many overlying the scalp, can be associated with underlying neuroectodermal defects.[1] These children should be evaluated by a dermatologist or a pediatrician.

Brown Birthmarks There are two main types of brown birthmarks. Although these can be difficult to distinguish at times, café-au-lait spots are generally hyperpigmented patches without surface texture and congenital pigmented nevi have some substance or surface change.

Café-au-Lait Spots Café-au-lait spots are evenly pigmented macules or patches (see Fig. 11.4). These lesions are sharply demarcated and may be single or multiple. Sizes range from a few millimeters to many centimeters, occasionally covering large portions of the trunk. These lesions are more common, more numerous, and darker brown in black infants. Five or more café-au-lait spots of 5 cm or larger in a young child are suggestive of neurofibromatosis.[2] Café-au-lait spots can also be associated with other neurocutaneous syndromes, in particular McCune-Albright syndrome (polyostotic fibrous dysplasia). Café-au-lait spots with this syndrome often exhibit very irregular borders and generally do not cross the midline. However, one or two café-au-lait spots in an otherwise normal infant do not constitute cause for concern.

Pigmented Congenital Nevi Congenital melanocytic nevi occur in 1% to 2% of the population (for further discussion, see Ch. 11, Brown Lesions). When small, these nevi are essentially harmless, conferring an almost immeasurably small risk of the development of cutaneous melanoma. However, when larger, they are associated not only with a significant and sometimes remarkable risk of melanoma transformation, but they are also sometimes associated with underlying leptomeningeal involvement and neurologic abnormalities (Fig. 19.1).

Vascular Birthmarks Vascular abnormalities are even more common than pigmented birthmarks. There are two primary varieties: the flat, stable nevus flammeus, and the palpable, rapidly growing capillary hemangioma.

Nevus Flammeus The nevus flammeus is an extremely common finding in newborns, particularly visible in light-complexioned children. These lesions consist of permanently dilated but otherwise normal blood vessels. A high percentage of white babies exhibit the most common types of nevus flammeus, a poorly demarcated pink or red flush to the skin on the upper eyelids and glabella (angel kisses) or at the nape of the neck (stork

Figure 19.1 This dark brown, infiltrated plaque represents a giant congenital nevus that covers the upper arm and most of the trunk. The involved arm is smaller in diameter because of underlying spinal cord involvement, which eventually progressed to affect respiratory muscles.

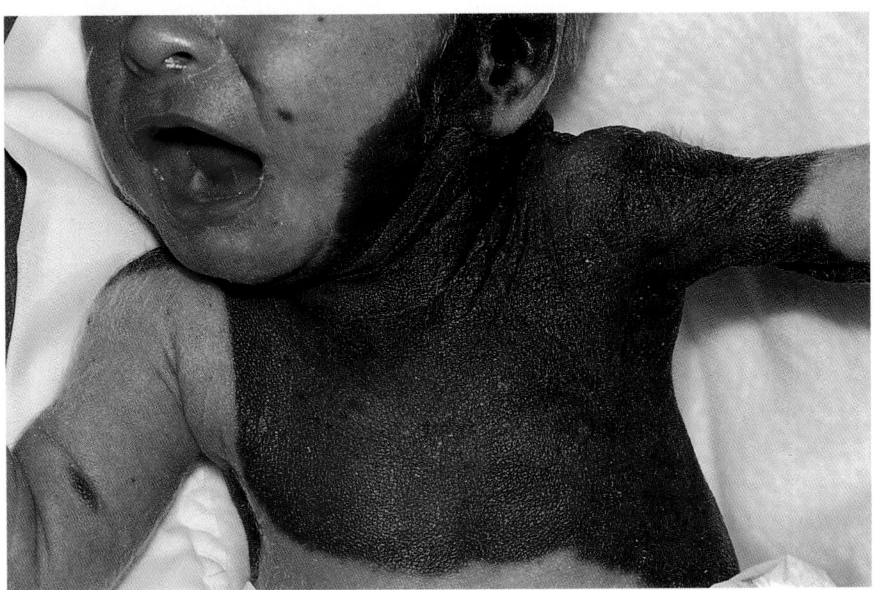

bites). These have no medical significance, and angel kisses generally fade within a few weeks or months, although some pinkness occasionally persists. Although stork bites also fade at times, they often persist into adulthood.

Less often, a nevus flammeus occurs in some other area as a sharply demarcated, evenly pink or red patch (port-wine stain). These are often located in a dermatomal distribution or over the upper lateral aspect of the face. When distribution of the first branch of the trigeminal nerve is involved, especially the upper eyelid and forehead, a nevus flammeus can be a marker for the Sturge-Weber syndrome. This syndrome includes underlying leptomeningeal involvement and intracranial calcification that usually produce seizure disorders. Other common complications of Sturge-Weber syndrome include mental retardation, hemiparesis, and glaucoma. A nevus flammeus located over the spine can indicate underlying neuroectodermal abnormalities, including tethering of the spinal cord.

Otherwise, sequelae of a nevus flammeus are minimal or absent. The lesion does not expand out of proportion to the growth of the skin. However, after puberty, blood vessels within the nevus flammeus often dilate further, becoming distended and tortuous. The lesion may become purple, elevated, and lumpy. Rarely, a nevus flammeus involving an extremity can produce hypertrophy of the affected limb. Even more uncommon is the development of an underlying vascular malformation that can produce complications from an increased cardiac output.

Capillary Hemangiomas Capillary hemangiomas, although sometimes present at birth, more often occur during the first few weeks of life. These common lesions occur in up to 12% of white infants.[3] They often begin as a pink or a bright red macule that enlarges, sometimes very rapidly. Occasionally, the hemangioma can actually be preceded by a blanched macule. These hemangiomas are usually single, but they can occasionally be multiple. Individual lesions can enlarge very rapidly over several months, with growth slowing and then stopping by the time the child is about 1 year of age. Lesions typically remain stable for several months to years, followed by slow resolution. About one-half have resolved by 5 years of age and 90% have involuted by 9 years of age.[4] Some lesions, particularly those with deep and large vascular channels ("cavernous" hemangiomas), do not completely resolve. In those that involute, the ultimate cosmetic result is excellent, although scarring and redundant skin occasionally complicate clearing. Therefore, surgical removal is generally discouraged, as significant scarring can occur from surgery and because of risk associated with general anesthesia in infants undergoing surgery.

However, complications can occur that require aggressive treatment. The most common significant complications result from a mass effect of the tumor, producing dysfunction (Fig. 19.2). For example, a hemangioma on the eyelid can obstruct vision or deform the globe causing abnormal vision. Either of these situations can produce

Figure 19.2 This lobular, bright red tumor is a typical capillary hemangioma occurring in an area at high risk of complications. The extra-auditory canal is obstructed and chronic otitis is a problem in this child.

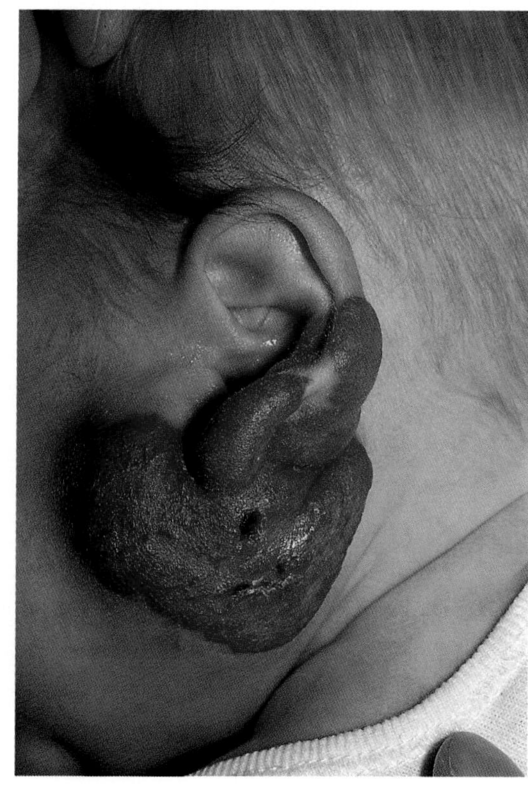

amblyopia and permanent blindness. A hemangioma around the mouth or nose can interfere with eating or breathing. A hemangioma in the genital area can necrose and ulcerate due to maceration from feces and urine. In addition, larger hemangiomas can ulcerate simply because of their size and fragility, producing pain, local infection, and bleeding. Perhaps the most common "complication" is parental aversion and fear of psychological consequences for the child. However, there is no evidence that a hemangioma confers the risk of poor self esteem.[5] Still, a parent wants the tumor removed despite risks and the likelihood of a poorer final outcome. Rarely, hemangiomas, particularly large ones, trap platelets, resulting in local or disseminated intravascular coagulation, called the Kasabach-Merritt syndrome.

When complications occur that require intervention, prednisone at 2 to 4 mg/kg/day is the standard therapy. In addition, intralesional injections of triamcinolone acetonide have been reported useful, especially in the setting of periorbital hemangiomas. However, doses have been high, and benefit may have derived from the systemic effect of the corticosteroid. In addition, loss of sight has occurred, from complications such as perforation of the globe, infection, and retinal artery emboli.[4] A less aggressive therapy that is sometimes used is cryotherapy. Although small lesions can reasonably be excised surgically, these lesions are generally not important to treat. Flashlamp pulsed-dye laser surgery appears promising for the treatment of hemangiomas; this therapy may someday become first-line therapy rather than observation for lesions that are cosmetically unacceptable to parents.[6] Finally, systemic α-interferon (α-IFN) has been shown to produce regression in complicated capillary hemangiomas.[7]

Rarely, infants exhibit large numbers of small hemangiomas, called neonatal hemangiomatosis. Benign neonatal hemangiomatosis is cutaneous only, but diffuse neonatal hemangiomatosis is a grim disease that involves the viscera. The organs most frequently affected are the liver, lungs, central nervous system, and gastrointestinal tract. These infants generally do not survive, with the leading cause of death from heart failure related to arteriovenous shunting in the liver. However, central nervous system and lung involvement can prove fatal as well. Any infant with large numbers of cutaneous hemangiomas should immediately be evaluated clinically for hepatosplenomegaly, signs of shunting, or heart failure. Any infant with multiple cutaneous hemangiomas and any significant physical abnormalities should be quickly evaluated by both a dermatologist and a pediatrician. An ill infant should be admitted to the hospital with immediate consultation with these specialists, since supportive therapy may quickly become essential.

Red, Scaling Rashes

Three primary red, scaling rashes occur in early childhood. Atopic dermatitis and seborrheic dermatitis are frequently clinically indistinguishable, with similar first-line therapy. However, seborrheic dermatitis is self-limiting, whereas atopic dermatitis is chronic.

Diaper Dermatitis Diaper dermatitis (napkin dermatitis) is a very common irritant eruption due to occlusion of urine, feces, and perspiration next to skin. This occurs in nearly all infants at some time; it is also common in other populations of incontinent people.

Diaper dermatitis presents as pink plaques that become redder and macerated as the rash worsens. Although scale is present, it is difficult to detect because of the wet environment. Lesions are more prominent on convex surfaces, such as the mons, vulva, and scrotum, where wet diapers are held directly against the skin. Skin folds are relatively protected from urine and feces and are thus somewhat spared. However, secondary *Candida albicans* infection is common, and yeast preferentially affects skin folds. Therefore, prominent, erythematous skin fold plaques, especially with peripheral pustules, collarettes, or papules, indicates a yeast superinfection. Far less often, seborrhea in a very young infant plays a role in diaper dermatitis. These children also exhibit cradle cap and other areas of red papules with a glazed surface or yellowish scale.

Although dangerous skin diseases such as Langerhans' cell histiocytosis (histiocytosis X) can produce a diaper eruption, these conditions are extremely rare, and they are not immediately life-threatening. However, infants who do not respond to therapy for common diaper dermatitis should be evaluated by their pediatrician or a dermatologist.

The first line of care is to keep the area dry. Although a time-honored instruction is to leave the infant undiapered, this is practically very difficult. Generally, very prompt diaper changes suffice, although even this is difficult for families whose child spends time in daycare.

For very mild diaper dermatitis, with skin folds relatively unaffected, hydrocortisone cream 1% applied sparingly twice daily and compulsive diaper changes eliminate pinkness within a day or two. For more inflammatory disease, including those with skin fold involvement, collarettes, or pustules, a topical antifungal medication should be added 2 to 4 times per day. Choices include nystatin ointment, clotrimazole or miconazole creams (available over the counter as creams marketed for vaginal candidiasis or tinea cruris), or prescription creams such as econazole, ketoconazole, or sulconazole (for further discussion, see Ch. 3, Medical Therapy). If the infant shows very significant inflammation or maceration, ointments rather than creams should be used, because the alcohols in creams sting. Hydrocortisone is easily available as an ointment, although the only anticandidal agent available in a soothing ointment is nystatin. For the very rare circumstance of extreme exudation, oral therapy is preferred. Fluconazole at 3 to 5 mg/kg/day can be used for a few days, in combination with a tepid bath as a soak 2 or 3 times a day.

A thick layer of zinc oxide paste or Desitin ointment helps protect the skin from urine and feces, especially when the infant has diarrhea or is extremely inflamed. This should be applied over the medications and with each diaper change.

Lotrisone (clotrimazole and betamethasone dipropionate) is often, and inappropriately, used for diaper dermatitis. This topical corticosteroid is far too potent for the genital area, particularly in a child, whereas hydrocortisone is quite safe. Unfortunately, hydrocortisone is not available in combination with an anticandidal agent. However, both hydrocortisone and clotrimazole are available over the counter, and these medications are adequate for children whose diapers are changed frequently.

DIAPER DERMATITIS

Clinical Manifestations

Red scaling or macerated plaques under the diaper area of an incontinent person. When the dermatitis is irritant only, the skin folds are relatively spared. When yeast is playing a role, skin fold erythema is remarkable, and satellite collarettes or pustules are often seen at the edges of the plaques.

Management in the Emergency Department

1. *Frequent diaper changes*
2. *Hydrocortisone cream (mild) or ointment (more severe) 1% or 2.5% applied twice a day until clear*
3. *Nystatin ointment or clotrimazole cream to diaper area 4 times a day until clear if skin folds significantly involved or satellite lesions present*
4. *Parent education (see the patient handout on p. 338, Diaper Rash)*

Seborrheic Dermatitis Seborrheic dermatitis is a relatively common scaling eruption that usually appears at about 1 to 2 months of age. This disease is especially common in babies whose parents are unaware of or afraid to remove the buildup of scale in the scalp (cradle cap). In some children, this retained scale initiates inflammation that can become widespread.

Infants exhibit poorly demarcated, pink, coalescing papules and plaques with a yellowish scale (Fig. 19.3). These are typically concentrated over the scalp and face as well as skin folds, but lesions may become generalized in babies. Those skin lesions often have a slightly shiny or "glazed" appearance. The scalp is always involved.

Seborrheic dermatitis is most easily confused with atopic dermatitis. However, atopic dermatitis is excruciatingly itchy, and seborrhea may or may not itch. Also, seborrheic dermatitis is characterized by yellowish scalp scale. A therapeutic trial of scalp debridement and hydrocortisone cream 1% or 2.5% clears seborrhea, whereas eczema generally recurs. Although other conditions, including

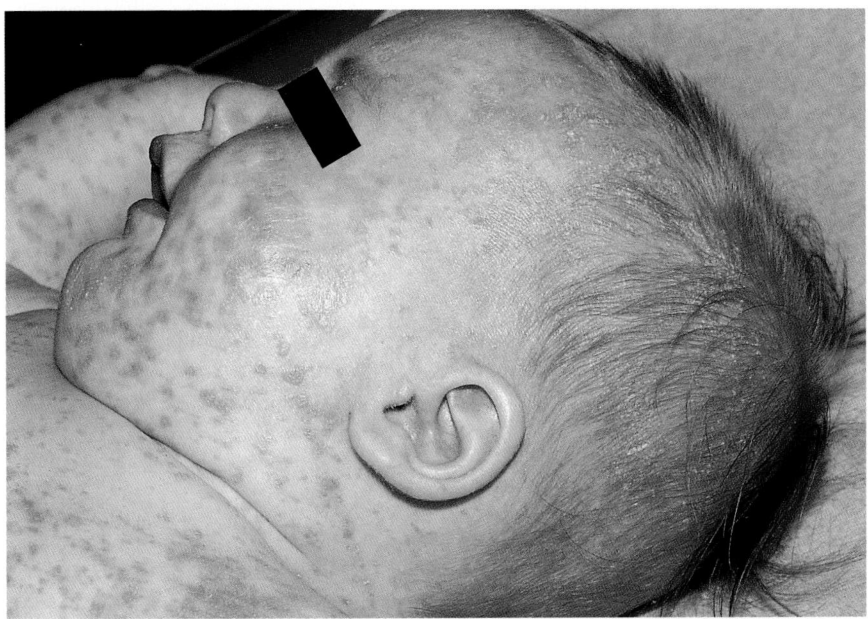

Figure 19.3 Seborrheic dermatitis is always associated with adherent scalp scale, and more severe disease produces red, scaling plaques that can extend to all areas. A glazed appearance to the plaques is common.

psoriasis and widespread dermatophyte infections are theoretical considerations, they rarely occur during the neonatal period.

The therapy for seborrheic dermatitis is very rewarding and children improve rapidly. First, scalp scale must be removed. This can be done by the application of mineral oil or baby shampoo to the scalp for 30 to 60 minutes to soften scale. The scalp should then be shampooed vigorously with baby shampoo and scale is then gently removed with fingernails or a soft brush. In addition, hydrocortisone 1% or 2.5% cream should be applied to all affected areas twice a day. If the baby has sufficient scalp hair to make the application of a cream difficult, hydrocortisone lotion can be substituted in that area.

After patients are clear, recurrences can be prevented by taking care to prevent the accumulation of scale in the scalp. After several months, when maternal circulating hormones have been eliminated, seborrheic dermatitis is not generally a problem until after puberty.

INFANTILE SEBORRHEIC DERMATITIS

Clinical Manifestations

1. *Poorly demarcated, pink, coalescing papules and plaques with a yellowish scale concentrated over scalp, face, and skin folds*
2. *Skin lesions might have a "glazed" appearance*

Management in the Emergency Department

1. *Removal of cradle cap: Apply shampoo or mineral oil to the scalp until the scale is soft; then remove scale mechanically with fingernails or soft brush; keep scalp clear with regular shampoos*
2. *Hydrocortisone cream 1% or 2.5% bid until clear*
3. *Patient education (see the patient handout on p. 362, Seborrheic Dermatitis in Babies)*

Atopic Dermatitis Atopic dermatitis, or eczema, is an inflamed, scaling, and excoriated or lichenified eruption produced by rubbing or scratching (for further discussion of this disease, see Ch. 15, Eczematous Diseases; see Figs. 15.1 to 15.4). Black children often appear hyperpigmented rather than red. Because this eruption is produced and exacerbated by rubbing and scratching, the areas of involvement reflect this. The cheeks and dorsal arms can easily be rubbed against bed clothes and these areas tend to be affected early.

The differentiation of atopic dermatitis and seborrheic dermatitis can usually be made by the later age of onset (atopic dermatitis usually occurs after 3 months of age), by the greater prominence of itching in infants with atopic dermatitis, and by the presence of heavy yellow scale in the scalp of those with seborrheic dermatitis.

Fortunately, treatment of these diseases is similar. Important facets of therapy include topical hydrocortisone ointment 1% or 2.5% bid, lubrication, nighttime sedation, and infection control.

ATOPIC DERMATITIS/ECZEMA/NEURODERMATITIS

Clinical Manifestations

Poorly demarcated, inflamed, scaling plaques with evidence of rubbing or scratching in the form of excoriations or lichenification.

Management in the Emergency Department

1. *Corticosteroids:*
   - *Mild to moderate eczema: hydrocortisone ointment 1% or 2.5% ointment applied sparingly bid*
   - *Moderate to severe or recalcitrant eczema: triamcinolone 0.1% ointment applied sparingly twice daily*
   - *Severe eczema: add prednisone 1 mg/kg/day for 1 week to a topical corticosteroid ointment*
2. *Moisturization with Vaseline petroleum jelly or Eucerin cream (not lotion) over corticosteroid and whenever the skin dries*
3. *Nighttime diphenhydramine at sedating doses, starting at twice the usual antihistamine dose for the child's age, increasing dose until the child sleeps well*
4. *Treat superinfections with cephalexin or dicloxacillin*

(Continues)

(Continued)

5. *Decrease irritants, such as frequent bathing, scratchy fabrics, and heat*
6. *Patient education (see the patient handouts on p. 331, Atopic Dermatitis, Eczema, and Neurodermatitis and p. 368, Topical Cortisone Creams, Ointments, and Solutions)*
7. *Follow-up evaluation in 1 month with regular health care provide for mild or moderate eczema, or in 1 week with a dermatologist for severe eczema treated with oral corticosteroids*

CHILDHOOD EXANTHEMS

Although some diseases characterized by a fever and rash are easy to diagnose, such as well-developed varicella, others can be discouragingly nonspecific. For the clinician faced with a toxic child who has a fever and rash, clues to the specific diagnosis for an early identification of life-threatening diseases such as meningococcemia, Rocky Mountain spotted fever, and Kawasaki disease are critical. Unfortunately, most red exanthems do not have specific clinical or histologic findings that allow a diagnosis in the emergency department. However, a differential diagnosis can be generated, so that appropriate empiric therapy can be instituted to enhance the probability of a good outcome, and follow-up testing can be planned.

These exanthems (a rash in response to an infection) are discussed according to morphology rather than on the basis of etiology. Many of these diseases are accompanied by an enanthem (oral mucous membrane involvement).

Red Exanthems

Viral The red rashes associated with infections are the least specific. For many of these diseases, the diagnosis must be made by correlating the timing of the eruption and associated constitutional signs with local epidemiology and laboratory studies (Table 19.1).

Roseola The clinical signs of roseola (exanthem subitum) occur in almost one-third of children at some time, and about 85% of adults exhibit sero-

TABLE 19.1 Fever and Red Rashes

DISEASE	LOCATION OF RASH	RASH MORPHOLOGY	ASSOCIATED FINDINGS	COMMON AGE	DIAGNOSIS
Viral exanthems[a]					
Roseola (exanthem subitum)	Head and trunk, occasionally pharynx	Nonspecific pink, nonscaling, 2–3 mm, blanchable irregular macules and papules	Preceding high fever that resolves just before rash appears, mild constitutional symptoms	6 mo–3 yr	Acute/convalescent serology; isolation of virus from peripheral blood mononuclear cells[b]
Erythema infectiosum (fifth disease)	Cheeks, then extremities	Bright red, nonscaling "slapped cheeks," light, reticular, nonscaling erythema over extremities	Uncommonly, mild fever, headache, malaise	5–15 yr	Acute/convalescent serology[b]
Rubella (German measles, 3-day measles)	Face and neck, later extending to trunk and extremities; oral mucosa (Forscheimer spots)	Pink macules coalescing into morbilliform eruption	Prodrome of malaise, eye pain, headache, posterior cervical lymphadenopathy, sore throat	Preschool[c]	Acute/convalescent serology, rubella IgM
Rubeola (measles)	Prodrome: mouth (Koplik spots), conjunctivae; then hairline, face, and extending to neck, trunk, and extremities	Pink macules becoming confluent, sometimes purpuric	Prodrome of cough, coryza, fever; adenopathy, sore throat may occur with rash	Preschool[c]	Acute/convalescent serology
Gianotti-Crosti syndrome (papular acrodermatitis of childhood)	Extremities, especially knees, elbows, cheeks, buttocks	Pink or skin-colored firm, monomorphous papules or nodules; sometimes flat-topped, sometimes edematous papules that appear almost vesicular	Usually none	1–6 yr	Clinical proof of recent infection with any virus known to produce this
Bacterial exanthems					
Scarlet fever (scarlatina)	Trunk, extending peripherally; oral mucous membrane	Pink, sandpapery eruption, with accentuation in skin folds, Pastia's lines; flushed face, circumoral pallor; red (sometimes exudative) oropharynx, white then red strawberry tongue; late desquamation	Preceding fever, rigors, sore throat and mouth, headache, abdominal pain	6–18 yr	Throat culture positive for group A streptococcus
Staphylococcal scalded skin syndrome (SSSS)	Mouth and nose, then becoming generalized, but sparing mucous membranes	Red macular erythema around mouth, then generalizing and developing a sandpapery texture before the upper epidermis wrinkles and detaches; radial fissuring around mouth	Fever, skin pain, irritability, anorexia	Under 5 yr	Clinical, culture that yields *Staphylococcus aureus* from nasopharynx, eye or site of skin infection

(Continues)

TABLE 19.1 (Continued)

DISEASE	LOCATION OF RASH	RASH MORPHOLOGY	ASSOCIATED FINDINGS	COMMON AGE	DIAGNOSIS
Toxic shock syndrome (TSS)	Trunk, extending peripherally; oral mucosa and conjunctivae	Nonscaling generalized red flush, accentuation in skin folds; late peeling of fingertips	Diarrhea/vomiting, abdominal pain, hypotension, fever, myalgias, headache, sore throat, periorbital/joint edema`	Adults	Clinical case definition criteria (see boxed list on p. 184, Criteria for Toxic Shock Syndrome) identification of *Staphylococcus aureus*
Acute meningococcemia	Anywhere	Scattered pink papules, often not large numbers; may become purpuric, vesiculopustular; purpura fulminans with severe disease	Abrupt onset headache, malaise, fever, myalgias, nausea/vomiting	Half-children, half-adults	Organisms identified in cerebro-spinal fluid, smears from skin lesions
Lyme disease (erythema migrans)	Site of tick bite, sometimes other areas	Red, flat-topped plaque or plaques, often with peripheral accentuation of inflammation, giving an annular appearance	Flu-like symptoms of fever, malaise, headache, vomiting, local lymphadenopathy, arthralgia	All ages	Clinical
Rickettsial exanthem					
Rocky Mountain spotted fever	Hands, feet, extending centripetally; conjunctivae	Pinpoint pink macules becoming petechial; conjunctival hyperemia; purpura fulminans with severe disease	Periorbital edema, fever, chills, frontal headache, photophobia, myalgias, arthralgias, diarrhea/vomiting	All ages	Clinical suspicion; direct Immunofluorescent skin biopsy for organism (many false-negatives)
Other					
Kawasaki disease (mucocutaneous lymph node syndrome)	Anywhere; oropharynx, lips, face, hands, and feet	Polymorphous; generally red or pink, nonscaling macules, papules, plaques or patches	Fever, acute nonpurulent cervical lymphadenopathy, edema of hands and feet, coronary artery aneurysms	Under 5 yr	Clinical case definition criteria (see Table 19.2)
Juvenile rheumatoid arthritis (JRA)	Trunk, proximal extremities	Small, pink, nonscaling, blanchable papules, often with peripheral pallor, evanescent	Arthritis, sometimes constitutional symptoms of fever, malaise, serositis	Under 16 yr	Clinical case definition
Systemic lupus erythematosus (SLE)	Face, eyelids, posterior nail folds	Erythematous flushing over malar area, lid margins, posterior nailfold sometimes with scale	Arthritis, serositis, kidney or central nervous system involvement with dysfunction, low peripheral white blood cells, platelets, photosensitivity	Adults and children	Clinical case definition, positive serologies

[a]Any virus can produce a nonspecific erythematous, nonscaling macular or papular eruption.
[b]Diagnosis usually made on clinical grounds alone.
[c]Seen in nonimmunized people, usually preschool children.

logic evidence of past exposure. This disease is caused by human herpesvirus 6.[8]

This viral exanthem can usually be diagnosed by its rather characteristic onset. Most common in toddlers, roseola begins with the sudden onset of a high fever that spikes in the late afternoon for 2 to 4 days. Otherwise, children are not particularly ill. The rash begins up to 2 days after the fever resolves. The pink, nonscaling, blanchable, barely palpable papules are small and are located primarily on the trunk and head. Although the eruption usually lasts one or two days, it can be very evanescent in some children. Also, some children with roseola do not develop a rash at all.

The diagnosis of this disease is made on the basis of the clinical course and, when desired, by documenting rising antibody titers or by isolation of the virus from peripheral blood mononuclear cells during the acute disease.

Treatment is symptomatic only. Acetaminophen (Tylenol) minimizes constitutional symptoms associated with the fever.

Erythema Infectiosum Erythema infectiosum (fifth disease) is a very common viral exanthem that has the distinction of being diagnosable from the rash. This common disease is caused by human parvovirus B19, and antibodies to this virus can be detected in about one-half of adults.[9]

The rash is characterized by bright red, nonscaling patches on the cheeks (the "slapped cheek" appearance) (Fig. 19.4). This erythema is usually accompanied within the next day or two by a faint, pink eruption that can occur anywhere but is most common over the arms, legs, and buttocks. Classically, this eruption becomes reticular over the extremities. The rash characteristically waxes and wanes, becoming much more prominent with fever, sunlight, or any other exposure to heat. This reticulate erythema can sometimes be long-lasting, reappearing for weeks, and sometimes longer.

Children with erythema infectiosum are generally well, although some may experience preceding mild fever and symptoms of an upper respiratory tract infection. By the time the rash appears, children are no longer infectious.

Therapy consists of reassurance only.

Rubella Because of childhood immunizations, rubella (German measles) is now rare. However, it remains important because of its ability to produce congenital malformations and illness in newborns.

Although very young children often have no prodrome, adolescents and adults frequently expe-

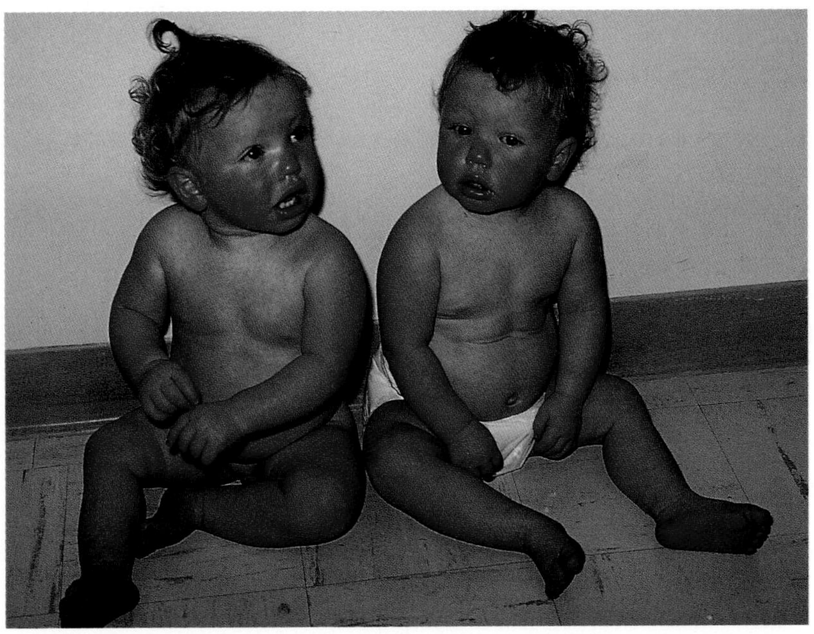

Figure 19.4 Bright red "slapped" cheeks are characteristic of erythema infectiosum. (Photograph courtesy of Ronald E. Hansen, MD, Tucson, Arizona)

rience malaise, sore throat, headache, eye pain, and fever preceding the eruption. The rash typically begins as pink, nonspecific, nonscaling macules and papules that become confluent, producing a morbilliform eruption. Beginning over the head and neck, it progresses over the next day or two to involve the trunk and extremities. A more specific finding are Forscheimer spots—discrete, tiny, red, sometimes petechial macules over the posterior palate. In addition, posterior cervical lymphadenopathy is common. The eruption lasts 2 to 4 days and it is asymptomatic, requiring no therapy.

Congenital rubella is a different disease. The classic skin manifestations, present at or shortly after birth, are "blueberry muffin spots." These blue-purple papules represent extramedullary hematopoiesis. Of more importance are the common findings of microcephaly and growth retardation. Although the blueberry muffin spots disappear spontaneously, some children later develop a skin rash more characteristic of classic rubella.

Rubeola Although uncommon since childhood vaccinations were implemented, rubeola (measles) is still seen in people vaccinated before the age of 15 months or in preschool children in lower socioeconomic areas.

Cough, upper respiratory symptoms, conjunctivitis, and constitutional symptoms appear 10 to 12 days after exposure to the virus. Patients also develop a characteristic enanthem of Koplik spots, well-demarcated, bluish gray macules with surrounding erythema over the mucous membranes of the mouth. This is followed a day or two later by the representative, but not pathognomonic rash of measles. Pink, confluent macules over the face and neck become purplish and extend to the neck, then to the trunk and extremities over the next few days. Systemic symptoms peak on the second or third day of the exanthem and then recede. Complications of measles include bacterial pneumonia, subacute sclerosing panencephalitis, and postinfectious encephalomyelitis.

Atypical measles can occur in patients inoculated with killed measles vaccine, which was available during 1963 to 1967. These patients present with fever, cough, and constitutional symptoms, and a rash very different from that seen with typical measles. This eruption begins with red papules over the extremities, progressing to alarmingly purpuric papules, petechiae, and vesicles that can mimic Rocky Mountain Spotted Fever.

Therapy for measles consists of symptomatic treatment and the recognition and treatment of bacterial superinfections.

Gianotti-Crosti Syndrome Gianotti-Crosti syndrome (papular acrodermatitis of childhood) is an uncommon eruption that is a nonspecific reaction to any of several virus infections. When first recognized in Italy, Gianotti-Crosti syndrome was found to be a marker for hepatitis B infection. More recently in the United States, viral studies in patients with this eruption have yielded positive results for Epstein-Barr virus, respiratory syncytial virus, hepatitis A, echovirus types 7 and 9, cyto-

Figure 19.5 Lichenoid (shiny, flat-topped) papules and nodules most concentrated over the extremities, especially the elbows and knees, are typical of Gianotti Crosti syndrome.

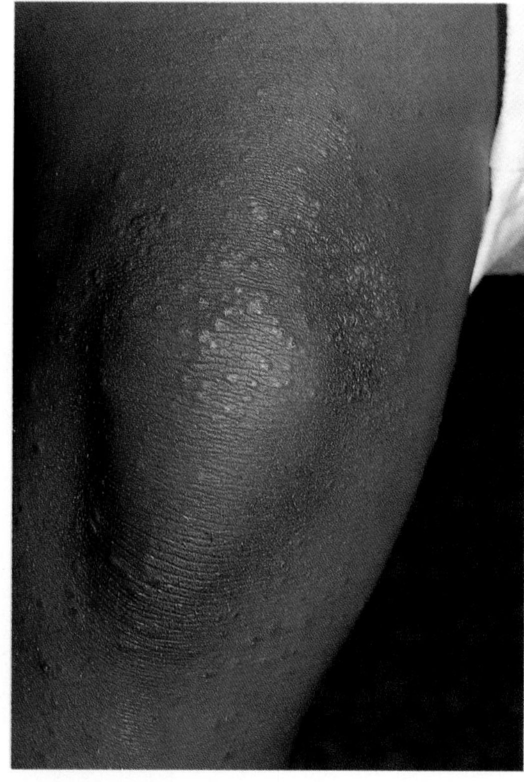

megalovirus, and coxsackievirus types A16, B4, and B5.[10,11]

These children exhibit pink or skin-colored firm, nodular or flat-topped papules concentrated primarily over the extremities, especially dense on the knees and elbows (Fig. 19.5). The buttocks and cheeks are also characteristically affected. Scale is subtle. This rash is generally seen in children who seem otherwise well.

No specific therapy is useful, but reassurance is often greatly appreciated because the eruption can last up to 6 weeks. Some clinicians believe that topical corticosteroids can exacerbate the rash. Because of the occasional association with hepatitis B, the clinician should consider evaluating the child for the presence of hepatitis B surface antigen, which is identifiable 10 days after the eruption appears.

Bacterial

Scarlet Fever Scarlet fever (scarlatina) is a generalized exanthem produced by toxins elaborated by group A β-hemolytic streptococci. The severity of the disease depends partly on the toxin elaborated. Occurring almost exclusively in children younger than 10 years but older than 2 years, this disease is re-emerging after years of relative quiescence.

Children with scarlet fever present with fever, rigors, sore throat (sometimes with purulent tonsillitis), headache, abdominal pain, vomiting, myalgias, malaise, and bright red oral mucous membranes and palatal petechiae. Often, a white coating of the tongue with red, prominent papillae occurs (a "white strawberry tongue"). Several days later, this white coating desquamates, leaving erythematous mucosae with prominent papillae (a "red strawberry tongue"). The exanthem begins a day or two after the onset of illness, beginning as a pink, fine eruption on the trunk and a predisposition for skin folds such as the antecubital fossae and areas of pressure. The texture is often described as "sandpapery," and distinctive linear petechiae sometimes occur within the rash on flexural skin folds (Pastia's lines). Although the face is typically flushed with circumoral pallor, the characteristic fine, papular exanthem generally spares this area, and it may spare the lower extremities.

The rash fades over several days, but this is followed by peeling of the hands, fingers, and skin folds. Desquamation of fine scale from the trunk is usual.

The differential diagnosis includes the other red exanthems discussed in this section, but the texture of the rash, the presence of Pastia's lines, and the prominent pharyngeal and oral findings are usually very helpful. The diagnosis can be confirmed by laboratory testing, including a rapid streptococcal test, although this test produces an unacceptable number of false-negative results. Otherwise, cultures and rising antibody titers are diagnostic.

Therapy for scarlet fever includes oral or parenteral antibiotics with penicillin, but erythromycin or cephalosporins can be used in those allergic to penicillin. Supportive care, including bed rest and acetaminophen, can make the child more comfortable during the illness.

Complications include infection and abscess of the tonsils, otitis, cervical lymphadenopathy, and osteomyelitis. Poststreptococcal rheumatic fever and glomerulonephritis are also possible.

Staphylococcal Scarlet Fever Not surprisingly from the name of this disease, *Staphylococcus aureus* can cause a disease similar to classic scarlet fever. Although staphylococcal scarlet fever (staphylococcal scarlatina) is also characterized by an abrupt fever, headache, and generalized sandpapery rash, staphylococcal scarlet fever spares the mucous membranes. This condition often shares features of toxic shock syndrome and staphylococcal scalded skin syndrome (SSSS), and it may actually represent mild forms of either.

The diagnosis can be made by the identification of a staphylococcal infection. Therapy consists of the oral administration of a cephalosporin or a penicillinase-resistant penicillin such as dicloxacillin, as well as supportive and comfort care.

Toxic Shock Syndrome Although first described in children, toxic shock syndrome is a life-threatening disease that affects all ages and both genders, but occurrence before the age of 15 years is uncommon. Toxic shock syndrome results from toxins produced by certain strains of *Staphylococcus aureus*, and the infection itself can be mild or severe. Common sites of the infection in children include the skin and nasopharynx.

The rash consists of generalized, flat, nonscaling, blanchable erythema that is most marked over the trunk, with the extremities becoming involved later. Like scarlet fever, the eruption can then develop a sandpapery texture and prominence of the erythema in flexual skin folds. Also like scarlet fever, oral and conjunctival mucous membranes may be red, and a strawberry tongue can occur. Diarrhea, fever, malaise, and myalgias are usual, and hypotension is regularly present. Headache and confusion are common. The diagnosis is made by the application of specific criteria (see boxed list on p. 184, Criteria for Toxic Shock Syndrome).

Therapy includes both intravenous antistaphylococcal antibiotics and control of hypotension and the possible complications of renal, heart, and respiratory failure. With prompt recognition and therapy, this serious disease is now associated with a good prognosis.

Acute Meningococcemia About one-half of patients with acute meningococcemia are children, but this disease does not require special consideration in children. It is listed here only because it produces fever and a red rash, placing it in the differential diagnosis, and because of its extremely grave prognosis when untreated (for further discussion, see Ch. 16, Purpura; see Figs. 16.4 and 16.6).

Staphylococcal Scalded Skin Syndrome SSSS is generally considered a blistering condition. However, the first day or two are characterized by nonscaling erythema that may become sandpapery, mimicking the red exanthems. A more complete discussion is included under Blistering Diseases, in this chapter.

Lyme Disease Lyme disease (erythema chronicum migrans, erythema migrans) is a disease of both adults and children, but it is mentioned here because it is a prominent cause of fever with an erythematous rash in some parts of the world, and because of the long-term morbidity that occurs when it is untreated.

A red macule or papule develops up to 1 month after the bite of a deer tick infected with *Borrelia burgdorferi*. The lesion enlarges into a flat, nonscaling plaque that is often, but not always, annular, with the periphery redder than the center of the lesion (see Fig. 13.7). There are sometimes multiple lesions. Occasionally, a malar rash and conjunctivitis occur. Associated symptoms are a flu-like illness that often includes fever, headache, pharyngitis, malaise, and vomiting. Untreated patients can develop cardiac, neurologic, and joint complications. The diagnosis is made on clinical grounds and the likelihood of this disease appearing in a particular locality. Available serologic tests are poorly standardized, and results are variable (for further discussion, see Ch. 13, Vascular Reactions and Other Flat-Topped, Nonscaling Patches and Plaques).

Therapy consists of a 10- to 14- day course of antibiotics, including oral penicillin V 250 to 500 mg qid or amoxicillin 500 mg tid. For children older than 8 years, tetracycline 250 to 500 mg qid, or minocycline or doxycycline 50 to 100 mg bid.[12] Those with neurologic symptoms may require intravenous antibiotics.

Rickettsial

Rocky Mountain Spotted Fever Like acute meningococcemia, Rocky Mountain Spotted Fever occurs in both children and adults, and it does not require special consideration in children. It is also listed here because it produces fever and a red rash, and because early recognition and therapy are extremely important (for further discussion, see Chap 16, Purpura; see Fig. 16.3).

Red Rashes, Other and Unknown

Kawasaki Disease Although the etiology of Kawasaki disease (mucocutaneous lymph node syndrome) is unknown, this disease presents with a fever and rash, most closely mimicking an infectious disease. This condition is found most often in children who exhibit the major histocompatibility antigens HLA Bw22 and Bw22J2. The importance of this disease derives from the frequent complication of coronary artery aneurysms in inadequately managed patients.

Kawasaki disease occurs in very young children, with 80% of affected patients under the age of 4 years.[13] More common in Japanese and Korean children, the presenting signs include fever of undocumented cause, injection of the vessels of the conjunctivae, prominent, red papillae on the tongue, erythema of the pharynx, red, cracked lips, cervical lymphadenopathy, and a nonspecific rash. This rash is usually red and nonscaling, and may be morbilliform, resemble erythema multiforme, or a toxic erythema, but even pustular lesions have been reported. Other characteristic changes include edema of the hands and feet, palmar and plantar erythema, and intense erythema in the diaper area.[14] Arthralgias and arthritis, hydrops of the gallbladder, and aseptic meningitis associated with extreme irritability are common findings. Desquamation of the hands and feet are regular findings, but these occur too late in the course of the disease to be helpful in diagnosis and management. However, desquamation of the diaper area occurs earlier and can be a useful sign. The diagnosis of Kawasaki disease is made by the identification of a minimum number of criteria from those that define the disease (Table 19.2).

Appropriate and early therapy for Kawasaki disease improves the prognosis remarkably. Without therapy, up to 20% of children develop coronary artery aneurysms, but appropriate therapy reduces this number to about 3%. This therapy includes intravenous γ-globulin, 2 g, infused over 12 hours one time.[15] In addition, aspirin—not other nonsteroidal medications or acetaminophen—should be administered at a dose of 80 to 100 mg/kg/day qid for 2 weeks.[15] This is followed by doses at 3 to 5 mg/kg once daily until the absence of coronary aneurysms is verified at about 6 to 8 weeks after onset of the illness. Prednisone worsens the prognosis.

About 1% to 2% of children die of cardiac complications including myocardial infarction, arrhythmias, heart failure, valvular insufficiency, and pericardial effusions. Aneurysms can be identified as early as the second week of illness, and risk factors include male gender, age younger than 1 year, longer duration of fever, and recurrence of fever after apparent defervescence. Children with a diagnosis of Kawasaki disease should be evaluated with a two-dimensional echocardiogram at onset and at the third week of illness, as well as 3 to 4 weeks later, when aspirin can be stopped, following a normal echocardiogram.

Juvenile Rheumatoid Arthritis Usually misdiagnosed initially as an infection, juvenile rheumatoid arthritis (JRA) presents with daily spiking fever and arthritis, sometimes associated with constitutional symptoms, serositis, uveitis, and rash. The rash classically consists of discrete, small, pink, blanching, and often evanescent papules.

Criteria developed by the American College of Rheumatology can aid in the diagnosis. These

TABLE 19.2 Diagnostic Criteria for Kawasaki Disease

1. Fever ≥39.4°C persisting 5 days or longer
2. Changes of distal extremities
   - Acute: erythema of palms and soles, edema
   - Late: desquamation of fingertips
3. Polymorphous exanthem
4. Injection of conjunctival vessels
5. Inflammation of lips and mouth: erythema, cracking of lips; strawberry tongue, injection of oral and pharyngeal mucosae
6. Nonpurulent cervical lymphadenopathy

[a]At least five signs must be present for the diagnosis of Kawasaki disease, or four signs in the presence of coronary artery aneurysm detected on two-dimensional echocardiography or angiography. (From Japan Kawasaki Disease Research Committee.)

include age younger than 16 years, arthritis not produced by other discernible disease or fever, and duration of signs lasting longer than 6 weeks. The presence of constitutional signs as well as age of onset, gender predominance, and prognosis differ among the types of JRA, that is, pauciarticular, polyarticular, and systemic diseases.

The task in the emergency department is to rule out significant infection as a cause of these symptoms and to refer the patient to a pediatrician for further workup.

Systemic Lupus Erythematosus Systemic lupus erythematosus (SLE) can present with the same constellation of a red, flat, blanching rash in association with malaise, myalgias, and fever noted in most of the infectious diseases discussed in this section (see Fig. 13.14). It is included here for the sake of completeness, although SLE is not exclusively a pediatric disease. However, SLE can be a serious disease, and this diagnosis should be considered in a patient with fever and rash with no obvious infectious etiology, particularly if symptoms have been more chronic than would be expected with an infection (for further discussion, see Ch. 14, Papulosquamous Diseases: Red, Scaling, Well-Demarcated Papules and Plaques).

Bistering Diseases

Some infections characteristic of childhood produce blistering. In addition to HSV infection (for further discussion, see Ch. 14, Vesicular Diseases), several other diseases are important to include in the different diagnosis.

Hand-Foot-and-Mouth-Disease Hand-foot-and-mouth disease is a common childhood vesicular exanthem, most often produced by coxsackievirus A16. Because several different viruses can cause this disease, hand-foot-and-mouth disease can occur more than once in the same child. Many children experience a mild prodrome of fever and malaise before the development of superficial erosions on the tongue and buccal mucosa, and sometimes the palate and pharynx. Small oval vesicles generally occur on the hands and feet as well, often with some blisters that align in palmar and plantar creases (see Fig. 4.14). Very young children frequently exhibit red papules, erosions, or crusts concentrated over the diaper area.

The diagnosis of hand-foot-and-mouth disease is made by the distribution of these vesicles and papules. Primary HSV infection (herpes stomatitis) is a theoretical consideration in the differential diagnosis, but HSV is far more painful, and the scattered palmar and plantar lesions are not seen. Varicella can be differentiated by its more generalized distribution and by the identification of some characteristic, intact vesicles with a central crust. Hand-foot-and-mouth disease is a minor illness that, at most, produces soreness of the mouth and other affected areas. Reassurance, cool, bland liquids, and acetaminophen are the only treatment indicated.

HAND-FOOT-AND-MOUTH DISEASE

Clinical Manifestations

Oral erosions in association with oval vesicles over the hands and feet; erythematous papules common over the buttocks and diaper area of small children.

Management in the Emergency Department

1. *Reassurance*
2. *Pain management for oral lesions, including cool, bland liquids and topical anesthetics*

Blistering Dactylitis Blistering dactylitis is classically produced by group A β-hemolytic streptococci, although group B streptococci and *Staphylococcus aureus* have also been associated with this finding.[16] Most often, tense bullae arise from red skin, covering the distal fingerpad of school-age children. As can occur with any blister as it ages, blister fluid can become cloudy.

The diagnosis can be confirmed by a Gram stain that reveals gram-positive cocci in the blister fluid, although other diseases to consider include friction or thermal blisters and HSV infection.

Therapy consists of oral penicillin, cephalosporin, or erythromycin.

Varicella Varicella (chickenpox), a well-known viral vesicular exanthem, is easily recognized in its fully developed form (for further discussion, see

Ch. 4, Vesicular Diseases). One to 3-mm red papules, vesicles on a pink base, crusts surrounded by an intact vesicle, and crusts without a peripheral vesicle are scattered over the skin surface, prominently affecting the scalp, face, and genital area early in the course of the disease (see Figs. 4.12 and 4.13). Oral lesions are common. Fever and malaise are usual, although very young children often exhibit minimal constitutional symptoms.

The diagnosis is made by the clinical picture and awareness that chickenpox is "going around." Very early disease can easily be confused with insect bites, hand-foot-and-mouth disease, or, less often, allergic contact dermatitis.

Therapy consists of nighttime sedation to allow sleeping in spite of pruritus, control of constitutional signs with acetaminophen (never aspirin, because of the risk of Reye syndrome), and control of any secondary staphylococcal skin infections.

VARICELLA

Clinical Manifestations

Scattered vesicles, pustules, and crusts in all stages of evolution, usually accompanied by symptoms of an upper respiratory tract infection.

Management in the Emergency Department

1. *Nighttime sedation with hydroxyzine (HCl) or diphenhydramine for control of itching*
2. *Oral cephalexin, dicloxacillin, or erythromycin for those patients with signs of secondary bacterial infection*
3. *Specific antiviral medication: Consider oral acyclovir at 20 mg/kg up to 800 mg 5 times a day if the child is seen within the first 24 hours*
4. *Avoid aspirin for fever—acetaminophen*
5. *Parent education (see the patient handout on p. 370, Varicella [chicken pox])*

Staphylococcal Scalded Skin Syndrome Although SSSS can present as an eruption disturbingly similar to that of the very dangerous toxic epidermal necrolysis (TEN), this disease is usually minor. The morphologic similarity is reflected in the outdated names of toxic epidermal necrolysis, Ritter type (SSSS), and toxic epidermal necrolysis, Lyell type (also called drug-induced TEN). However, whereas drug-induced TEN produces full-thickness epidermal necrolysis with sloughing of the entire epidermis, SSSS is associated with toxin-induced detachment of the stratum corneum only. Most of the protective epidermis is left intact, so that the dermis is not exposed. Fluid loss and secondary infection are far lesser threats to children with SSSS as compared to those with TEN.

Usually, these two diseases can be fairly easily differentiated. Children with SSSS are typically not seriously ill, although they are generally febrile and irritable. The earliest skin changes include pink macules over the lower face, followed by generalized painful, nonscaling erythema. The skin may develop a sandpapery texture, followed a day or two later by detachment of the stratum corneum. Tense bullae are not seen; rather, sheets of stratum corneum wrinkle and separate, beginning in the skin folds and exposing wet epithelium. Characteristic radial fissuring and crusting around the mouth are very helpful diagnostically (Fig. 19.6). Unlike drug-induced TEN, mucous membrane involvement is absent. If the diagnosis is not clinically obvious, a shave biopsy of skin that includes intact skin and the edge of a detached area can be submitted for frozen-section examination. A punch biopsy is inappropriate because the rotary motion of a punch shears the fragile epithelium. TEN and SSSS can be differentiated rapidly and definitively by this biopsy.

The blisters of SSSS are not produced by direct infection, but rather by the toxin exfoliatin, which is elaborated by specific phage types of *Staphylococcus aureus* infecting any area of the body. Nasopharyngeal sites, conjunctivae, and skin infections are most common, but Gram stains and cultures of blistered skin do not yield the organism.

Treatment of SSSS includes an antistaphylococcal antibiotic, although the course of the disease is not particularly affected if this medication is given late. Effective antibiotics include cephalexin- and penicillinase-resistant penicillins. If the child appears well, he can be discharged, but ill and anorectic children require hospitalization for analgesia, sedation, and hydration. The skin should be treated with great care, including the avoidance of

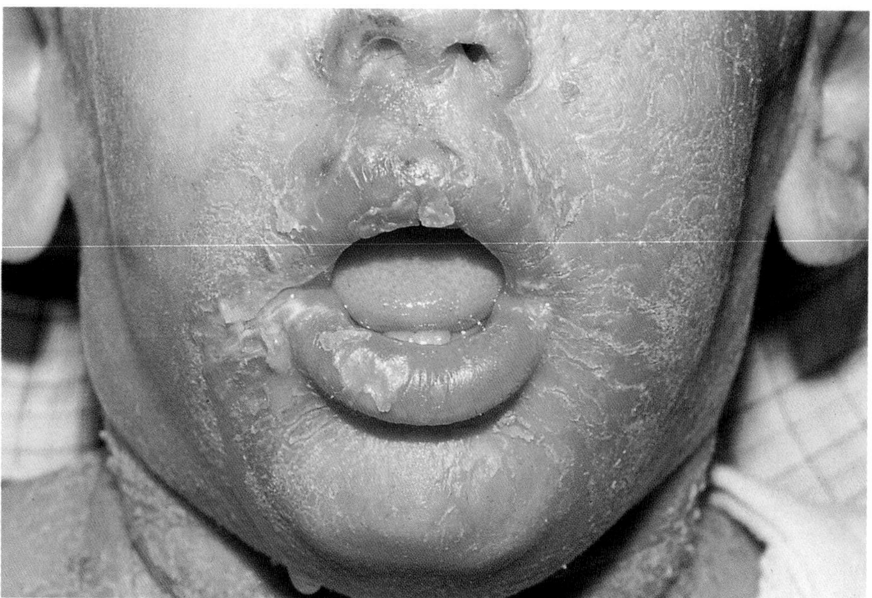

Figure 19.6 Radial fissuring and crusting around the mouth and nose is a very helpful diagnostic sign for staphylococcal scalded skin syndrome.

tape, topical medications, and friction from clothing and sheets. Lubrication should not be used until the skin has exfoliated, and the wet epithelium has begun to scale and crack.

CHILD ABUSE

A major cause of longlasting morbidity, and sometimes death, is child abuse. Although sexual abuse occurs roughly equally in all economic and cultural classes, physical abuse is more prevalent in lower socioeconomic groups. These parents and caretakers usually have fewer options and support systems. In addition, this group of people often obtain general health care in an urgent care system, so that the clinician in an emergency department is frequently the only person in a position to identify and interrupt abuse patterns. This subject is serious and deserving of coverage beyond the scope of this text. Standard emergency medicine textbooks treat this subject in more detail. The following discussion is limited to the identification of potential cutaneous signs of abuse.

Physical Abuse

Young children are uncoordinated and often have a poorly refined sense of self-preservation. This results in frequent accidents and injuries. Although a diagnosis of injury due to intentional trauma rather than an accident can be difficult, specific signs can suggest the circumstances.

Linear, Angular, or Bizarre-Shaped Lesions Linear or angular lesions, or lesions of any bizarre shape are indicative of external causation (Fig. 19.7). While this does not signify intentional injury, it does establish that the injury was due to contact with an object. Rectangular lesions are suspicious for belt buckles, and linear lesions suggest a belt or stick. One of the most specific signs of intentional injury are loop marks on the skin from a doubled over belt, rope, or cord. Blisters or erosions in a splatter or drip pattern indicate thermal or chemical liquid burns.

Unusual Distribution of Lesions An unusual distribution of lesions should raise suspicion of

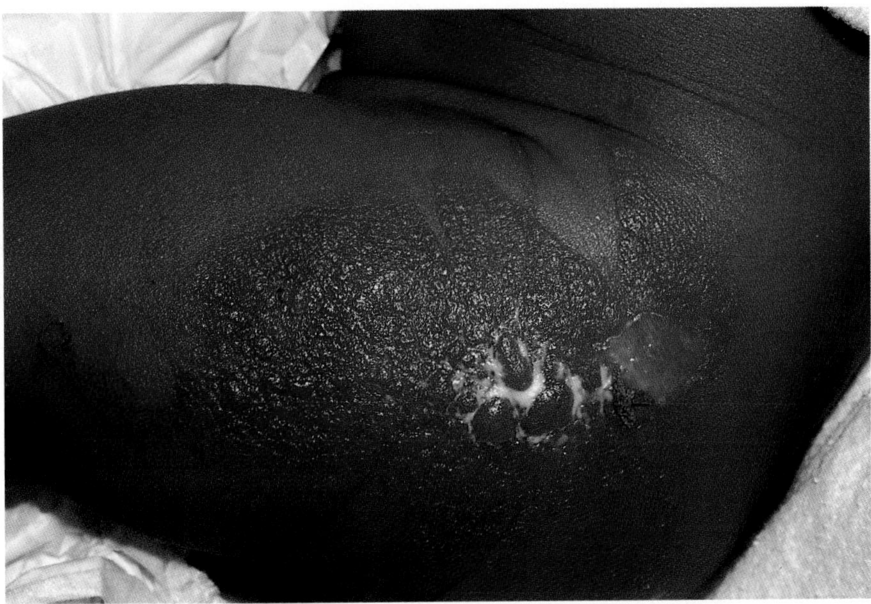

Figure 19.7 This pattern of blistering, with sharp borders that spare the protected skin fold, is diagnostic of a burn.

physical abuse. Some areas of the skin surface are especially susceptible to accidental trauma. Skinned knees, bumped chins, and bruised extensor surfaces of the limbs are examples. However, other areas are usually protected during falls, such as the medial thighs. Or, some areas are unlikely to be burned from spills of hot liquid, such as the feet or buttocks. The genital area is an especially likely site of intentional trauma, even in the absence of sexual abuse. This area is not visible to the casual observer, and frustration with toilet training or excessive masturbation sometimes makes this area a target.

Unusually Numerous Injuries Unusually numerous injuries for the reported accident should also suggest the possibility of deliberate injury. A fall from a chair or a table should not produce multiple, generalized contusions, abrasions, or lacerations. Also, especially frequent episodes of "typical" accidents can indicate abuse.

Age of Injury Incompatible With History If the age of the injury does not correlate with the history, or if there are injuries of different ages, the clinician should consider intentional trauma a possibility. However, the age of injuries can be difficult to acertain. Although the color of bruises correlates roughly with their age, other factors such as the depth, location, and natural skin color play a role as well. Conventional wisdom holds that newer bruises are purple or blue, with green and yellow predominating after the first few days or week, and residual brown color then often lasting up to 2 weeks. However, newer, more objective and controlled data from photographs show that the colors of bruises are very variable.[17] Although yellow color does not appear before 18 hours, red, purple, and blue colors can occur at any time during the duration of a contusion. Different bruises produced at the same time can be different colors.

Unusually Severe Injury Incompatible With History An injury that appears unusually severe for the history can be another indication of nonaccidental injury. For example, serious burns are unlikely in a child who stepped into a tub of hot water and immediately jumped out. This explanation suggests that the child was forcibly held in hot water. However, although first reports of child abuse emphasized the severity of injuries, 60% of intentional injuries are moderate and nonspecific.[18]

Other Injuries Incompatible With History Similarly, other injuries incompatible with the history can denote intentional trauma. A hot liquid spilled on a child should not encompass areas not in the expected path of the spill. A fall from a bicycle should not leave a linear imprint on a buttock, whereas this is typical of a belt or switch.

Skin Diseases That May Mimic Intentional Trauma Some skin diseases erroneously raise the suspicion of intentional trauma. Mongolian spots, poorly demarcated blue patches found most often over the buttocks and back of infants of darker-skinned races, can be misdiagnosed as bruises. These spots often occur around wrists and ankles, mistakenly suggesting that these areas have been bound tightly. Berloque dermatitis is erythema or hyperpigmentation resulting from the interaction of a photosensitizing chemical and sunlight. This condition can leave linear marks and handprints not produced by trauma. These chemicals are found in some colognes, hair dressings, and in some citrus fruits such as limes. A common scenario is a family picnic where adults are squeezing limes for drinks, and when they pick up their child, lime juice on their hands is deposited on the child's arms. Interaction with sunlight causes inflammation or hyperpigmentation in the pattern of a handprint.

Purpura from coughing, tourniquets, or self-inflicted injury from games can also occur and mimic child abuse. The distribution and a reasonable history usually allows for the correct diagnosis.

By law, when cutaneous injuries suggest the possibility of child abuse, protective services must be notified. Any suspicion should be reported; proof is certainly not required and is the responsibility of social services professionals. Chronic abuse patterns are often identified retrospectively following serious injury or death of a child.

Sexual Abuse

Childhood sexual abuse, often defined as unwanted sexual contact by a person 5 or more years older than the child, is very common. About 20% of girls in all socioeconomic groups and cultures are sexually abused, with some surveys reporting even higher rates.[19,20] A fewer but significant number of boys are also abused. This form of abuse can be very difficult to detect, and a high index of suspicion is usually essential.

Presence of a Sexually Transmitted Disease The presence of a sexually transmitted disease is usually a sign of sexual abuse in a prepubertal child. Diseases such as gonorrhea and syphilis are always indications of sexual contact. However, genital warts in very young children can be, but usually are not, a sign of sexual abuse. This viral infection can be transmitted to the infant during delivery through an infected birth canal, and the incubation and latent period can be months to years. In addition, the wart virus can be transferred to the young child by fingers of a caretaker during bathing or diaper change. Associated sexual abuse is more likely in older children, but these children can also develop genital warts from latent viral infection or from nonsexual contact.[21] However, because genital warts can sometimes be transmitted sexually, the possibility of sexual abuse should be considered in these children. Molluscum contagiosum in the genital area, although a sexually transmitted disease in adults, is so very common in children that sexual transmission should not be a serious consideration in the absence of other signs of abuse. A genital HSV infection is generally considered a sign of sexual contact, but this infection in small children has not been studied, and its specificity for sexual abuse is not documented.

Genital Injury A genital injury is suggestive of sexual abuse, particularly tears of the introitus or anus. However, these injuries heal extremely quickly, so the absence of injury should not dissuade the examiner from a diagnosis of sexual abuse. Perineal and buttock trauma are far from specific, as these are common targets of intentional nonsexual trauma. Evidence of attempted penetration are more indicative. Lichen sclerosus (et atrophicus) is an uncommon skin disease of the vulva and, less often, the penis that results in cutaneous fragility[22,23] (for further discussion, see Ch. 9, White Lesions). The skin is hypopigmented, and purpura and erosions result from very minor trauma such as scratching or rubbing with toilet paper (see Fig. 9.7). Obvious genital injuries can occur as a result of subtle lichen sclerosus and in the absence of sexual abuse, a circumstance of which the examiner should be aware. Perianal streptococcal disease is a relatively common cause of chronic, nonspecific perianal erythema, sometimes associated with scale or fissures. This diagnosis can be confirmed by a skin culture, and it should not be confused with sexual abuse. Other diseases that have caused confusion include Crohn's disease and cicatricial pemphigoid.

Other signs of sexual abuse have been suggested, including anal fissures, and a reflex relaxation of the anal sphincter during an examination. Many of these signs are not specific and can be seen in normal, nonabused children. Tears in the hymen can imply sexual activity, but the appearance of the hymen of small children is very variable. Not only is there individual variation, but normal changes occur with age as well.

As is true for physical abuse, any suggestion of sexual abuse must be reported to protective services. For some diseases, such as genital warts or suspicious trauma, the input of a child's pediatrician or family doctor may allay misgivings. Otherwise, reporting is essential. Because children are not under the direct care of their parents at all times, and because of the media attention given to misconduct at daycare facilities and by babysitters, most parents of unabused children will share your concern if they are approached with tact and consideration.

Physical and sexual abuse of children are emotionally loaded issues, have severe legal and criminal implications, and must be treated seriously and with great care. The safety and emotional wellbeing of many children depend on this approach.

PHYSICAL ABUSE

Cutaneous Clinical Manifestations

Linear or angular lesions, or lesions of any bizarre shape

An unusual distribution of lesions

Unusually numerous injuries

Age of the injury inconsistent with the history

Injuries of different ages

(Continues)

(Continued)

An injury that appears unusually severe for the history

Injuries incompatible with the history

SEXUAL ABUSE

Clinical Manifestations

Sexually transmitted disease

Genital injury

SUSPECTED PHYSICAL AND SEXUAL ABUSE

Management in the Emergency Department

1. *Pain control and treatment of injuries*
2. *Social and medical history*
3. *Physical examination, with evaluation of entire skin surface including genitalia*
   - *Documentation of abnormalities, written and photographic*
   - *For suspected sexual abuse, genital examination for the presence of sperm, semen, acid phosphatase; testing for sexually transmitted disease*
4. *Consultation with regular health care provider*
5. *Consider skeletal radiographs for old injuries*
6. *Immediate telephone report to local child protective services, followed by written report*
7. *Immediate protection of child, including hosptalization, if required*

Please see patient information handouts for this chapter on pages 338, 362, 368, and 370.

REFERENCES

1. Serna MJ, Vazquez-Doval J, Vanaclocha V et al: Occult spinal dysraphism; a neurosurgical problem with a dermatologic hallmark. Pediatr Dermatol 10:149, 1993
2. Fienman NL, Yakovac WC: Neurofibromatosis in childhood. J Pediatr 76:339, 1970
3. Wagner AM, Hansen RC: Neonatal skin and skin disorders. p. 263. In Schachner LA,

Hansen RC (eds): Pediatric Dermatology. 2nd Ed. Churchill Livingstone, New York, 1996

4. Rabinowitz LG, Esterly NB: Vascular birthmarks and other abnormalities of blood vessels and lymphatics. p. 953. In Schachner LA, Hansen RC (eds): Pediatric Dermatology. 2nd Ed. Churchill Livingstone, New York, 1996
5. Dieterich-Miller CA, Cohen BA, Liggett J: Behavioral adjustment and self-concept of young children with hemangiomas. Pediatr Dermatol 9:241, 1992
6. Garden JM, Bakus AD, Passer AS: Treatment of cutaneous hemangiomas by the flashlamp-pumped dye laser: prospective analysis. J Pediatr 120:555, 1992
7. Ezekowitz RAB, Mulliken JB, Folkman J: Interferon alfa-2a therapy for life-threatening hemangiomas of infancy. N Engl J Med 326: 1456, 1992
8. Yamanishi K, Okuno T, Shiraki K et al: Identification of human herpesvirus-6 as a causal agent for exanthem subitum. Lancet 1:1065, 1988
9. Anderson LJ: Role of parvovirus B19 in human disease. Pediatr Infect Dis J 6:711, 1987
10. Lowe L, Hebert AA, Duvic M: Gianotti-Crosti syndrome associated with Epstein-Barr virus infection. J Am Acad Dermatol 20:336, 1989
11. Draelos ZK, Hansen MC, James WE: Gianotti-Crosti syndrome associated with infections other than hepatitis B. JAMA 256:2386, 1986
12. Galen WK, Rogers M, Cohen I, Smith MHD: Bacterial infections. p. 1169. In Schachner LA, Hansen RC (eds): Pediatric Dermatology. 2nd Ed. Churchill Livingstone, New York, 1996
13. Melish M, Hicks R: Kawasaki syndrome: clinical features, pathophysiology, etiology and therapy. J Rheumatol, suppl 24. 17:2, 1990
14. McCuaig C, Moroz G: Perineal eruption in Kawasaki's syndrome. Arch Dermatol 123:430, 1987
15. Leung DYM: Kawasaki syndrome. Curr Opin Rheumatol 5:41, 1993
16. Woroszylski A, Duran C, Tamayo L et al: Staphylococcal blistering dactylitis: report of two patients. Pediatr Dermatol 13:292, 1996
17. Langlois NEI, Gresham GA: The aging of bruises: a review and study of the color changes with time. Forensic Sci Int 50:227, 1991
18. Warner JE, Hansen DJ: The identification and reporting of physical abuse by physicians: a review and implications for research. Child Abuse Negl 18:11, 1994
19. Springs FE, Friedrich WN: Health risk behaviors and medical sequelae of childhood sexual abuse. Mayo Clin Proc 67:527, 1992
20. Bagdley R, Allard HA, Proudfoot M et al: Occurrence in the Population. Sexual Offences Against Children. Vol. 1. Canadian Government Publishing Centre, Ottawa, 1984
21. Obalek S, Misiewicz J, Jablonska S et al: Childhood condyloma acuminatum: association with genital and cutaneous human papillomaviruses. Pediatr Dermatol 10:101, 1993
22. Bays J, Jenny C: Genital and anal conditions confused with child sexual abuse trauma. Am J Dis Child 144:1319, 1990
23. Barton PG, Ford MJ, Beers BB: Penile purpura as a manifestation of lichen sclerosus et atrophicus. Pediatr Dermatol 10:129, 1993

SUGGESTED READINGS

General

Franz TJ, Lehman PA, Franz S et al: Comparative percutaneous absorption of lindane and permethrin. Arch Dermatol 132:901, 1996

Gerber MA, Shapiro ED, Burke GS et al: Lyme disease in children in Southern Connecticut. N Engl J Med 335:1270, 1996

Schachner LA, Hansen RC: Pediatric Dermatology. 2nd Ed. Churchill Livingstone, New York, 1996

Birthmarks

Dawson HA, Atherton DJ, Mayou B: A prospective study of congenital melanocytic naevi: progress report and evaluation after 6 years. Br J Dermatol 134:617, 1996

Esterly N (ed): Special symposium. Management of congenital melanocytic nevi: a decade later. Pediatr Dermatol 13:321, 1996

Maceyko RF, Camisa C: Kasabach-Merritt syndrome. Pediatr Dermatol 8:133, 1991

Morelli JG: On the treatment of hemangiomas. Pediatr Dermatol 10:84, 1993

Exanthems

Baialecki C, Feder HM, Grant-Kels JM: The six classic childhood exanthems: a review and update. J Am Acad Dermatol 21:891, 1989

Bligard CA: Kawasaki disease and its diagnosis. Pediatr Dermatol 4:75, 1987

Leung DYM: Kawasaki syndrome. Curr Opin Rheumatol 5:41, 1993

Prose NS, Resnick SD: Cutaneous manifestations of systemic infection in children. Curr Probl Dermatol 5:87, 1993

Childhood Abuse

Abel GG, Rouleau JL: Sexual abuses. Psychiatr Clin North Am 18:139, 1995

Berkowitz CD: Pediatric abuse. New patterns of injury. Emerg Med Clin North Am 13:321, 1995

Wissow LS: Child abuse and neglect. N Engl J Med 332:1425, 1995

CHAPTER 20

Cutaneous Signs of Immunosuppression and AIDS

Patients who are immunosuppressed are well known to experience infections more often than those who are immunocompetent and to experience more aggressive infections and malignancies. In these patients, the clinical appearance and course of the disease may be atypical. For the most part, these differences are discussed under the respective diseases throughout this book.

However, in addition to these well-known hallmarks of immunosuppression, patients with acquired immunodeficiency syndrome (AIDS) exhibit specific tumors, characteristic infections, and the sudden onset or extreme worsening of some noninfectious inflammatory diseases. Anyone who presents with these infections, tumors, or unusually severe exacerbations of these inflammatory diseases should be considered a possible patient with AIDS.

INFECTIONS

Certainly, some of the most well-recognized cutaneous signs of immunosuppression are infections. Cutaneous infections are rarely life-threatening in these patients, but they can be painful, atypical, and sometimes unusually recalcitrant to therapy. Although clinicians other than dermatologists and infectious disease physicians generally are concerned chiefly with bacterial infections, the latter infections are usually typical in appearance; most are caused by the same organisms that occur in immunocompetent patients. These infections are less likely to produce diagnostic or therapeutic problems, and the occurrence of bacterial infections in patients presenting to the emergency department generally does not raise the specter of immunosuppression. Therefore, bacterial infections are not discussed in this chapter.

Viral Infections

Extensive or severe cutaneous viral infections are extremely common in immunosuppressed people. Chronic, ulcerative herpes simplex virus (HSV) infection, facial mollusca contagiosa, and a second episode of varicella or herpes zoster should all suggest the presence of AIDS.

Herpes Simplex Virus Infection Infection with the HSV, including herpes labialis and genital herpes, is extraordinarily common in the general population. With immune suppression, latent infection is much more likely to activate and to become chronic rather than recurrent. Also, HSV infections in immunosuppressed patients do not present as grouped vesicles, erosions, or crusts as they do in immunocompetent patients. Rather, HSV infection often becomes ulcerative, rather than superficially erosive. Ulcers usually extend beyond the original borders of the infection, producing large plaques, often with arcuate borders representing coalescent smaller ulcers that originated as blisters. Nearly always, at least part of the ulcer touches a mucous membrane where the initial outbreak began (Fig. 20.1).

However, individual lesions are often larger as well as deeper. Especially common in the genital area, ulcerative HSV infection in an AIDS patient is often confused with other ulcerative sexually transmitted diseases (STDs), such as syphilis, chancroid, and granuloma inguinale. Cytomegalovirus infection can also produce chronic genital ulcerations in

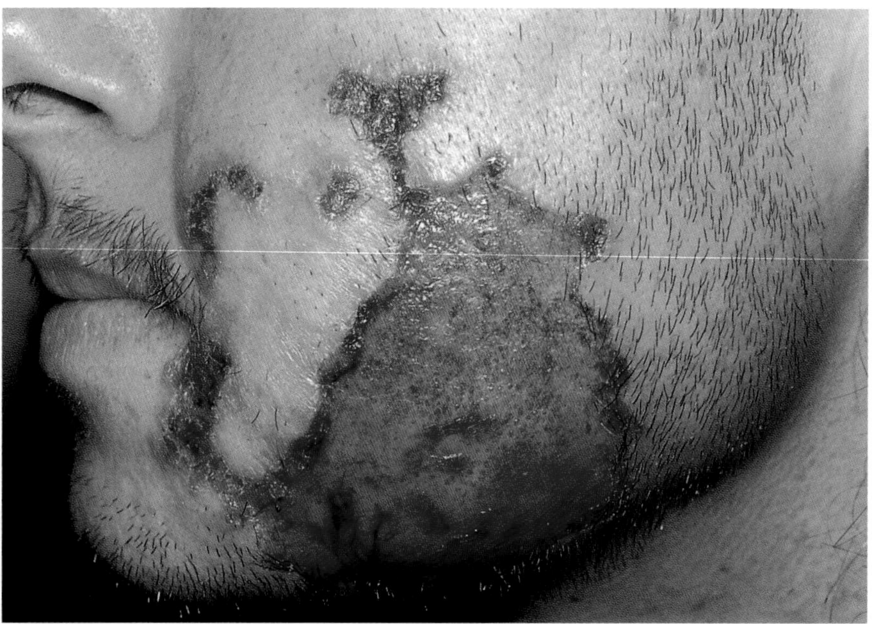

Figure 20.1 This large ulcerative plaque produced by an acyclovir-resistant form of herpes simplex virus (HSV) infection shows the characteristic morphology of HSV infection in an immunosuppressed patient: very large size, extension from a mucous membrane, and well-demarcated, irregular borders. This patient had a similar, large sacral ulceration.

immunosuppressed patients. Although the possibilities of these diseases should not be overlooked, HSV infection is far more common than these other diseases, and genital ulcerations in AIDS patients are nearly always due to HSV infection. In addition, ulcerations with HSV infection are usually larger, more numerous, and longer lasting than the ulcerations of other STDs.

A herpetic whitlow (HSV infection of the fingertip) can also appear atypical in AIDS patients. Punched-out ulcerations can occur in this location as well, while keratotic, crusted, or purulent lesions are seen as well. At times, multiple fingers are affected. HSV infection should be considered in any AIDS patient with an unusually severe or recalcitrant paronychia or when multiple fingers are involved.

HSV infection occasionally occurs on other areas of the skin surface; this diagnosis should be considered for any chronic ulcerative disease in an immunosuppressed patient. Although oral or anogenital sites account for the overwhelming majority of HSV infections, this diagnosis should be entertained for any punched-out ulcer in an immunosuppressed patient, especially a patient with AIDS.

Genital ulcers in a patient with AIDS are considered HSV infection until proved otherwise. Other, more exotic infections should be considered in the differential diagnosis of herpetic ulcers in immunosuppressed patients. However, most of these infections show more surrounding erythema, induration, and, often, pustulation. Generally, a typical herpetic ulcer in an immunosuppressed patient who is not toxic can be cultured and treated without submitting the patient to expensive and uncomfortable confirmatory biopsies and tissue cultures. Unresponsive ulcers that are culture negative require further investigation.

The management of HSV ulcers in immunosuppressed patients differs little from therapy in immunocompetent patients. However, immunosuppressed patients in general require longer therapy as well as ongoing suppressive therapy to prevent frequent and severe recurrences. AIDS patients definitely should receive suppressive therapy, since open wounds shed both HSV and human immunodeficiency virus (HIV). In addition, there is evidence that HSV potentiates the replication of HIV, theoretically both enhancing establishment of HIV infection in exposed people and amplifying an established infection.[1,2] The usual medications for treating HSV infection are acyclovir 200 mg PO 5 times a day, famciclovir 125 mg tid, or valacyclovir 500 mg tid, until complete healing has occurred. Acyclovir at 400 mg bid can then be continued indefinitely to prevent recurrences.

Occasionally, immunosuppressed patients, especially those with AIDS, experience an infection with an HSV that is resistant to the usual antiviral agents. This can be confirmed by a viral culture with sensitivities, which is available at some institutions. These patients should consult an infectious disease specialist. An HSV that is shown to be resistant to acyclovir is also resistant to famciclovir, valacyclovir, and ganciclovir.[3] Sometimes, topical therapy with trifuridine can produce some improvement.[4,5] Otherwise, foscarnet, a medication that is given only intravenously, is usually effective in these patients.[6] A very recent addition is cidofovir, which is beneficial both intravenously and topically in acyclovir- and foscarnet-resistant HSV infection.[7,8]

Varicella Zoster Infection Varicella zoster infection often produces atypical disease in immunosuppressed patients, particularly those with AIDS. These atypical presentations do not occur in otherwise healthy patients.

Patients with AIDS who have a history of childhood chickenpox occasionally experience a second episode of varicella.[9] This can present as typical varicella with small vesicles, pustules, and crusts, or individual lesions may be larger and more necrotic than usual. Also, patients who are HIV positive but without an AIDS-defining illness are more likely than immunocompetent patients to experience a classic episode of herpes zoster. Up to 23% of HIV patients with herpes zoster develop another episode of herpes zoster, usually occurring after their underlying disease has progressed to AIDS.[10,11] More than one episode of herpes zoster has also been reported in patients immunosuppressed due to other causes.

Herpes zoster in immunosuppressed patients often exhibits atypical lesions. Morphologic hallmarks of herpes zoster in an immunosuppressed patient include coalescing of vesicles into unusually large blisters, deeper ulcerative rather than erosive lesions, and, particularly in patients with AIDS, hyperkeratotic papules and plaques in a dermatomal distribution.

Another presentation of varicella zoster that occurs in very sick or immunodeficient patients is disseminated herpes zoster (Fig. 20.2). In this case, dermatomal herpes zoster is accompanied by generalized, scattered vesicles that resemble those of varicella. As occurs with varicella in immunodeficient patients, these individual, scattered lesions are occasionally larger and more necrotic than those seen with varicella in otherwise healthy individuals.

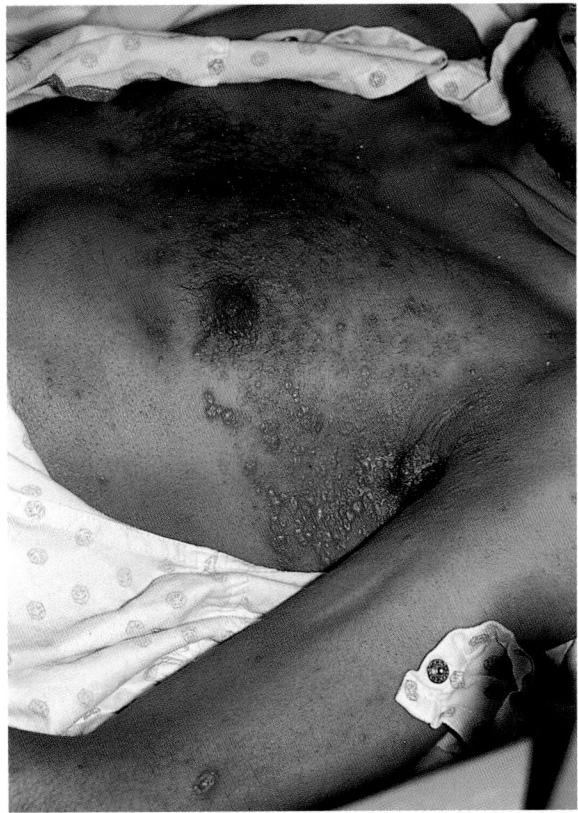

Figure 20.2 This patient with acquired immunodeficiency syndrome (AIDS) and disseminated herpes zoster has scattered large vesicles outside the affected dermatome.

The diagnosis of varicella zoster infection in immunosuppressed patients usually can be made clinically. The only disease easily confused with herpes zoster is HSV infection occurring in a dermatomal distribution. Varicella is most often confused with insect bites or folliculitis. Those occasional patients with larger and more necrotic lesions may mistakenly be believed to have multiple pyodermas or scattered vasculitic ulcers. Nearly always, a careful examination will show some blisters that allow for diagnosis without extensive laboratory testing.

Immunosuppressed patients with herpes zoster who appear otherwise well can be treated with oral antiviral therapy as outpatients. The medications used are acyclovir 800 mg 5 times a day, valacyclovir 1 g tid, or famciclovir 500 mg tid, until lesions heal. Patients should be instructed to return to the emergency department immediately if they become ill. Immunosuppressed patients with herpes zoster who are toxic, and most patients with disseminated herpes zoster or varicella, should be admitted for intravenous acyclovir therapy, 10 mg/kg tid. Although disseminated herpes zoster was once believed to be a dangerous disease itself, this condition is now associated with little direct morbidity but is considered a grim prognostic sign of end-stage underlying disease.

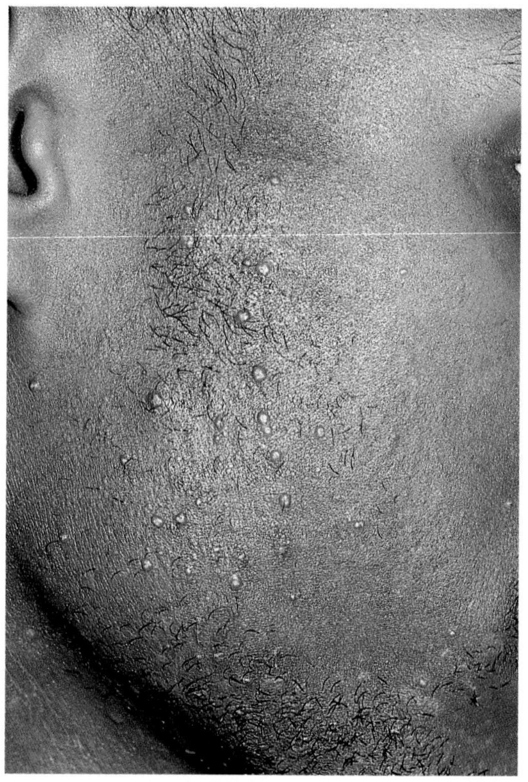

Figure 20.3 Numerous facial mollusca contagiosa are common in human immunodeficiency virus (HIV) disease.

Molluscum Contagiosum Mollusca contagiosa are common, virus-induced lesions that can occur anywhere in large numbers in children, but these are usually sexually transmitted in adults and confined to the genital area (see also Ch. 9, White Lesions). When an adult presents with these lesions over the face, immunosuppression in general, and HIV disease specifically, should be strongly suspected (Fig. 20.3).

These usually asymptomatic lesions are most often typical in appearance, even when occurring in an immunosuppressed patient (see Fig. 9.10). Skin-colored to white, discrete, dome-shaped papules range from solid-appearing lesions to pseudoblisters. Often, a central dell is present in some lesions. Immunosuppressed patients tend to exhibit very large numbers of lesions, and sometimes individual lesions are larger than typical. Other diseases can sometimes present similarly in patients with AIDS. Lesions of cutaneous cryptococcosis can appear nearly identical to large mollusca, as can histoplasmosis, coccidioidomycosis, and *Penicillium marnefi.* Therefore, a biopsy should be performed when there is any question of the correct diagnosis. Otherwise, these lesions are of cosmetic importance only.

Whereas some patients are not bothered by mollusca, others believe that this usually facial and very visible eruption is a constant reminder of AIDS, both to themselves and to others. Treatment, however, is an ongoing battle, since the patient's immune system continues to allow growth of new lesions. Light freezing with liquid nitrogen is often used, but drawbacks include pain (especially when used over multiple lesions) and dyspigmentation. Curettage is extremely effective, but this technique shares the disadvantage of pain and has the additional problem of being a relatively bloody procedure. Many dermatologists apply cantharidin (Cantharone) to the tip of each lesion. This painless chemical produces a blister and resolution of many of the lesions, although dyspigmentation sometimes occurs with this therapy as well. The greatest disadvantage of Cantharone is its unavailability in the United States. However, it can be ordered from several sources (e.g., Dormer Laboratories, Rexdale, Canada M9W5A3, and Omniderm, 997 Seguin, Hudson, Quebec, Canada JOP 1HO).

Patients should be warned that their mollusca will not be eliminated permanently with any of these treatments. Although individual lesions resolve, recurrences are usual.

Human Papillomavirus Infection Human papillomavirus (HPV) (genital warts) is extremely common in the general population, with up to 40% of patients exhibiting evidence of this virus with sophisticated testing, even in the absence of visible warts. Immunosuppressed patients are very likely to experience activation of subclinical infections, and the treatment of genital warts is the same as for immunocompetent patients (see Ch. 8, Skin-Colored Lesions).

However, immunosuppressed patients with genital warts often experience several complications. The first is an increase in the number and size of warts. Second, immunosuppressed patients rarely experience clearing of their warts with therapy. Although individual warts shrink or even disappear, recurrence is the rule. Finally, immunosuppressed patients with warts produced by HPV types associated with squamous cell carcinoma, such as HPV 16 and 18, are at risk of faster malignant transformation and earlier metastases of cervical and rectal carcinoma, as compared to immunocompetent patients.

Appropriate education regarding genital warts is important for all patients, but especially for immunosuppressed individuals. These patients should be aware of the recalcitrant nature of these lesions and of the necessity for careful surveillance for malignancy.

Oral Hairy Leukoplakia An occasional epithelial finding that is nearly specific for AIDS is oral hairy leukoplakia. This benign condition, produced by the Epstein-Barr virus, presents as white, corrugated plaques located primarily over the lateral tongue, although other oral mucosal surfaces can be affected.[12] Occasionally, oral hairy leukoplakia requires differentiation from a squamous cell carcinoma, which can also appear white when occurring on a mucous membrane. However, squamous cell carcinoma is usually less symmetric and exhibits an irregular surface, often with underlying induration. Oral warts, thrush, and lichen planus can also produce white lesions on the oral mucosa.

There is no good therapy, although spontaneous regression occasionally occurs. Also, high doses of oral acyclovir can produce temporary improvement.[13]

Fungal Infections

Mucocutaneous fungal infections are more common, and sometimes more severe, in immunosuppressed patients. Some of these infections, such as oral candidiasis, are associated especially with AIDS. Most cutaneous fungal infections in immunocompromised patients are superficial mucocutaneous infections. However, occasionally systemic fungal infections produce skin lesions.

Candidiasis Oral mucous membrane infection with *Candida albicans* is an AIDS-defining illness. Although oral thrush is found in other conditions and does not necessarily signify immunosuppression, its presence in the absence of dentures or antibiotics should raise the possibility of immunosuppression in general, and AIDS in particular. Most typically, oral thrush presents with white papules and plaques that can be removed from the surface of the epithelium with a tongue blade. However, oral candidiasis occasionally produces erosions; it is sometimes manifested as red, thin epithelium. These more unusual morphologies of oral candidiasis are usually missed by the examiner unless he or she has a high index of suspicion. Because a fungal preparation can be difficult for the nondermatologist to interpret, and because the atrophic, erythematous variant may exhibit a false-negative fungal preparation, cultures are indicated when there is a question or when the patient does not respond to therapy.

Candida is a frequent recurrent infection in uncircumcised men and in the vagina and over the modified mucous membrane of women with HIV disease. These infections usually have a typical appearance.

Patients with oral candidiasis, particularly those with a sore throat, suggesting esophageal involvement, are best treated with oral fluconazole 100 mg/day, until the mouth is clear. This medication is the treatment of choice because of hepatotoxicity associated with ketoconazole (Nizoral) and because both itraconazole (Sporanox) and ketoconazole are not well absorbed in the setting of gastric alkalinity, as occurs in some patients with AIDS. Patients who experience an immediate recurrence can be maintained on chronic, suppressive oral therapy, nystatin swish and spit, or clotrimazole vaginal troches, which are sugar free and are less likely to damage teeth than are oral troches. However, *Candida albicans* resistant to both oral and topical azole therapy is well described in patients with AIDS and should be considered in those patients who do not respond to standard therapy. These patients deserve referral to an infectious disease specialist.

The intermittent or chronic use of topical azoles or oral fluconazole 150 mg/week usually controls genital candidiasis, except for those women with non-*albicans Candida* infections such as *Torulopsis glabrata*. Non-*albicans Candida* infections are often resistant to azoles and may require nystatin vaginal suppositories and ointment, or boric acid capsules, prepared as 600 mg, inserted into the vagina twice daily.

Cutaneous Dermatophyte Infection Superficial dermatophyte infections such as tinea corporis, tinea cruris, and tinea pedis are often more extensive in immunosuppressed patients. Usually, the morphology of individual lesions is typical with annular, inflammatory plaques exhibiting peripheral scale that microscopically shows branching hyphae.

Sometimes, in addition to more extensive lesions, fungal infection in immunosuppressed patients may lose the annular appearance and exhibit solid plaques of scale. In addition, although tinea cruris normally affects only the inner thighs, patients who are immunosuppressed may experience extension of the fungal infection over the scrotum and penis or vulva. A superficial dermatophyte infection should be considered in any immunosuppressed patient exhibiting inflammatory scaling plaques.

Limited areas of tinea corporis in nonhairy locations can be treated with any topical azole, such as clotrimazole, miconazole, or econazole, or terbinafine. However, for extensive disease, for disease in areas with terminal hairs, and for plaques with fungal folliculitis, an oral antifungal agent such as griseofulvin or fluconazole is required (for details of therapy for dermatophyte infections, see Ch. 14, Papulosquamous Diseases: Red, Scaling, Well-Demarcated Papules and Plaques).

Onychomycosis Onychomycosis, or superficial dermatophyte infection of the nails, is a common condition in adults in general, and especially in men. These infections may be more common and more severe in immunosuppressed patients. In addition to the typical morphology of thickened nails lifted by underlying scale and fungal organisms, proximal white subungual onychomycosis is a peculiar finding that is almost specific for AIDS. The surface of the nail plate is smooth, with a normal texture, although the color is white[14] (Fig. 20.4). Superficial white onychomycosis, in which fungus infecting the surface of the nail plate imparts a white, rough surface, is not particularly indicative of immunosuppression.

Onychomycosis often does not require therapy. However, when the skin surrounding fungal nails becomes inflamed, fissures sometimes ensue, producing pain and providing a portal of entry for bacteria to produce cellulitis. Griseofulvin, fluconazole, and terbinafine are treatments of choice (for details of therapy, see Ch. 18, Diseases of the Hair and Nails).

Deep Fungal Infections Deep fungal infections are rare both in immunosuppressed patients and in immunocompetent patients. However, immunosuppressed patients are certainly more likely to develop deep fungal infections after exposure to offending organisms.

Cutaneous lesions of systemic fungal infection are generally multiple and superficial. These are usually edematous, indurated nodules or masses which often break down and drain. This appearance is shared by sporotrichosis and other deep

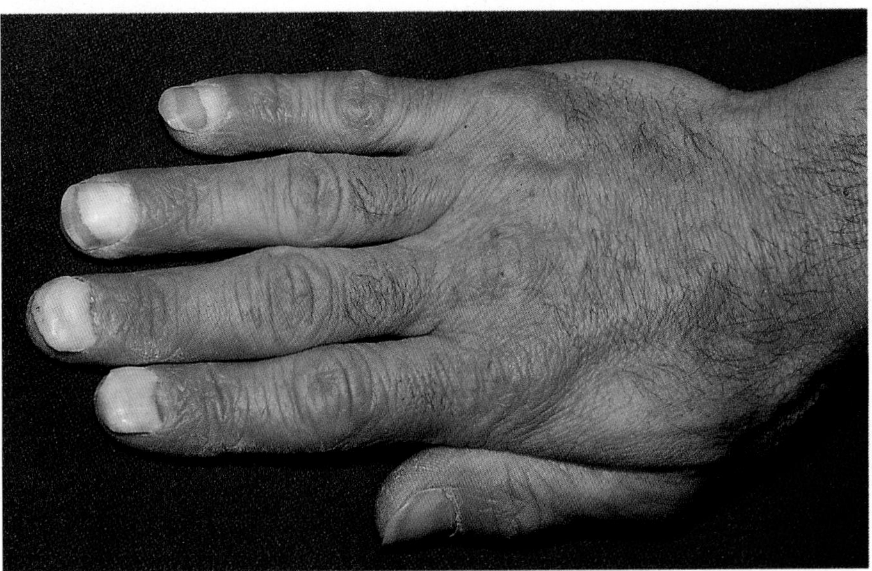

Figure 20.4 Proximal white subungual onychomycosis is nearly always seen in patients with AIDS.

fungal infections (for further discussion, see Ch. 12, Red Papules and Nodules). This appearance is also indistinguishable from some skin diseases caused by parasitic infections, such as scabies, or by acid-fast bacilli.

Immunosuppressed patients may exhibit smaller and less impressive lesions but in greater numbers, particularly patients with cryptococcal or histoplasmosis infections. Dome-shaped papules, pustulopapules, and crusts can occur and appear very nonspecific. A high index of suspicion is important. The diagnosis requires biopsy and either special stains or culture. Therapy depends on the diagnosis, and it should be directed by an infectious disease specialist.

BACTERIAL INFECTIONS

Although bacterial infections present with the same clinical findings in immunosuppressed patients as in immunocompetent patients, some infections are far more common and recalcitrant in those who are immunocompromised, especially those with AIDS.

Staphylococcal Folliculitis/Furunculosis

Because patients with AIDS have a predisposition to be itchy, these patients often develop eczema (atopic dermatitis, neurodermatitis). This scaling, excoriated eruption produced by scratching is nearly always colonized with *Staphylococcus aureus*. In the setting of immunosuppression, recurrent or chronic infection is usual. This can be manifested by purulence, exudation, and crusting, signs that are usually recognized and promptly treated by clinicians of all disciplines. However, low-grade infection of follicles is even more common but is more difficult to appreciate in the absence of a high index of suspicion. Exudation and crusting are often absent, because the infection lies within the follicle. Superficial infection of the follicular epithelium produces folliculitis, or "impetigo" of the follicle. A pustule may occur at the follicular orifice, but it is quickly removed with the fingernails. Thus, round erosions in association with eczema constitute the usual presentation of this condition in patients with AIDS.

Furunculosis represents deeper infection with involvement of the surrounding dermis, so that a nodule is present. As with folliculitis, a round erosion is often seen on the surface of these nodules, and less often a draining opening is present. Folliculitis and furunculosis exist on a spectrum, and often both types of lesions are present.

The diagnosis is usually made on the basis of the clinical presentation, but a confirmatory bacterial culture can be useful when doubt exists. The patient should be treated with an oral antistaphylococcal antibiotic, such as cephalexin (Keflex) or dicloxacillin. After control of new lesions is established with a dose of 500 mg qid, the patient can be continued on a dose of 500 mg bid until the skin is clear. Topical bactroban ointment (Mupirocin) inserted into the nares three times per day for the first week helps eliminate the carrier state. The eczema must be treated as well, because as long as the skin is scaling, *Staphylococcus aureus* will remain on the skin and re-establish itself within follicles (see Ch. 15, Eczematous Diseases). When both eczema and folliculitis/furunculosis are controlled, the antibiotic can be discontinued, but recurrence is usual and most patients require chronic therapy.

PARASITIC

Norwegian Scabies

Scabies occurring in immunosuppressed patients often presents atypically. Although otherwise healthy people with scabies normally host only 8 to 10 mites, immunocompromised people often exhibit confluent plaques that are teeming with mites.

Unlike typical scabies, where burrows occur between skin folds and between the fingers, and itching seems out of proportion to the degree of clinical inflammation, Norwegian scabies displays red plaques with dense yellow scale/crust. Although skin folds are often affected, lesions extend far beyond these protected, damp areas.

The diagnosis is easily made by microscopic examination of scale. Whereas scabies preparations are often negative in immunocompetent patients, making the clinician's experience crucial, in immunosuppressed patients, a casual examination of the yellow scale/crust normally yields several mites, as well as ova and feces.

The treatment of scabies in the United States at this time is permethrin 5% applied overnight to the patient and other members of the household (see also Ch. 15, Eczematous Diseases). Immunosuppressed patients often benefit from a repeat application several days later. Topical corticosteroids can help itching, and nighttime sedation can allow patients to rest at night despite intense pruritus. Bedclothes and clothing worn during the past 24 hours should be washed in hot water. Oral ivermectin is very effective, but it is not yet available in the United States.

OTHER INFECTONS

Bacillary Angiomatosis

Bacillary angiomatosis is a peculiar skin eruption produced by the rickettsia-like organism, *Rochalimaea henselae*, one of the organisms responsible for cat-scratch fever.[15] Clinically, patients present with tiny red or purple papules that enlarge to form larger papules and nodules. Lesions are generally clustered and may range from one or a few to thousands. Deeper cutaneous or subcutaneous indurated nodules sometimes occur, and these can ulcerate. Occasionally, more poorly demarcated plaques of bacillary angiomatosis mimic cellulitis.

Some affected patients experience visceral diseases, including mucosal surfaces, pulmonary involvement, and lesions of the heart, peritoneum, diaphragm, liver, and central nervous system. About one-third of patients experience bone marrow infection with resulting pain and osteolytic lesions on radiography.[16] Patients with visceral disease may experience fever, chills, and wasting.

The diagnosis is made on the basis of the clinical appearance and setting, in conjunction with serologic studies and blood, skin, or visceral cultures. Therapy consists of oral erythromycin 500 mg qid, sometimes for weeks or months, until lesions disappear. Alternative therapies include other macrolides, the tetracyclines, trimethoprim-sulfamethoxazole, or ciprofloxacin.

Syphilis

Syphilis in immunosuppressed patients requires special considerations (see also the discussion in Ch. 14, Papulosquamous Diseases: Red, Scaling, Well-Demarcated Papules and Plaques). The greatest clinical experience with syphilis in a setting of immunosuppression has been with AIDS patients.

First, syphilis serology (Venereal Disease Research Laboratory [VDRL] and rapid plasma reagin [RPR]) can produce false-negative results, although this is uncommon. Therefore, the clinician should not rule out this diagnosis solely on the basis of a negative serology if other signs point strongly to syphilis. A skin biopsy with Warthin-Starry or immunofluorescent stains may demonstrate the organism. In addition, syphilis can progress to tertiary disease, especially neurosyphilis, far more quickly than in immunocompetent people. Lumbar punctures should be performed in any AIDS patients with syphilis and with any abnormalities detected during neurologic examination. Ocular involvement is also more common in patients with AIDS.

Although most patients with AIDS exhibit skin lesions typical for syphilis, lesional morphology can differ in AIDS patients. Chancres may be larger and more painful, due to secondary infection. Individual lesions can be more infiltrative and nodular; sometimes larger psoriasiform plaques occur instead of smaller, oval, generalized papules (Fig. 20.5). Also, response to penicillin therapy is poor, compared to immunocompetent patients. Therefore, more vigorous therapy is indicated. Penicillin 2.4 million units IM should be administered weekly for 3 weeks, unless the lumbar puncture is abnormal. In that circumstance, intravenous therapy should be administered. Finally, syphilis can recur after therapy in AIDS patients without re-exposure.

Any immunosuppressed patient with syphilis should be followed carefully after therapy to ensure adequate response to therapy and evaluate

Figure 20.5 This patient with AIDS and secondary syphilis exhibits plaques suggestive of psoriasis, but the papules surrounding the large plaques and underlying infiltrated, indurated skin were not typical for psoriasis.

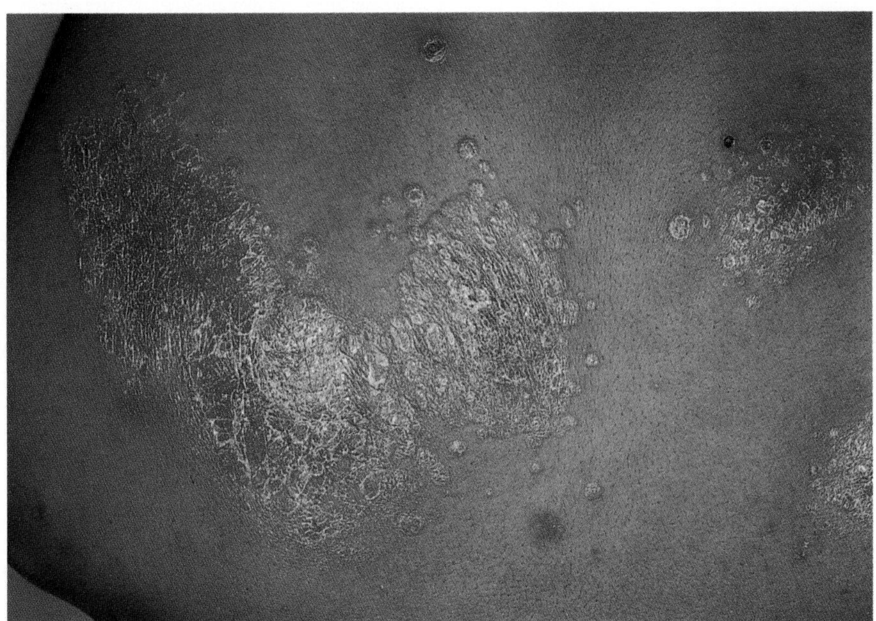

periodically for recurrence of disease. Often, the local public health department is best equipped to do this.

SKIN MALIGNANCIES

Any immunosuppressed patient is likely to experience more rapid transformation, growth, and metastasis of various malignancies, including squamous cell carcinomas. In addition, although no skin cancers are pathognomonic for AIDS, several cutaneous malignancies are extremely suggestive of this diagnosis.

Squamous Cell Carcinoma

Patients who are immunosuppressed by virtue of disease or medications are much more likely than immunocompetent people to develop squamous cell carcinomas, particularly in the setting of sun damage and warts. Patients with renal failure and organ transplants often experience major problems with rapid growth of actinic keratoses and morphologically atypical warts that can be impossible to differentiate clinically from squamous cell carcinomas. The usual presentation is one of skin-colored or red, keratotic nodules that are often confluent and occurring in a background of actinically damaged, scaling skin. Careful and regular skin examinations with frequent biopsies and excisional removals are generally required. These patients should be referred to a dermatologist on an urgent basis, since rapid growth and metastasis can occur.

In addition, invasive squamous cell carcinoma associated with genital human papillomavirus (HPV) infection is more common in immunosuppressed patients because of the patients' inability to contain the HPV and because of early malignant transformation. These squamous cell carcinomas occur primarily at the transition zones of glandular epithelium and squamous epithelium on the cervix and within the rectal canal. Papanicolaou smears should be performed on immunosuppressed women with anogenital warts at least every 6 months, with immediate colposcopy performed for any abnormalities. Anoscopy should be performed in immunocompromised men with perianal warts and biopsies performed of any abnormalities to evaluate for changes of dysplasia.

As the polymerase chain reaction (PCR) technique for typing HPV becomes more available, this test will probably be used routinely in immunocompromised patients to detect those warts caused by HPV 16, 18, 31, 33, or 35. These HPV types are the most likely to produce squamous cell carcinoma. In the absence of PCR, careful surveillance of all patients is indicated, but particularly of those with flat warts, pigmented warts, and warts that are atypical in any way. In addition, warts that show any suggestion of dysplasia should be treated with physically destructive modalities, such as electrocautery, laser, excision, or liquid nitrogen. The use of podophyllin and podofilox should be avoided, as these agents are theoretical carcinogens.

Kaposi Sarcoma

Kaposi sarcoma occurs worldwide in several different settings and in several different populations, but the strongest association in the United States is with AIDS. Still, patients who are otherwise predisposed to Kaposi sarcoma, such as men of Mediterranean or Jewish descent, sometimes develop this tumor when they are immunosuppressed by virtue of medication or illness. When, and if, this immunosuppression is reversed, the Kaposi sarcoma often regresses spontaneously.

Kaposi sarcoma was one of the first skin signs associated with AIDS. AIDS-associated Kaposi sarcoma is almost entirely confined to patients with sexually acquired AIDS, but the incidence of this tumor has decreased dramatically. Recent investigations have found a novel herpesvirus-like DNA sequence (human herpesvirus type 8) in 90% of Kaposi sarcoma of HIV patients,[17,18] and the sexual transmission of this Kaposi sarcoma-associated herpesvirus-like DNA sequence has been postulated.[18,19]

Occurring anywhere over the skin surface, including the face and oral mucosa, Kaposi sarcoma in white patients appears as purple or red-brown papules or plaques (Fig. 20.6). Black patients usually exhibit very dark brown or nearly black lesions. Visceral involvement of any organ

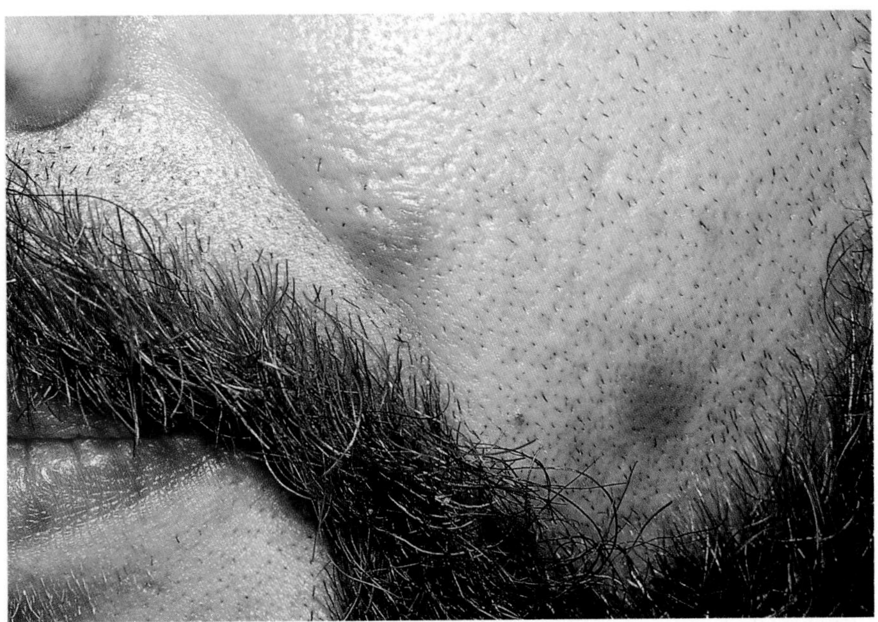

Figure 20.6 These brown-red nodules over the face are typical for AIDS-associated Kaposi sarcoma.

can occur, especially the lungs, gastrointestinal tract, and lymph nodes.

Histologically, this condition does not appear malignant but has both inflammatory and proliferative features. In addition, it often has a rather benign course, and patients are more likely to succumb to other complications from AIDS.

Lesions are usually nontender, but these tumors serve as a constant reminder of the patient's underlying AIDS. Although many patients do not develop serious complications of Kaposi sarcoma because of the indolent nature of this disease, enlarging skin tumors in the mouth can sometimes produce symptoms and dysfunction. Occasionally, Kaposi sarcoma can progress and extend aggressively, infiltrating skin and subcutaneous tissues to the extent that the lymphatics are blocked and tissue begins to necrose. Visceral involvement can produce problems as well. Even patients who do not medically require therapy for their tumors often prefer treatment for cosmetic reasons. There is no appropriate therapy in the emergency department, except for local care of any necrosing tumors and general supportive care. However, accepted therapies for skin lesions include cryotherapy, radiation therapy, α-interferon (α-IFN), and intralesional or intravenous chemotherapy with vinca alkaloids, such as vincristine or vinblastine.

Lymphoma

Patients with AIDS are at an increased risk of the development of lymphoma, primarily non-Hodgkin lymphoma. The age of onset in these patients is younger, and aggressive subtypes are more common. These patients generally present with advanced disease, and extensive visceral involvement is common. However, skin lymphoma is rare. Systemic B symptoms may be present but are difficult to differentiate from the constitutional symptoms of AIDS. Therapy is complicated by the underlying immunodeficiency, and the prognosis is grim.

Primary central nervous system lymphoma, a discrete entity, rather than evidence of systemic lymphoma occurs more often in HIV-positive individuals than among other patients. This multicentric condition can be difficult to differentiate from central nervous system infection or AIDS dementia, since the presenting symptoms include lethargy, confusion, memory loss, headaches, or cranial nerve palsy. There are no skin findings.

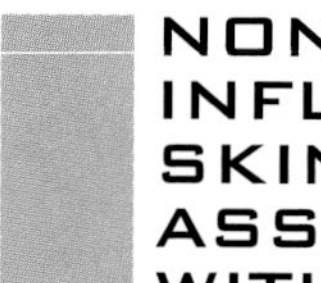

NONINFECTIOUS INFLAMMATORY SKIN DISEASES ASSOCIATED WITH AIDS

Despite the fact that AIDS patients are immunodeficient, these patients exhibit signs of hyperimmune responsiveness in some situations. Some common inflammatory diseases are more severe, and several inflammatory diseases are unique to AIDS. In general, AIDS patients seem to itch and to develop rashes very easily.

Seborrheic Dermatitis

Unusually severe seborrheic dermatitis (inflammatory dandruff) was one of the first recognized cutaneous markers for AIDS. However, typical seborrheic dermatitis and very severe disease in the presence of neurologic disease are very common findings and should not necessarily raise the suspicion of AIDS.

AIDS patients often exhibit, in addition to scalp scale, marked erythema and yellowish scale of the face, particularly at the hairline, and over the central face to include the eyebrows and naso-labial folds (Fig. 20.7). Occasionally, seborrheic dermatitis even affects the central back and chest, and even less often, the skin folds of the axilla and groin.

Sometimes, erythema and scale over the face are so marked as to suggest a diagnosis of psoriasis or fungal infection. However, negative fungal smears and an examination of other skin surfaces usually help rule out these diseases and confirm the diagnosis of seborrheic dermatitis.

Not only is seborrheic dermatitis more prevalent and more severe in patients with AIDS, but it is often more recalcitrant to therapy as well. Antiseborrheic shampoos and topical steroids are appropriate for patients with AIDS (for further discussion, see Ch. 15, Eczematous Diseases). However, those patients who do not respond to low-potency topical corticosteroids may require a mid-potency medication such as triamcinolone cream 0.1%. Topical ketoconazole cream and shampoo are more expensive alternatives.

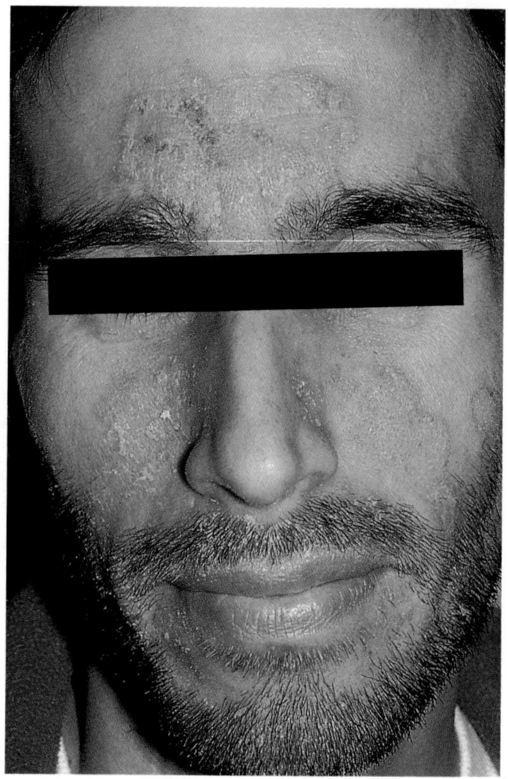

Figure 20.7 Extensive and inflammatory plaques of seborrheic dermatitis are common in patients with AIDS.

Psoriasis

New onset of psoriasis, sudden worsening of preexisting psoriasis, and psoriasis that is recalcitrant to therapy should raise suspicion for AIDS. Certainly, most patients with psoriasis are not HIV positive, so HIV testing is not routine for patients with psoriasis. However, the possibility of HIV disease should be considered, and questioning about risk factors in any patient with new onset of psoriasis or recent worsening of their disease is certainly warranted. Generally, patients with HIV-associated

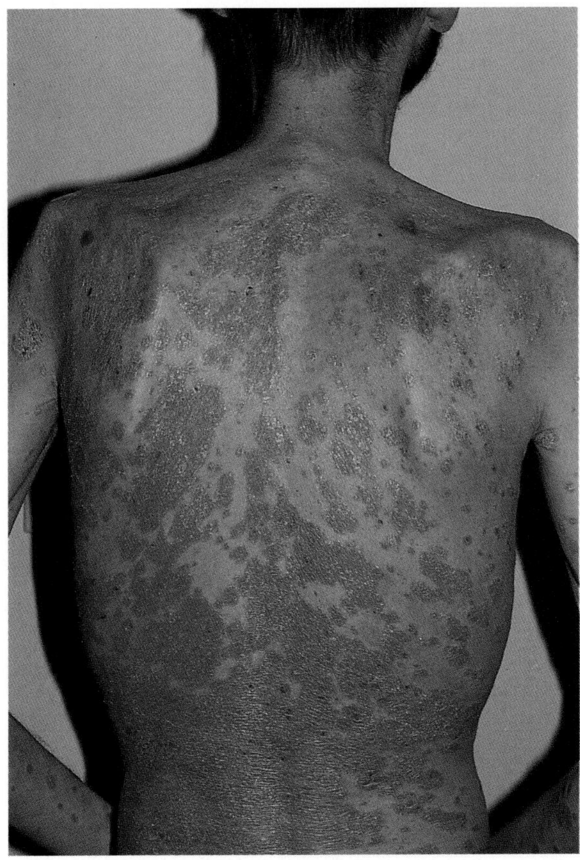

Figure 20.8 Extensive psoriasis in this wasted patient should raise the concern for AIDS.

psoriasis are not merely HIV positive; rather, they have advanced AIDS. Wasting and a history of AIDS-defining illnesses are common. Not only is typical, plaque-type psoriasis more common in these patients, but generalized erythrodermic psoriasis and pustular psoriasis are more common as well (Fig. 20.8). Psoriatic arthritis is six times more common in patients with AIDS than in other patients with psoriasis.[20]

Superficial fungal infections, seborrheic dermatitis, and atopic dermatitis are diseases that both mimic psoriasis and are more common in patients with AIDS. Also, these diseases often coexist. Fungal smears and an examination of other skin surfaces and nails for typical disease usually help to sort out the proper diagnosis or diagnoses.

Management of the patient with AIDS and psoriasis is similar to that of the immunocompetent patient (see Ch. 14). The only therapy appropriate for the Emergency Department is topical corticosteroids, such as triamcinolone ointment 0.1% applied bid, with follow-up evaluation by a dermatologist as soon as convenient. After first-line therapy with topical corticosteroids, and second-line therapy with ultraviolet (UV) light treatments, systemic medical therapy is usually modified. Although oral methotrexate is one of the most common medications used in immunocompetent patients with psoriasis, it is used only when absolutely necessary in patients with AIDS because of its own immunosuppressant effects. Instead, etretinate (Tegison) is often used in these patients. For many patients, treating the AIDS infection with antiviral agents produces improvement in psoriasis that parallels improvement in their HIV disease.[21]

Reiter Syndrome

Because pustular psoriasis and Reiter syndrome are closely related diseases (for further discussion, see Ch. 7, Pustular Diseases), the increased prevalence of Reiter syndrome in patients with AIDS is not surprising. The skin lesions of pustular psoriasis and Reiter syndrome are indistinguishable clinically and histologically. Classically, Reiter syndrome occurs in men and is associated with scaling, crusted plaques, often with pustules, over the palms, soles, and genitalia, particularly the glans penis.

The diagnosis is made by recognizing the presence of inflammatory arthritis, urethritis, and inflammatory eye disease. Therapy consists of topical corticosteroids when disease is mild or moderate, and of oral retinoids or exposure to UV light for more severe disease.

Vascular Hypersensitivity Reactions

Although immunosuppressed, patients with HIV disease often exhibit evidence of hypersensitivity reactions, such as urticaria, morbilliform medication reactions, erythema multiforme, and leukocytoclastic vasculitis.[22] This may be partially due to the compensatory increase in immunoglobulins found in these patients. In addition, these patients are exposed to more allergens in the form of infections and medications. Although common in patients with AIDS, hypersensitivity skin reactions do not differ in morphologic appearance, causes, or therapy (see also Ch. 13, Vascular Reactions and Other Flat-Topped, Nonscaling Patches and Plaques).

Atopic Dermatitis/Eczema

Eczema, also called neurodermatitis, atopic dermatitis, and lichen simplex chronicus, is skin eruptions produced by scratching (for further discussion, see Ch. 15, Eczematous Diseases). This condition is very common and often recalcitrant in patients with AIDS, since these patients have a predisposition to itch.

The clinical presentation and morphology of eczema are typical but often unusually widespread and severe in these patients. Patients with AIDS are even more likely than the average eczema patient to have underlying, predisposing skin conditions that initiate the itch-scratch cycle. The skin should be evaluated carefully for the presence of folliculitis, either bacterial or sterile, xerosis, scabies, and fungal infection. Optimal improvement does not occur unless these coexisting factors are addressed (for a detailed discussion of therapy, see Ch. 15).

Eosinophilic Folliculitis

Eosinophilic folliculitis, also called Ofugi disease, is an uncommon skin condition. In the United States, it is seen primarily in patients with AIDS. Patients exhibit red, nonscaling papules and nodules distributed especially over the face and upper trunk. These lesions may appear skin colored or hyperpigmented in dark-complexioned patients.

Eosinophilic folliculitis can be confused with insect bites or bacterial folliculitis. However, lesions are more numerous and more evenly scattered as compared with insect bites, and more monomorphous, lacking in pustules and crusts as compared to bacterial folliculitis.

The pathogenesis of eosinophilic folliculitis is believed to be infectious, but the organism is unknown. Both oral isotretinoin and metronidazole have been reported useful for this condition, as has UV light therapy.[23–25]

Lichenoid Photoeruptions of AIDS

Although classic lichen planus is uncommon in patients with AIDS, a lichenoid photoeruption is associated with AIDS, primarily in black patients.[26] Sometimes associated with the use of medications known to induce lichenoid medication reactions, this eruption often has no obvious etiology. This rash begins in a photosensitive distribution and presents as violaceous or hyperpigmented scaling, sharply demarcated plaques. Unlike lichen planus, mucous membrane involvement does not occur. Involved areas sometimes then develop depigmentation. This disease is often unsightly but is not otherwise dangerous, although patients report significant itching.

Lichenoid photoeruptions can resemble lichen planus, psoriasis, seborrheic dermatitis, and superficial dermatophyte infections. However, a slightly atypical appearance and distribution for these diseases in conjunction with a skin biopsy generally provide the correct diagnosis. The biopsies are not diagnostic of typical lichen planus.

Therapy consists of the discontinuation of any offending medications and sunscreens, as well as sunlight avoidance.

Aphthous Ulcers

Patients with AIDS sometimes develop unusually large aphthous ulcers, particularly of the mouth. These ulcers occur only over mucous membrane not attached to bone, such as the buccal mucosa, the tongue, and the inner aspect of the lips. Lesions are punched out and sharply demarcated, with little surrounding inflammation (Fig. 20.9). The borders of these large ulcers are often irregular, and the base of the ulcer may be white or red.

The etiology of aphthae is unknown, but they do not result from infection. However, atypical, ulcerative HSV infection must be ruled out in immunosuppressed patients. Generally, HSV infection affects the outer aspect of the lip, and often

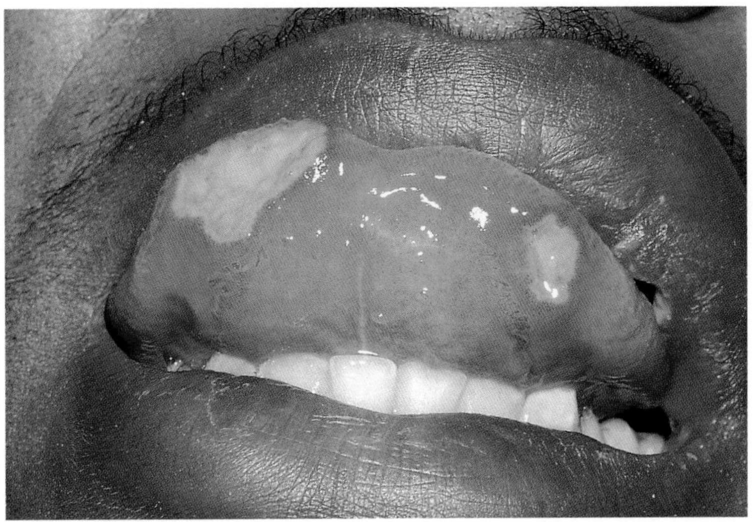

Figure 20.9 Large, deep, irregular aphthous ulcers can occur in immunocompetent people, but they occur more often in patients with AIDS.

the surrounding skin of the face, whereas aphthae never affect keratinized skin.

Therapy for large aphthae is difficult. Although prednisone induces healing, this immunosuppressant medication is best avoided in patients with AIDS, especially because of recurrence after discontinuation of the corticosteroids. A topical ultrapotent medication, such as clobetasol dipropionate (Temovate) cream under damp cotton ball occlusion, can be useful for some. Oral dapsone or colchicine are sometimes beneficial. Oral thalidomide can be extremely effective, but obtaining this medication is difficult although not impossible.

MISCELLANEOUS SKIN DISEASES OR SYMPTOMS ASSOCIATED WITH AIDS

Essential Pruritus

Some patients with AIDS described excruciating itching in the absence of specific skin lesions. These patients often exhibit excoriation, but no underlying rash or evidence of infection.

The usual causes of itching include subtle dermatoses, xerosis, anxiety or depression, and infestations, all of which should be considered and addressed. In addition, these patients are at risk of multiorgan disease. Renal failure, liver disease, and lymphomas are all possible causes of essential pruritus that can be ruled in or out with simple serum chemistries.

Many patients are found not to have any of these associated conditions. These patients are often best treated with nighttime sedation that at least allows them to sleep. Doxepin or amitriptyline can provide this while also helping the depression that so often accompanies unremitting pruritus. Moisturization of the skin can be beneficial, and patients deserve a trial of a topical corticosteroid, although often this is not beneficial. Recalcitrant patients sometimes improve with UV light therapy.

Ichthyosis

Ichthyosis refers to morphologic skin changes that resemble fish scale. This appearance can be extremely severe in some congenital genetic diseases, but more often it occurs as an interesting but trivial skin change. Mild ichthyosis can be inherited, and acquired ichthyosis occurs in several classic settings, including lymphoma and AIDS.

Patients rarely present to a physician with a complaint of this appearance to their skin. However, if the clinician notes these changes during a physical examination, particularly in association with other findings suggestive of AIDS, he or she should be aware of this association.

Therapy is generally unhelpful and unnecessary, unless ichthyosis is associated with pruritus. Moisturization, sometimes with a lubricant that contains lactic acid (LactiCare lotion) to dissolve scale, and topical corticosteroids are then used.

Hair Changes

Diffuse thinning of scalp and body hair occurs in many patients with AIDS, probably associated in part with poor nutrition. Early graying of hair can also occur. Very long eyelashes are also found in some patients with AIDS. No therapy is indicated for these cosmetic changes.

REFERENCES

1. Albrecht MA, DeLuca NA, Byrn RA et al: The herpes simplex virus immediate-early protein, ICP4, is required to potentiate replication of human immunodeficiency virus in CD4+ lymphocytes. J Virol 63:1861, 1989
2. Latchman DS: Herpes infection and AIDS. Nature 325:487, 1987
3. Birch CJ, Tachedjian G, Doherty RR et al: Altered sensitivity to antiviral drugs of herpes simplex virus isolates from a patient with the acquired immunodeficiency syndrome. J Infect Dis 162:731, 1990
4. Murphy M, Morley A, Eglin RP, Monteiro E: Topical trifuridine for mucocutaneous acyclovir-resistant herpes simplex II in AIDS patient, letter. Lancet 2:1040, 1992
5. Weaver D, Weissbach N, Kapell K et al: Topical trifluoridine (TFT) treatment of acyclovir-resistant (ACV-R) herpes simplex disease, abstract 507. In Program and Abstracts of the Thirty-first Interscience Conference on Antimicrobial Agents and Chemotherapy, Chicago, IL. American Society for Microbiology, 1991 Washington, DC
6. Saftin S: Treatment of acyclovir-resistant herpes simplex virus infections in patients with AIDS. J Acquired Immune Defic Syndr, suppl 1.5:s29, 1992
7. Snoeck R, Andrei G, Gerard M: Successful treatment of progressive mucocutaneous infection due to acyclovir- and foscarnet-resistant herpes simplex virus with (*S*)-1-(3-hydroxy-2-phosphonylmethoxypropyl)cytosine (HPMPC). Clin Infect Dis 18:570, 1994
8. Lalezari JP, Drew LW, Glutzer E et al: Treatment with intravenous (*S*)-1-[3-hydroxy-2-(phosphonylmethoxy)propyl]-cytosine of acyclovir-resistant mucocutaneous infection with herpes simplex virus in a patient with AIDS. J Infect Dis 170:570, 1994
9. Perronne C, Lazanas M, Leport C et al: Varicella in patients infected with the human immunodeficiency virus. Arch Dermatol 126:1033, 1990
10. Colebunders R, Man JM, Francis H et al: Herpes zoster in African patients: a clinical predictor of human immunodeficiency virus infection. J Infect Dis 157:314, 1988
11. Melbye M, Grossman RJ, Goedert JJ et al: Risk of AIDS after herpes zoster. Lancet 2:728, 1987
12. Snijders PJF, Schulten EAJM, Mullink H et al: Detection of human papillomavirus and Epstein-Barr virus in oral hairy leukoplakia. J Oral Pathol 137:659, 1990
13. Resnick LI, Herbst JHS, Ablashi DV et al: Regression of oral hairy leukoplakia following orally administered acyclovir therapy. JAMA 259:384, 1988
14. Weismann K, Knudsen EA, Pedersen C: White nails in AIDS/ARC due to *Trichophyton rubrum* infection. Clin Exp Dermatol 13:24, 1988
15. Cockerell CJ: Bacillary angiomatosis and related diseases caused by *Rochalimaea*. J Am Acad Dermatol 32:783, 1995
16. Conrad SE, Jacobs D, Gee J et al: Pseudoneoplastic infection of bone in acquired immuno-

deficiency syndrome. J Bone Joint Surg 73A: 774, 1991

17. Chang Y, Cesarman E, Pessin MS et al: Identification of herpesvirus-like DNA sequences in AIDS-associated Kaposi's sarcoma. Science 266:1865, 1994
18. Kedes DH, Operskalski E, Busch M et al: The seroepidemiology of human herpesvirus 8 (Kaposi's sarcoma-associated herpesvirus): distribution of infection in KS risk groups and evidence for sexual transmission. Nature Med 2:918, 1996
19. Lin J-C, Lin S-C, Mar E-C et al: Is Kaposi's sarcoma-associated herpesvirus detectable in semen of HIV-infected homosexual men? Lancet 346:1601, 1995
20. Obuch ML, Maurer T, Becker B et al: Psoriasis and human immunodeficiency virus infection. J Am Acad Dermatol 27:667, 1992
21. Duvic M, Crane MM, Conant M: Zidovudine improves psoriasis in human immunodeficiency virus-positive males. Arch Dermatol 130: 447, 1994
22. Coopman SA, Stern RS: Cutaneous drug reactions in human immunodeficiency virus infection. Arch Dermatol 127:714, 1991
23. Otley CC, Avram MR, Johnson RA: Isotretinoin treatment of human immunodeficiency virus-associated eosinophilic folliculitis. Arch Dermatol 131:1047, 1995
24. Smith KJ, Skelton HG, Yeager K: Metronidazole for eosinophilic pustular folliculitis in human immunodeficiency virus type 1-positive patients. Arch Dermatol 131:1089, 1995
25. Sadick NS: Acquired immunodeficiency syndrome. p. 651. In Sams WM Jr, Lynch PJ (eds): Principles and Practice of Dermatology. 2nd Ed. Churchill Livingstone, New York, 1996
26. Berger TG, Dhar A: Lichenoid photoeruptions in human immunodeficiency virus infection. Arch Dermatol 130:609, 1994

SUGGESTED READINGS

Adal KA, Cockerell CJ, Petrie WA: Bacillary angiomatosis, cat-scratch disease and other syndromes due to *Rochalimaea.* N Engl J Med 330: 1509, 1994

Buchness MR: Treatment of skin diseases in HIV-infected patients. Dermatol Clin 13:321, 1995

Itin PH, Rufli T: Oral hairy leukoplakia. Int J Dermatol 31:301, 1992

Itin PH, Lautenschlager S, Fluckiger R: Oral manifestations in HIV-infected patients: diagnosis and management. J Am Acad Dermatol 29:749, 1993

James W: AIDS: A ten-year perspective. Dermatol Clin 9:391, 1991

Murakawa GJ, Kerschmann R, Berger T: Cutaneous *Cryptococcus* infection and AIDS. Report of 12 cases and review of the literature. Arch Dermatol 132:545, 1996

Obuch ML, Maurer T, Becker B et al: Psoriasis and human immunodeficiency virus infection. J Am Acad Dermatol 27:667, 1992

Orkin M: Scabies in AIDS. Semin Dermatol 12:9, 1993

Rosental D, LeBoit PE, Klumpp L: Human immunodeficiency virus-associated eosinophilic folliculitis. Arch Dermatol 127:206, 1991

Sadick NS, Pahwa S: Cutaneous diseases associated with human immunodeficiency virus infection. Curr Opin Infect Dis 5:673, 1992

Sadick NS, McNutt NS, Kaplan MH: Papulosquamous dermatoses of AIDS. J Am Acad Dermatol 22:1270, 1990

Schwartz JJ, Myskowski PL: Molluscum contagiosum in patients with human immunodeficiency virus infection. J Am Acad Dermatol 27:583, 1992

Spach DH: Bacillary angiomatosis. Int J Dermatol 32:19, 1992

Webster GF, Cockerell CJ, Friedman-Kien AG: The clinical spectrum of bacillary angiomatosis. Br J Dermatol 126:535, 1992

APPENDIX

Instructional to Patient Handouts

A major role in the outcome of therapy for skin diseases lies in day to day care of the skin and appropriate patient expectations. Although a topical corticosteroid is firstline therapy for eczema, a topical steroid alone does not produce maximal improvement. Unfortunately, people generally retain very little of what they are told in a stressful situation such as an emergency department. Also, much patient education regarding therapy is discounted by both the patient and the clinician when the therapy is not a prescription medication. These handouts are designed to explicitly tell patients, in clear lay terms, the cause (when possible) of their skin problem, the steps needed for maximal improvement, and the reasons behind specialized skin care.

The handouts are also designed to address the patients' expectations. Whereas clinicians are aware of the joke that dermatology patients never get well and they never die, patients persist in the belief that a cure should be possible. Very often, I see a patient referred because their eczema always returns when therapy is stopped. No one ever made the chronic and recurring nature of eczema clear to the patient. Hopefully, these handouts will allow your patients to understand that, for many of them, control of their disease is considered success.

Acne

You have acne, a condition in which hair pores become blocked with dead skin and cause pimples. Usually, people with acne have blackheads, whiteheads, red bumps, and pus bumps. Sometimes these can scar. Although most people with acne are teenagers, adults sometimes have acne too.

Acne is not related to diet, germs, or dirt. It is related to hormones and to the use of heavy creams, greases, makeup, and stress. Therefore, you *do not* need to change the foods you eat, and you should not scrub your skin often or use harsh, antibacterial soaps. However, you *should* use only light moisturizers and makeup that has the word "noncomedogenic" on the label (meaning it does not worsen acne).

Acne improves very slowly with treatment, so you will probably not notice much improvement for the first 1 or 2 months. This is normal, so you should continue your medications, even if you do not seem to be improving at first. Also, once your skin is clear, you must continue with these medications, or your acne will return. You and your regular health care provider will decide how long you should be treated.

You have probably been given a prescription for a medication called Retin-A cream. This medication unblocks pores and helps clear blackheads and whiteheads. Because it can be irritating, use very small amounts of the medication until your skin has adjusted to it. It should be applied once a day, just before bedtime, to clean, dry skin. It should be rinsed off in the morning, and you should apply a sunscreen every day, because Retin-A can make your skin more sensitive to sunlight. If your skin becomes irritated, decrease the frequency of application to every other day, until your skin is used to the medication.

For red bumps and pus bumps, you may have been given an antibiotic. Because acne is not an infection and antibiotics improve skin by means other than killing bacteria, your skin will not improve immediately. Either apply or take the antibiotic twice a day according to instructions. Be sure to take your medication on an empty stomach (no food—clear liquids only—from 2 hours before, until 1 hour after, your medicine), if these are the instructions. You should continue to use the medication for about 2 months.

Acne Keloidalis

You have a type of skin rash called acne keloidalis. In spite of its name, this is not acne, and you do not have keloids. This condition causes bumps over the back of the scalp, and hair loss in this area. Sometimes the bumps drain, become inflamed, and can itch or hurt.

Although the cause of acne keloidalis is not known, this is not an infection. There is no medication that can cure this problem, but treatment often helps control it. Even though acne keloidalis is not an infection, some types of antibiotics can be helpful when used continuously. Also, cortisone applied to the skin can help somewhat. Sometimes, scraping the bumps off the surface of the skin by a dermatologist and injecting cortisone will remove bumps at least temporarily. The only cure for acne kelodalis is surgery—the involved skin will be removed, leaving only underlying fat, and the area allowed to gradually heal.

Acute Urticaria

You have urticaria, which is sometimes called hives. This itchy rash is an allergic reaction. Often it is an allergy to a medication, to an infection, or even to an insect bite or sting. Sometimes the cause of the allergy cannot be found.

The hives usually disappear 1 or 2 weeks after the cause of the allergy has disappeared. Even when the cause of the hives cannot be discovered, the bumps usually go away in several weeks at most.

The best treatment for hives is an antihistamine, and there are many different choices. Diphenhydramine (Benadryl), which is over the counter, or hydroxyzine (Atarax) are good choices at night, because they will help you to sleep, even if you are still itchy. Antihistamines are better at preventing new hives than at getting rid of those already on your skin. So don't wait to get the hives before you take the medicine—be sure to take it regularly.

If the antihistamine that your health care provider has given you does not greatly improve your hives within 3 days, or if you find in 3 weeks that you still get hives when you stop taking the medicine, you should follow up with your regular health care provider. Sometimes different types of antihistamines work in different patients, and trying other medications may be beneficial.

Adult Seborrheic Dermatitis (Seborrhea, Inflammatory Dandruff)

You have a very common skin condition called seborrheic dermatitis. Seborrheic dermatitis occurs when skin in the scalp, and sometimes on the face and ears, grows more quickly than usual. As new skin cells multiply, old skin forms scale that builds up in the scalp. This buildup of scale can be irritating and can also cause redness. Usually, seborrheic dermatitis is worst at the edges of the scalp and in and behind the ears. Sometimes, the eyebrows and creases at the sides of the nose can show redness and scale too. Occasionally, seborrheic dermatitis can even affect the chest and back.

Seborrheic dermatitis is not dangerous. Some doctors believe that it may be related to a yeast infection, while other doctors believe it is simple irritation from buildup of scale. All doctors believe that you cannot pass this to another person.

Although there is no cure for seborrheic dermatitis, there are medications that control the redness and scaling. First, the scale should be removed from your scalp. The best way to do this is with vigorous shampooing with a shampoo that helps dissolve scale or slow down the growth of new scale. Examples include T-Gel, T-Sal, Ionil T Plus, and Zincon shampoos (all available without a prescription) or Selsun shampoo (available only with a prescription). The shampoo should be *scrubbed* into your scalp with your fingernails, and then left on for 5 minutes. Then, scale should be scrubbed off your scalp and the shampoo rinsed off. You can then apply a conditioner if you wish. You should do this daily or every other day until your seborrheic dermatitis is controlled, and then once or twice a week as needed to keep your skin clear. If you are black, shampooing this often will dry your hair and make it likely to break off. Therefore, wash your hair twice a week, following the above instructions, until your skin is under control, and then weekly or as seldom as you can and still stay clear. Although moisturizing your hair helps protect it, try to avoid getting moisturizers on the skin of your scalp, because they can worsen seborrheic dermatitis.

(continues)

A cortisone lotion (betamethasone valerate is a very common type) will also help clear your skin more quickly. This medication should be applied to the skin of your scalp (not your hair, and not your face or ears) once or twice daily, as needed to control your skin. A milder cortisone cream (hydrocortisone 1%, which is available without prescription, or hydrocortisone 2.5%, which is available by prescription) can be applied to the face and ears twice a day as needed.

Although these treatments do not cure seborrheic dermatitis, they usually control the scaling. Seborrheic dermatitis often comes and goes, and stress makes it worse in some people. Use these treatments as needed when the seborrheic dermatitis is a problem.

Alopecia Areata

You have a kind of hair loss called alopecia areata. This occurs because your immune system, that part of your body that normally fights off infections, has become overactive and is fighting off your hair. No one knows why this happens, but it is not an infection so you did not catch it from anyone, and you cannot pass it on to others.

Usually, alopecia areata only causes one or a few bald patches that come and go. Eventually, the bald patches usually go away permanently. Occasionally, patches can be large, and rarely the whole scalp can lose hair. When this happens, regrowth of the hair is unlikely.

The only effective treatment is cortisone, and improvement is temporary. Some patients improve with cortisone creams (such as triamcinolone), but often cortisone must be injected into the skin of the scalp. Local cortisone injections must be repeated about every 4 to 6 weeks, or the hair will fall out again. Although cortisone taken by mouth is possible, the side effects are usually too dangerous for this treatment to be practical.

There is no other therapy that is useful. Special shampoos and diets are not beneficial. Permanents, straighteners, and coloring can damage fragile hair that remains or regrows, so that the hair loss may be more obvious.

Aphthous Ulcers (Canker Sores)

You have aphthous ulcers, also called aphthae. These sores are common. They are not dangerous, but they can be very painful. These ulcers are not an infection. You did not catch them from anyone and you cannot pass them on. The cause is not known. There is no cure for aphthous ulcers, but some people get these sores only once or twice in their lives. However, other people get several sores every month.

The most reliable treatment for aphthous ulcer is cortisone. Cortisone heals the ulcers, but it does not keep you from getting more ulcers in the future. The safest way to use cortisone is in a gel or salve. This is usually very helpful, especially when used immediately when ulcers begin to appear. For large and very painful ulcers, cortisone pills (prednisone) by mouth are more beneficial. Unfortunately, the dangerous side effects of prednisone, when it is used often or for long periods of time, prevent it from being very useful to people who have frequent bouts of aphthous ulcers.

If you get frequent aphthous ulcers, you should see a dermatologist who can try other types of medication by mouth to help prevent new ulcers from coming.

Atopic Dermatitis, Eczema, and Neurodermatitis

You have a skin problem called eczema. Atopic dermatitis, eczema, neurodermatitis, and dermatitis are different names for the same disease. Eczema is an itchy, scaly skin rash that occurs in people like you who have sensitive skin. Normal mild irritations of daily living, such as soap, water, stress, rubbing from clothes, and sweat, cause irritation in sensitive skin. Although some people feel irritation as soreness, people with eczema usually feel irritation as an itch. Scratching feels really good to most people with eczema, but scratching irritates the skin even more. The itching causes the scratching, and the scratching worsens the itching.

There is no cure for eczema. However, cortisone creams put on the skin to decrease itching and irritation, and very careful skin care to minimize irritation, usually control the problem.

Eczema is usually not an allergic reaction to a particular thing, but instead a reaction to irritation. If your doctor thinks you're allergic to something that is touching your skin, she or he will talk to you about it, and if you feel that there is an allergy to a particular substance, let your doctor know.

The treatment of eczema includes:

1. *Avoid irritation to your skin:* Washing the skin is the most common and harshest irritation for skin. Washing dissolves the natural oils in the skin and allows tiny, invisible cracks and breaks that itch. Therefore, bathing (either shower or bath) should be limited to three times a week, avoiding hot water and harsh soaps. Dove soap is the least expensive mild soap. Also, a moisturizer should be applied immediately after bathing to help replace those natural oils that were washed away.

Rough fabric, new, stiff fabrics, and wool should be avoided. Overheating can worsen itching, and sweat can be very irritating, so patients with eczema should stay as cool as comfortable. This is especially important for children who are too small to tell their parents that they are hot.

(continues)

It is especially difficult to protect the hands and feet from irritation, since shoes tend to trap heat and sweat against the skin, and hands handle all kinds of rough and irritating chemicals and objects. Overwashing of the hands is especially common.

2. *Use a cortisone ointment or cream:* This medication helps soothe irritation and inflammation and also helps stop the itching. Although cortisones are extremely useful in the treatment of eczema, simply applying the cortisone without attention to moisturizing the skin and avoiding excessive washing and irritation often do not improve eczema very much. Cortisones are applied very sparingly—more does *not* work better than less—and they are applied only to the areas of scaling, redness, or itching. The cortisone should be used until the skin feels normal to the touch, and then often it can be discontinued.

3. *Keep your skin moisturized:* This is important because flaking and cracking of the skin are very irritating and worsen itching. Covering the cracks with a moisturizer soothes the skin and decreases itching. Also, when moisturizers are applied over the cortisone, they help push the cortisone into the skin and make it work much better.

The best moisturizers are those that are very stiff and that do not pour. The greasier the moisturizer, the better it works. Moisturizers should be applied both immediately after the cortisone and as often as necessary, to keep the skin from feeling and looking dry. People with severe eczema may need five or six applications a day until their skin improves. Moisturizers that pour from a bottle have been mixed with alcohols (which are irritating) and water. Good moisturizers to try are plain Vaseline petroleum jelly, Eucerin *cream* (not lotion), Aquaphor, and even vegetable shortening like Crisco from the grocery store. Moisturizers are available over the counter. Vaseline and vegetable shortening are the least expensive.

4. *Take medication at night:* Medication at night to make you sleep without scratching is important. As long as the skin is being scratched, it will not heal. You can take an antihistamine such as diphenhydramine (Benadryl) that is available over the counter. The usual dose is one to three 25-mg capsules. Or, your health

(continues)

care provider may have given you a prescription for a different medication.

5. *Take an antibiotic:* When your skin gets infected from scratching, you should take an antibiotic. Signs of infection are weeping and crusting of the skin.

Treatment of your eczema will be a lot of work. It is important to follow these instructions carefully until the eczema is much better. You should see your regular health care provider in a week if you are receiving prednisone, or in a month if you are doing well and using creams only. Your health care provider will decide when to decrease the frequency of cortisone use, moisturizing, and nighttime medication. However, even after your eczema is controlled, your skin may worsen from stress and new irritations. If you understand how to treat your skin, and you have the medications at home ready to use, you will be able to treat your skin quickly.

Atypical Moles (Dysplastic Nevi)

You have moles that are abnormal in appearance. These moles are a sign that you may have an increased risk of malignant melanoma, a very dangerous type of skin cancer.

Normal moles are smaller than a pencil eraser in diameter, and they have distinct and regular borders. Also, in normal moles the color is evenly brown. Moles that are unusually large and that have irregular borders and uneven color are abnormal, even though they may not be cancerous. People who have large numbers of very irregular moles have a greater risk of melanoma skin cancer, and people who have family members with either atypical moles or melanoma are at even greater risk.

Fortunately, people with atypical moles know that they have an increased risk of melanoma, so they can be followed carefully by a dermatologist. Melanomas can usually be diagnosed early, when they can be easily removed in the doctor's office, before there is a chance for spread to other parts of the body. You need to see a dermatologist, and you should have your immediate family examined also, since the tendency for melanoma is sometimes inherited. Not only do family members need to be aware of their own risk, but your own risk also depends partly on whether atypical moles are of the inherited variety.

The usual treatment of atypical moles is careful examination, with the frequency depending on many factors, including the appearance and number of your moles and whether atypical moles are found in other family members. Sometimes, moles are photographed, so that changes can be identified early. Any moles that change or that look especially abnormal will probably need to be removed. However, it is not practical to remove every mole, since more will appear and removal of moles does not remove your risk of melanoma.

Chronic Urticaria

You have urticaria, which is sometimes called hives. This itchy rash is an allergic reaction. Often, it is an allergy to a medication, to an infection, or even to an insect bite or sting. But, when a person has had hives for more than a month, the cause is usually never discovered. The best way to find the cause is good detective work on your part and by your health care provider. A careful physical examination is also important. Blood and urine tests are not very helpful in finding the cause of urticaria when it has been present for more than 1 month.

Hives cannot be cured when the cause is not known. Still, the hives can be controlled in most people with medication that treats allergic reactions. The best treatment for hives is an antihistamine, and there are many different choices. Diphenhydramine (Benadryl), which is available over the counter, or hydroxyzine (Atarax) are good choices at night, because they will help you to sleep, even if you are still itchy. Antihistamines are better at preventing new hives than at getting rid of those already on your skin. So, don't wait to get the hives before you take the medicine—be sure to take it regularly.

If the antihistamine that your health care provider has given you does not greatly improve your hives within 3 days, or if you find in 3 weeks that you still get hives when you stop taking the medicine, you should follow up with your regular health care provider. Sometimes different types of antihistamines work in different patients, and trying other medications may be beneficial.

People who have hives for more than a month usually continue to get them, at least off and on, for a long time. By the end of 1 year, about one-half of people will no longer have hives, and most other people gradually have fewer and fewer problems with this as the years go by.

Contact Dermatitis

You have contact dermatitis—irritation of the skin because of something that has touched it. Sometimes this is an allergy to something like nickel in jewelry or leather in a watchband. At other times this rash is caused by irritation of the skin, but it is not an allergy to anything. Chapping from overwashing is a common cause of this kind of contact dermatitis.

If you or your doctor know what touched your skin to cause the dermatitis, you should try to avoid it in the future. If you do not know what caused your rash, you should see a dermatologist for an examination or tests to try to find the cause.

Otherwise, you should use the cortisone cream or ointment your doctor has given you, twice a day, on the dermatitis. Cover it with a moisturizer such as Vaseline petroleum jelly or Eucerin *cream* (not lotion). If you are itchy at night, you may have been given medicine to help you sleep, or you can take one to three tablets of diphenhydramine (Benadryl), which is available over the counter.

Cutaneous Lupus Erythematosus

You have, or may have, lupus erythematosus of the skin. This is a skin problem in which your body's immune system, the part of your body that fights off infections, mistakenly attacks your own skin. Often, lupus erythematosus only causes skin disease. However, lupus erythematosus sometimes causes other complications such as joint aches and kidney problems. This disease must be discovered by a careful history and physical examination, as well as laboratory tests on urine and blood.

Lupus erythematosus of the skin is not a curable problem, but there are medications that usually control the spots. Cortisone creams can help but usually do not make the areas completely disappear. Your regular health care provider or dermatologist can give you medication by mouth (usually hydroxychloroquine) that is especially good for lupus erythematosus of the skin.

Diaper Rash

Your baby has a diaper rash. This is caused by irritation from urine and stool held against the skin. Sometimes, a yeast infection worsens a rash, because yeast grows well in warm, damp areas.

Usually, a diaper rash is easy to clear up when treatment is begun early. Most important, your baby's diapers should be changed frequently. Even though new disposable diapers do not feel very wet after your baby has urinated, they should still be changed quickly. Check you baby every hour during the day for wetness, and more often if she or he has diarrhea. If the rash is very red and weeping, leave the diapers off as much as possible, until the area begins to heal.

Second, when irritation first appears, apply hydrocortisone 1% cream or ointment twice daily, and pay even more attention to changing the diapers. If the area becomes very red, and if the creases of the skin are also red, apply a medicine for yeast infection. You may have been given a prescription for yeast medicine, or you can buy it without a prescription at your pharmacy as clotrimazole or miconazole cream, sold to women for a vaginal yeast infection. If the skin becomes very inflamed, your baby will need prescription medication.

If your baby has a very bad rash, or if your baby has diarrhea, you should apply a thick layer of either zinc oxide paste or Desitin cream (both are available without a prescription at your pharmacy) over the medicated creams and after each diaper change, to protect the skin from stool and urine. Be sure that other caretakers and babysitters have a supply of medication and understand the importance of proper care.

A diaper rash is usually very easy to treat if you begin treatment as soon as redness first occurs, and if you change the baby's diapers as soon as they become soiled.

Dissecting Cellulitis of the Scalp

You have a skin condition called dissecting cellulitis of the scalp, which causes boils to appear in the scalp. Although red boils often drain pus, this problem is not caused by an infection. Instead, dissecting cellulitis of the scalp is a type of acne that occurs in these areas. This is not caused by dirt or lack of bathing. Sometimes this problem runs in families.

Although this problem is not curable, it is usually improved with treatment. Even though dissecting cellulitis of the scalp is not an infection, antibiotics taken by mouth are sometimes the best treatment. The antibiotics most likely to be effective are those that not only kill irritating germs on the skin, but that also help inflammation by other means. However, this method (and all safe methods) of decreasing inflammation is slow, and antibiotics normally take 1 to 2 months to improve dissecting cellulitis of the scalp. If antibiotics by mouth do not improve your problem, your health care provider may recommend other medications or injections into the areas, to improve the skin.

Dyshidrosis (Pomphylox, Hand or Foot Dermatitis)

Dyshidrosis refers to small blisters that occur over the hands or feet, or both, because of swelling in the skin. Sometimes blisters over the thick skin of the hands and feet appear as brown dots, rather than as blisters. Most often, these are very itchy. This condition most often, but not always, affects people with a tendency toward allergies, including medication allergies, hay fever, asthma, or hives. Often people rub this itchy rash, and the skin becomes inflamed, scaling, crusted, and sometimes weeping and painful.

The tendency toward sensitive, easily inflamed skin is incurable. However, it is very treatable, and most people do well as long as they use soothing cortisone creams as needed and take care not to irritate their skin.

Although no one knows what causes dyshidrosis to show up at a particular time in a patient's life, anything that irritates the skin is known to make this problem worse. Therefore, be very careful with your skin. One of the most common irritating activities is handwashing. Soap and water remove natural oils from the skin and cause irritation that worsens or triggers dyshidrosis. You should stop to consider whether handwashing is important each time you go to wash your hands, because sometimes people wash simply from habit. Harsh chemicals used for housecleaning or hair care also can worsen dyshidrosis.

Your doctor has given you a cortisone cream or ointment. This should be used regularly but sparingly twice daily and covered with a heavy, healing cream moisturizer to help seal irritating, tiny cracks in the skin. Common creams are Eucerin *cream* (not lotion), Aquaphor, or Vaseline petroleum jelly. When your skin has improved, you can switch to a cosmetically nicer, thinner lotion. You should follow up with your personal doctor or, if you are not doing well, a dermatologist in about a month, to evaluate your skin for both response to therapy and side effects. Often, a less potent cortisone can be substituted. If you have severe dyshidrosis and were given cortisone by mouth or injection, you will probably be asked to come for a follow-up visit much sooner.

Epidermal Cysts

You have an epidermal cyst (sebaceous cyst), a very common benign tumor caused by a hair pore or follicle that is blocked. This causes the hair follicle to become filled with dead surface scale and oils, making a large bump, or knot.

An epidermal cyst is not dangerous. A cyst needs no treatment unless you want it to be surgically removed for cosmetic or personal reasons. Occasionally, if the cyst is squeezed or bumped, it can leak its dead surface scale and oils into surrounding skin. This can cause irritation, redness, and pain. Because healing is more difficult, and the scar will be larger if the cyst is removed while it is irritated, removal should be delayed until inflammation has resolved. Sometimes your doctor can inject cortisone into an inflamed cyst with a needle, or lance it to let out pus, and hasten healing of the inflammation.

Female-Pattern Alopecia (Androgenic Alopecia)

You have a type of thinning hair that is inherited from your parents and grandparents. Although this is usually much less obvious when it occurs in women as compared to inherited hair loss in men, it can still be unattractive.

The only usual therapy is a medication called minoxidil applied to the scalp twice a day. Minoxidil helps to regrow hair in more than one-half of women, but it must be used continually, or hair loss will recur.

Fever Blisters (Herpes Simplex Virus Infection of the Lip)

The herpes simplex virus produces blisters, scabs, or sores on the skin. Infection is most common on the lip, where it is called a fever blister. Most adults have been exposed to this virus, which is spread by skin-to-skin contact. A fever blister begins as small blisters; then the blisters break, leaving sores or scabs.

After the skin heals, the herpesvirus does not disappear but moves to the base of the nerve under the skin. The herpesvirus can then become active again and cause blisters or sores to recur occasionally. This can happen as seldom as every year or two, or as often as once a month. Outbreaks become less and less frequent as years go by.

An HSV infection is painful and annoying, but it is not dangerous. However, it can be passed from one person to another. You should not kiss another person or share drinking glasses or eating utensils when your lip is affected.

If given very early, medications such as acyclovir, famciclovir, and valacyclovir decrease the duration and severity of a fever blister. Also, if you have very frequent fever blisters, these medications, taken daily, can prevent outbreaks. Other ways to prevent outbreaks include protecting your lips from sun, as sunlight can cause outbreaks. You should wear a lip balm with sunscreen when you are going to be in the sun. Be ready for outbreaks when you get colds or flu, or if you are under emotional stress.

Follicular Degeneration Syndrome

You have a common type of scarring of the scalp that causes hair loss called the follicular degeneration syndrome. This occurs almost always in black people, and most often in black women. Although the cause is not known, this type of hair loss seems related to acne, where inflammation causes bumps and scarring. It does not seem to be caused by an infection. You did not catch this from anyone, and you cannot give it to anyone else. Also, antibiotics will not cure it. This never turns into cancer or any other important medical problem, but it can cause severe and unsightly scarring.

There is no cure for the follicular degeneration syndrome, but medication used every day can help stop further hair loss and scarring. Antibiotics such as those used for acne can decrease inflammation, even when it is not caused by an infection. Also, a cortisone solution helps soothe the skin.

These medications take 1 to 2 months to help, and they must be used continually, since they only control—but do not cure—the follicular degeneration syndrome.

Genital Herpes Simplex Virus Infection

You have been told that you have a herpes infection. This diagnosis makes some people frightened or embarrassed, partly because of information they have heard or read. You should know that almost all adults have been exposed to this virus, which is spread by skin-to-skin contact.

A herpes infection is painful and annoying, but it is not dangerous. The herpes simplex virus (HSV) produces blisters, scabs, or sores on the skin. Sometimes this infection occurs on the lips, where it causes a fever blister. At other times it occurs in the genital area.

A herpes infection begins as small blisters. However, over thin, moist skin, such as the entrance to the vagina or on the head of the penis, the blisters may break quickly and form sores, and you may never even see the blisters. Over drier skin, the blisters break to form scabs.

After the skin heals, the herpesvirus does not disappear, but moves to the base of the nerve under the skin. Then, the herpesvirus can become active again and cause blisters or sores to recur occasionally. This can happen as seldom as every year or two, or as often as once a month. Most people experience a herpes outbreak three or four times a year, and outbreaks become less and less frequent as years go by.

Herpes can be passed from one person to another. You should avoid sexual contact when you have any sores, blisters, or crusts. Herpes infections are most often passed to another person when the skin is actively sore or blistered. However, some people shed herpesvirus even when there are no symptoms of herpes infection. The likelihood of spreading herpes infection during this shedding when the skin looks and feels normal is unknown, but it is probably small. A condom decreases the chance of spread of herpes. A patient with genital herpes has a responsibility to tell sexual partners about this infection.

There are several aspects to the treatment of herpes infection.

1. Medications taken by mouth (acyclovir, famciclovir, or valacyclovir) speed healing when given within the first 2 or 3 days of an

(continues)

outbreak. These can sometimes make an outbreak very mild if given at the first sign of tingling, burning, or itching, even before skin sores are visible. Medications applied to the skin have not been shown to be useful in scientific studies, although some people strongly believe that ether, Blistex, or other treatments are helpful to them. If you have frequent outbreaks, you may want to ask your health care provider to consider giving you a prescription for acyclovir, 400-mg tablets, twice a day. This medicine stops outbreaks and decreases shedding of the herpesvirus between outbreaks in women with genital herpes. These medications have no significant side effects.

2. The skin should be treated gently when it is sore from a herpes infection. You should not scrub it or use disinfectants. Rinsing the area with clear water daily, and the application of Vaseline petroleum jelly to crusted areas to prevent cracking is usually sufficient care. If you are having a painful outbreak, your doctor has probably given you an oral medication for pain. You should not need this pain medication for more than a few days.

Women with genital HSV infection should inform their gynecologists, because this virus can be transmitted to a baby during delivery. If the doctor is aware of the mother's history, steps can be taken to ensure the baby's safety.

Many people do not know when or from whom they caught herpes because the time from exposure to an outbreak can be days or sometimes years. It is also very difficult to trace the source of a viral infection, because some viruses can be inactive for months or even years after exposure. If you have genital herpes, you should not automatically assume that your sexual partner has been unfaithful. Although this is certainly possible, he or she may have had herpes for years and not been aware of it. Or your sexual partner may have caught it from you.

Finally, if you have questions or find yourself very upset about your diagnosis, you should consider joining a support group. For many people, herpes is an annoying, trivial condition. Other people are much more upset and depressed. There are many people with

(continues)

herpes. With the available medications and good emotional support, herpes should not be a major life trauma.

For more information, call:
National Herpes Hotline (919) 361-8488 9 AM–7 PM Eastern time
To order publications about herpes, call:
American Social Health Association Resource Center
(800) 230-6039 9 AM–7 PM Eastern time

Genital Warts

You have been told that you have genital warts (venereal warts). These warts are caused by a viral infection. This infection is usually transmitted through sexual intercourse, but some people, especially small children, may catch the infection in other ways. Because the wart bumps can take months or years to appear after a person is exposed to the virus, sometimes it can be very difficult to discover where you caught this infection.

Usually, these warts are not important medically, although sometimes they may itch or feel irritated. However, genital warts can grow inside the vagina and on the cervix, the opening to the uterus or womb. When this happens, a Papanicolaou (Pap) smear can show an abnormality, and sometimes the wart can lead to cancer of the cervix. For this reason, you (if you are a woman) or your female sexual partner should see a gynecologist now, and regularly, for a Pap smear. Any changes your doctor finds on the Pap smear will allow early treatment, to prevent the development of cancer.

There are several ways to treat genital warts. A common treatment is podofilox, a medicine you apply at home twice a day for 3 consecutive days each week. Or, medications can be applied every week or two in your doctor's office. The warts can be frozen to produce blisters by using a very cold liquid (liquid nitrogen) in the doctor's office, or warts can be burned off with an electric needle or a laser. No therapy will remove these warts permanently with a single treatment. The wart virus can continue to live silently in the skin even after the wart bumps disappear. This causes no harm, but it explains how warts can recur either soon after treatment or, sometimes, many years later, even if you have not been re-exposed.

For more information, you can call:
STD Hotline
(800)-227-8922 (Monday to Friday, 8 AM to 11 PM Eastern time)

Or, to order printed material, call:
American Social Health Association HealthLine
(800)-972-8500 anytime

Herpes Zoster Infection (Shingles)

Herpes zoster infection, also called shingles, is caused by the chickenpox virus. When a person has chickenpox, he or she is never completely cured of the virus. The virus lives at the base of nerves under the skin, and the body's immune system usually keeps the infection confined there. However, sometimes the virus becomes active again, and produces blisters.

Pain is usually the first sign of shingles, followed by blisters most often located over one side of the chest and back, or on one side of the face or neck. However, shingles can occur almost anywhere on the body.

The blisters of shingles usually heal in about 3 weeks. Several medications can hasten healing slightly if given within the first 2 to 3 days. These medications are acyclovir (Zovirax), famciclovir (Famvir), and valacyclovir (Valtrex).

Occasionally, the pain of shingles lasts after the skin has healed. This is called *postherpetic neuralgia.* People over about 60 years of age are at greatest risk of this. Postherpetic neuralgia can be treated with oral medications for pain, a cream called Zostrix, and tricyclic antidepressants such as amitriptyline (Elavil). These tricyclic antidepressants are not used for their antidepressant actions, but rather for their beneficial effects on healing inflamed nerves. Postherpetic neuralgia usually disappears within 6 months.

Hidradenitis Suppurativa

You have a skin condition called hidradenitis suppurativa, which causes boils to appear in either the armpits or the genital area, or both. Although red boils often drain pus, this problem is not caused by an infection. Instead, hidradenitis suppurative is a type of acne that occurs in these areas. This is not caused by dirt or lack of bathing. Sometimes this problem runs in families.

Although this problem is not curable, it can be improved with treatment. Even though hidradenitis suppurativa is not an infection, antibiotics taken by mouth are sometimes the best treatment. The antibiotics most likely to be effective are those that not only kill irritating germs on the skin, but that also help inflammation by other means. However, this method (and all safe methods) of decreasing inflammation is slow, and antibiotics normally take 1 to 2 months to improve hidradenitis suppurativa. If antibiotics taken by mouth do not improve your problem, your health care provider may recommend birth control pills with high doses of estrogen (if you are a woman), or surgery to remove the affected skin.

Insect Bites

Insect bites can cause red bumps in people who are allergic to them, but they cause no visible skin changes in people who are not allergic. Therefore, only one or two people in a family usually get red bumps from insect bites, even though everyone may have been bitten. Children are especially likely to react to insect bites. Although red bumps are the most common sign of insect bites, people who are very allergic and people with tender skin, such as children, may develop blisters over the bites as well.

Most often, insect bites are itchy. The most common insects to cause bites are fleas and mosquitos. Flea bites are usually painless, so people are often unaware of being bitten. Mosquito bites are often noticed by adults but are sometimes overlooked by busy children until the bumps and itching appear. Horseflies and deerflies can cause insect bites, but the bite is painful, so most people notice and remember being bitten.

The treatment of insect bites includes avoidance of the insects in the future. Defleaing an animal rids the animal of the fleas, but then fleas may be more likely to bite people. Be sure to deflea the house and yard as well. Susceptible people should wear an insect repellant such as Off, Cutter, or 6–12 until the fleas are gone. People sensitive to mosquito bites should avoid being outdoors in the evening, when mosquitos are most active. Insect repellents can be useful for the prevention of the bites as well. Removal of obvious breeding areas of standing water can be helpful.

Insect bites, especially flea bites, can sometimes be very long lasting, with bumps persisting for several weeks. This is especially common when the spots are being scratched. Also, bites can become infected when scratched often, especially in children. You may have been given a cortisone cream to put on the bumps to help stop the itching, or an antibiotic if your bites look infected. If you have problems sleeping at night because of itching, you can take diphenhydramine (Benadryl), an over-the-counter medication. Adults may need 50 or 75 mg, and children may need two or three times the child's dose printed on the bottle.

Often, brown spots remain after the bumps heal. This is just a temporary color change, and scarring generally does not occur except when bites become infected.

Lichen Planus

You have a skin disease called lichen planus. Although the cause is not known for sure, many doctors believe that this is an autoimmune disease. In this disease, your body's immune system, the part of your body that fights off infections, mistakenly attacks your own skin. Lichen planus is not an infection, so you cannot give it to other people. It is not caused by foods or an allergy to something that touches the skin. Sometimes, certain medications can cause skin spots that look like lichen planus.

When lichen planus shows up as red spots on the skin, it usually goes away on its own within about 3 years. When it shows up in the mouth as sore areas, lichen planus usually does not go away. However, there are medicines that can help keep lichen planus under control.

The most common medicine used for lichen planus is cortisone cream or gel. This is applied to the skin twice a day, or to the inside of the mouth 4 times a day. Often, holding a damp cotton ball on the lichen planus for a few minutes after the cortisone is applied can make it work better.

You should see your regular health care provider in about 1 month. You should call for an earlier appointment if your skin is getting worse on the treatment you have been given.

Male-Pattern Alopecia (Androgenic Alopecia)

You have male-pattern alopecia, or baldness, the most common type of hair loss. You inherited this tendency from your parents, and male hormone then allows hair loss to occur. Although women inherit the same tendency for hair loss, androgenic alopecia occurs less often and less severely because they have less male hormone.

There are several treatments for male-pattern alopecia. Minoxidil, a medicine that was originally taken by mouth for high blood pressure, can induce regrowth in some people. If the scalp has been bald long enough that the skin is shiny, regrowth is unlikely. In people who have some hair remaining, or even have very fine "fuzz," about one-third regrow hair, one third do not have worsening of hair loss, and one third continue to lose hair. About 6 months is required to tell if the medication is working, and sometimes the effect can be subtle. Unfortunately, the medication must be used continuously, or hair that would have been lost will fall out when medication is stopped. Hair transplants are expensive, but permanent. A piece of hairless scalp skin can be surgically removed, so that the skin that has hair is stitched together. Finally, there are a number of different artificial hair alternatives.

Pityriasis Rosea

You have a common rash called pityriasis rosea. Although the cause of this rash is not known, many doctors believe that it is a mild virus infection. Pityriasis rosea does not make people feel sick.

There is no treatment that makes the rash go away, but pityriasis rosea goes away on its own. The rash is always gone within 3 months, and usually sooner. Sunlight exposure can make the rash better, and itchy people can get some relief from itching with a cortisone cream and moisturizers. If you are very itchy, you should take diphenhydramine (Benadryl) 25-mg capsules (available without a prescription) at bedtime. You can take from one to three capsules to help you sleep.

Sometimes, temporary brown spots remain after the rash has gone. This color change will go away completely, but it may take several months.

Pityriasis "Tinea" Versicolor

You have a common fungus infection of the skin, called pityriasis versicolor. This minor infection usually appears as brown, pink, or even light patches over the chest and back. Often, the infection is only seen in summer, and it seems to go away each winter. Some people have itching with this skin problem, but most people have no symptoms.

This rash can be treated in several ways. You may have been given a medication to apply to the area, or you may have been given pills. Both types of treatment are very effective. However, the color change in your skin may take several weeks to improve. Also, because some people seem especially susceptible to this fungus infection, you may wish to treat your skin once every 2 months to avoid catching it again. In the future, if you see pityriasis versicolor returning, it can be treated with clotrimazole cream, a medication available over the counter.

Poison Ivy and Poison Oak

Rashes caused by poison ivy and poison oak occur because of an allergy to those or similar plants. Although no one gets a rash after the first exposure to poison ivy or poison oak, most people eventually develop an allergy to these plants if they are exposed often enough. You may be unaware of where and when you were exposed to poison ivy or poison oak. You may not have recognized the plant, or the plant oils may have been transferred to you from the fur of a dog, or from the bottom of shoes.

The rash breaks out 1 to 4 days after exposure. The first rash is itchy red bumps, which then turn into small water blisters. Although scratching the rash makes it worse simply because of irritation, blister fluid that touches other skin will not cause the rash to spread there. However, until you take a warm soapy bath or shower, any remaining oil can spread from one area to another and cause new blisters.

The treatment of poison ivy and poison oak requires attention to several different factors. First, you should try to discover where and how you were exposed to the plant, so that you can avoid it in the future. Second, if you have not had a warm soapy shower, do it. Third, be sure your clothes have been washed and that shoes that have been touched by poison ivy or oak are cleaned, top and bottom, and not lying on clothes.

Your doctor has probably given you cortisone, in either a cream or ointment form, if your rash is mild, or by pill or injection if your rash is more severe. Use your cortisone as directed, since discontinuing it too soon allows the rash to worsen. If your rash is very severe, you may be given cortisone to take orally (prednisone) or an injection to improve the skin initially, and an ointment or cream as a safe way to prevent worsening of the rash after initial improvement. Use the cream or ointment until your skin feels normal to the touch. The cortisone should be used regularly but sparingly twice daily and covered with a heavy, healing cream moisturizer to help seal irritating, tiny cracks in the skin. Common creams are Eucerin *cream* (not lotion), Aquaphor, or Vaseline petroleum jelly. When your skin has improved, you can switch to a cosmetically nicer, thinner lotion.

Prednisone (Cortisone Pills)

You have been given cortisone (prednisone, prednisilone) to take by mouth. This medication is useful for inflammation of almost any cause. It is often given for skin disease when the skin is blistered or weeping, or if skin disease is especially severe. Usually, the prednisone pills are given for 5 to 14 days to get the skin started healing, and then cortisone creams are prescribed to finish the healing. Cortisone creams are more trouble, but medication applied to the skin is safer than pills taken by mouth.

Prednisone given for 2 weeks or less usually does not cause important medical complications. Generally, the only side effect during the first few days can be mood changes. Although most people feel especially content and energetic, some people can become depressed, and occasionally people (especially older patients) can become confused and disoriented. If this happens to you, stop your medication and let your doctor know.

Other side effects that can occur during the first few days include increased appetite and swelling of the feet and legs. After several days, the immune system is less effective in fighting infections. If you develop symptoms of an infection, such as fever or cough, or red, painful swelling of the skin, you should call your doctor.

Be sure that your doctor knows if you have high blood pressure, diabetes, problems with your immune system, or any known infections. Prednisone sometimes can complicate these problems, so that you may need to be followed with laboratory tests or frequent office follow-up visits.

Side effects of cortisone taken by mouth for months include softening and weakening of the bones, weight gain, loss of muscle, thinning and bruising of the skin, stretch marks, hair loss, and an increased risk of infection.

The body normally makes small amounts of cortisone that are necessary for good health, but when you take cortisone by mouth for long periods, the body "forgets" how to make cortisone. Therefore, if you have been taking cortisone for 3 weeks or longer, you will be instructed how to gradually reduce your dose instead of suddenly stopping the medicine, so that your body can slowly regain its ability to make this chemical.

Any time you have problems or questions about your prednisone, ask your doctor.

Psoriasis

You have psoriasis, a common skin problem that can occur at any age. The cause of psoriasis is not known, but it sometimes runs in families. Psoriasis is not an infection and no one can catch it from you. Usually, psoriasis only affects the skin, but sometimes people with psoriasis have arthritis as well.

Psoriasis usually causes patches of red, scaling skin. Psoriasis is most likely to affect the scalp, elbows, and knees, but it can occur anywhere on the skin surface. Some people only have one or two patches, whereas other people may have many areas of psoriasis.

There is no cure for psoriasis, but many treatments can be helpful. The main treatments for psoriasis are as follows:

1. *Medications that are applied to the skin:* These are the safest and least expensive treatments, but they usually only work for mild cases of psoriasis. These medications include cortisone creams and ointments, coal tar products, a vitamin D medicine (Dovonex), and anthralin, a very strong medicine that helps very thick plaques of psoriasis. Shampoos with tar or salicylic acid (T-Sal, T-Gel, Ionil T Plus) can help psoriasis of the scalp.

2. *Ultraviolet light treatments:* Sunlight usually helps to clear psoriasis. When the weather permits, you should lie out in the sun—taking care not to burn. Wear a strong sunscreen, with a sun protection factor (SPF) number of at least 15 on areas not affected by psoriasis. Artificial sunlight (similar to but not the same as a tanning booth) is available at many dermatologists' offices. Either ultraviolet light alone or in combination with medication clears most people of their psoriasis. Side effects include the risk of sunburn and, after years, an increased risk of skin cancers and wrinkling. This type of treatment is otherwise very safe and effective, but it is also expensive and time consuming, because treatments must be continued from one to three times every week.

3. *Medications taken by mouth:* There are several medications that can be taken by mouth for psoriasis, but these are generally used only if creams and ultraviolet light do not work or cause side

(continues)

effects for that patient. The most often used oral medication is methotrexate, a drug generally used for cancer. Methotrexate works very well for psoriasis, but it can cause liver damage and decrease the body's ability to make blood cells. Etretinate (Tegison) is a medication similar to vitamin A that improves psoriasis. It causes bone and muscle aches in some people, and dry skin in everyone. It also causes birth defects if you should get pregnant. These medicines are usually only given to patients by dermatologists because they require frequent blood tests to avoid side effects.

Otherwise, using a good moisturizer, such as plain Vaseline or Eucerin cream can make psoriasis look and feel better. If you are very itchy, one to three capsules of diphenhydramine (Benadryl) 25 mg, available over the counter, can help you sleep at night.

Some things can make your psoriasis worse. These include sunburn, infections, stress, and some medications. Because so many people have psoriasis, a national foundation has been formed that publishes a regular newsletter and provides information on local support groups.

To join this foundation or obtain further information, call or write:

National Psoriasis Foundation
6600 SW 92nd Ave, Suite 300
Portland, OR 97223-7195

(503) 244-7404

Rosacea

You have a skin disease called rosacea. Sometimes this problem is called "adult acne" because the bumps and pimples can resemble acne, and the treatment is similar. No one knows the cause of rosacea, but it is not an infection, and it is not caused by dirt. Hot and spicy foods and drinks as well as drinking alcohol can make it worse.

Rosacea is not a curable problem, but it usually is easily controlled with medication. The most common medication used is called metronidazole (Metrogel), and it is applied to the skin twice daily. Normally, 1 to 2 months is required for rosacea to go away. You will probably need to continue using your medication, or the bumps will come back.

You should see your regular health care provider in about 2 months for a follow-up visit.

Scabies

You have a condition called scabies, which is a skin infection caused by a very small mite. Although this is not a dangerous infection, it is very itchy, and it can be passed to other people. Fortunately, scabies can be cured, although itching often continues for a week or two after treatment.

You should apply the medicine prescribed for you to all areas of your body from the neck down, taking care even to put the medicine under your fingernails. Everyone who is living in your house should apply the medication to themselves at the same time, because even people who are not itchy can have scabies and not know it. Anyone living in your house who is either too young to walk or too ill to be out of bed should apply the medicine to their scalp and ears as well as to the rest of the body. The medicine should be washed off in the morning. One treatment almost always cures scabies.

However, the scabies mite can live in clothing and bedsheets for about a day. Therefore, clothes, towels, and bedclothes should be washed in hot water at the same time everyone in your home applies their medicine. If this is done, you will not catch scabies from sleeping in a bed that still has some living mites on the sheets.

If your skin is very inflamed, your health care provider may have given you a cortisone cream to apply to your skin to help with itching. This should be applied sparingly to areas of the rash twice a day. If you have problems sleeping because of itching, diphenhydramine (Benadryl), an over-the-counter medicine, can help you sleep at night in doses of 25 to 75 mg (one to three pills).

If your itching is not much better in 2 weeks, and gone in 1 month, you should see a dermatologist or your regular health care provider.

Seborrheic Dermatitis in Babies

Seborrheic dermatitis is a rash that is common in small babies. This red, scaling rash is likely to occur when a baby has cradle cap. Cradle cap is a layer of dead skin and scale that sticks to the scalp.

Treatment for seborrheic dermatitis is to remove the cradle cap, and to apply a mild cortisone cream to the rash. To remove the cradle cap, wet the scalp with baby shampoo or mineral oil for 10 to 15 minutes. After the scale has softened, remove it gently with fingernails or a soft brush. You may need to repeat this several times to completely remove the scale. Then, you will need to keep scale from building up again on the scalp by carefully shampooing the scalp several times a week.

Either hydrocortisone cream 1% (available over the counter) or hydrocortisone cream 2.5% (available by prescription) applied twice a day will heal the rash. Once the rash has disappeared, the medicine can be stopped. The rash does not return as long as the scalp stays clear of scale. Also, babies lose the tendency to develop cradle cap and seborrheic dermatitis after the first few months.

Skin Cancer

You have been told that you have a skin cancer called a basal cell carcinoma or a squamous cell carcinoma. These skin cancers are usually low-grade skin cancers that do not often spread, or metastasize, to other parts of the body, such as the lymph nodes, liver, or lungs. However, they grow until they are removed surgically or by radiation treatments, and they can cause local destruction, especially around the eyes, nose, mouth, or ears. Skin cancers on the lip are especially dangerous because these *can* spread to other parts of the body.

These skin cancers are generally produced by years of exposure to sunlight, including the time you spent outdoors as a child. You may have not gotten much sunlight during the past few years, but your skin never "forgets" sun exposure.

You should see a dermatologist, family doctor, or surgeon in the next few weeks for further evaluation and treatment. If your possible cancer is on your lip, or is a possible cancer from a mole, you need to seek follow-up attention immediately.

Sunburn

Sunburns are not only painful, but they can be dangerous, especially for children. Blistering sunburns before puberty are an important risk factor for malignant melanoma, a deadly form of skin cancer that often strikes even young people. Sunburns can also cause permanent spotting of the skin, and sun exposure of any kind gradually builds up in the skin over a lifetime, causing wrinkling and less dangerous skin cancers.

Because you are a person who can get a bad sunburn, you should protect yourself in the future to prevent sunburns. Fortunately, good sunscreens and clothing are available and will help protect you when used properly. You should use a sunscreen with a sun protection factor (SPF) of at least 15, and many recommend the higher SPF numbers of 45 or 50. The sunscreen should be applied heavily (about 1 ounce, or one-quarter of a usual 4-ounce bottle for your whole body). It should be applied at least 30 minutes before sun exposure. And, it should be reapplied after swimming or sweating heavily. Wearing long sleeves and a hat and avoiding exposure to the sun between 10 AM and 3 PM are other ways to protect yourself.

You should consider protecting yourself year-round on a daily basis, *not* just when you are at risk of a sunburn, such as in summer or on a sunny day. Applying a sunscreen to your face, ears, hands, and arms will help protect you from the long-term damage of skin cancer and wrinkles.

Once you have a sunburn, there is no good treatment. Cortisones taken by mouth or by spray to the skin can be helpful if started very soon after the burn. Cool water and medication, such as aspirin, ibuprofen, naproxen, or ketoprofen (all over the counter), can help alleviate pain. Medication such as over-the-counter diphenhydramine (Benadryl), 1 or 2 tablets at bedtime, may help you sleep.

Syphilis

You have syphilis, an infection passed by sexual contact. The first sign of syphilis is an ulcer that usually appears on the genitals or the mouth. Sometimes, especially in women, the ulcer can be inside where you cannot see it. This ulcer heals on its own, and several weeks later a rash appears. This rash goes away quickly after you are treated, or slowly if you are not treated. Disappearance of the rash does not mean that syphilis is gone. The infection often remains in the body for years doing silent damage that can eventually cause death. Because of this risk, it is very important to keep your appointments for blood tests to make sure that the infection is cured. It is also important to help the Health Department to warn and treat any sexual partners you have had, and to track down any of their other sexual partners.

The treatment for the rash of syphilis is an antibiotic, usually penicillin unless you are allergic to it. The rash goes away very quickly after treatment.

Tinea Capitis (Ringworm of the Scalp)

Your child has a fungus infection of the scalp. Although this is not dangerous, the infection can cause scaling, crusting, itching, and hair loss, and it can spread to other children. Ringworm is very common, and it is not caused by dirt or not bathing enough.

Because the fungus lives deep in the hair pores (follicles), creams and shampoos cannot get to the fungus to kill it, and medication by mouth is needed to cure the infection. Several different medications can be used, but they must be continued until the scalp looks completely normal. This usually takes one to two months.

Sometimes the infection can cause scabbing and pus. Children who have this kind of reaction often need other medications for the first week or two, to stop the inflammation and prevent permanent hair loss. If your child is treated with cortisone (prednisone) taken by mouth, you should follow up with your child's regular health care provider in a week, so that a decision can be about which medications to continue.

Tinea Cruris (Jock Itch) and Tinea Pedis (Athlete's Foot)

Jock itch and athlete's foot are fungus infections that are most common in men. These infections are usually red, scaling patches of skin that can be itchy. Often, people with athlete's foot also have infection in the toenails that makes the nail thicken and come loose.

Usually, these infections can be cleared or greatly improved with a cream or solution applied to the skin. Sometimes, especially when the infection is oozing or there are scabs, medication taken by mouth is necessary. Toenails with fungus infection require medicine taken by mouth over many months to clear.

Some people, such as you, are more susceptible to catching a fungus infection. Since fungus grows in many places and you are often exposed to it, you are likely to catch it again. Wearing shoes that don't breathe, sharing towels with someone who has athlete's foot or jock itch, and taking showers in public places where your wet feet are exposed to other people's fungus makes you especially likely to catch a fungus infection again. Keep your medication handy and use it as soon as you see early signs of skin fungus returning.

Usually, only susceptible people catch fungus infections. So, men do not often spread their fungus infection to women or family members unless they are susceptible too.

Topical Cortisone Creams, Ointments, and Solutions

You have been given a cortisone cream, ointment, or solution for your skin condition. Cortisones (also called corticosteroids or steroids) decrease skin inflammation. This type of steroid is not related to body-building steroids.

Cortisone creams are used for many different skin conditions, including eczema, dermatitis, allergic rashes, psoriasis, seborrhea (dandruff), lichen planus, and many other causes of dry, itchy skin. Sometimes, when used with moisturizers and nighttime medications to control itching, cortisones applied to the skin cure the problem. In other cases, cortisones must be used continuously, because the rash is temporarily cleared or improved, but is not cured, with cortisone cream.

Your cortisone cream should be applied very sparingly, only to the affected area twice daily until either the skin completely clears, or until you see a doctor at a follow-up visit. A moisturizer should be applied over the cortisone cream, except on the face, scalp, armpits, and groin. Good choices of moisturizers are thick creams, such as Eucerin cream (*not* lotion), Aquaphor, or Vaseline petroleum jelly. Thinner lotions have water, and alcohols added to make them easier to spread, but this also makes them less effective if your skin is very dry or scaling.

You should make an appointment with your doctor or dermatologist as directed. Cortisone creams used for prolonged periods without careful follow-up can result in thin skin, stretch marks, and dermatitis. People who are applying cortisone creams over large areas, or applying the cream to very inflamed skin, can absorb the cortisone into their bloodstream and get side effects. This is not a problem for short periods, but you should be re-evaluated within the next month or two if you are using any prescription cortisones continuously to control your skin problem.

Traction Alopecia

You have hair loss called traction alopecia. When hair is pulled into a tight hairstyle and left in place for days or weeks, the hair roots can be damaged. Usually, hair around the edges of the face is most affected. When traction alopecia is mild, the hair in these areas loosens and falls out, but it will grow again when the hair style is changed. If traction alopecia is severe, permanent damage occurs and hair loss is permanent.

To prevent permanent hair loss and allow new hair to grow, a hairstyle that does not pull the hair should be used. For example, loose braids should be substituted for tight braids.

Varicella (Chickenpox)

Chickenpox is a viral infection that causes small bumps and blisters. Very young children sometimes do not feel sick or have fever, but older children and adults often have symptoms of a cold, fever, or cough with the blisters, and they may become very sick.

Chickenpox is spread through the air and is a highly contagious infection. People with chickenpox are most contagious just before and just after the blisters appear. Chickenpox is probably not contagious when new blisters are no longer appearing, but most schools and child care facilities require all blisters to be scabbed over before an infected child is allowed to return.

Medication (acyclovir, Zovirax) can hasten healing of chickenpox if given within the first 24 hours of a rash, but most people do not see a doctor quickly enough to take advantage of this therapy. Often, brothers and sisters or close friends of the child with chickenpox know they have been exposed and can get to a doctor quickly enough to benefit from the medication.

Otherwise, the treatment of chickenpox includes control of itching. Because there is no good anti-itch therapy, soaking in a bathtub with Aveeno, a soothing over-the-counter medication, can be useful, and nighttime medicine to induce sleep makes itching more bearable. Your health care provider may prescribe Benadryl (diphenhydramine) or Atarax (hydroxyzine HCl), in higher doses than generally prescribed, as a good sleeping medication. People with chickenpox can be given up to four times the dose normally recommended to make them sleep. If you or your child cannot get to sleep after using the prescribed or suggested dose of medication, contact your doctor about adjusting the dose or changing the medication.

Sometimes, the blistered skin becomes infected, with red, crusted bumps and pus. Your health care provider may prescribe an antibiotic taken by mouth to heal these areas and reduce scarring.

Adults and children who are in poor general health should be followed especially carefully if they become infected with chickenpox. Occasionally, this can be a dangerous disease and anyone with chickenpox who has a bad cough, shortness of breath, or feels unusually sick should consult a doctor.

(continues)

The chickenpox rash lasts about a week. Once a person has had chickenpox, they never get it again, although they are at a slight risk of an episode of shingles later in life. Shingles is chickenpox localized to one area of the skin. Chickenpox should become much less common as more children receive chickenpox vaccinations.

Vascular Reactions: Erythema Multiforme, Erythema Nodosum, Morbilliform Eruptions

You have a rash caused by an allergic reaction. Often it is an allergy to a medication, to an infection, or even to an insect bite or sting. This is not an allergy to something that has touched your skin; instead, it is something internal. Sometimes the cause of the allergy cannot be found.

This rash usually disappears 1 or 2 weeks after the cause of the allergy has disappeared. Even when the cause of the rash cannot be discovered, the bumps usually go away within several weeks at most.

The best treatment, when possible, is to avoid whatever caused the rash. This is sometimes easy, as in the case of some medications. But, avoidance can be difficult if the cause is not known. If your rash is not itchy or painful, no other treatment is needed and there is no safe and effective treatment. The kind of rash that you have is usually annoying, but it is not dangerous.

If you are itchy, the best treatment for hives is an antihistamine, and there are many different choices. Diphenhydramine (Benadryl), which is available over the counter, or hydroxyzine (Atarax) are good choices at night, because they will help you to sleep, even if you are still itchy.

If your rash starts to blister or if it worsens a lot, you should either call your regular health care provider or return to the emergency department.

Vitiligo

You have a skin condition called vitiligo, with white patches appearing on the skin. These patches are caused by the disappearance of the cells called melanocytes that make the tan color of skin. No one knows the exact cause of vitiligo. Many believe that the body's own immune system, that part of the body that fights infection, becomes overactive and fights the melanocytes.

Vitiligo is not a dangerous disease. Although it is not usually associated with other medical problems, some patients may have thyroid problems, and your doctor may want to check this. The white areas of skin often do not enlarge, but sometimes the areas can continue to grow.

There are several treatments for vitiligo. Most important is protection of the white skin from the sun, since natural skin color and the ability to make a protective tan are now gone. A sunscreen with a sun-protection factor (SPF) of at least 15 should be applied every day to any skin not covered by clothing. Sometimes, especially in children, a cortisone cream will slowly enable normal skin color to return. Other treatments may include a solution applied to the skin, or pills taken by mouth, before exposure to ultraviolet light in a dermatologist's office. Sometimes skin grafting can be beneficial. Otherwise, excellent coverup makeups are available. These include Dermablend and Lydia O'Leary's Covermark. These coverups are available at department stores, and colors are blended to match your natural skin color. These coverups are waterproof and, with expert application, the results are excellent.

Warts

You have a skin virus infection that causes warts. This virus is passed from one person to another by skin-to-skin contact, but most people are not aware of being exposed to the wart virus. The virus is very common and can be transmitted any time there is a break in the skin and the virus is present. Depending on the location of the wart and exactly which wart virus is present, warts can appear differently.

Warts on the hands are most common in children, but they can occur in other places as well, including the knees. A plantar wart is any wart located on the bottom of the foot. Flat warts are small, barely raised warts, most common over the backs of the hands, over the face, and over the lower legs of women who shave their legs.

Warts are not dangerous. They are only important because they are unattractive. Occasionally, a wart forms in an area that causes pain from pressure, as often happens with plantar warts on the bottom of the foot. In addition, because warts are viral infections, they sometimes spread to other areas of the skin, if left untreated. However, because they are not dangerous, whether to treat your warts is up to you.

Warts in children usually go away without treatment. This can happen within weeks or within years (there is no way to predict this). Leaving warts to go away of their own accord is a very reasonable "treatment." Otherwise, warts have to be destroyed for removal, because there are no good medications that kill the wart virus itself. The most common treatments are acids applied to the warts at home, and liquid nitrogen treatments in a doctor's office, where extremely cold liquid is sprayed or applied to the warts. This painful treatment causes a blister that, after healing, removes much or all of the wart along with it. Often, several treatments spaced about 1 month apart are required.

If you choose to treat your warts at home, you must take care to do it properly, to get good results. The area of the wart should be soaked with warm water until the wart is soft and white. Medication is applied to the wart with a cotton-tipped swab (if liquid) or by an adhesive patch cut to the size of the wart. A piece of adhesive tape

(continues)

is applied over the sticky patch to ensure that it stays in place. Each night the medication and any dead wart are removed after soaking and sanding the surface with an emery board or a pumice stone, and medication is reapplied. In most cases, the wart will disappear after 1 to 3 months of nightly treatment. Any new warts that appear during treatment should be tended to as well.

GLOSSARY

Acne surgery — socially acceptable popping of zits in a dermatologist's office (see *Zit*)

Actinic — produced by ultraviolet light exposure. In its most common dermatologic usage, this refers to conditions induced by chronic sun exposure.

Acuminate — pointed tip, seen often in some warts and in keratosis pilaris.

Alopecia — thinning of the hair or balding, either from increased hair loss or decreased growth.

Antibiotic medication — medications used by dermatologists not only to eradicate bacteria but also for unrelated anti-inflammatory effects of the medication.

Antifungal medication — medication that eliminates a fungus. Some medications, such as the azoles, eliminate both yeast and dermaotphyte forms. Others, such as nystatin, are only effective against yeast forms, and still others, such as griseofulvin, are only active against dermatophytes.

Annular — papule, plaque, macule, or patch with central clearing and peripheral accentuation. This is often used by nondermatologists as a synonym for tinea corporis (ringworm), but it is also a usual presentation of granuloma annulare, erythema migrans, and some forms of cutaneous lupus erythematosus.

Arcuate — scalloped pattern formed by coalescing annular or round lesions.

Atopic — an allergic diathesis; tendency for cutaneous irritation to produce itching.

Atrophic — thinned. Epidermal atrophy is manifested by a loss of skin markings, shininess, and visible dermal telangiectasias. Dermal atrophy is characterized by laxity, wrinkling, purpura, and, when severe, palpable or visible loss of tissue.

Balanitis — inflammation of the glans penis and prepuce.

Black — skin color produced either by increased melanin or by necrosis/old hemorrhage. Skin diseases that are black and not produced by necrosis/old hemorrhage are categorized with brown lesions morphologically.

Blister — superficial papule or nodule containing loculated fluid. If pierced, fluid drains and the lesion collapses. A blister that sloughs the roof becomes a round, well demarcated erosion.

Blue — skin color produced either by a foreign body (i.e., tattoo) or by melanin in the dermis; skin diseases that are blue are categorized with brown lesions morphologically.

Bulla — a blister larger than 1.5 cm. Flaccid bullae result from a superficial blister that breaks easily. A tense bulla is produced by a deeper blister that breaks less easily.

Chronic cutaneous lupus erythematosus — discoid lupus erythematosus.

Cigarette paper texture — fine crinkling due to thinning of the epidermis.

Collarette — the round peripheral scale remaining after a blister roof is shed.

Contact dermatitis — inflammation with vesiculation or scale/crust due to direct contact with an irritant (such as overwashing) or an allergen (such as poison ivy).

Cream — a topical vehicle containing water, fats, and alcohols. This is a white preparation that "rubs in" (evaporates) rather than leaving a greasy residue, but can be irritating. Preservatives and stabilizers are present, and this vehicle is less moisturizing than an ointment.

Crust — scale and exudate, sometimes with blood. A scab.

Cryosurgery — destruction by freezing.

Depigmented — complete lack of pigment, resulting in milk-white skin that shows a bright white color with a Wood's lamp (black light). Depigmentation generally results from different disorders than those producing hypopigmentation, a decrease in pigment that leaves the skin lighter than the patient's normal skin color, but not white.

Dermatophyte — fungus (often called tinea) that causes superficial infection of skin, hair, or nail in its hyphal form, as distinct from fungal yeast infections, and deep, usually systemic, fungal infections such as histoplasmosis or coccidioidomycosis.

Dermographism — the property of a wheal occurring in skin following a firm stroke with a fingernail or the cap of a pen, representing low-grade or subclinical urticaria.

Ditzel — see *Lesion*.

Dosepak — methylprednisolone packaged in a daily premeasured dose that provides an automatic taper. However, these are expensive, higher doses are tapered more rapidly than desirable for skin diseases, and the total course is longer than needed.

Dusky erythema — brown-red.

Ecchymoses — large areas of superficial cutaneous purpura.

Eczematized — excoriated or lichenified from scratching or rubbing.

Electrodessiccation — also called hyfrecation, electrocautery, and electrosurgery by dermatologists, and known by patients as "burning off with an electric needle."

Enanthem — oral lesions occurring in response to an infection.

Ephelides — freckles.

Erosion — loss of part or all of the surface epithelium, leaving the dermis intact (see *Ulcer*).

Exanthem — rash or keratinized skin in response to an infection.

Excoriation — erosions, usually linear or angular, produced by scratching or picking.

Factitial — produced by the patient. This can be done deliberately for secondary gain, from habit or compulsion, or because of psychosis.

Filiform — thin, finger-like, or hair-like papillae.

Fissure — linear crack in the skin, ranging from an obvious erosion to a fine red line.

Fungal preparation, fungal smear — preparation of skin scale placed on a microscope slide and treated with potassium hydroxide (KOH) to dissolve epithelial cells, so that fungal elements can be identified more easily.

Gel — vehicle that is alcohol-based, and although a clear gel when at room temperature, it becomes a liquid when warmed to body temperature. It is drying and irritating, but useful for hairy areas and oral mucous membrane skin. It has the same uses and properties as lotions, solutions, and liquids.

Guttate — drop-like. Used to describe the pattern of a disease. For example, guttate psoriasis appears as scattered round scaling papules rather than large plaques over the typical distribution of the elbows, knees, and scalp.

Gyrate erythema — inflammation with an annular, arcuate, or serpiginous pattern that occurs as a reaction to a systemic illness. Examples include erythema annulare centrifugum and erythema marginatum.

Horn, cutaneous — extreme hyperkeratosis, or retained scale that piles up to form a hard column, or horn. These are most often produced by warts, squamous cell carcinomas, seborrheic keratoses, or actinic keratoses. They should be biopsied to include a sample of underlying skin, unlike a skin tag.

Hyfrecation — also called electrosurgery by dermatologists and "burning off with an electric needle" by patients.

Hyperkeratotic — retained scale that is thick and gives the surface a hard texture.

Hyperpigmented — darker brown than surrounding normal skin. The darker color can occur from increased quantities of melanin or from dermal hemosiderin. Also, black skin can appear hyperpigmented when the cause is actually erythema in a setting of dark natural skin color.

Hypopigmented — a decrease in melanin that leaves the skin lighter than the patient's normal skin color but not white. This is in contrast to depigmentation, a complete lack of pigment that results in milk-white skin.

Immunobullous disease — blistering diseases produced by autoimmune mechanisms. Examples are bullous pemphigoid and pemphigus vulgaris.

Immunofluorescent biopsy, direct — a skin biopsy that is examined with fluorescein-tagged antibodies against human antibodies, making the identification of the patient's autoantibodies possible.

Intertrigo, intertriginous — pertaining to skin folds, such as the axillae and groin.

Keratinized skin — skin that is dry and has a layer of stratum corneum, as distinguished from mucous membrane skin that is wet and lacks sweat glands and hair follicles.

Keratolytic — substance that dissolves scale, such as lactic acid, tretinoin, or salicylic acid.

Keratosis — generic term for a benign keratotic or scaling tumor, especially an actinic keratosis or seborrheic keratosis when the clinician cannot differentiate due to either irritation of the lesion or ignorance.

Keratotic — rough surfaced due to retained scale.

Kerion — tinea capitis that is unusually inflamed, boggy, and purulent due to an exaggerated immunologic response to the fungal organism.

Koebner phenomenon — the precipitation of a disease as a result of injury or inflammation, especially psoriasis, lichen planus, and vitiligo. For example, the common location of psoriasis over the elbows is at least partially explained by the chronic low grade trauma associated with elbows resting on tables.

KOH preparation — lesional skin scale applied to a microscope slide and treated with potassium hydroxide (KOH) to dissolve epithelial cells so that fungal elements can be identified more easily.

Koplik spots — bluish-gray inflamed oral mucous membrane macules that accompany measles (rubeola).

Lentigo — hyperpigmented macule produced by increased melanin in the epidermis, often produced by chronic sun exposure. Also known as age spots or liver spots, and erroneously called freckles.

Lesion — medical term for "thing," calculated to fool others into thinking the speaker knows what the "thing" really represents.

Lichenification — thickening of the epidermis and stratum corneum from rubbing, recognized by an accentuation of skin markings and shine due to adherent surface scale.

Lichenoid — when used as a clinical morphologic term, this means flat-topped and shiny with adherent scale. When this term is used as a histologic descriptive term, lichenoid refers to a mononuclear infiltrate in a band-like distribution in the upper dermis, extending to and damaging the basal cell layer.

Livedo — net-like pattern of reticulate erythema produced either by vascular instability associated with estrogen, cold intolerance, or vasculitis of medium or larger arterioles.

Lotion — a vehicle that contains primarily water and alcohol, and exhibits the same properties as gels, liquids, and solutions. This is irritating and drying, but useful for hairy areas.

Maceration — softening, fragility, and erosion produced by chronic moisture, colonizing organisms, and friction.

Macule — a skin lesion smaller than about 1.5 cm that exhibits color change only, lacking in scale, crust, or elevation. For example, a freckle is a macule.

Maculopapular — composed of macules and papules. This term is often used by clinicians who feel that this expression covers all descriptive possibilities. Generally, they either do not know the difference between a macule and a papule, or they cannot decide which is the active lesion.

Mohs surgery — specialized skin cancer surgery that employs a frozen section technique and horizontal skin sections to examine all margins during the procedure for a very high cure rate.

Mole — nevocellular or pigmented nevus. Often erroneously used to describe any brown papule, including seborrheic keratoses.

Morbilliform — irregular, macular, faint erythema, usually due to a medication allergy or a virus infection.

Mucous membrane — wet, thin skin lacking the protective stratum corneum. This skin lines the mouth, nose, eyes, and vagina. Modified mucous membrane skin that is partially keratinized covers the lips, the inner labia majora, the labia minora, the glans penis, and the inner prepuce.

Nail pit — tiny pits in the surface of the nail plate, associated with psoriasis (and, much less often, alopecia areata).

Nevus — a cutaneous hamartoma. Most common is a pigmented nevus (mole), but other nevi (indicated by a prefix) include a collagen nevus (hamartoma of collagen), smooth muscle nevus (overgrowth of the arrector pili), the nevus sebaceous, and epidermal nevus (papillomatous proliferation of the epidermis).

Nikolsky sign — fragility of the skin that allows friction from rubbing to remove the surface of the epithelium. This is a classic finding in skin affected with pemphigus vulgaris.

Nodule — a papule that is at least roughly spherical.

Oil drop spot — a brownish-pink spot under nails, produced by psoriasis.

Ointment — a vehicle consisting of oils only, often petrolatum (Vaseline petroleum jelly). A good but greasy moisturizer, soothing because of lack of alcohols, stabilizers, and preservatives. It usually confers some occlusion, so that medication is often better absorbed.

Onycholysis — lifting of the nail from the underlying skin. This is most often seen with a fungal nail infection, but this also occurs with other conditions such as psoriasis, manipulation, and allergy to nail polish.

Palpable purpura — term denoting the classic presentation of leukocytoclastic vasculitis. Neutrophilic inflammation of the vessel produces palpable edema, and destruction of the vessel allows for extravasation of red blood cells.

Panniculitis — inflammation of the fat manifested by poorly demarcated, subcutaneous inflamed nodules or plaques; associated with infection, erythema nodosum, thrombophlebitis, pancreatic fat necrosis, lupus erythematosus, and other diseases.

Papilla — small projection.

Papillomatous — confluent papillae.

Papule — a skin lesion smaller than about 1.5 cm that is palpable because of scale, induration, or elevation.

Papulosquamous disease — any skin disease that is inflammatory, scaling, and sharply demarcated. Psoriasis, tinea, lichen planus, subacute and chronic cutaneous lupus erythematosus, pityriasis rosea, and secondary syphilis are the most common of these diseases.

Pastia's lines — petechiae and accentuation of rash in flexural creases of patients with scarlet fever.

Patch — a skin lesion larger than about 1.5 cm that is not palpable, exhibiting color change only.

Petechiae — a pinpoint area of cutaneous purpura.

Pedunculated — attached by a stalk, such as a skin tag.

Photoallergic — an increased sensitivity to light induced only in patients who develop a hypersensitivity to a chemical, manifested by epidermal edema or vesiculation.

Photosensitivity — increased sensitivity to the sun; occurring from disease such as lupus erythematosus, medication, or poor natural protection such as an unusually light normal complexion.

Phototoxic — a medication that produces an increased sensitivity to sunlight in every exposed patient, manifested by an exaggerated sunburn.

Pityriasis — fine scale that is subtle and often unappreciated unless the surface is scuffed with a fingernail or a scalpel blade, revealing the powdery scale.

Pityriasis versicolor — more appropriate name for "tinea" versicolor, which is not dermatophyte.

Polymerase chain reaction (PCR) technique — a sophisticated and sensitive technique for amplifying DNA so that minute amounts can be detected. Especially useful in dermatology for the identification of virus infections.

Polymorphous — no consistent morphology; can look like anything.

Postherpetic neuralgia — residual pain following a herpes zoster (shingles) — not herpes simplex — infection.

Plaque — a skin lesion larger than about 1.5 cm that is palpable because of scale, induration, or elevation.

Pruritus — a frequently misspelled word for itching.

Psoriasiform — when used as a clinical morphologic term, this means heavily scaling, thickened, and well-demarcated, mimicking psoriasis. When this term is used as a histologic descriptive term, psoriasiform refers to regular thickening and downward proliferation of the rete ridges of the epidermis.

Punched-out — well-demarcated and round borders of an ulcer or an erosion. When referring to an ulcer, the sides are perpendicular as one would expect if the defect had been produced by a skin punch biopsy, rather than sloped.

Purpura — hemorrhage into the skin.

Pustule — a skin lesion within or just under the epidermis filled with loculated pus, or exudate with neutrophils. A needle stick drains the lesion.

PUVA — therapy with oral or topical *p*soralen (a photosensitizing chemical) with *u*ltraviolet *A* *l*ight.

Rash — multiple lesions (see *Lesion*).

Reticulate — interlacing, net-like pattern.

Rhus dermatitis — an acute allergic dermatitis to a plant, usually poison ivy, poison oak, or poison sumac.

Ringworm — tinea (a dermatophyte fungal infection) that forms an annulus.

Satellite lesion — extension of a process with discrete lesions separated from the main abnormality by normal skin. For example, metastatic melanoma can produce small "satellite" islands of tumor near, but not confluent with, the original cutaneous melanoma, and a plaque of candidiasis within a skin fold can develop small "satellite" pustules or erosions scattered around the primary area of infection.

Sebaceous cyst — misnomer for an epidermal, or epidermoid, cyst.

Skin tag — a soft, pedunculated papule or nodule. These can be produced by friction in a skin fold, particularly in an obese patient, by an intradermal nevus, by a seborrheic keratosis in a damp area, or by a neurofibroma. None of these causes is important and a biopsy is generally not necessary, unlike a cutaneous horn.

Solution — a liquid vehicle that contains alcohol and water with little or no oil. A solution exhibits the same properties as gels and liquids. It is irritating and drying, but useful for hairy areas and the oral mucosa, but too irritating for other mucosal surfaces.

Scale — excess stratum corneum that is visible either because there is increased production due to proliferation of the epidermis, or the stratum corneum is not shed normally and accumulates.

SPF (sun protection factor) — a measure of the potency of a sunscreen. An SPF of 2 reports that the sunscreen protects the skin from sunburn for twice the duration of noontime ultraviolet B usually required to produce burning. Accordingly, an SPF of 15 reports that skin protected by this sunscreen can withstand fifteen times the duration of noonday sunlight before burning.

Spongiotic vesicle — a vesicle formed by edema within the epidermis that loculates. These form in acute eczema or dermatitis, such as the vesicular allergic contact dermatitis of poison ivy. Spongiotic vesicles are morphologically characteristic and show confluent, small, cobblestoned blisters.

Steroid-sparing medication — medication that either confers anti-inflammatory or immunosuppressive effects, so that systemic corticosteroid dosing can be decreased. Common examples include methotrexate, azathioprine, dapsone, and other anti-inflammatory antibiotics such as tetracycline.

Strawberry tongue — prominent, red lingual papillae reminiscent of a strawberry. This can occur over a white coated tongue (white strawberry tongue) or on a red tongue (red strawberry tongue). A strawberry tongue is characteristic of several diseases, including scarlet fever and Kawasaki disease.

Target lesion (targetoid) — euphemism for lesions of classic erythema multiforme that show a central accentuation of inflammation, surrounding pallor, and peripheral erythema.

Tinea — a superficial dermatophyte, or fungus that produces infection in its hyphal form. Also used as a misnomer in the terms tinea versicolor (a yeast infection better termed pityriasis versicolor) and tinea amiantacea (nonfungal scale/crust, from eczema, trauma, and bacterial infection).

Tzanck smear — a microscopic examination of a stained smear of the base of a blister. The results can be useful in the rapid diagnosis of herpes or pemphigus.

Ulcer — loss of surface epithelium and at least a portion of the dermis, as compared with an erosion, which leaves the dermis intact.

Undermined — the borders of an ulcer that overhang the ulcer edges. Characteristic of pyoderma gangrenosum.

Urticarial — morphologically similar to urticaria. Pink, nonscaling, flat-topped papules and plaques. Early inflammatory changes in several diseases produce "urticarial" plaques, including bullous pemphigoid and herpes zoster before blisters appear.

Vascular reaction — a red, nonscaling, flat-topped eruption with individual lesions that tend to become confluent; occurring as a hypersensitivity response to a systemic allergen such as infection or medication. Common vascular reactions include urticaria and erythema multiforme.

Vasculitis — the destruction of blood vessels by inflammatory cells, producing purpuric papules, nodules, or blisters. A hyperimmune reaction.

Verrucous — warty. Papillomatous surface.

Vesicle — a superficial papule smaller than about 1.5 cm containing loculated fluid. If pierced, fluid drains and the lesion collapses. A vesicle that sloughs the roof becomes a round, well demarcated erosion.

Violaceous — deep red, purple-red.

Vulgaris — common. As acne vulgaris (common acne), psoriasis vulgaris (common psoriasis), pemphigus vulgaris (common pemphigus), and verruca vulgaris (common warts).

Wheal — an edematous papule or plaque. The fluid is not loculated, so that piercing the lesion produces a few drops of serosanguinous fluid only.

Wood's light — an ultraviolet light that, like a "black light," highlights depigmented areas of vitiligo (but not hypopigmented areas), and areas of subtle hyperpigmentation. It is also useful for the identification of erythrasma, but it is no longer useful in the evaluation of tinea in the United States.

Yeast — a fungus that produces infection in its budding form.

Zit — inflammatory papule or pustule of acne.

INDEX

Note: Page numbers follwed by f indicate figures; those followed by t indicate tables.

D

E

Q

R

S

T

U